MEDICAL RADIOLOGY
Diagnostic Imaging

Editors:
A. L. Baert, Leuven
K. Sartor, Heidelberg

Springer-Verlag Berlin Heidelberg GmbH

A. H. Chapman (Ed.)

Radiology and Imaging of the Colon

With Contributions by

W. Atkin · I. Baeli · G. L. Beets · R. G. H. Beets-Tan · J. Bruzzi · D. F. Caroline · A. H. Chapman
E. M. Danse · G. P. Economou · R. Edwards · H. Fenlon · R. Ferrari · A. A. Ghiatas · A. Gillams
S. Gryspeerdt · J. A. Guthrie · S. Halligan · N. Hennessy · M. C. Hill · S. Hodgson · F. Iafrate
N. Kritikos · A. Laghi · P. Lefere · A. Lowe · F. Maccioni · J. Macpherson · F. Mangiapane
D. Marin · C. Miglio · J. Northover · P. Paolantonio · R. Passariello · R. J. Peck · B. Rembacken
I. Robertson · P. J. A. Robinson · B. P. Saunders · N. Scott · M. Sheridan · S. J. Skehan
P. Taourel · R. F. Thoeni · M. Tischkowitz · D. Tolan · S. Trenna · K. Tung · B. E. Van Beers

Foreword by

A. L. Baert

With 303 Figures in 456 Separate Illustrations, 77 in Color and 21 Tables

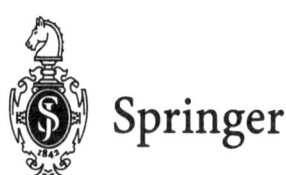

Springer

Anthony H. Chapman, MD
Department of Clinical Radiology
St. James's University Hospital
Beckett Street
Leeds, West Yorkshire LS9 7TF
UK

Medical Radiology · Diagnostic Imaging and Radiation Oncology
Series Editors: A. L. Baert · L. W. Brady · H.-P. Heilmann · M. Molls · K. Sartor

Continuation of Handbuch der medizinischen Radiologie
Encyclopedia of Medical Radiology

ISBN 978-3-642-62314-1

Library of Congress Cataloging-in-Publication Data
Radiology and imaging of the colon / A. H. Chapman (ed.) ; with contributions by J. F.
Adell ... [et al.] ; foreword by A. L. Baert.
    p. ; cm. -- (Medical radiology)
  Includes bibliographical references and index.
  ISBN 978-3-642-62314-1   ISBN 978-3-642-18834-3 (eBook)
  DOI 10.1007/978-3-642-18834-3
    1. Colon (Anatomy)--Diseases--Diagnosis. 2. Colon (Anatomy)--Imaging. 3. Colon
(Anatomy)--Radiography. 4. Diagnostic imaging. I. Chapman, A. H. (Anthony Hugh) II.
Adell, J. F. (Jean François) III. Series.
    [DNLM: 1. Colonic Diseases--radiography. 2. Diagnostic Imaging. WI 520 R1287 2004]
RC804.R6R344 2004
616.3'40757--dc22   2003061306

http//www.springeronline.com
© Springer-Verlag Berlin Heidelberg 2004
Originally published by Springer-Verlag Berlin Heidelberg New York in 2004
Softcover reprint of the hardcover 1st edition 2004

Cover-Design and Typesetting: Verlagsservice Teichmann, 69256 Mauer

21/3150xq – 5 4 3 2 1 0 – Printed on acid-free paper

To my wife *Jennifer*

For her forbearance.

ANTHONY CHAPMAN

Foreword

The radiological study of the colon has completely changed during the past decade. The emphasis has shifted largely from the classical double-contrast barium enema to more recent methods such as CT colonography, MR colonography, endorectal ultrasound, colonic scintigraphy and PET.

This exhaustive volume covers all these new modalities as well as all aspects of colonic pathology. Particular attention is given to neoplasm screening, detection and staging. Interventional methods such as stent placement are also well covered. The eminently readable text is complemented by numerous superb illustrations.

The editor, A. H. Chapman, is a world-renowned expert in the field with a lifelong dedication to imaging of the colon. The authors of individual chapters were invited to contribute on the strength of their long-standing experience and major contributions to the radiological literature on the topic.

I would like to thank and to congratulate most sincerely the editor and the authors for their superb efforts in producing this outstanding volume, a much-needed update of our knowledge of colon radiology and imaging.

This book will be of great interest for general and gastrointestinal radiologists but also for abdominal surgeons and gastroenterologists. I am confident that it will encounter the same success with the readers as the previous volumes published in this series.

Leuven   ALBERT L. BAERT

Preface

It is over 80 years since the double-contrast barium enema was first popularised by Fisher in Germany, and until recently this examination has been the mainstay of colonic radiology. The 1930s saw the barium enema being refined, but after that radiology in this field seemed to stand still, with the exception of some advances in angiography and nuclear medicine. By the early 1990s the impact of colonoscopy was being felt and there was concern that radiology would soon have little to offer. It was at this time that David Vining took his idea of virtual colonoscopy to Bowman Gray and with the financial support offered by the then chairman, Douglas Maynard, developed his technique. His presentation at the 1994 annual meeting of the Society of Gastrointestinal Radiologists caused great excitement, with the audience bursting into spontaneous applause. Thanks to subsequent dramatic improvements in computer processing, virtual colonoscopy has become part of everyday practice in major hospitals throughout the world. MR colonography is now being developed and although the same resolution has yet to be achieved, it has the added advantage of avoiding the risks of radiation. Both of these examinations have rekindled interest in faecal tagging, as it is apparent that if perfected this would enable the colon to be imaged with little or no bowel cleansing and allow these examinations to have a role in colon cancer screening. The race is now on; in a number of countries the introduction of national screening programmes for those at normal risk is under serious consideration. One problem is the difficulty in recognising flat adenomas and carcinomas using virtual colonoscopy, barium enema or routine colonoscopy. However, technical advances in colonoscopy are now helping with the identification and management of these lesions whose importance has only recently been recognised in the West.

Mesorectal excision for rectal carcinoma is a surgical advance in the past decade that has reduced the risk of local recurrence. This operation relies on MR scanning to identify the mesorectal fascia for accurate pre-operative staging. Less recognised is the value of MR and trans-abdominal ultrasound in the diagnosis of colitis. PET scanning is now showing its value for colon cancer staging and for the diagnosis of recurrent disease, and we have also seen the introduction of the metallic self-expanding stent, a device now regularly used as a temporising or palliative measure in patients with left-sided colonic obstruction.

This book concentrates on these recent developments and on some of the clinical issues that impact on today's radiologist, such as colon cancer screening, the pathology of colonic polyps and the importance of the flat adenoma. I have not attempted to be comprehensive but have included some chapters on conventional radiology that I hope will also be of interest, such as scintigraphy and aspects of angiographic, barium and plain-film radiology of the colon.

I am indebted to Professor Baert and Springer-Verlag for providing me with the opportunity to assemble this book and to the many authors who have so generously given their time to contribute chapters.

Leeds, UK   ANTHONY H. CHAPMAN

Contents

1 Screening for Colorectal Cancer
WENDY ATKIN and JOHN NORTHOVER 1

2 Screening Those at High Risk for Colorectal Cancer
MARC TISCHKOWITZ and SHIRLEY HODGSON 13

3 The Significance of the Flat Adenoma
BJORN REMBACKEN 25

4 The Pathology of Large Bowel Polyps
NIGEL SCOTT and ANTHONY H. CHAPMAN 31

5 An Introduction to Imaging Colonic Neoplasms
ALISON GILLAMS 51

6 Virtual Colonography
JOHN BRUZZI and HELEN FENLON 61

7 Dietary Faecal Tagging
PHILIPPE LEFERE and STEFAN GRYSPEERDT 71

8 MR Colonography
ANDREA LAGHI, ISABELLA BAELI, PASQUALE PAOLANTONIO, FRANCO IAFRATE,
DANIELE MARIN, CARLO MIGLIO, ROBERTO PASSARIELLO 81

9 Self-Expanding Metal Colonic Stents
STEPHEN HALLIGAN 89

10 Endorectal Ultrasound in Rectal Carcinoma
MICHAEL C. HILL 97

11 Rectal Tumours – MRI
REGINA G. H. BEETS-TAN and GEERARD L. BEETS 111

12 Staging and Follow-Up of Colorectal Cancer
J. ASHLEY GUTHRIE 125

13 Positron Emission Tomography in the Management of Colon Cancer
STEPHEN J. SKEHAN 137

14 Sonography of Appendicitis in Adults: Current Status
ETIENNE M. DANSE, BERNHARD E. VAN BEERS, PATRICE TAOUREL 147

15 CT of Appendicitis
   ABRAHAM A. GHIATAS and NICK KRITIKOS 157

16 CT of Diverticulitis
   ABRAHAM A. GHIATAS and GEORGIA P. ECONOMOU 165

17 Diagnosing Inflammatory Bowel Disease –
   Is There Still a Case for Barium Enema?
   MARIA SHERIDAN 171

18 Ultrasound of Colitis
   ROBERT JAMES PECK 177

19 CT of Colitis
   RUEDI F. THOENI 185

20 MRI of Colitis
   FRANCESCA MACCIONI 201

21 Colonic Scintigraphy
   PHILIP J. A. ROBINSON 215

22 CT Angiography of Splanchnic Vessels
   ANDREA LAGHI, RICCARDO FERRARI, FILIPPO MANGIAPANE, SIMONA TRENNA,
   DANIELE MARIN, ROBERTO PASSARIELLO 227

23 Diagnosis and Management of Acute Colonic Bleeding
   IAIN ROBERTSON and RICHARD EDWARDS 235

24 Colonic Lymphoma
   NIKLAS HENNESSY, JENNY MACPHERSON, KEN TUNG 243

25 Colorectal Trauma
   DINA F. CAROLINE and ANTHONY H. CHAPMAN 251

26 The Diagnosis and Management of Colonic Obstruction
   and Pseudo-Obstruction
   ANDREW LOWE and ANTHONY H. CHAPMAN 263

27 Barium Radiology of Unusual Colonic Morphology
   DAMIAN TOLAN and ANTHONY H. CHAPMAN 279

28 New Developments in Colonoscopy
   BRIAN P. SAUNDERS 301

Subject Index 315

List of Contributors 321

1 Screening for Colorectal Cancer[1]

Wendy Atkin and John Northover

CONTENTS

1.1 The Disease as a World Health Issue *1*
1.2 Natural History in Relation to Potential for Early Detection *2*
1.3 Appropriate Groups for Prophylactic Treatment or for Asymptomatic Screening *2*
1.4 Treatment Options Following Diagnosis by Screening *3*
1.5 Effectiveness of Screening Options in Terms of Incidence/Mortality Reduction *3*
1.5.1 Faecal Occult Blood Test (FOBT) *3*
1.5.2 Flexible Sigmoidoscopy (FS) *5*
1.5.3 Colonoscopy screening *6*
1.5.4 Imaging Techniques *6*
1.5.5 DNA Based Stool Tests *7*
1.6 Acceptability of Screening Methods *7*
1.7 Morbidity Associated with Screening and the Subsequent Management Process *8*
1.8 Costs of the Screening Process *8*
1.9 Cost-Effectiveness of Different Screening Strategies *9*
1.10 Conclusions *9*
References *10*

1.1
The Disease as a World Health Issue

The large bowel is world-wide the fourth commonest site for cancer after lung, stomach and breast and the fourth cause of cancer death after lung, stomach and liver cancer. There were 943,000 new cases diagnosed and 510,000 large bowel cancer deaths in 2000 (Parkin

W. Atkin, MD
Deputy Director, Colorectal Cancer Unit, Cancer Research UK, Honorary Reader in Epidemiology, Imperial College of Science, Technology and Medicine, London, St. Mark's Hospital, Northwick Park, Watford Road, Harrow, Middlesex HA1 3UJ, UK
J. Northover, MD
Professor of Intestinal Surgery, Imperial College of Science, Technology and Medicine, London, Director, Colorectal Cancer Unit, Cancer Research UK, Chair, Department of Surgery, St Mark's Hospital, Northwick Park, Watford Road, Harrow, Middlesex HA1 3UJ, UK

[1] This chapter is published with the permission of the BMJ Publishing Group as a similar review has been published in: Williams C. (ed) (2003) Evidence Based Oncology. BMJ Books.

et al. 2001). Highest incidence rates occur in North America, Northern Europe and Australasia where the disease ranks second after lung cancer. Lowest rates are found in sub-Saharan Africa and India. There have been marked increases in incidence rates in Asian populations adopting a Western lifestyle, such as the Chinese of Shangai and Hong Kong, Singaporeans and Japanese, and in Eastern Europe (Coleman et al. 1993). In higher risk areas rates are increasing more slowly, and in some countries have stabilised. In the UK, incidence rates of colorectal cancer increased during the 1970s and 1980s, but in the 1990s rates have stabilised and then fallen slightly in older men and women (Quinn et al. 2001) (Figs. 1.1.and 1.2). In

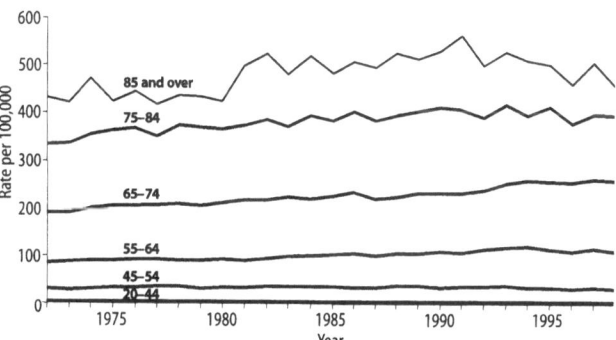

Fig. 1.1. SEER age-adjusted incidence rates for England and Wales between 1973 and 1999 (*http://seer.cancer.gov/faststats/html/inc_colorect.html*)

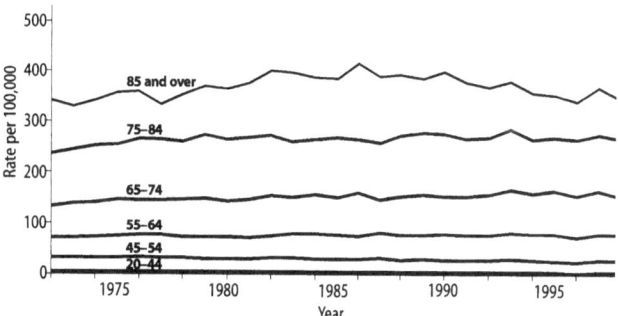

Fig. 1.2. Age-specific incidence rates for colorectal cancer for England and Wales between 1971 and 1997. [Taken from Quinn et al. (2001), with kind permission from Her Majesty's Stationery Office]

the US a pronounced decrease in incidence and mortality rates in white men and women began in the 1980s, but only very small reductions have been recorded in black men and women. Some researchers (INCIARDI et al. 2000; RABENECK et al. 2001) have speculated that the increased use of sigmoidoscopy and polypectomy have played an important role, although there is some evidence that the increased consumption of fruit and vegetables, non-steroidal anti-inflammatory drugs and hormone replacement therapy may also be playing a part.

In the US and the UK the estimated probability at birth of eventually developing colorectal cancer is 6% and the probability of dying from the disease is around 3%. Cancer of the colon is equally frequent in men and women while cancer of the rectum occurs 20–50% more frequently in men (PARKIN et al. 2001).

1.2
Natural History in Relation to Potential for Early Detection

Survival rates in the US improved substantially during the 1980s and now exceed 60% of all cases diagnosed (SEER Cancer stats 1973–1999). In the 1980s, UK survival rates were 8% lower for colon and 4–6% lower for rectal cancer than the average for Europe (40%) (GATTA et al. 2000). The wide differences in colorectal cancer survival across Europe in the 1980s (GATTA et al. 2000) were found to depend largely on the stage at diagnosis in different countries. Five-year survival rates for localised disease are 85%–90%, compared with 55%–60% for regional disease and only 5%–8% for cases with distant disease at primary diagnosis (WINGO et al. 1998).

Epidemiological, pathological and molecular genetic studies (MUTO et al. 1975; MORSON et al. 1983; JASS 1989; VOGELSTEIN et al. 1988) have provided convincing evidence that most colorectal cancers arise in adenomatous polyps and that their ablation arrests the development of cancer at that site (ATKIN et al. 1992). People with familial adenomatous polyposis (FAP) typically develop hundreds or thousands of adenomas in their teens and have an almost 100% risk of developing cancer by age 40. In sporadic bowel cancer the risk of developing metachronous adenomatous polyps or colorectal cancer increases with the number of adenomas detected initially (WINAWER et al. 1993a; MORSON et al. 1990). It is not uncommon to see a focus of malignancy within a large adenoma or

to see remnant adenomatous tissue adjacent to a carcinoma in early stage cancers; this finding is rarely seen in advanced cancers, suggesting that the invasive tissue overgrows the adenomatous element soon after progression to malignancy. The chance of finding a focus of malignancy within an adenoma grows with increasing adenoma size, and with more advanced histology (tubular $\rightarrow$ tubulovillous $\rightarrow$ villous) and dysplasia (MUTO et al. 1975). Molecular genetic studies (VOGELSTEIN et al. 1988) have provided further evidence for the concept of the adenoma-carcinoma sequence by demonstrating that the adenoma accumulates genetic mutations as it enlarges, and as dysplasia progresses and moves on to malignancy.

The average duration of the adenoma-carcinoma sequence can be deduced from the difference in the average age at diagnosis of adenomas and of cancers; in both FAP and sporadic disease the estimate is around 10 years (MUTO et al. 1975; WINAWER et al. 1987). In a retrospective study (STRYKER et al. 1987) in which patients with unresected ≥1cm colon polyps that were followed radiologically, the cumulative risk of developing cancer was 2.5% at 5 years, 8% at 10 years and 24% at 25 years. The progression of the disease may be faster for flat or depressed adenomas; these have been reported frequently in Japanese colons (MUTO et al. 1985; SUZUKI et al. 1997) but less frequently in Western patients (HART et al. 1998; REMBACKEN et al. 2000). The proportion of cancers that develop from flat or depressed adenomas is unknown.

1.3
Appropriate Groups for Prophylactic Treatment or for Asymptomatic Screening

A number of groups have an increased risk of developing colorectal cancer. Those at highest risk are those with either of the dominantly inherited conditions, FAP and hereditary non-polyposis colorectal cancer (HNPCC). Prophylactic colectomy is performed in teenagers and young adults affected by FAP since the cumulative risk of developing cancer by age 40 approaches 100%. In HNPCC the lifetime risk of colorectal cancer in mutation carriers is 80% (DUNLOP et al. 1997), so close surveillance is advised; prophylactic colectomy may be offered to those developing their first cancer, or who have widespread synchronous or recurrent adenomas. Other groups at moderately increased risk include those with long-standing ulcerative colitis or Crohn's disease (ITZKOWITZ 1997), individuals with a personal history of colorectal cancer or large, villous or multiple adenomas (ATKIN et al. 1992) and those with a 'non-dominant' family history of colorectal cancer. It has been estimated using life-table methods (LOVETT 1976; JOHN et al. 1993) that risk is increased 2–3 fold in those with a single affected first degree relative (FDR) and 5–6 fold in those with two FDRs.

At least 75% of colorectal cancers develop in people with no known risk factors apart from older age. Colorectal cancer is infrequent below age 40, but incidence increases rapidly from age 50, with an approximate doubling with each decade of life. It is probably not worth screening asymptomatic average risk people below age 50 years. The age at which to stop screening is more contentious. Fifty percent of all cases are diagnosed at age ≥70, and 25% at ≥80 years. Of course, with increasing age, life expectancy decreases, as does the number of life-years saved as a result of screening-initiated treatment of the disease (LAW et al. 1999). Therefore most colorectal cancer screening initiatives have focused on the age-group 50–74 years.

The intervals at which to offer screening depend on the target lesion and the screening modality. If the test predominantly detects early cancer rather than adenomas, it will need to be offered at least every 2 years, the period thought to be the average time for an asymptomatic cancer to become symptomatic. If, on the other hand, the test is able to detect adenomas sensitively, the test can be applied much less frequently as adenomas progress slowly to cancer.

those which are sufficiently large and sessile to make endoscopic removal impossible or ill-advised require surgical excision. There is a variety of methods available for endoscopic polypectomy. The main aims are to remove the lesion completely without perforating the bowel wall or causing bleeding. The method used in individual cases will depend largely on the size and shape of the polyp. It is desirable to retain all or part of the polyp for histological examination.

Within 3 years of removal of adenomas, around 30%–50% of people will have a further neoplasm identified at repeat examination (WINAWER et al. 1993). Some lesions are truly metachronous, while others found at repeat endoscopy are adenomas missed at the initial examination (HIXSON et al. 1991; REX et al. 1997a). On this basis, it is customary to offer colonoscopic surveillance at 3-yearly intervals to all patients following adenoma detection (WINAWER et al. 1995). Because adenomas are very common and colonoscopy is costly and not without risk, it is gradually becoming accepted that people with adenomas should be stratified according to their risk of being found to have an advanced adenoma or cancer at follow-up (ATKIN et al. 1992; GROSSMAN et al. 1989; NOSHIRWANI et al. 2000). This risk is increased if adenomas are multiple, large or have villous histology, in contrast to single, small, tubular adenomas (ATKIN et al. 1992; SPENCER et al. 1984; LOTFI et al. 1986) Long term follow-up data from the National Polyp Study (ZAUBER et al. 1999) suggest that subsequent surveillance intervals can be extended to 6 years in the low risk group; in the context of a mass screening programme it may be appropriate to offer no follow-up surveillance to this group (ATKIN et al. 2001).

1.4
Treatment Options Following Diagnosis by Screening

Around 20% of cancers detected during endoscopic screening (ATKIN 2002) will be malignant polyps that have only invaded locally and can be removed during endoscopy or by local surgical excision (LE). The others will require open abdominal surgery. At least 50% of colorectal cancers detected at screening will be localized, and then treated by endoscopic polypectomy, LE or open radical resection (ATKIN 2002; HARDCASTLE et al. 1996). This compares with around 10% Dukes' stage A cases amongst patients presenting after symptom onset (HARDCASTLE et al. 1996).

The vast majority of adenomatous polyps are small enough to be removed safely at endoscopy. Only

1.5
Effectiveness of Screening Options in Terms of Incidence/Mortality Reduction

1.5.1
Faecal Occult Blood Test (FOBT)

Haemoccult is the most extensively examined method for colorectal cancer screening. It is a qualitative guaiac-based test designed to detect an elevated level of blood in stool, assumed to be shed from a bleeding neoplasm. The hematin component of haemoglobin in the faecal blood catalyses the oxidation of guaiac after the addition of hydrogen peroxide to produce a blue colour. The test sensitivity is around 30%–50% for colorectal cancers but <20% for adenomas (AHLQUIST et al. 1993) (Table 1.1). It has high specificity of around 98% (HARDCASTLE et al. 1996; KRONBORG et al. 1996). In practice, this translates into about one case of cancer and three or four with adenomas for every 10 positive tests.

The test requires collection of two samples from each of three consecutive stools, which are smeared onto cards and mailed to a laboratory for processing. Colonoscopy is recommended if any of the six card

'windows' is positive as up to 50% will be found to have a cancer or large adenoma (≥ 1 cm). False positive results may be caused by components of the diet, including vegetables and some fruits, red meat, aspirin or horseradish; dietary restriction is sometimes advised before and during testing, but when requested tends to reduce compliance rates (THOMAS et al. 1989; ROZEN et al. 1999). Occasionally a positive result is due to a bleeding lesion proximal to the colon.

Table 1.1. Prevalence of adenomas and adenocarcinomas in average risk persons undergoing screening by flexible sigmoidoscopy, faecal occult blood testing or colonoscopy

First Author	Year	Screen	Subjects (n)	Adenomas (n)	(%)	Adenomas ≥1cm (n)	(%)	Cancers (n)	(%)	Mean age or age range	% Male	Type of test
Flexible sigmoidoscopy												
MEYER	1980		122	9	7.4		92	1	0.8	56.6	79	
WINNAN	1980		342	34	9.9					53	86	
SPENCER	1983		508	55	10.8					60	45	
ROSEVELT	1984		825	57	6.9			3	0.4	59		
MCCALLUM	1984		1015	78	7.7					20-89	76	
UJSZASZY	1985		3863	305	7.9	171	4.4	11	0.3			
WARDEN	1986		632	49	7.8					60		
ROZEN	1987		1176	38	3.2			4	0.3	52	42	
NEALE	1987		718	18	2.5					40		
YAO	1988		365	37	10.1			3	0.8	63	45	
SCHERTZ	1989		1236	137	11.1			15	1.2		61	
SHIDA	1989		1573	134	8.5	28	1.8	3	0.2		81	
REX used colonoscope	1990		500	60	12.0			1	0.2	55	93	
RIFF	1990		329	26	7.9	13	4.0	0		63		
CAUFFMAN	1992		1000	53	5.3			1	0.1	61	47	
FOLEY	1992		900	165	18.3	41	4.6	8	0.1	53	61	
WHERRY	1994		4005	217	5.4			11	0.3	55	66	
CANNON-ALBRIGHT	1994		406	48	11.8			0		52	51	
OLYNYK	1996		342	56	16.3	19	5.6			55-59		
VERNE	1998		1116	76	6.8			4	0.4		51	
PAILLOT	1999		450	22	4.9	9	2.0	0			40	
COLLETT	2000		2605	352	13.5	51	2.0	10	0.4	55-64	59	
LIEBERMAN	2000		3121	554	17.7	128	4.1			63	97	
IMPERIALE	2000		1994	229	11.5	26	1.3			60	59	
HOFF	2002		8840	1408	15.9					55-64		
Faecal occult blood testing												
KEWENTER	1994	P & R	41338	419	1.0	238	0.6	81	0.2	60-64		H II-U
HARDCASTLE	1996	P	44838	357	0.8	311	0.7	104	0.2	40-74		H II-U
		R (3-6 times)	88158	353	0.4	271	0.3	132	0.1			
KRONBORG	1996	P	20672			68	0.3	37	0.2	45-75		HII
		R 1	18781			61	0.3	13	0.1			Biennial -U
		R 2	17279			41	0.2	24	0.1			
		R 3	15845			44	0.3	21	0.1			
		R 4	14203			56	0.4	25	0.2			
LIEBERMAN	2001	P	2885	116	4.0	25	0.9	12	0.4	63		H II-R
NAKAMA	2001	P	17432					39	0.2	>40		I
Colonoscopy												
LIEBERMAN	2000	P	3121	1141	36.5	264	8.5	30	1.0	62.9		
IMPERIALE	2000	P	1994	354	17.8			12	0.6	59.8		

P, prevalence; *R*, rescreening; *H II–U*, unhydrated Haemoccult test; *H II-R*, rehydrated Haemoccult test; *I*, immunochemical test

FOBT has been shown in three large randomised trials (in Minnesota, USA (MANDEL et al. 1993; MANDEL et al. 1999); Odense, Denmark (KRONBORG et al. 1996; JORGENSEN et al. 2002) and Nottingham, UK (HARDCASTLE et al. 1996) to reduce CRC mortality by up to 20% if offered biennially, and possibly up to 33% if offered every year. In the US study (MANDEL et al. 2000) CRC incidence rates were reduced respectively by 20% and 17% in the annually and biennially screened groups, but this was apparent only 18 years after inception of screening. No incidence reduction has been observed in either of the two European studies (JORGENSEN et al. 2002), both of which offered the test at 2-yearly intervals; however, both cohorts have been followed for only 13 years so far and at that stage no effect on incidence was discernible in the US data. In the US trial (MANDEL et al. 1993) the majority of the test samples were rehydrated to increase sensitivity by inducing hemolysis through adding a drop of water to each sample during processing; this led to an increase in the positivity rates from 2% to 10% and a cumulative colonoscopy rate at 13 years of 38% in the annual and 29% in the biennially screened groups (compared with only 4% in the Danish study; JORGENSEN et al. 2002). It has been suggested that the reduction in cancer incidence rate observed in the US study was in part due to the serendipitous incidental detection of adenomas in the excess colonoscopies (LANG and RANSOHOFF 1998).

Haemoccult is a relatively insensitive test; in a case-control study (SELBY et al. 1993), only 36% of FOBTs performed within the year prior to diagnosis of fatal colorectal cancer yielded positive results. This represents the maximum efficacy of the test even if 100% compliance rates are achieved. Immunochemical tests for haemoglobin or other blood components show greater sensitivity for both CRC and adenomas but at the expense of lower specificity. Immunochemical tests are used routinely in Japan (SAITO 1996) but there is only limited experience elsewhere (ROZEN et al. 2000; CASTIGLIONE et al. 2000).

The feasibility and acceptability of FOBT screening are now being examined in demonstration pilot projects in Australia (*http://www.health.gov.au/ pubhlth/strateg/cancer/bowel/index.htm*) and in the UK (STEELE et al. 2001). The UK pilot covers two populations (one in Scotland, one in England) each with around 200,000 people in the age-range 50–69 years. A guaiac test similar to Haemoccult is being offered on a single occasion. Following the results of this 2-year study a decision will be made on whether to offer this form of screening in a programme within the National Health Service.

1.5.2
Flexible Sigmoidoscopy (FS)

The 60-cm flexible sigmoidoscope routinely examines the sigmoid colon and rectum, where two thirds of colorectal cancers and adenomas are located; the examination is usually without sedation or analgesia and performed in an endoscopy unit. A single phosphate enema, self-administered around one hour before leaving home for the test, is required to clear the distal bowel (ATKIN et al. 2000). The technique is sensitive for the detection of both adenomas and colorectal cancers within its reach. Those with 'high risk' adenomas (see below) may be referred for subsequent examination of the rest of the colon by colonoscopy.

The detection rates of distal adenomas and cancers at screening FS in different studies are shown in Table 1.1. Prevalence rates of distal adenomas increase with age during the 50s but level off after age 60 (ATKIN et al. 1993). Distal adenoma prevalence rates in men are approximately double those in women (ATKIN 2002).

Evidence from case-control and cohort studies indicates that screening by FS reduces incidence and mortality rates of distal CRC (SELBY et al. 1992; NEWCOMB et al. 1992; MULLER and SONNENBERG 1995a; GILBERTSEN and NELMS 1978) by around 60%. Without randomised trial evidence, most countries have been unwilling to introduce endoscopic screening. Three RCTs are in progress (UK, ATKIN et al. 2001, Italy, SEGNAN et al. 1999, and the US, PROROK et al. 2000) to address this issue.

A 5-year interval is recommended by several professional organisations in the US (WINAWER et al. 1997; SMITH et al. 2001), although the protection afforded by a single FS may last for up to 10 years (SELBY and FRIEDMAN 1988) or even longer depending on the age at which it is undertaken (ATKIN et al. 1993). The UK and Italian trials are examining the efficacy of a single FS screen at around age 60 years while the US trial is examining the efficacy of 5-yearly screening.

In the UK and Italian trials small polyps are removed during FS, a practice that has been shown to be safe (ATKIN 2002). Colonoscopy is offered only to those found to have adenomas with features associated with increased risks of synchronous or metachronous cancer (≥ 3 adenomas, size ≥ 1 cm, villous histology, severe dysplasia or malignancy). On these criteria only 5% of people screened are offered colonoscopy compared with 24% if all people found to have any type of polyp are referred.

The three randomised trials all reached their recruitment targets but several more years of follow-up will be required to determine fully the effects on incidence and mortality. Meanwhile a population experiment has been in progress in Northern California where for the past decade the Health Maintenance Organisation, Kaiser Permanente, has been offering FS screening at 10 yearly intervals to its members aged over 50 years (LEVIN and PALITZ 2002). The uptake rate has been 70%. Colorectal cancer incidence rates have fallen steadily in California and the decrease in left sided tumours is about twice that of right sided tumours (24.3% vs. 11.6%) (INCIARDI et al. 2000).

1.5.3
Colonoscopy screening

A limitation of FS screening is that it does not examine the proximal colon, where 40% of adenomas and cancers occur. The finding of a distal adenoma is associated with an increased likelihood of having adenomas in the proximal colon so colonoscopy in people with distal neoplasia should enable detection of some proximal disease. A recent study (LIEBERMAN et al. 2000) suggested that around 70% of all advanced colorectal neoplasia will be detected with this strategy.

Around 50% of proximal neoplasia occurs without a distal marker lesion, so some experts in the US (NEUGUT and FORDE 1988; REX et al. 2000) have advocated colonoscopy screening to avoid missing these lesions. Existing data suggest that there is only a moderate additional reduction in incidence and mortality rates with primary colonoscopy compared with flexible sigmoidoscopy and selective colonoscopy. In a case-control study by MULLER and SONNENBERG (1995a,b) odds ratios for the development of colon cancer were 0.47 (CI 0.37–0.58) following colonoscopy compared with 0.56 (CI 0.46–0.67) following flexible sigmoidoscopy; odds ratios for colorectal cancer death were respectively 0.24 (CI 0.17–0.35) and 0.38 (CI 0.29–0.49). KAVANAGH et al. (1998) examined prospectively the risk of CRC in 24,000 people, 3000 of whom had undergone endoscopic screening 8 years previously, 18% by colonoscopy and the remainder by flexible sigmoidoscopy. There was an 80% reduction in stage C and D cancers of the distal large bowel among the screened group, but no reduction in either early or late stage proximal cancer. Data from the National Polyp Study (WINAWER et al. 1993b) suggest that there is a 75% reduction in colorectal cancer incidence rates following colonoscopic polypectomy. However, this might be due solely to a distal effect. WINAWER and ZAUBER (2001) suggested that a randomised trial is

required to examine the efficacy of colonoscopy and a pilot study is in progress.

For the motivated individual, whole colon screening by colonoscopy may give the greatest reassurance, but it may not be suitable for mass population screening because of the personal commitment required of the screenee, the considerable provider resources required, and the morbidity likely to result from widespread delivery of colonoscopy. Bowel preparation for colonoscopy requires participants to take a laxative and consume a liquid-only diet on the day before screening. The procedure can be painful so sedation and analgesia are usually necessary. As a result colonoscopy screening requires of the screenee at least 36 hours of commitment and time off work, compared with only a couple of hours for flexible sigmoidoscopy. Complication rates are also higher (see below). Flexible sigmoidoscopy can be performed competently by nurses (MAULE 1994; SCHOENFELD et al. 1999), while colonoscopy requires the skills of an experienced endoscopist; therefore offering colonoscopy at 10 yearly intervals in the US presents manpower problems that have yet to be resolved. It is not seen as a viable screening tool in many other countries.

1.5.4
Imaging Techniques

In the pre-colonoscopy era, barium enema (BE) was the only method available to examine areas of the bowel proximal to the distal sigmoid colon, apart from surgery. The advent of double contrast barium enema improved the ability to detect polyps. There has been a long debate on the relative merits of barium enema and colonoscopy (THOENI and PETRAS 1982; KEWENTER et al. 1995). Proponents of BE have stressed its relative safety, while critics have stressed its relative insensitivity compared with colonoscopy. In a study of 2193 consecutive colorectal cancers from 21 Indiana hospitals (REX et al. 1997b), colonoscopy correctly identified 95% of cancers and barium enema only 83%. Barium enema has been shown to be relatively insensitive for the detection of polyps compared with colonoscopy (WINAWER et al. 2000), detecting only 21%, 42% and 46% respectively of polyps ≤5mm, 6–10 mm or >10mm in size.

Computed tomography (CT) and magnetic resonance (MR) colonography are new techniques for imaging the bowel that may find application in screening. Virtual colonoscopy (CT colonography), first described by VINING et al. (1994), applies complex image rendering techniques to a spiral CT pneumocolon to create 3D graphical images of the colon that simulate colonoscopy (Fig. 1.3). These techniques require satisfactory bowel cleansing and temporary paralysis of the colon using a muscle relaxant. The technology is advancing rapidly and the performance characteristics are improving. Differentiation of faeces from mural lesions can be difficult, but it has been reported (CALLSTROM et al. 2000; LAUENSTEIN et al. 2002) that oral contrast, taken the day before screening, may obviate the need for bowel preparation by differentiating faeces from polyps. The techniques appear to have high sensitivity for colorectal cancer and large polyps, but are less sensitive for flat lesions and for smaller polyps (FENLON 2002). A major limitation at present is the time required to interpret the output (around 15–20 min) although computer algorithms under development (SUMMERS et al. 2001) may allow automatic detection and label suspicious regions, alerting the radiologist to the presence of a lesion. If accuracy improves, if costs can be reduced, and if bowel preparation becomes unnecessary, there may be a role for these methods in screening average risk people.

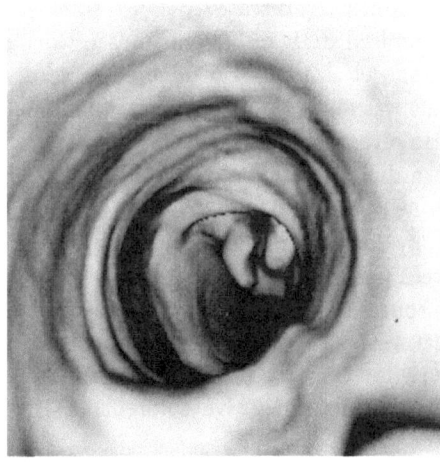

Fig. 1.3. Virtual colonoscopy. 3D rendering of spiral CT data, giving an intraluminal view of a colon cancer

1.5.5
DNA Based Stool Tests

Stool tests have the advantage that they are non-invasive and, despite the universal distaste for handling faecal material, are potentially more convenient for the participant. The past decade has seen enormous advances in the ability to detect the tiny amounts of DNA present in stool, derived from cells shed from neoplastic lesions. DNA extraction from stool presents special problems as human DNA is often degraded and food digestion products and bacterial contaminants inhibit the polymerase chain reaction. The quantity and quality of the DNA extracted from stool are generally increased in the presence of colorectal neoplasia, probably because there is less efficient degradation by apoptosis of neoplastic cells compared with that of fully differentiated cells. However, several recent studies have reported that it is now possible, although still technically difficult, to extract epithelial DNA from 100% of stool samples, including those with no neoplasia. Mutations in several genes have been examined including k-ras, APC, p53 and BAT26 (AHLQUIST et al. 1999; RENGUCCI et al. 2001; DONG et al. 2001; TRAVERSO et al. 2002a).

Using a panel of DNA markers, three research groups (AHLQUIST et al. 1999; RENGUCCI et al. 2001; DONG et al. 2001) have reported high sensitivity for cancers and large adenomas. Data so far suggest that, with the exception of k-ras, these markers are highly specific and therefore represent a significant improvement over FOBT. However a large National Cancer Institute study is in progress to examine the sensitivity and specificity of these markers in 10,000 average risk men and women aged over 50 years, all of whom will be examined by colonoscopy as a gold standard for comparison. It has been suggested (TRAVERSO et al. 2002b) that BAT26 might be a useful test for the detection of proximal cancers in combination with FS screening. Whether stool-based DNA tests will replace or supplement existing screening methods has yet to be determined.

1.6
Acceptability of Screening Methods

In the Nottingham trial of FOBT (HARDCASTLE et al. 1996), 60% of participants completed at least one screening test, and 38% completed all (3–6) the biennial screening tests they were offered. These results are similar to experience in Burgundy (France) (TAZI et al. 1997) where, during the first five successive rounds of screening, 69% completed at least one round and 37% completed all five. In the Danish trial (JORGENSEN et al. 2002), 67% completed the first test. In this study only compliers with the first test were invited for subsequent tests, leading to 93% compliance in the later rounds. Experience in Nottingham and in France suggests that higher compliance rates are achieved in non-compliers when they are invited at subsequent rounds.

Reported compliance rates with FS screening are highly variable. In a US Army screening initiative

(WHERRY and THOMAS 1994), attendance was 95%, perhaps related to FS screening being a requirement for overseas posting (WHERRY and THOMAS 1994)! An attendance rate of 81% was achieved in Norway (HOFF et al. 1985, 1996), 38% in Ireland (FOLEY et al. 1992), and in the UK (VERNE et al. 1998) 49% complied with an invitation to undergo FS screening by their own GP (VERNE et al. 1998). Lower rates were observed in studies in Australia (12%) (OLYNYK et al. 1996) and in Italy (29%) (SENORE et al. 1996). These rates are still higher than the 6% compliance in a study inviting physicians, dentists and their spouses to undergo colonoscopic screening (REX et al. 1991).

In a survey undertaken in 1999 among Americans aged over 50 years (CDC 2001), 40% reported ever having FOBT and 44% ever having a sigmoidoscopy. Compliance with the recommended US screening strategy was 21% for FOBT (test within previous year) and 34% for sigmoidoscopy (test within previous 5 years); 44% had had either sigmoidoscopy or FOBT during the recommended period.

1.7
Morbidity Associated with Screening and the Subsequent Management Process

The main complications of screening are associated with colonoscopy, flexible sigmoidoscopy and surgery. Generally flexible sigmoidoscopy is a much lower risk procedure than colonoscopy, particularly the perforation rate. In the UK flexible sigmoidoscopy screening trial (ATKIN 2002) there was only one perforation in 40,000 examinations despite removal of more than 19,000 polyps. A similar low perforation rate was reported in a 10-year study from the Mayo Clinic (ANDERSON et al. 2000) (two perforations in 49,500 FS), and in a screening programme in Northern California (LEVIN et al. 2001) (2 perforations in 109,000 examinations, all of which included polypectomy). In contrast, there is a higher risk of perforation at colonoscopy: in the UK Flexible Sigmoidoscopy trial there were four perforations in 2377 examinations (1:600), all following polypectomy, a rate similar to that reported in the Nottingham FOBT trial (five in 1474 (1:300) colonoscopies) (ROBINSON et al. 1999), and in a series from the Mayo Clinic (20 in 10,486 (1:500) colonoscopies) (ANDERSON et al. 2000). However, in one screening colonoscopy study in average risk men, there were no perforations reported in over 3000 examinations (LIEBERMAN et al. 2000).

Haemorrhage, the next most important complication, is most likely to follow polypectomy. WAYE et

al. (1996), using data from several prospective studies, estimated the rate to be 1:81 if polypectomy had been performed and 1:1352 if it had not. In the UK flexible sigmoidoscopy trial there were only 12 bleeds in 40,000 (1:3300) FS examinations (eight following 19,000 (1:2400) polypectomies) and nine cases in 2377 (1:260) colonoscopies (all following polypectomy). Risk of bleeding following polypectomy is minimised by discontinuing any anticoagulant therapy several days beforehand.

Endoscopic procedures can induce transient bacteraemia, but prophylactic antibiotics are only needed for patients who are immunosuppressed or who have an implanted mechanical heart valve. Inadequately disinfected endoscopic equipment poses a potential risk of infectious transmission; cases of hepatitis acquired through endoscopy have been reported (BRONOWICKI et al. 1997; KARSENTI et al. 1999).

Cardiac morbidity secondary to laxative or sedative use has been reported in up to 15% of people undergoing colonoscopy (ECKARDT et al. 1999). In the FOBT trials the observed reduction in colorectal cancer mortality was of the same order as the increase in mortality from ischaemic heart disease (AHLQUIST 1997). In a small randomised study of FS screening in Norway (THIIS-EVENSEN et al. 1999), a 5% increased cardiac mortality rate was observed in the group undergoing screening. However, in the series from Northern California myocardial infarction was no more frequent at one day, one week or one month following flexible sigmoidoscopy than the remainder of the post-examination 52 week period (LEVIN et al. 2001).

Another source of morbidity and mortality is the surgical treatment of early cancers and adenomas too large to be removed endoscopically. Data are scarce but the mortality from elective colorectal surgery varies between 1 and 7%.

1.8
Costs of the Screening Process

The most commonly used FOBT test (Haemoccult) itself costs less than £1. However, testing needs to be offered at one or two yearly intervals and test positive individuals are examined by colonoscopy. Positivity rates with the un-rehydrated FOBT are around 2% at the initial screen and 1–1.5% in subsequent rounds (HARDCASTLE et al. 1996; KRONBORG et al. 1996). Positivity rates with the rehydrated test vary between 4 and 10% (MANDEL et al. 1993); it has been estimated that cumulative colonoscopy rates over a lifetime of screening make such testing prohibitively expensive (FRAZIER et al. 2000).

The costs of colonoscopy, flexible sigmoidoscopy and polypectomy vary enormously, not only between countries but also between different providers within the same country (Whynes, personal communication). In some countries, FS costs nearly as much as colonoscopy: clearly, therefore, colonoscopy, which examines the colon more extensively, would be more cost-effective. In other settings, such as in the UK NHS and in managed care, FS is 3–5 times less costly than colonoscopy. Accurately costing these procedures is obviously essential in modelling the cost-effectiveness of different screening regimens.

The predicted lifetime costs for cases of localised, regional and disseminated cancer have been estimated to be of the order of $22,000, $44,000 and $58,000 (costs estimated from Group Health Cooperative, Seattle, Washington). However, a recent study (RAMSEY et al. 2002) suggests that the lifetime costs of early cancers may be greater than late cancers because of the long follow-up for early cases and high mortality in late cases.

1.9
Cost-Effectiveness of Different Screening Strategies

Many different CRC screening strategies based on FOBT, sigmoidoscopy and colonoscopy have been proposed in the US (SMITH et al. 2001; LEVIN and MURPHY 1992; LIEBERMAN et al. 2001). US strategies include FOBT (un-rehydrated or rehydrated) at annual or 2-yearly intervals, sigmoidoscopy at 3, 5 or 10 yearly intervals or just once at around age 55–60, and colonoscopy at 10 yearly intervals or just once at age 60 or 65 years. In estimating cost-effectiveness, most studies (FRAZIER et al. 2000; EDDY et al. 1987; WAGNER et al. 1991) have used a state-transition Markov model, which simulates the evolution from normal epithelium→adenomatous polyp→malignancy under various assumptions.

There is general agreement that the cost-effectiveness of all strategies for CRC screening (except those using rehydrated FOBT) compare favourably with those for other cancers, including breast and cervix. The net cost of un-rehydrated FOBT is higher than expected since the test is not associated with a decrease in cancer incidence rates (JORGENSEN et al. 2002) and thereby the cost of treating the disease. By contrast, endoscopic screening, by detecting the disease in the premalignant phase, reduces incidence and avoids the cost of future

cancer treatment. Several studies (ATKIN et al. 1993; FRAZIER et al. 2000; LOEVE et al. 2000) have shown that the net cost of flexible sigmoidoscopy screening are close to zero and become cost-saving under some assumptions. Similar claims have been made for a single colonoscopy (SONNENBERG and DELCO 2002).

Increasing the interval or reducing the number of screening examinations profoundly reduce costs (MARSHALL et al. 1996). Decreasing the age at which screening is first offered increases the number of life-years saved but at much greater cost. EDDY (1990) showed that delaying the start of screening from age 40 to 50 reduces costs of FOBT by a factor of two and this became the basis for the US recommendations (LEVIN and MURPHY 1992). Similarly, a single colonoscopy at age 60 saves more lives but is more cost-effective when offered after age 70, when it becomes cost-saving (SONNENBERG and DELCO 2002).

There is some controversy about the threshold at which to offer colonoscopy to look for synchronous proximal neoplasia following detection of an adenoma at sigmoidoscopy. The chance of finding advanced neoplasia or colorectal cancer is increased in those with multiple or advanced distal adenomas at FS (ATKIN et al. 1992; ZARCHY and ERSHOFF 1994). Offering colonoscopy only for high risk adenomas rather than for any adenoma potentially increases the feasibility of the screening regimen when resources are limited by reducing their referral rate from 12% to 5% (ATKIN 2002). This strategy will inevitably miss some advanced proximal adenomas as only around 25% of proximal cancers occur in the presence of a distal marker (LEMMEL et al. 1996; DINNING et al. 1994). Thus sigmoidoscopy is inevitably an inefficient method of detecting proximal neoplasia whatever threshold is used.

The factor that most profoundly affects the costs of all screening regimens is the nearly universal practice of offering 3-yearly surveillance colonoscopy following detection of any adenoma (RANSOHOFF 1999). Depending on the frequency of screening and the proportion of people entering into surveillance, this component can account for up to one half of the costs of screening programmes (WAGNER et al. 1991; MARSHALL et al. 1996; RANSOHOFF et al. 1999).

1.10
Conclusions

Randomised trials have demonstrated that early detection of colorectal cancer by screening can reduce disease-specific mortality. Evidence from case-control studies is highly suggestive that removal of adenomas reduces colorectal cancer incidence rates. The US is the only country that has advocated endoscopic screening for the purpose of detecting the neoplasia in the pre-malignant phase, and is the only country in which incidence rates are falling.

There are many methods now available for colorectal cancer screening, with adequate evidence of benefit. The precise choice of screening regimen within a particular health care setting will depend on issues of acceptability, safety, feasibility and cost-effectiveness. Whatever method is chosen, it will be necessary to perform colonoscopy to a high standard. It is therefore essential that training and quality assurance programmes are in place before screening is implemented.

References

Ahlquist D (1997) Fecal occult blood testing for colorectal-cancer – can we afford to do this? Gastroenterol Clin North Am 26:41–55

Ahlquist D, Wieand H, Moertal C et al (1993) Accuracy of fecal occult blood screening for colorectal neoplasia: a prospective study using Hemoccult and Hemoquant. J Am Med Assoc 269:1262–1267

Ahlquist D, Clin M, Rochester M et al (1999) Detection of altered DNA in stool: feasibility for colorectal neoplasia screening. Gastroenterology 116 [Suppl 1]:A661

Anderson M, Pasha T, Leighton J (2000) Endoscopic perforation of the colon: lessons from a 10-year study. Am J Gastroenterol 95:3418–3422

Atkin W (2002) UK Flexible Sigmoidoscopy Screening Trial Investigators. Single flexible sigmoidoscopy screening to prevent colorectal cancer; baseline findings of a UK multicentre randomised trial. Lancet 359:1291–1300

Atkin W, Morson B, Cuzick J (1992) Long-term risk of colorectal cancer after excision of rectosigmoid adenomas. N Engl J Med 326:658–662

Atkin W, Cuzick J, Northover J et al (1993) Prevention of colorectal cancer by once-only sigmoidoscopy. Lancet 341:736–740

Atkin W, Hart A, Edwards R et al (2000) Single-blind, randomised trial of the efficacy and acceptability of oral Picolax vs self-administered phosphate enema in bowel preparation for flexible sigmoidoscopy screening. BMJ 320:1504–1509

Atkin W, Edwards R, Wardle J et al (2001) Design of a multicentre randomised trial to evaluate flexible sigmoidoscopy in colorectal cancer screening. J Med Screen 8:137–144

Bronowicki J, Venard V, Botte C et al (1997) Patient-to-patient transmission of hepatitus-c virus during colonoscopy. N Engl J Med 337:237–240

Callstrom M, Johnson C, Reed J et al (2000) CT colonography of the unprepped colon: an early feasibility study of "virtual preparation". Gastroenterology 118 [Suppl 2]:A257

Castiglione G, Zappa M, Grazzini G et al (2000) Screening for colorectal cancer by faecal occult blood test: comparison of immunochemical tests. J Med Screen 7:35–37

CDC (2001) Trends in screening for colorectal cancer – United States, 1997 and 1999. MMWR 50:162–166

Coleman M, Esteve J, Damiecki P et al (1993) Trends in cancer incidence and mortality. International Agency for Research on Cancer, Lyon

Dinning J, Hixson L, Clark L (1994) Prevalence of distal colonic neoplasia associated with proximal colon cancers. Arch Intern Med 154:853–856

Dong S, Traverso G, Johnson C et al (2001) Detecting colorectal cancer in stool with the use of multiple genetic targets. J Natl Cancer Inst 93:858–865

Dunlop M, Farrington S, Carothers A et al (1997) Cancer risk associated with germline DNA mismatch repair gene-mutations. Hum Mol Genet 6:105–110

Eckardt V, Kanzler G, Schmitt T et al (1999) Complications and adverse effects of colonoscopy with selective sedation. Gastrointest Endosc 49:560–565

Eddy D (1990) Screening for colorectal cancer. Ann Intern Med 113:373–384

Eddy D, Nugent F, Eddy J et al (1987) Screening for colorectal cancer in a high-risk population. Results of a mathematical model. Gastroenterology 92:682–692

Fenlon H (2002) Virtual colonoscopy. Br J Surg 89:1–3

Foley D, Dunne P, Dervan P et al (1992) Left-sided colonoscopy and haemoccult screening for colorectal neoplasia. Eur J Gastroenterol Hepat 4:925–936

Frazier A, Colditz G, Fuchs C et al (2000) Cost-effectiveness of screening for colorectal cancer in the general population. JAMA 284:1954–1961

Gatta G, Capocaccia R, Sant M et al (2000) Understanding variations in survival for colorectal cancer in Europe: a EUROCARE high resolution study. Gut 47:533–538

Gilbertsen V, Nelms J (1978) The prevention of invasive cancer of the rectum. Cancer 41:1137–1139

Grossman S, Milos M, Tekawa I et al (1989) Colonoscopic screening of persons with suspected risk factors for colon cancer. II. Past history of colorectal neoplasms. Gastroenterology 96:299–306

Hardcastle J, Chamberlain J, Robinson M et al (1996) Randomised controlled trial of faecal-occult-blood screening for colorectal cancer. Lancet 348:1472–1477

Hart A, Kudo S, Mackay E et al (1998) Flat adenomas exist in asymptomatic people – important implications for colorectal-cancer screening programs. Gut 43:229–231

Hixson L, Fennerty M, Sampliner R et al (1991) Prospective blinded trial of the colonoscopic miss-rate of large colorectal polyps. Gastrointest Endosc 37:125–127

Hoff G, Foerster A, Vatn M et al (1985) Epidemiology of polyps in the rectum and sigmoid colon. Histological examination of resected polyps. Scand J Gastroenterol 20:677–683

Hoff G, Sauar J, Vatn M et al (1996) Polypectomy of adenomas in the prevention of colorectal-cancer – 10 years follow-up of the telemark polyp study. 1. A prospective, controlled population study. Scand J Gastroenterol 31:1006–1010

Inciardi J, Lee J, Stijnen T (2000) Incidence trends for colorectal cancer in California: Implications for current screening practices. Am J Med 109:277–281

Itzkowitz S (1997) Inflammatory bowel-disease and cancer. Gastroenterol Clin North Am 26:129–139

Jass J (1989) Do all colorectal cancers arise in pre-existing adenomas? World J Surg 74:45–51

John DS, McDermott F, Hopper J et al (1993) Cancer risk in

relatives of patients with common colorectal cancer. Ann Intern Med 118:785–790

Jorgensen O, Kronborg O, Fenger C (2002) A randomised study of screening for colorectal cancer using faecal occult blood testing: results ater 13 years and seven biennial screening rounds. Gut 50:29–32

Karsenti D, Metman E, Viguier J et al (1999) Transmission of hepatitis C virus by colonoscopy: study of 97 "presumed" risk patients. Gastroenterol Clin Biol 23:985–986

Kavanagh A, Giovannucci E, Fuchs C et al (1998) Screening endoscopy and risk of colorectal cancer in United States men. Cancer Causes Control 9:455–462

Kewenter J, Brevinge H, Engaras B et al (1995) The value of flexible sigmoidoscopy and double-contrast barium enema in the diagnosis of neoplasms in the rectum and colon in subjects with a positive hemoccult: results of 1831 rectosigmoidoscopies and double-contrast barium enemas. Endoscopy 27:159–163

Kronborg O, Fenger C, Olsen J et al (1996) Randomised study of screening for colorectal cancer with faecal-occult-blood test. Lancet 348:1467–1471

Lang C, Ransohoff D (1998) What can we conclude from the randomized controlled trials of fecal occult blood test screening? Eur J Gastroenterol Hepatol 10:199–204

Lauenstein T, Goehde S, Ruehm S et al (2002) MR colonography with barium-based fecal tagging: initial clinical experience. Radiology 223:248–254

Law M, Morris J, Wald N (1999) The importance of age in screening for cancer. J Med Screening 6:16–20

Lemmel G, Haseman J, Rex D et al (1996) Neoplasia distal to the splenic flexure in patients with proximal colon-cancer. Gastrointest Endosc 44:109–111

Levin B, Murphy G (1992) Revision of American Cancer Society recommendations for the early detection of colorectal cancer. CA A Cancer J Clin 42:296–299

Levin T, Palitz A (2002) Flexible sigmoidoscopy; an important screening option for average-risk individuals. Gastrointest Endosc Clin North Am 12:23–40

Levin T, Conell C, Shapiro J et al (2001) Complications of screening sigmoidoscopy. Gastroenterology 120 [Suppl 1]:A65

Lieberman D, Weiss D, Bond J et al (2000) Use of colonoscopy to screen asymptomatic adults for colorectal cancer. N Engl J Med 343:162–168

Lieberman D, Weiss D, Group VACS (2001) One-time screening for colorectal cancer with combined fecal occult-blood testing and examination of the distal colon. N Engl J Med 345:555–560

Loeve F, Brown M, Boer R et al (2000) Endoscopic colorectal cancer screening: a cost-saving analysis. J Natl Cancer Inst 92:557–563

Lotfi A, Spencer R, Ilstrup D et al (1986) Colorectal polyps and the risk of subsequent carcinoma. Mayo Clin Proc 61:337–43

Lovett E (1976) Family studies in cancer of the colon and rectum. Br J Surg 63:533–537

Mandel J, Bond J, Church T et al (1993) Reducing mortality from colorectal cancer by screening for fecal occult blood. N Engl J Med 328:1365–1371

Mandel J, Church T, Ederer F et al (1999) Colorectal cancer mortality: effectiveness of biennial screening for fecal occult blood. J Natl Cancer Inst 91:434–437

Mandel J, Church T, Bond J et al (2000) The effect of fecal occult blood screening on the incidence of colorectal cancer. N Engl J Med 343:1603–1607

Marshall J, Fay D, Lance P (1996) Potential costs of flexible sigmoidoscopy-based colorectal cancer screening. Gastroenterology 111:1411–1417

Maule W (1994) Screening for colorectal cancer by nurse endoscopists. N Engl J Med 330:183–187

Morson B, Bussey H, Day D et al (1983) Adenomas of large bowel. Cancer Surv 3:451–477

Morson B, Williams C, Fruhmorgen P et al (1990) Colorectal adenomas: risk of cancer and results of follow-up. Gastroenterol Int 3:57–62

Muller A, Sonnenberg A (1995a) Prevention of colorectal cancer by flexible sigmoidoscopy and polypectomy. A case-controlled study of 32,702 veterans. Ann Intern Med 123:904–910

Muller A, Sonneberg A (1995b) Protection of colorectal cancer by endoscopy against death from colorectal cancer: A case-controlled study among veterans. Arch Intern Med 155:1741–1748

Muto T, Bussey H, Morson B (1975) The evolution of cancer of the colon and rectum. Cancer 36:2251–2270

Muto T, Kamiya J, Sawada T et al (1985) Small "flat adenoma" of the large bowel with special reference to its clinicopathologic features. Dis Colon Rectum 28:847–851

Neugut A, Forde K (1988) Screening colonoscopy: has the time come? Am J Gastroenterol 83:295–297

Newcomb P, Norfleet R, Storer B et al (1992) Screening sigmoidoscopy and colorectal cancer mortality. J Natl Cancer Inst 84:1572–1575

Noshirwani C, VanStolk U, Rybicki L et al (2000) Adenoma size and number are predictive of adenoma recurrence: implications for surveillance colonoscopy. Gastrointest Endosc 51:433–437

Olynyk J, Aquilia S, Fletcher D et al (1996) Flexible sigmoidoscopy screening for colorectal-cancer in average-risk subjects – a community based pilot project. Med J Aust 165:74–76

Parkin D, Bray F, Devesa S (2001) Cancer burden in the year 2000. The global picture. Eur J Cancer 37:4–66

Prorok P, Andriole G, Bresalier R et al (2000) Design of the Prostate, Lung, Colorectal and Ovarian (PLCO) Cancer Screening Trial. Contr Clin Trials 21 [Suppl 6]:273S–309S

Quinn M, Babb P, Brock A et al. (2001) Cancer trends in England and Wales 1950–1999, National Statistics London. Stationary Office

Ramsey S, Berry K, Etzioni R (2002) Lifetime cancer-attributable cost of care for long term survivors of colorectal cancer. AM J Gastroenterol 97:440–445

Rabeneck L, El-Serag H, Sandler R (2001) Incidence and survival of coloretal cancer in the US: 1989–1997. Gastroenterology 120 [Suppl 1]:A65

Ransohoff D (1999) Economic impact of surveillance. Gastrointest Endosc 49:S67–S71

Rembacken B, Fujii T, Cairns A et al (2000) Flat and depressed colonic neoplasms: a prospective study of 1000 colonoscopies in the UK. Lancet 355:1211–1214

Rengucci C, Maiolo P, Saragoni L et al (2001) Multiple detection of genetic alterations in tumors and stool. Clin Cancer Res 7:590–593

Rex D, Lehman G, Hawes R et al (1991) Screening colonoscopy in asymptomatic average-risk persons with negative fecal occult blood tests. Gastroenterology 100:64–67

Rex D, Cutler C, Lemmel G et al (1997a) Colonoscopic miss rates and adenomas determined by back-to-back colonoscopies. Gastroenterology 112:24–28

Rex D, Rahmani E, Haseman J et al (1997b) Relative sensitivity of colonoscopy and barium enema for detection of colorectal cancer in clinical practice. Gastroenterology 112:17–23

Rex K, Johnson A, Lieberman A et al (2000) Colorectal cancer prevention 2000: screening recommendations of the American College of Gastroenterology. Am J Gastroenterol 95:868–877

Robinson M, Hardcastle J, Moss Set al (1999) The risks of screening: data from the Nottingham randomised controlled trial of faecal occult blood screening for colorectal cancer. Gut 45:588–592

Rozen P, Knaani J, Samuel Z (1999) Eliminating the need for dietary restrictions when using a sensitive guaiac fecal occult blood test. Dis Dis Sci 44:756–760

Rozen P, Knaani J, Samuel Z (2000) Comparative screening with a sensitive guaiac and specific immunochemical occult blood test in an endoscopic study. Cancer 89:46–51

Saito H (1996) Screening for colorectal-cancer by immunochemical fecal occult blood testing. Jpn J Cancer Res 87:1011–1024

Schoenfeld P, Cash B, Kita J et al (1999) Effectiveness and patient satisfaction with screening flexible sigmoidoscopy performed by registered nurses. Gastrointest Endosc 49:158–162

Segnan N, Sciallero S, Bonelli L et al (1999) Multicentre randomised controlled trial of "once only" flexible sigmoidoscopy screening in Italy-score. Endoscopy 31 [Suppl 1]:E9

Selby J, Friedman G (1988) Sigmoidoscopy and mortality from colorectal cancer: the Kaiser-Permanente multiphasic evaluation study. J Clin Epidemiol 41:427–434

Selby J, Friedman G, Quesenberry CP Jr, Weiss N (1992) A case-control study of screening sigmoidoscopy and mortality from colorectal cancer. N Engl J Med 326:653–657

Selby J, Friedman G, Quesenberry C et al (1993) Effect of fecal occult blood testing on mortality from colorectal cancer. A case-control study. Ann Intern Med 118:1–6

Senore C, Segnan N, Rossini F et al (1996) Screening for colorectal cancer by once only sigmoidoscopy: a feasibility study in Turin, Italy. J Med Screen 3:72–78

Smith R, vonEschenbach A, Wender R et al (2001) American Cancer Society guidelines for the early detection of cancer: update of early detection guidelines for prostate, colorectal and endometrial cancers. Cancer J Clin 51:38–75

Sonnenberg A, Delco F (2002) Cost-effectiveness of a single colonsocopy in screening for colorectal cancer. Arch Intern Med 162:163–168

Spencer R, Melton L, Ready R et al (1984) Treatment of small colorectal polyps: a population-based study of the risk of subsequent carcinoma. Mayo Clin Proc 59:305–310

Steele R, Parker R, Patnick J et al (2001) A demonstration pilot trial for colorectal cancer screening in the United Kingdom: a new concept in the introduction of healthcare strategies. J Med Screen 8:197–203

Stryker S, Wolff B, Culp C et al (1987) Natural history of untreated colonic polyps. Gastroenterology 93:1009–1013

Summers R, Johnson C, Pusunik L et al (2001) Automated polyp detection at CT colonography: Feasibility assessment in a human population. Radiology 219:51–59

Suzuki Y, Honma T, Yoshida H et al (1997) Prospective follow-up-study of flat-elevated colorectal adenomas by magnifying colonoscopy. Gastrointest Endosc 45:377

Tazi M, Faivre J, Dassonville F et al (1997) Participation in fecal occult blood screening for colorectal cancer in a well defined French population: results of five screening rounds from 1988 to 1996. J Med Screen 4:147–151

Thiis-Evensen E, Hoff G, Sauar J et al (1999) Population-based surveillance by colonoscopy: effect on the incidence of colorectal cancer. Telemark Polyp Study I. Scand J Gastroenterol 34:414–420

Thoeni R, Petras A (1982) Detection of rectal and rectosigmoid lesions by double-contrast barium enema examination and sigmoidoscopy. Radiology 142:59–62

Thomas W, Pye G, Hardcastle J et al (1989) Role of dietary restriction in Haemoccult screening for colorectal cancer. Br J Surg 76:976–978

Traverso G, Shuber A, Levin B et al (2002a) Detection of APC mutations in fecal DNA from patients with colorectal tumors. N Engl J Med 346:311–320

Traverso G, Shuber A, Olsson L et al (2002b) Detection of proximal colorectal cancers through analysis of faecal DNA. Lancet 359:403–404

Verne J, Aubrey R, Love S et al (1998) Population based randomised study of uptake and yield of screening by flexible sigmoidoscopy compared with screening by faecal occult blood testing. BMJ 317:182–185

Vining D, Gelfand D, Bechtold R et al (1994) Technical feasibility of colon imaging with helical CT and virtual reality. Am J Roentgenol 162 [Suppl]:104

Vogelstein B, Fearon E, Hamilton S et al (1988) Genetic alterations during colorectal-tumor development. N Engl J Med 319:525–532

Wagner J, Herdman R, Wadhwa S (1991) Cost effectiveness of colorectal cancer screening in the elderly. Ann Intern Med 115:807–817

Waye J, Kahn O, Auerbach M (1996) Complications of colonoscopy and flexible sigmoidoscopy. Gastrointest Endosc Clin North Am 6:343–377

Wherry D, Thomas W (1994) The yield of flexible fiberoptic sigmoidoscopy in the detection of asymptomatic colorectal neoplasia. Surg Endosc 8:393–395

Winawer S, Zauber A (2001) Colonoscopic polypectomy and the incidence of colorectal cancer. Gut 48:753–756

Winawer S, Zauber A, Diaz B (1987) The National Polyp Study: temporal sequence of evolving colorectal cancer from normal mucosa. Gastrointest Endosc 33:167

Winawer S, Zauber A, O'Brien M et al (1993a) Randomized comparison of surveillance intervals after colonoscopic removal of newly diagnosed adenomatous polyps. N Engl J Med 328:901–906

Winawer S, Zauber A, Ho M et al (1993b) Prevention of colorectal cancer by colonoscopic polypectomy. N Engl J Med 39:1977–1981

Winawer S, St John D, Bond J et al (1995) Guidelines for the prevention of colorectal cancer: update based on new data. World Health Organization collaborating center for the prevention of colorectal cancer. Z Gastroenterol 33:574–576

Winawer S, Fletcher R, Miller L et al (1997) Colorectal-cancer screening – clinical guidelines and rationale. Gastroenterology 112:594–642

Winawer S, Stewart E, Zauber A et al (2000) A comparison of colonoscopy and double-contrast barium enema for surveillance after polypectomy. N Engl J Med 342:1766–1772

Wingo P, Ries L, Parker S et al (1998) Long-term cancer patient survival in the United States. Cancer Epidemiol Biomarkers Prev 7:269–270

Zarchy T, Ershoff D (1994) Do characteristics of adenomas on flexible sigmoidoscopy predict advanced lesions on baseline colonoscopy? Gastroenterology 106:1501–1504

Zauber A, Winawer S, Bond J et al (1999) Long term National Polyp Study (NPS) data on post-polypectomy surveillance. Endoscopy 31:E13 (abstract)

2 Screening Those at High Risk for Colorectal Cancer

Marc Tischkowitz and Shirley Hodgson

CONTENTS

2.1   Introduction   13
2.2   Hereditary Non-polyposis Colorectal Cancer
        (HNPCC)   13
2.2.1   Diagnostic Criteria and Clinical Features   13
2.1.2   Genetics of HNPCC   15
2.2.3   Screening in HNPCC Carriers   16
2.3   Familial Adenomatous Polyposis (FAP)   16
2.3.1   Clinical Features   16
2.3.2   Genetics   17
2.3.3   Screening in FAP   17
2.4   Other Rare Genetic Conditions Predisposing
        to Colorectal Cancer   17
2.4.1   Juvenile Polyposis Syndrome (JPS)   17
2.4.2   Peutz-Jeghers Syndrome (PJS)   18
2.5   Non-syndromic Familial Colorectal Cancer   18
2.6   Other Increased Risk Groups   19
2.6.1   Previous History of Adenomatous Polyps   19
2.6.2   Previous History of Colorectal Cancer   19
2.6.3   Inflammatory Bowel Disease   19
2.7   Non-endoscopic Screening Modalities in
        Individuals at High Risk for Colorectal Cancer   19
2.7.1   Faecal Occult Blood Testing (FOBT)   19
2.7.2   Barium Enema   19
2.7.3   Computed Tomographic Colonography   20
2.8   Conclusion   20
        References   20

2.1 Introduction

Colorectal cancer (CRC) is the second commonest malignancy in the United Kingdom and is a major cause of morbidity and mortality. Prognosis is closely related to stage at presentation and this underlies the importance of early detection. The major risk factor for developing CRC is advancing age, the incidence of CRC being very low in young people and increasing

M. Tischkowitz, MD
Clinical Research Fellow, Division of Medical and Molecular Genetics, Guy's Hospital, St. Thomas Street, London SE1 9RT, UK
S. Hodgson, MD
Professor of Cancer Genetics, Department of Medical Genetics, St George's Hospital, Tooting, London SW17 0RE, UK

rapidly with age, approximately trebling with each decade between 40 and 70. Nevertheless, approximately 10%–15% of CRC occurs in individuals with a family history of cancer (those with one or more parents, siblings or children with the disease), suggesting a genetic susceptibility, but in the absence of any clearly defined genetic syndrome (WINAWER et al. 1997). A further 5% of cases are thought to arise in individuals with a genetic syndrome, predisposing to the development of CRC, and such families are obvious targets for screening strategies (Table 2.1). The two commonest autosomal dominant CRC predisposition syndromes are hereditary non-polyposis colorectal cancer (HNPCC) and familial adenomatous polyposis (FAP) and the molecular genetics, clinical presentation, and screening practices in these syndromes will be discussed in this chapter. Other, rarer CRC predisposition syndromes and the management of non-syn-

Table 2.1. Risk Factors and known gene for CRC

Risk category	Risk factor	Gene
Average risk:	Age> 50 years	
High risk:	Familial adenomatous polyposis	APC, MYH
	Gardner syndrome	
	HNPCC	MSH2, MLH1, MSH3, MSH6, PMS1, PMS2
	Juvenile polyposis	SMAD4, BMPR1
	Cowden syndrome	PTEN
	Ruvalcaba-Myhre-Smith syndrome	PTEN
	Gorlin syndrome	PTCH
	Peutz-Jeghers	LKB1
Moderate risk:	Family history of CRC	Possibly multiple lower penetrance genes
	Previous History of CRC/polyps	
	Inflammatory bowel disease	
	Chronic ulcerative colitis	
	Chronic Crohn's disease	NOD2/CARD15

dromic familial CRC, where familial clustering of CRC in the absence of these conditions may be due to other, lower penetrance genes, will also be covered.

2.2
Hereditary Non-polyposis Colorectal Cancer (HNPCC)

HNPCC is thought to account for around 1% of cases of CRC (SAMOWITZ et al. 2001), although this may be as high as 3%, particularly in countries such as Finland where there are founder mutations (AALTONEN et al. 1998; SALOVAARA et al. 2000). These occur when a population is largely composed of descendants of a small number of individual founders, one or more of whom carried that mutation.

2.2.1
Diagnostic Criteria and Clinical Features

HNPCC was originally described by LYNCH and KRUSH (1967) as an autosomal dominantly inherited predisposition to CRC in the absence of florid polyposis with two main forms, Lynch I (no family history of other cancers) and Lynch II (with other cancers in the family, e.g. endometrial). In 1991 the International Collaborative Group on HNPCC developed a set of diagnostic criteria, which subsequently

became known as the Amsterdam Criteria, which were required to make the diagnosis of HNPCC (VASEN et al. 1991) (Table 2.2); families must have at least three relatives over two generations with colorectal cancer, one a first degree relative of the other two, with at least one case being diagnosed below the age of 50 years. This was intended to create a standard definition to ensure research groups had a consistent approach in the study of the disease. To allow for more flexibility in the clinical setting, modified Amsterdam criteria were subsequently developed which allows the inclusion of extracolonic tumours and smaller families (BELLACOSA et al. 1996) (Table 2.2). The Bethesda criteria were developed which incorporated data about site and histopathology of CRC (Table 2.2) and these criteria are more sensitive but less specific than the Amsterdam criteria in diagnosing HNPCC (RODRIGUEZ-BIGAS et al. 1997). The lifetime risk of developing CRC in affected individuals with HNPCC is 70%–80% for males and 40%–65% for females (VASEN et al. 1996; DUNLOP et al. 1997), with a mean age of onset of CRC at 44 years compared to 62 years in the general population. At total of 1% of CRC in HNPCC occurs below the age of 20 with 92% of cases occurring by age 60 (VASEN et al. 1994, 1996). Affected females in HNPCC kindreds have a 40%–60% lifetime risk of developing endometrial cancer, depending on the mutation, compared to the population risk of 3% (VASEN et al. 1996; AARNIO et al. 1999) and risks for cancers of the small intestine, ureter, stomach, ovary and kidney are also increased (WATSON and LYNCH

Table 2.2. Clinical criteria for HNPCC

Amsterdam criteria (VASEN et al. 1991) (all of the criteria must be met):
1. At least three family members with colorectal cancer, two of whom are first-degree relatives
2. At least two generations affected
3. At least one individual less than 50 years old at diagnosis

Modified Amsterdam criteria (BELLACOSA et al. 1996) (any of the criteria must be met):
1. Very small families, which cannot be further expanded, can be considered as HNPCC even if only two colorectal cancers are found (in the presence of the other criteria)
2. In families with two first-degree relatives affected by colorectal cancer, the presence of a third relative with an early-onset unusual neoplasm or endometrial cancer is sufficient to consider the family as HNPCC

Bethesda criteria (RODRIGUEZ-BIGAS et al. 1997) (any of the criteria must be met):
1. Individuals with cancer families that meet the Amsterdam Criteria
2. Individuals with two HNPCC-related cancers, including synchronous and metachronous or associated extracolonic cancers (endometrial, ovarian, hepatobiliary or small bowel cancers and transitional cell carcinoma of renal pelvis or ureter)
3. Individuals with colorectal cancer and a first-degree relative with colorectal cancer and/or HNPCC – related extracolonic cancer and/or a colorectal adenoma; one of the cancers diagnosed at age <45 years, and the adenoma diagnosed at age <40 years
4. Individuals with colorectal cancer or endometrial cancer diagnosed at age <45 years
5. Individuals with right-sided colorectal cancer with an undifferentiated pattern (solid/cribiform) on histopathology diagnosed at age <45 years
6. Individuals with signet-ring-cell-type colorectal cancer diagnosed at age <45 years
7. Individuals with adenomas diagnosed at age <40 years

1993) (Table 2.3). There is a high incidence of multiple tumours with 18% presenting with synchronous tumours and 40%–50% developing further primary malignancy over a 10–15 year follow-up period (MECKLIN and JARVINEN 1993). Mucinous tumours tend to be more common, there is a preponderance of right sided locations in the colon and several studies have indicated that tumours have a generally better overall prognosis (SANKILA et al. 1996; MYRHOJ et al. 1997; WATSON et al. 1998), although this is not a uniform finding (BERTARIO et al. 1999).

Table 2.3. Observed/expected ratios of other cancers in HNPCC families (WATSON and LYNCH 1993)

Tumour type	Observed/expected ratio
Small intestine	25
Ureter	22
Stomach	4.1
Ovary	3.5
Kidney (mainly transitional cell tumours of renal pelvis and ureter)	3.2

2.1.2
Genetics of HNPCC

Approximately 70% of families with HNPCC have mutations in one of six known genes *MLH1*, *MSH2*, *PMS1*, *PMS2*, *MLH3* and *MSH6* (FISHEL et al. 1993; LEACH et al. 1993; BRONNER et al. 1994; NICOLAIDES et al. 1994; PAPADOPOULOS et al. 1994; AKIYAMA et al. 1997; MIYAKI et al. 1997; WU et al. 2001). Of these, mutations in *MLH1* and *MSH2* are the most common (Table 2.4), between them accounting for around 60% of all cases (which equates to 90% of all identified mutations) with *MSH6* accounting for a further 7% (BERENDS et al. 2002). Mutation screening for these three genes is now available through clinical genetics specialists, but mutations in the other three genes are infrequently found so these are not routinely screened.

Some of these genes were initially localised by linkage studies using microsatellite DNA markers. Microsatellite DNA markers are small runs of repeats of very simple DNA sequence, e.g. (ATATATATATA) and are useful tools in genetic mapping. The microsatellites provided clues to the function of the genes mutated in HNPCC, since analysis of colorectal and other tumours from HNPCC carriers showed that the length of the microsatellites differed between the tumour and germline DNA, so-called microsatellite instability (MSI) (AALTONEN et al. 1993; PELTO-

MAKI et al. 1993). Tumours that display MSI are also described as having "mismatch repair" or being "replication error positive". This phenomena is a consequence of defective function of the mutated HNPCC gene protein products, which are normally involved in maintaining DNA fidelity during replication.

Over 80% of tumours in people with HNPCC have MSI (AALTONEN et al. 1993) compared to 15% of sporadic tumours (THIBODEAU et al. 1993). MSI can also be detected in other tumours associated with HNPCC such as endometrial cancers. Another way to look for loss of function of the HNPCC genes is to use monoclonal antibodies (immunohistochemistry) to identify the protein products of the HNPCC genes in tumours; loss of expression of a specific protein corresponding to an HNPCC gene product implies a defect in that HNPCC gene (LEACH et al. 1996). Whether the probability of HNPCC being present is best determined by microsatellite marker analysis or immunohistochemistry as a screening test remains to be established (DE LA CHAPELLE 2002; LINDOR et al. 2002).

The HNPCC genes appear to act as tumour suppressors; heterozygote cells (which have one normal copy and one mutated copy of a HNPCC gene) have normal or near normal mismatch repair. Loss or mutation of the normal gene copy leads to a drastic reduction in DNA replication fidelity and consequent accumulation of mutations in other tumour suppressor genes and oncogenes, thereby accelerating the multiple genetic steps leading to cancer development.

The fact that MSI is observed in 15%–20% of sporadic tumours and 3%–5% of sporadic adenomas suggests that it can develop through acquired genetic events in the absence of an inherited mutation of one of the HNPCC genes. This has implications if tumour MSI status is to be used as a screening method to identify HNPCC mutation carriers as a proportion of tumours with MSI will not be due to germline HNPCC gene mutations.

Table 2.4. Frequency of mutations detected in HNPCC

Gene	Chromosome	Frequency in HNPCC (%)	Reference
MSH2	2p21-22	30	FISHEL et al. (1993) LEACH et al. (1993)
MLH1	3p21	30	PAPADOPOULOS et al. (1994) BRONNER et al. (1994)
MSH6	2p16	7	AKIYAMA et al. (1997) MIYAKI et al. (1997)
PMS1	2q31.1	<5	NICOLAIDES et al. (1994)
PMS2	7p22	<5	NICOLAIDES et al. (1994)
MLH3	14q24.3	<5	WU et al. (2001)

2.2.3
Screening in HNPCC Carriers

Individuals with HNPCC have a 50:50 risk of handing on the condition to each of their children (male or female), so first-degree relatives of affected individuals should be screened for HNPCC-related cancers.

Colonoscopic screening in HNPCC families has been shown to reduce the incidence of colorectal cancers; one study showed a 7.4% reduction in cancer incidence in 133 members of HNPCC kindreds undergoing 3-yearly colonoscopies or barium enemas compared to 118 HNPCC controls (JARVINEN et al. 1995). As less than 2% of colorectal cancers in HNPCC occur below the age of 20, the current consensus is that colonoscopy screening programmes should start between 20 and 25 years of age. Sigmoidoscopy is not recommended because of the high incidence of right-sided tumours.

The optimum frequency of colonoscopic screening is unknown and varies from annually to every 2 years between centres. There is evidence that adenomas in HNPCC carriers progress to carcinomas at a faster rate than in the general population, probably as a result of accelerated accumulation of somatic mutations (JASS et al. 1994) and a study of 225 colorectal cancer patients from HNPCC families found that 10.2% had developed colorectal cancer within 5 years of partial colonic resection for a first tumour or normal colonoscopy (LANSPA et al. 1994). A second study in the Netherlands of 394 at risk members from 51 HNPCC families found an unexpectedly high occurrence of advanced cancers within 3.5 years of a negative screening procedure and recommended that the interval between screening procedures be reduced to 1–2 years in proven gene carriers (VASEN et al. 1995). A 15-year prospective randomised study of 3-yearly colonoscopic screening in HNPCC families showed that screening more than halved the risk of CRC and reduced overall mortality by 65% by the complete prevention of CRC deaths (JARVINEN et al. 2000). Colonoscopy is thus an effective screening tool in HNPCC families and when combined with genetic testing to identify mutation carriers and genetic registers to maintain contact with individuals, it becomes an efficient and cost effective method to reduce morbidity and mortality due to CRC (DUNLOP 2002a).

It is probable that women with HNPCC should be offered screening for endometrial cancer by annual pelvic ultrasound scan or endometrial Pipelle biopsy, although the efficacy of this has not yet been confirmed (DOVE-EDWIN et al. 2002). There is also an argument for sub-total colectomy as treatment for any CRC detected in an individual with HNPCC, or even for prophylactic colectomy in HNPCC mutation carriers (DECOSSE 1995; SYNGAL et al. 1998), and consideration of prophylactic hysterectomy (and oophorectomy) in female carriers (AARNIO et al. 1995).

In families in which the mutation causing HNPCC has been identified, it is possible to offer a genetic test to at-risk relatives of affected individuals, allowing identification of individuals who have not inherited the mutation, and who can thus be released from surveillance, and those who have, and who therefore require follow-up and management as appropriate.

2.3
Familial Adenomatous Polyposis (FAP)

2.3.1
Clinical Features

FAP is characterised by profuse colonic adenomatous polyposis, with affected individuals developing hundreds of polyps by the second decade and in the absence of prophylactic colectomy, over 90% will have developed CRC by the age of 45 (GUILLEM et al. 1992; KING et al. 2000). In addition to colonic polyps, 80% will have duodenal adenomas (CHURCH et al. 1992; CAMPBELL et al. 1994; WALLACE and PHILLIPS 1998) and there is a 5%–10% lifetime risk of small bowel carcinoma (OFFERHAUS et al. 1992; WALLACE and PHILLIPS 1998). There is also an increased risk of hepatoblastoma, medulloblastoma, papillary carcinoma of the thyroid and desmoid tumours. Desmoids tumours are often found in the small bowel mesentery and occur predominantly in female FAP patients. These benign but treatment-resistant lesions can cause significant morbidity and mortality, and management is difficult; they often recur after surgical resection and treatment with anti-estrogens and salicylates have limited success (CLARK et al. 1999).

Approximately two thirds of individuals with FAP will have flat, oval, pigmented retinal lesions, so-called congenital hypertrophy of the retinal pigment epithelium (CHRPE). These do not cause any clinical problems but are present from birth and can be a useful adjunct to diagnosis in at-risk individuals (TIRET et al. 1997). Gardner syndrome refers to FAP in the context of extracolonic manifestations, including dental abnormalities, osteomas and soft tissue tumours.

2.3.2
Genetics

FAP is autosomally dominantly inherited with a disease prevalence of 1 in 8500; about a third of cases arise sporadically as new mutations. It is caused by germ-line mutations in the adenomatous polyposis coli (*APC*) gene located on chromosome 5q21(Groden et al. 1991; Kinzler et al. 1991). It is a large gene and the clinical phenotype can vary with the location of a mutation; mutations at either end of the gene cause a variant of FAP with few polyps, called attenuated FAP (Spirio et al. 1993; Gardner et al. 1997; Giardiello et al. 1997). Mutations in the mutation cluster region cause a severe disease (Lamlum et al. 1999), and although a large number of *APC* mutations have been described, there are two common ones within this region.

2.3.3
Screening in FAP

At-risk individuals (e.g. children of those affected) are offered at least annual surveillance for the development of colorectal polyps from early teenage onward. If the causative mutation is known in the family then predictive genetic testing should be offered, as this is clearly useful to prevent unnecessary screening of unaffected individuals and concentrate resources on those harbouring a mutation (Terdiman et al. 1999). For those individuals who carry the mutation, prophylactic colectomy is the treatment of choice when polyps become established. Where the mutation is not known entry into a screening programme is advised; during teenage years sigmoidoscopy suffices, since in classical FAP, polyps almost always occur initially in the rectum and sigmoid colon. Current guidelines recommend yearly sigmoidoscopy from ages 14–19 years and 5-yearly colonoscopy with dye spray by an experienced endoscopist from age 20 with yearly sigmoidoscopy or colonoscopy in the intervening years (The Polyposis Registry, St Mark's Hospital 2001); individuals with no polyps by age 25 have a less than 10% chance of developing them, and surveillance intervals can be increased in those free of polyps after 35 years (Dunlop 2002a). The two main surgical options are colectomy with ileorectal anastomosis (which preserves the rectum) and proctocolectomy. If the rectum is preserved, surveillance of the rectal stump is necessary since the cumulative risk of rectal cancer rises to 10% by age 50, and restorative proctocolectomy or conversion to ileostomy should be considered after 35 years of age. Regular surveillance of the upper gastrointestinal (GI) tract is also necessary, as duodenal carcinoma is the major cause of death in FAP patients treated with colectomy. The favoured method is side viewing video duodenoscopy, performed by an endoscopist experienced in FAP (The Polyposis Registry, St Mark's Hospital, 2001). In attenuated FAP, prophylactic colectomy may be avoided providing regular screening is performed and this should be by colonoscopy rather than sigmoidoscopy as recto-sigmoid sparing of adenomas can occur (Spirio et al. 1993).

Recently Al-Tassan et al. (2002) identified bi-allelic mutations in the MYH gene (which is involved in base excision repair of oxidative damage to DNA) in cases of attenuated polyposis. These individuals have an autosomal recessive inheritance pattern of 30–300 adenomatous polyposis in the colon with increased colorectal cancer risk, and this may account for about a third of such cases. This has important implications for genetic counselling and management (Sieber et al. 2003).

2.4
Other Rare Genetic Conditions Predisposing to Colorectal Cancer

2.4.1
Juvenile Polyposis Syndrome (JPS)

This uncommon condition tends to be sporadic although 20%–50% have a family history showing autosomal dominant inheritance (Desai et al. 1995). It is characterised by hamartomatous polyps developing throughout the gastrointestinal tract and by adulthood 50–200 polyps may be present, commonly in the rectosigmoid region. Germline mutations in *SMAD4* and *BMPR1A* together account for approximately 60% of cases (Houlston et al. 1998; Howe et al. 1998; Woodford-Richens et al. 2000) and affected individuals can have extracolonic manifestations. Juvenile polyps may also occur in Cowden syndrome or Ruvalcaba-Myhre-Smith syndrome (due to inherited mutations in the *PTEN* gene) and Gorlin syndrome (due to inherited mutations in the *PTCH* gene). JPS is associated with a 20%–50% lifetime risk of developing CRC (Jass et al. 1988; Desai et al. 1995) and there is also an increased risk of upper gastrointestinal malignancies. Based on these risks, current surveillance recommendations include 3-yearly upper and lower endoscopy in affected individuals and first-degree relatives.

2.4.2
Peutz-Jeghers Syndrome (PJS)

This is another rare condition characterised by hamartomatous polyposis throughout the GI tract, particularly in the upper jejunum (TOMLINSON and HOULSTON 1997). It is autosomal dominant and can be due to mutations in *LKB1* (HEMMINKI et al. 1998) which are identified in 50%–60% of cases (YLIKORKALA et al. 1999). Affected individuals have characteristic melanin flecks on the lips and mucocutaneous borders. In addition to an increased risk of CRC, there are also increased risks of developing other malignancies, including pancreatic, breast and ovarian carcinomas, and a rare ovarian neoplasm, sex cord tumour with annular tubules (SCTAT). SCTAT has features of both granulosa cell tumours and Sertoli cell tumours and has also been occasionally reported in testicular tumours. Surveillance is problematic in view of these diverse malignancies but, for the GI tract, 2 yearly upper and lower endoscopy is recommended together with a small bowel examination by barium follow-through (DUNLOP 2002a).

2.5
Non-syndromic Familial Colorectal Cancer

In addition to the highly penetrant syndromic causes of CRC described above, there are a large number of families where the there is a weaker family history of CRC. It is estimated that 1% of the population will have two first-degree relatives affected with CRC or have a relative with CRC under the age of 45 years (St. JOHN et al. 1993; SLATTERY and KERBER 1994), and 25% of CRC occurs in younger individuals or those with a family history of CRC (WINAWER et al. 1997). First-degree relatives of cases of CRC have a between two-and three-fold increased risk of developing CRC which rises to four- or five-fold in cases diagnosed under 45 years (ROZEN et al. 1987; BONELLI et al. 1988; KUNE et al. 1989; STEPHENSON et al. 1991; FUCHS et al. 1994). Whilst a few of these families may harbour HNPCC mutations and some will be due to chance, the majority are likely to be

due to inheritance of one or more yet to be discovered lower penetrance genes whose combined effects result in a continuum of risk between the normal population and high risk CRC syndromes. Evidence to decide optimum surveillance methods and frequencies for this heterogeneous group is still lacking and current guidelines are based on using average risk CRC screening methods and increasing the screening intensity according to individual risk based on family history (WINAWER et al. 1997). Guidelines based on family history criteria for screening, and the age to start and frequency of colonoscopic surveillance are still being debated in the absence of firm evidence of cost-benefit (BURT 2000), and funding and management issues have still to be resolved. Surveillance recommendations are based on the premise that colonoscopy will allow the detection and removal of adenomas in at-risk individuals with consequent reduction of CRC risk. Since the risk of CRC in individuals with a family history of the condition appears to develop 10 years earlier than in the general population, it would seem reasonable to initiate colonoscopic surveillance at 45 years of age in such individuals (when the risk of CRC is about 50/100,000 per annum, equivalent to the risk in men in the general population at 50–55 years of age and women at 55–59 years of age) (ROZEN et al. 1987; GUILLEM et al. 1992). The adenocarcinoma sequence is thought to take 5–10 years in the absence of HNPCC (MUTO et al. 1975), so 5-yearly colonoscopies are probably adequate, unless adenomas are detected, in which case the frequency could be increased to 3-yearly. Such surveillance can be offered to individuals with a family history which does not conform to HNPCC criteria, but who have two first-degree relatives or one first- and one second-degree relative with CRC on the same side of the family and those with one first-degree relative diagnosed below 45 years of age. Individuals with a single first-degree relative diagnosed above 45 years of age or with no first-degree but one or two second-degree relatives with CRC could be reassured and excluded from surveillance. Such criteria remain arbitrary and protocols will require careful long-term audit before they are accepted for the development of cost-effective strategies recommended for funding nationally. Suggested guidelines have recently been published for the management of individuals with a family history of colorectal cancer (DUNLOP 2002b). One colonoscopy at 35 years and one at 55 years if the first is clear has been recommended for those at sufficiently increased risk.

2.6
Other Increased Risk Groups

2.6.1
Previous History of Adenomatous Polyps

Evidence from the National Polyp Study showed that subsequent colonoscopic screening in individuals who have previously undergone colonoscopic removal of one or more adenomatous polyps reduced the rates of CRC by 76%–90% compared to non-surveillance reference groups (WINAWER et al. 1993), although it is likely that a significant part of this reduction is from having the polyp removed in the first place. Current guidelines recommend one follow-up colonoscopy 3 years after removal of the initial polyp (WINAWER et al. 1997).

2.6.2
Previous History of Colorectal Cancer

Individuals previously diagnosed with CRC (in the absence of HNPCC) not only have a risk of recurrence but also a risk of a second (metachronous) tumour. It is therefore recommended that patients have a follow-up screening procedure 1 year after resection, a further examination at 3 years and subsequently every 5 years (WINAWER et al. 1997). As the local anatomy may be distorted following surgery, this needs to be taken into account when choosing the most suitable screening modality.

2.6.3
Inflammatory Bowel Disease

Patients with a long-standing history of inflammatory bowel disease are at increased risk of developing CRC (SHARAN and SCHOEN 2002). Recently, mutations in the NOD2/CARD15 gene have been shown to be associated with susceptibility to Crohn's disease (HAMPE et al. 2001; HUGOT et al. 2001; OGURA et al. 2001), but genotype-phenotype studies have not shown an increased risk of CRC in mutation carriers, due to the small numbers studied. Colonoscopy is the preferred screening method for these patients as CRC can arise from flat infiltrating lesions not seen with barium enemas. However, questions remain regarding the frequency of surveillance, type of sampling, and effectiveness of colonoscopy regarding detection of dysplasia (WINAWER et al. 1997; SHARAN and SCHOEN 2002).

2.7
Non-endoscopic Screening Modalities in Individuals at High Risk for Colorectal Cancer

Most of the screening protocols discussed in this chapter have involved either sigmoidoscopy or colonoscopy. However, colonoscopy is a costly, uncomfortable, operator-dependent procedure and complications due to perforation, ileus or haemorrhage occur in about 1 in 300 procedures and death in 1–3/10,000 (WAYE et al. 1992; KEWENTER and BREVINGE 1996). Could alternative screening modalities be considered which would offer similar accuracy with fewer disadvantages?

2.7.1
Faecal Occult Blood Testing (FOBT)

This has been suggested as a possible adjunct to other screening modalities. Randomised prospective studies have shown a 15%–33% reduction in CRC mortality using FOBT in population-risk individuals (HARDCASTLE et al. 1996; KRONBORG et al. 1996; MANDEL et al. 2000), but the estimated 30%–50% sensitivity (RANSOHOFF and LANG 1997) is too low to consider FOBT as an effective single screening modality in high-risk individuals, particularly since a positive FOB is unlikely to occur as a result of adenomas before malignant transformation. Nevertheless, technological advances which improve the accuracy of the test together with the possible use of specific molecular markers (AHLQUIST 2000) may make this a more acceptable modality in the future.

2.7.2
Barium Enema

Barium enema is generally considered less sensitive than colonoscopy for detecting colonic polyps or CRC with one direct comparison study in normal risk individuals showing a sensitivity to detect CRC of 81.8% for single contrast barium enema, 85.2% for double contrast barium enema versus 95% for colonoscopy (REX et al. 1997). The most important factor for the difference was the better ability of colonoscopy to detect Duke's A lesions. Nevertheless, barium enema could be considered as an alternative screening measure in those individuals unable to tolerate a colonoscopy.

2.7.3
Computed Tomographic Colonography

Computed tomographic (CT) colonography or virtual colonoscopy uses thin-section helical CT to generate high resolution, two-dimensional axial colonic images which are then reconstructed into three-dimensional images simulating those of actual colonoscopy (HARA et al. 1996; VINING 1996). In a direct comparison of this technique with normal colonoscopy in 100 high-risk individuals (age>50, previous history of polyps, positive FOBT or family history), CT colonography identified all three cancers, 91% of polyps >10 mm in diameter, 82% of polyps 6–9 mm in diameter and 55% of polyps <5 mm diameter (FENLON et al. 1999). Similar results have been published from other studies (FLETCHER et al. 2000; YEE et al. 2001; LAGHI et al. 2002) showing that virtual colonoscopy has a similar sensitivity to conventional colonoscopy for lesions >5 mm in diameter.

CT colonography is safe with no complications reported in any of the studies so far. It is also acceptable and well tolerated by patients and, as no sedation is required, patients can leave immediately after the procedure. Furthermore, it allows for whole colon examination even when conventional colonoscopy is incomplete because of stenosing lesions or uncooperative patients, which may occur in 10%–20% of procedures (THIIS-EVENSEN et al. 1999). This is of great importance in high-risk individuals where synchronous tumours may be present. Finally, CT colonography can detect the presence of bowel wall invasion, lymphadenopathy and liver metastases which allows more accurate tumour staging and the detection of other extracolonic findings such as uterine tumours or desmoid tumours which could be an advantage in syndromic CRC risk groups (HARA et al. 2000).

The main problems with CT colonography relate to residual stool or fluid as a result of inadequate bowel preparation, which can either simulate or disguise the presence of a lesion (JOHNSON and DACHMAN 2000). Lesions may also be missed due to incompletely distended bowel segments (JOHNSON and DACHMAN 2000) and flat lesions are more likely to be missed. Although the radiation dose is approximately 20% lower than double contrast barium enema (HARA et al. 1997) the dose is significant and the long-term health consequences of repeat radiation exposure from regular screening in the high-risk CRC group are unclear and need to be addressed. For example, while FAP cell lines exposed to gamma radiation have similar radiosensitivity compared to control cell lines (BRAS et al.

1995), studies on the Apc1638N FAP mouse model have shown that female mice exposed to a single dose of 5 Gy total body X-irradiation have an increased incidence of mammary tumours and desmoids (VAN DER HOUVEN VAN OORDT et al. 1997, 1999). Magnetic resonance colonography would circumvent this issue but CT colonography is currently preferred because of better image quality and shorter examination and interpretation times (PAPPALARDO et al. 2000).

CT colonography has shown promising results so far and improvements in technology will make this procedure a cheaper, more accurate and potentially a better screening modality than conventional colonoscopy and there is clearly a need for further screening trials in specific groups with a high-risk of CRC.

2.8
Conclusion

Around 25% of all CRCs occur in individuals at increased risk of developing CRC of which a small proportion occur in highly penetrant CRC predisposition syndromes. Screening has been shown to be effective in reducing morbidity and mortality form CRC in these high-risk individuals. The current favoured methods of screening are endoscopic but significant advances in molecular stool screening together with the advent of new technologies such a CT colonography may lead to more accurate, patient-acceptable screening procedures in the future.

References

Aaltonen LA, Peltomaki P, Leach FS et al (1993) Clues to the pathogenesis of familial colorectal cancer. Science 260:812–816

Aaltonen LA, Salovaara R, Kristo P et al (1998) Incidence of hereditary nonpolyposis colorectal cancer and the feasibility of molecular screening for the disease. N Engl J Med 338:1481–1487

Aarnio M, Mecklin JP, Aaltonen LA et al (1995) Life-time risk of different cancers in hereditary non-polyposis colorectal cancer (HNPCC) syndrome. Int J Cancer 64:430–433

Aarnio M, Sankila R, Pukkala E et al (1999) Cancer risk in mutation carriers of DNA-mismatch-repair genes. Int J Cancer 81:214–218

Ahlquist DA (2000) Molecular stool screening for colorectal cancer. Using DNA markers may be beneficial, but large scale evaluation is needed. BMJ 321:254–255

Akiyama Y, Sato H, Yamada T et al (1997) Germ-line mutation of the hMSH6/GTBP gene in an atypical hereditary nonpolyposis colorectal cancer kindred. Cancer Res 57:3920–3923

Al-Tassan N, Chmiel NH, Maynard J et al (2002) Inherited variants of MYH associated with somatic G:C-->T:A mutations in colorectal tumors. Nat Genet. 30:227–232

Bellacosa A, Genuardi M, Anti M et al (1996) Hereditary nonpolyposis colorectal cancer: review of clinical, molecular genetics, and counseling aspects. Am J Med Genet 62:353–364

Berends MJ, Wu Y, Sijmons RH et al (2002) Molecular and clinical characteristics of MSH6 variants: an analysis of 25 index carriers of a germline variant. Am J Hum Genet 70:26–37

Bertario L, Russo A, Sala P et al (1999) Survival of patients with hereditary colorectal cancer: comparison of HNPCC and colorectal cancer in FAP patients with sporadic colorectal cancer. Int J Cancer 80:183–187

Bonelli L, Martines H, Conio M et al (1988) Family history of colorectal cancer as a risk factor for benign and malignant tumours of the large bowel. A case-control study. Int J Cancer 41:513–517

Bras A, Cristovao L, Coelho C et al (1995) Normal genetic response to gamma irradiation in familial adenomatous polyposis. Eur J Cancer 31A:1506–1510

Bronner CE, Baker SM, Morrison PT et al (1994) Mutation in the DNA mismatch repair gene homologue hMLH1 is associated with hereditary non-polyposis colon cancer. Nature 368:258–261

Burt RW (2000) Colon cancer screening. Gastroenterology 119(3):837–853

Campbell WJ, Spence RA, Parks TG (1994) Familial adenomatous polyposis. Br J Surg 81:1722–1733

Church JM, McGannon E, Hull-Boiner S et al (1992) Gastroduodenal polyps in patients with familial adenomatous polyposis. Dis Colon Rectum 35:1170–1173

Clark SK, Neale KF, Landgrebe JC et al (1999) Desmoid tumours complicating familial adenomatous polyposis. Br J Surg 86:1185–1189

De La Chapelle A (2002) Microsatellite instability phenotype of tumors: genotyping or immunohistochemistry? The jury is still out. J Clin Oncol 20:897–899

DeCosse JJ (1995) Surgical prophylaxis of familial colon cancer: prevention of death from familial colorectal cancer. J Natl Cancer Inst Monogr 17:31–32

Desai DC, Neale KF, Talbot IC et al (1995) Juvenile polyposis. Br J Surg 82:14–17

Dove-Edwin I, Boks D, Goff S et al (2002) The outcome of endometrial carcinoma surveillance by ultrasound scan in women at risk of hereditary nonpolyposis colorectal carcinoma and familial colorectal carcinoma. Cancer 94:1708–1712

Dunlop MG (2002a) Guidance on gastrointestinal surveillance for hereditary non-polyposis colorectal cancer, familial adenomatous polyposis, juvenile polyposis and Peutz jegher syndrome. Gut 51 [Suppl V]:v21–v27

Dunlop MG (2002b) Guidance on large bowel surveillance for people with two first-degree relatives with colorectal cancer or one first degree relative diagnosed with colorectal cancer under 45y. Gut 51 [Suppl V]:v17–v20

Dunlop MG, Farrington SM, Carothers AD et al (1997) Cancer risk associated with germline DNA mismatch repair gene mutations. Hum Mol Genet 6:105–110

Fenlon HM, Nunes DP, Schroy PC 3rd et al (1999) A comparison of virtual and conventional colonoscopy for the detection of colorectal polyps. N Engl J Med 341:1496–1503

Fishel R, Lescoe MK, Rao MR et al (1993) The human mutator gene homolog MSH2 and its association with hereditary nonpolyposis colon cancer. Cell 75:1027–1038

Fletcher JG, Johnson CD, Welch TJ et al (2000) Optimization of CT colonography technique: prospective trial in 180 patients. Radiology 216:704–711

Fuchs CS, Giovannucci EL, Colditz GA et al (1994) A prospective study of family history and the risk of colorectal cancer. N Engl J Med 331:1669–1674

Gardner RJ, Kool D, Edkins E et al (1997) The clinical correlates of a 3' truncating mutation (codons 1982–1983) in the adenomatous polyposis coli gene. Gastroenterology 113:326–331

Giardiello FM, Brensinger JD, Luce MC et al (1997) Phenotypic expression of disease in families that have mutations in the 5' region of the adenomatous polyposis coli gene. Ann Intern Med 126:514–519

Groden J, Thliveris A, Samowitz W et al (1991) Identification and characterization of the familial adenomatous polyposis coli gene. Cell 66:589–600

Guillem JG, Forde KA, Treat MR et al (1992) Colonoscopic screening for neoplasms in asymptomatic first-degree relatives of colon cancer patients. A controlled, prospective study. Dis Colon Rectum 35:523–529

Hampe J, Cuthbert A, Croucher PJ et al (2001) Association between insertion mutation in NOD2 gene and Crohn's disease in German and British populations. Lancet 357: 1925–1928

Hara AK, Johnson CD, Reed JE et al (1996) Detection of colorectal polyps by computed tomographic colography: feasibility of a novel technique. Gastroenterology 110:284–290

Hara AK, Johnson CD, Reed JE et al (1997) Reducing data size and radiation dose for CT colonography. AJR Am J Roentgenol 168:1181–1184

Hara AK, Johnson CD, MacCarty RL et al (2000) Incidental extracolonic findings at CT colonography. Radiology 215: 353–357

Hardcastle JD, Chamberlain JO, Robinson MH et al (1996) Randomised controlled trial of faecal-occult-blood screening for colorectal cancer. Lancet 348:1472–1477

Hemminki A, Markie D, Tomlinson I et al (1998) A serine/threonine kinase gene defective in Peutz-Jeghers syndrome. Nature 391:184–187

Houlston R, Bevan S, Williams A et al (1998) Mutations in DPC4 (SMAD4) cause juvenile polyposis syndrome, but only account for a minority of cases. Hum Mol Genet 7: 1907–1912

Howe JR, Roth S, Ringold JC et al (1998) Mutations in the SMAD4/DPC4 gene in juvenile polyposis. Science 280: 1086–1088

Hugot JP, Chamaillard M, Zouali H et al (2001) Association of NOD2 leucine-rich repeat variants with susceptibility to Crohn's disease. Nature 411:599–603

Jarvinen HJ, Mecklin JP, Sistonen P (1995) Screening reduces colorectal cancer rate in families with hereditary nonpolyposis colorectal cancer. Gastroenterology 108: 1405–1411

Jarvinen HJ, Aarnio M, Mustonen H et al (2000) Controlled 15-year trial on screening for colorectal cancer in families with hereditary nonpolyposis colorectal cancer. Gastroenterology 118:829–834

Jass JR, Williams CB, Bussey HJ et al (1988) Juvenile polyposis – a precancerous condition. Histopathology 13:619–630

Jass JR, Smyrk TC, Stewart SM et al (1994) Pathology of hereditary non-polyposis colorectal cancer. Anticancer Res 14:1631–1634

Johnson CD, Dachman AH (2000) CT colonography: the next colon screening examination? Radiology 216:331–341

Kewenter J, Brevinge H (1996) Endoscopic and surgical complications of work-up in screening for colorectal cancer. Dis Colon Rectum 39:676–680

King JE, Dozois RR, Lindor NM et al (2000) Care of patients and their families with familial adenomatous polyposis. Mayo Clin Proc 75:57–67

Kinzler KW, Nilbert MC, Su LK et al (1991) Identification of FAP locus genes from chromosome 5q21. Science 253: 661–665

Kronborg O, Fenger C, Olsen J et al (1996) Randomised study of screening for colorectal cancer with faecal-occult-blood test. Lancet 348:1467–1471

Kune GA, Kune S, Watson LF (1989) The role of heredity in the etiology of large bowel cancer: data from the Melbourne Colorectal Cancer Study. World JSurg 13:124–129; discussion 129–131

Laghi A, Iannaccone R, Carbone I et al (2002) Detection of colorectal lesions with virtual computed tomographic colonography. Am J Surg 183:124–131

Lamlum H, Ilyas M, Rowan A et al (1999) The type of somatic mutation at APC in familial adenomatous polyposis is determined by the site of the germline mutation: a new facet to Knudson's ‚two-hit' hypothesis. Nat Med 5: 1071–1075

Lanspa SJ, Jenkins JX, Cavalieri RJ et al (1994) Surveillance in Lynch syndrome: how aggressive? Am J Gastroenterol 89: 1978–1980

Leach FS, Nicolaides NC, Papadopoulos N et al (1993) Mutations of amutS homolog in hereditary nonpolyposis colorectal cancer. Cell 75:1215–1225

Leach FS, Polyak K, Burrell M et al (1996) Expression of the human mismatch repair gene hMSH2 in normal and neoplastic tissues. Cancer Res 56:235–240

Lindor NM, Burgart LJ, Leontovich O et al (2002) Immunohistochemistry versus microsatellite instability testing in phenotyping colorectal tumors. J Clin Oncol 20: 1043–1048

Lynch HT, Krush AJ (1967) Heredity and adenocarcinoma of the colon. Gastroenterology 53:517–527

Mandel JS, Church TR, Bond JH et al (2000) The effect of fecal occult-blood screening on the incidence of colorectal cancer. N Engl JMed 343:1603–1607

Mecklin JP, Jarvinen H (1993) Treatment and follow-up strategies in hereditary nonpolyposis colorectal carcinoma. Dis Colon Rectum 36:927–929

Miyaki M, Konishi M, Tanaka K et al (1997) Germline mutation of MSH6 as the cause of hereditary nonpolyposis colorectal cancer. Nat Genet 17:271–272

Muto T, Bussey HJ and Morson BC (1975) The evolution of cancer of the colon and rectum. Cancer 36:2251–2270

Myrhoj T, Bisgaard ML, Bernstein I et al (1997) Hereditary non-polyposis colorectal cancer: clinical features and survival. Results from the Danish HNPCC register. Scand J Gastroenterol 32:572–576

Nicolaides NC, Papadopoulos N, Liu B et al (1994) Mutations of two PMS homologues in hereditary nonpolyposis colon cancer. Nature 371:75–80

Offerhaus GJ, Giardiello FM, Krush AJ et al (1992) The risk of upper gastrointestinal cancer in familial adenomatous polyposis. Gastroenterology 102:1980–1982

Ogura Y, Bonen DK, Inohara N et al (2001) A frameshift muta-

tion in NOD2 associated with susceptibility to Crohn's disease. Nature 411:603–606

Papadopoulos N, Nicolaides NC, Wei YF et al (1994) Mutation of amutL homolog in hereditary colon cancer. Science 263: 1625–1629

Pappalardo G, Polettini E, Frattaroli FM et al (2000) Magnetic resonance colonography versus conventional colonoscopy for the detection of colonic endoluminal lesions. Gastroenterology 119:300–304

Peltomaki P, Lothe RA, Aaltonen LA et al (1993) Microsatellite instability is associated with tumors that characterize the hereditary non-polyposis colorectal carcinoma syndrome. Cancer Res 53:5853–5855

Ransohoff DF, Lang CA (1997) Screening for colorectal cancer with the fecal occult blood test: a background paper. American College of Physicians. Ann Intern Med 126:811–822

Rex DK, Rahmani EY, Haseman JH et al (1997) Relative sensitivity of colonoscopy and barium enema for detection of colorectal cancer in clinical practice. Gastroenterology 112:17–23

Rodriguez-Bigas MA, Boland CR, Hamilton SR et al (1997) A National Cancer Institute Workshop on Hereditary Nonpolyposis Colorectal Cancer Syndrome: meeting highlights and Bethesda guidelines. J Natl Cancer Inst 89:1758–1762

Rozen P, Fireman Z, Figer A et al (1987) Family history of colorectal cancer as amarker of potential malignancy within a screening program. Cancer 60:248–254

Salovaara R, Loukola A, Kristo P et al (2000) Population-based molecular detection of hereditary nonpolyposis colorectal cancer. J Clin Oncol 18:2193–2200

Samowitz WS, Curtin K, Lin HH et al (2001) The colon cancer burden of genetically defined hereditary nonpolyposis colon cancer. Gastroenterology 121:830–838

Sankila R, Aaltonen LA, Jarvinen HJ et al (1996) Better survival rates in patients with MLH1-associated hereditary colorectal cancer. Gastroenterology 110:682–687

Sharan R, Schoen RE (2002) Cancer in inflammatory bowel disease. An evidence-based analysis and guide for physicians and patients. Gastroenterol Clin North Am 31: 237–254

Sieber OM, Lipton L, Crabtree M et al (2003) Multiple colorectal adenomas, classic adenomatous polyposis, and germline mutations in MYH. N Engl J Med 348:791–799

Slattery ML, Kerber RA (1994) Family history of cancer and colon cancer risk: the Utah Population Database. J Natl Cancer Inst 86:1618–1626

Spirio L, Olschwang S, Groden J et al (1993) Alleles of the APC gene: an attenuated form of familial polyposis. Cell 75:951–957

St John DJ, McDermott FT, Hopper JL et al (1993) Cancer risk in relatives of patients with common colorectal cancer. Ann Intern Med 118:785–790

Stephenson BM, Finan PJ, Gascoyne J et al (1991) Frequency of familial colorectal cancer. Br J Surg 78:1162–1166

Syngal S, Weeks JC, Schrag D et al (1998) Benefits of colonoscopic surveillance and prophylactic colectomy in patients with hereditary nonpolyposis colorectal cancer mutations. Ann Intern Med 129:787–796

Terdiman JP, Conrad PG, Sleisenger MH (1999) Genetic testing in hereditary colorectal cancer: indications and procedures. Am JGastroenterol 94:2344–2356

The Polyposis Registry, St Mark's Hospital, London, UK (2001)

Protocol for the management of patients with polyposis. A guide for medical staff

Thibodeau SN, Bren G, Schaid D (1993) Microsatellite instability in cancer of the proximal colon. Science 260:816–819

Thiis-Evensen E, Hoff GS, Sauar J et al (1999) Population-based surveillance by colonoscopy: effect on the incidence of colorectal cancer. Telemark Polyp Study I. Scand JGastroenterol 34:414–420

Tiret A, Taiel-Sartral M, Tiret E et al (1997) Diagnostic value of fundus examination in familial adenomatous polyposis. Br J Ophthalmol 81:755–758

Tomlinson IP, Houlston RS (1997) Peutz-Jeghers syndrome. J Med Genet 34:1007–1011

Van der Houven van Oordt CW, Smits R, Williamson SL et al (1997) Intestinal and extra-intestinal tumor multiplicities in the Apc1638N mouse model after exposure to X-rays. Carcinogenesis 18:2197–2203

Van der Houven van Oordt CW, Smits R, Schouten TG et al (1999) The genetic background modifies the spontaneous and X-ray-induced tumor spectrum in the Apc1638N mouse model. Genes Chromosomes Cancer 24:191–198

Vasen HF, Mecklin JP, Khan PM et al (1991) The International Collaborative Group on Hereditary Non-Polyposis Colorectal Cancer (ICG-HNPCC). Dis Colon Rectum 34:424–425

Vasen HF, Taal BG, Griffioen G et al (1994) Clinical heterogeneity of familial colorectal cancer and its influence on screening protocols. Gut 35:1262–1266

Vasen HF, Nagengast FM, Khan PM (1995) Interval cancers in hereditary non-polyposis colorectal cancer (Lynch syndrome). Lancet 345:1183–1184

Vasen HF, Wijnen JT, Menko FH et al (1996) Cancer risk in families with hereditary nonpolyposis colorectal cancer diagnosed by mutation analysis. Gastroenterology 110:1020–1027

Vining DJ (1996) Virtual endoscopy: is it reality? Radiology 200:30–31

Wallace MH, Phillips RK (1998) Upper gastrointestinal disease in patients with familial adenomatous polyposis. Br J Surg 85:742–750

Watson P, Lynch HT (1993) Extracolonic cancer in hereditary nonpolyposis colorectal cancer. Cancer 71:677–685

Watson P, Lin KM, Rodriguez-Bigas MA et al (1998) Colorectal carcinoma survival among hereditary nonpolyposis colorectal carcinoma family members. Cancer 83:259–266

Waye JD, Lewis BS, Yessayan S (1992) Colonoscopy: a prospective report of complications. J Clin Gastroenterol 15:347–351

Winawer SJ, Zauber AG, Ho MN et al (1993) Prevention of colorectal cancer by colonoscopic polypectomy. The National Polyp Study Workgroup. N Engl J Med 329:1977–1981

Winawer SJ, Fletcher RH, Miller L et al (1997) Colorectal cancer screening: clinical guidelines and rationale. Gastroenterology 112:594–642

Woodford-Richens K, Bevan S, Churchman M et al (2000) Analysis of genetic and phenotypic heterogeneity in juvenile polyposis. Gut 46:656–660

Wu Y, Berends MJ, Sijmons RH et al (2001) A role for MLH3 in hereditary nonpolyposis colorectal cancer. Nat Genet 29:137–138

Yee J, Akerkar GA, Hung RK et al (2001) Colorectal neoplasia: performance characteristics of CT colonography for detection in 300 patients. Radiology 219:685–692

Ylikorkala A, Avizienyte E, Tomlinson IP et al (1999) Mutations and impaired function of LKB1 in familial and non-familial Peutz-Jeghers syndrome and a sporadic testicular cancer. Hum Mol Genet 8:45–51

3 The Significance of the Flat Adenoma

Bjorn Rembacken

CONTENTS

3.1   Background   25
3.2   Classification of Colorectal Adenomas   25
3.3   What Is the Relevance of Non-polypoid
      Adenomas?   27
3.4   Potential Benefit from Removing Colorectal
      Polyps   27
3.5   Cancer Incidence After Colonoscopy Screening and
      Reasons for the Relative Failure of Surveillance   27
3.6   Reasons for the Relative Failure of Surveillance   28
3.6   Detection of Non-polypoid Adenomas   28
3.7   Detection of Flat and Depressed Adenomas
      by Barium Enema and CT Colonography   29
3.8   Conclusion   29
      References   29

3.1
Background

The importance of flat adenomas and their relationship to colorectal cancer has been increasingly recognised in the last 20 years. Japanese endoscopists were the first to report that flat and depressed adenomas were common in the colon and that some harboured high-grade dysplasia. Until then it had been thought that all significant colorectal adenomas were polypoid.

However, the finding of non-polypoid adenomas was not entirely unexpected as MORSON (1974) had estimated that up to two thirds of all colorectal carcinomas arose from adenomatous polyps but was unable to explain the origin of the remainder. In addition, 12 years earlier, SPRATT et al. (1962) had given a detailed description of 20 early colonic carcinomas some of which were flat.

Non-polypoid adenomas has now become recognised outside Japan. A few years ago, we reported on our experience of flat and depressed adenomas in Leeds (REMBACKEN et al. 2000). Of the 321 adeno-

B. REMBACKEN, MD
Consultant Gastroenterologist, The General Infirmary at Leeds, Great George Street, 15 Wayland Close, Adel, Leeds LS1 3EX, UK

mas found in 1000 consecutive patients attending for colonoscopy, 63% of the lesions were polypoid, 36% were flat-topped mucosal elevations and 0.6% of lesions were depressed. Thirty-seven of these adenomas harboured high-grade dysplasia or early invasive cancer. Flat, elevated or depressed lesions accounted for over half (20/37) of these early colonic malignancies.

The findings from Leeds are very similar to that of the largest series to date, from the Akita Red Cross Hospital in Japan. Of 17850 colonic neoplastic lesions, 55% were polypoid. 42.7% were flat mucosal elevations and 2.3% were depressed.

3.2
Classification of Colorectal Adenomas

Before discussing the relevance of flat and depressed adenomas, the classification used to describe colorectal adenomas should be considered.

The system currently used to describe the appearance of colorectal adenomas was first developed in Japan (JAPANESE SOCIETY FOR CANCER OF THE COLON AND RECTUM 1997). The relative frequency distribution of the different types of colorectal polyps as reported by KUDO (1996) is listed in Table 3.1. In this classification system, colonic polyps are sub-classified into pedunculated polyps (type Ip lesions), sub-pedunculated polyps (type Isp lesions), and sessile polyps (type Is lesions). Flat lesions are subdivided into flat-topped mucosal elevations (type IIa), completely flat lesions (type IIb) and depressed lesions (type IIc).

At endoscopy, type IIa lesions are only slightly elevated (Fig. 3.1), i.e. lower than type I lesions, but do not appear completely flat as type IIb lesions do. The term "flat adenoma" may be confusing as completely flat mucosal lesions are extremely rare in the colorectum. At colonoscopy, type IIc lesions usually appear as shallow mucosal depressions, often surrounded by a rim of reactive epithelium (Fig. 3.2).

Table 3.1. Relative frequency of macroscopic types of early adenomas

Macroscopic type		Proportion of all colonic adenomas	Proportion of lesions invading into the submucosa
Ip, Isp and Is		57%	2%
IIa		39%	1%
IIa+IIc		2%	16%
IIc		2%	16%

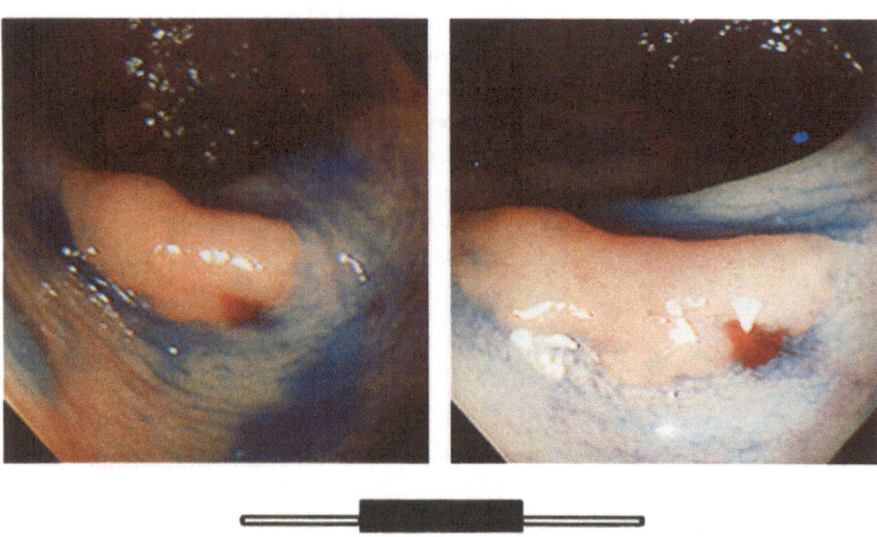

Fig. 3.1. Colonoscopy. A slightly elevated lesion (type IIa)

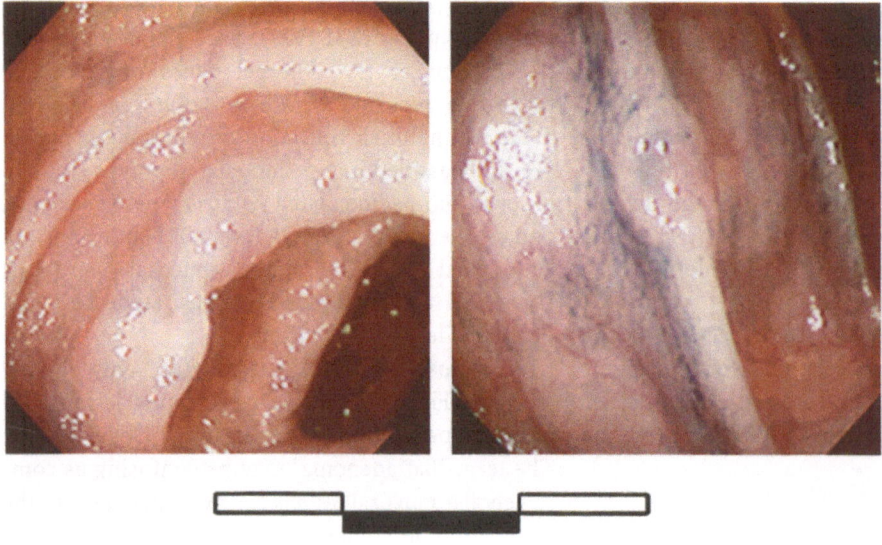

Fig. 3.2. Colonoscopy. A shallow mucosal depression surrounded by a rim of reactive epithelium (type IIc lesion)

There are also lesions combining these features such as "IIa +IIc type lesions", with a superficial elevated portion and a shallow central depression. In the colon and rectum, this central depression is often situated above the level of the normal surrounding mucosa (Fig. 3.3).

3.3
What Is the Relevance of Non-polypoid Adenomas?

Although non-polypoid colorectal adenomas are now widely recognised, controversy remains over the relevance of these lesions. What proportion of colorectal cancer arises from flat and depressed adenomas? This question has implications for screening programmes. If fast-growing flat and depressed lesions are more common than previously thought, it could have important implications for cancer prevention programmes. Flat and depressed lesions are difficult to detect and may progress from precursor adenoma to cancer too quickly to be detected by screening programmes.

WILSON and JUNGNER (1968) stipulated that a well understood natural history of the disease and a long prodromal phase are fundamental prerequisites for any screening protocol. Although flat and depressed lesions are common in the colon, we do not know what proportion of advanced colorectal carcinomas arises from these precursors.

3.4
Potential Benefit from Removing Colorectal Polyps

MORSON (1974) proposed that most colonic cancer arise from polypoid precursors over a 10–15 year period. St Mark's Hospital analysed the characteristics of 2489 polyps with respect to risk of harbouring cancer. The risk of malignancy was only 1.3% in polyps smaller than 1 cm, but rose to 9.5% in polyps of 1–2 cm in diameter and 46% in lesions larger than 2 cm in diameter. In this series, 60% of polyps were smaller than 1 cm, 23% were 1–2 cm and 17% were larger than 2 cm in diameter.

The understanding that it is mainly the larger polyps that carry a significant risk of harbouring early cancer is good news for colorectal cancer surveillance. Barium enema, colonoscopy, flexible sigmoidoscopy and CT colonography could all be expected to detect the majority of large polyps and therefore remove most early cancers.

3.5
Cancer Incidence After Colonoscopy Screening and Reasons for the Relative Failure of Surveillance

The hypothesis that removing all colorectal polyps should virtually eliminate the risk of colorectal

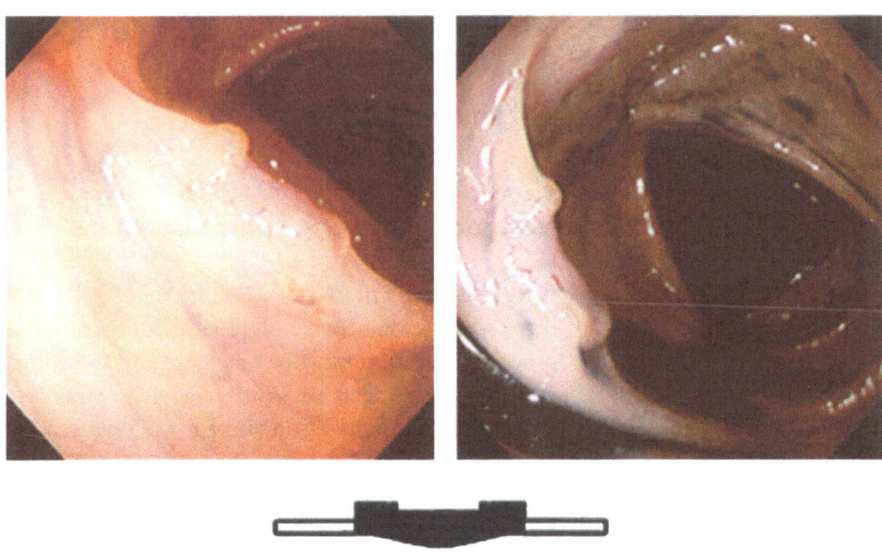

Fig. 3.3. Colonoscopy. A lesion with a superficial elevated portion and a shallow central depression. The central depression is situated above the level of the normal surrounding mucosa (IIa + IIc type lesion)

cancer for up to 10 years has been put to the test in a couple of large prospective trials.

In the National Polyp Study (WINOWER et al. 1993), 1418 patients underwent between two and three colonoscopies to clear their colons of polyps and were then followed over 3 years. Using the background risk of cancer in age and sex matched individuals, patients had 76% reduced risk of developing colorectal cancer.

In the larger retrospective Veterans Affairs Study, data from 32.702 patients who had previously undergone a colonoscopy was examined. Compared with the background population risk, a previous colonoscopy provided 47% (95% CI 37–58) protection against colorectal cancer (MULLER and SONNENBERG 1995).

3.6
Reasons for the Relative Failure of Surveillance

The relatively high cancer incidence after colonoscopy in the National Polyp Study and Veterans Affairs Study is surprising and disappointing. The expressed aim of colorectal cancer screening is to eradicate the disease completely (ATKIN and NORTHOVER 2003). What are the possible reasons for the failure of colonoscopy, with clearance of polyps, to provide near total protection against the subsequent development of colorectal cancer?

There are three possibilities, all which may contribute to the less than expected benefit of colonoscopy. Firstly, colonoscopy may be less effective than anticipated in detecting colonic polyps. Secondly, a substantial proportion of cancers may not arise from polyps and are missed at colonoscopy. A final possibility is that some precursor lesions are particularly aggressive and transform from adenoma to carcinoma much faster than the 10–15 years proposed by MORSON (1974).

It is unlikely that colonoscopy is inherently a poor method of colonic examination. REX et al. (1997a) determined that colonoscopy could be expected detect more than 95% of polyps larger than 1 cm in diameter and 87% of smaller lesions. This low "polyp miss rate" was supported by the American "Prostate Lung Colorectal and Ovarian Cancer Screening Trial" (DORIA-ROSE et al. 2002) which reported the yield of repeat flexible sigmoidoscopy 3 years after a negative examination and found that of 9317 subjects examined only 0.8% of patients (70/9317) had polyps ≥1 cm in diameter, lesions which had presumably been missed at the initial examination.

Furthermore, Japanese endoscopists are successful in reducing the cancer risk to near zero. A retrospective Japanese multicenter study (FUJII et al. 2002) evaluated the incidence of new lesions after colonoscopy and removal of all adenomas larger than 5 mm. During a median 5-year follow-up period, only 5.5% of patients developed either a >1 cm polyp or a lesion with high-grade dysplasia. Only seven patients of the 5309 individuals developed a cancer within 5 years of the colonoscopy. Another Japanese study, looked at the cancer rate after a clearing colonoscopy in 24 881 patients undergoing "annual medical health checkups between 1983 and 2000," (YAMAJI et al. 2002). There were only 13 cases of colorectal cancer during a mean follow-up of 5.5 years (ten Dukes' A, one Dukes' B, and two Dukes' C).

Why are Japanese endoscopists able to reduce the risk of subsequent cancer by more than 95% compared to the 50–75% risk reduction achieved in the West? The most likely explanation for the success of Japanese screening is that Japanese colonoscopists are more aware of non-polypoid adenomas and remove flat and depressed premalignant lesions, which in the West would go unrecognised.

Finally, there is evidence that some flat and depressed adenomas are more aggressive than polypoid adenomas. MUTO et al. (1991) reported a higher frequency of aneuploidy in non-polypoid adenomas compared to the polypoid type. WOLBER and OWEN (1991) reported that flat adenomas were 10 times more likely to contain high-grade dysplasia than polypoid adenomas. RUBIO et al. (1997) contrasted the histological findings of 90 flat adenomas found in Sweden with 141 flat adenomas resected in Tokyo. 24.8% of Japanese flat adenomas contained severe dysplasia and 13.3% of flat lesions detected in Sweden.

3.6
Detection of Non-polypoid Adenomas

It is certainly more difficult to detect flat and depressed lesions than polyps at colonoscopy. The bowel preparation must be adequate and the endoscopist must be alert to subtle changes in mucosal coloration, vascularization and surface texture.

Most early cancers are missed in the rectum and caecum. This is significant as most neoplastic lesions in these sites are flat or sessile rather than polypoid. With inadequate bowel preparation these lesions are easily missed. In our own data from Leeds, of 144 rectal lesions, 77 (53%) were flat or sessile and 67

Table 3.2. Published polyp detection rates with CT colonography

	Number of patients in study	Detection rates for 5-9 mm polyps	Detection rates for ≥1cm polyps
LAGHI et al. (2002b)	165	82%	92%
ARNESEN et al. (2002)	96	66%	77%
FENLON et al. (1999)	87	82%	91%
HARA et al. (1997)	70	66%	75%
LAGHI et al. (2002a)	65	85%	93%
GLUECKER et al. (2002)	51	33%	82%
PESCATORE et al. (2000)	50	71%	62%
KAY et al. (1999)	38	67%	90%
HARA et al. (1996)	10	71%	100%

were polypoid. In the caecum, 69/110 lesions (63%) were flat or sessile and 41 were polypoid.

Within Westernised countries, there are large variations in detection rates of colonic adenomas. A recently multicenter study from Europe reported polypectomy rates varying between 14% and 35% between different centres (WIETLISBACH et al. 2002). Similarly, in a British study, the polypectomy rate varied between 9% and 15% between different endoscopists (ATKIN et al. 2001). A Norwegian study found that the level of experience was not a predictor of better adenoma detection in a study of 8840 flexible sigmoidoscopies (HOFF et al. 2002).

If the level of experience of the endoscopist is not important, training in dye spraying and recognition of non-polypoid adenomas will probably be required to achieve the near 100% protection against subsequent colorectal cancer achieved in Japan.

The published polyp detection rates of CT colonography have been more encouraging (Table 3.2).

It appears that in enthusiastic centres at least, CT colonography has a good polyp detection rate. Unfortunately, outside of single centres the polyp detection rates is lower. The preliminary findings of a multicenter study of CT colonography, has recently been reported. In the 418 patients examined, 36% of small polyps (5–9 mm) and 47% of larger polyps (≥1 cm) were detected by CT colonography (COTTON et al. 2002). Furthermore, flat lesions have been highlighted as a particular problem for CT colonography. In a Mayo Clinic study of CT colonography in 70 patients, one flat adenoma was reportedly missed (HARA et al. 1997). REX et al. (1997) at the Indiana University also reported significant problems with detection of flat adenomas, particularly in the right hemi-colon.

3.7
Detection of Flat and Depressed Adenomas by Barium Enema and CT Colonography

There have been many studies comparing the polyp detection rate of barium enema with colonoscopy but none directly addressed the problem of flat and depressed adenomas. However, it is likely that barium enemas will be poor at detecting non-polypoid lesions as the barium enema has been found to be significantly inferior to colonoscopy in the detection of polyps. In a British study, colonoscopy was able to detect five times as many large polyps, (≥1 cm) as barium enema (1.6% vs. 7.7%) (SMITH and O'DWYER 2001). WINAWER et al. (2000) studied 580 patients in the National Polyp Study who were willing to undergo both a barium enema and a colonoscopy. Barium enemas detected only 56% of <6 mm in diameter and 46% of polyps 1 cm or larger in diameter.

3.8
Conclusion

From the discussion above we can begin to answer the question "what is the significance of the flat adenoma". The evidence suggests that these lesions give rise to between 25%–50% of colorectal cancers in Western populations. It appears that the majority of these lesions are missed at colonoscopy.

References

Arnesen RB, Adamsen S, Raaschou HO et al (2002) CT colonography (virtual colonoscopy) compared with colonoscopy in 231 paired examinations. Gastrointest Endosc 55: AB91

Atkin WS, Northover JMA (2003) Population based endoscopic screening for colorectal cancer. Gut 52:321–322

Atkin WS, Cook CF, Patel R et al (2001) Variability in yield of adenomas in average risk individuals undergoing flexible sigmoidoscopy screening. Gastroenterology [Suppl] 1:A66

Cotton PB, Durkalski VL, Palesch YY et al (2002) Comparison of virtual colonoscopy and colonoscopy in the detection of polyps/masses. Gastrointest Endosc 55:AB98

Doria-Rose VP, Levin TR, Selby JV et al (2002) Incidence of colorectal cancer following negative screening sigmoidoscopy. Gastroenterology 122:A17

Fenlon HM, Nunes DP, Paul C et al (1999) A comparison of virtual and conventional colonoscopy for the detection of colorectal polyps. NEJM 341:1496–1503

Fujii T, Sano Y, Liishi H et al (2002) Colorectal cancer screening in Japan-results of the multicenter retrospective cohort study. Gastroenterology 122:A481

Gluecker TH, Dorta G, Keller W et al (2002) Performance of multidetector computed tomography colonography compared with conventional colonoscopy. Gut 51:207–211

Hara AK, Johnson D, Reed JE et al (1996) Detection of colorectal polyps by computed tomographic colography: feasibility of a novel technique. Gastroenterology 110:284–290

Hara AK, Johnson CD, Reed JE et al (1997) Detection of colorectal polyps with CT colography:initial assessment of sensitivity and specificity. Radiology 205:59–65

Hoff G, Bretthauer M, Grotmol T et al (2002) Differences in detection rates of colorectal polyps and adenomas among endoscopists in population-based flexible sigmoidoscopy screening. Gastrointest Endosc 55:AB214

Japanese Society for Cancer of the Colon and Rectum (1997) Japanese classification of colorectal carcinoma, 1st English edn. Kanehara, Tokyo

Kay CL, Kulling D, Hawes RH et al (1999) Virtual endoscopy – comparison with colonoscopy in the detection of space-occupying lesions of the colon. Endoscopy 32:226–232

Kudo S (1996) Early colorectal cancer:detection of depressed types of colorectal carcinoma, 1st edn. Igaku-Shoin, Tokyo, pp 81–93

Laghi A, Iannaccone R, Carbone I et al (2002a) Computed tomographic colonography (virtual colonscopy): blinded prospective comparison with conventional colonoscopy for the detection of colorectal adenomas. Endoscopy 34:441–446

Laghi A, Iannaccone R, Carbone I et al (2002b) Detection of colorectal lesions with virtual computed tomographic colonography. Am J Surg 183:124–131

Morson B (1974) The polyp-cancer sequence in the large bowel. Proc R Soc Med 67:451–457

Muller AD, Sonnenberg A (1995) Protection by endoscopy against death from colorectal cancer in the general population. Arch Intern Med 155:1741–1748

Muto T, Masaki T, Suzuki K (1991) DNA ploidy pattern of flat adenomas of the large bowel. Dis Colon Rectum 34:696–698

Pescatore P, Glucker T, Delarive J et al (2000) Diagnostic accuracy and interobserver agreement of CT colonography (virtual colonoscopy). Gut 47:126–130

Rembacken BJ, Fujii T, Cairns A et al (2000) Flat and depressed colonic neoplasms: a prospective study of 1000 colonoscopies in the UK. Lancet 355:1211–1214

Rex DK, Cutler CS, Lemmel GT et al (1997) Colonoscopic miss rates of adenomas determined by back-to-back colonoscopies. Gastroenterology 112:24–28

Rex DK, Vining D, Kopecky K (1997) Screening for colon polyps using spiral CT with and without virtual colonoscopy (abstract). Gastrointest Endosc 45:AB116

Rubio C, Watanabe T, Masaki T (1997) Histological differences between flat tubular colorectal adenomas in Japan and Sweden. In Vivo 11:93–94

Smith GA, O'Dwyer PJ (2001) Sensitivity of double contrast barium enema and colonoscopy for the detection of colorectal neoplasms. Surg Endosc 15:649–652

Spratt JS, Lauren V, Ackerman LV (1962) Small primary adenocarcinomas of the colon and rectum. JAMA 179:337–346

Wietlisbach V, Burnand B, Vader JP et al (2002) Variations in technical performance and quality of use of colonoscopy throughout Europe: the EPAGE multicenter study. Gastrointest Endosc 55:AB82

Wilson J, Jungner G (1968) WHO publication. WHO, Geneva

Winawer SJ, Stewart ET, Zauber AG et al (2000) A comparison of colonoscopy and double-contrast barium enema for surveillance after polypectomy. N Engl J Med 342:1766–1772

Winawer SJ, Zauber AG, Ho MN et al (1993) Prevention of colorectal cancer by colonoscopic polypectomy. N Engl J Med 329:1977–1981

Wolber RA, Owen DA (1991) Flat adenoma of the colon. Hum Pathol 34:981–986

Yamaji Y, Okamoto M, Yoshida H et al (2002) Clinical features of invasive colorectal cancers which could not be prevented even by vigorous colonoscopy and polypectomy. Gastroenterology 122:A479

4 The Pathology of Large Bowel Polyps

NIGEL SCOTT and ANTHONY H. CHAPMAN

CONTENTS

4.1 Introduction 31
4.2 Neoplastic Polyps 32
4.2.1 Benign Neoplastic Polyps 32
4.2.2 Malignant Neoplastic Polyps 38
4.3 Non-Neoplastic Polyps 39
4.3.1 Hamartomatous Polyps 39
4.3.2 Metaplastic Polyps 40
4.3.3 Benign Lymphoid Polyps 41
4.3.4 Inflammatory Polyps 41
4.3.5 Polyps Related to Mucosal Prolapse 42
4.3.6 Inflammatory Fibroid Polyps 43
4.3.7 Other Non-Neoplastic Polyps 43
4.4 Polyposis Syndromes 43
4.4.1 Familial Adenomatous Polyposis 43
4.4.2 Metaplastic Polyposis 45
4.4.3 Juvenile Polyposis 45
4.4.4 Peutz-Jeghers Polyposis 45
4.4.5 Cronkhite-Canada Syndrome 46
4.4.6 Malignant Lymphomatous Polyposis 46
4.4.7 Other Polyposis Syndromes 46
4.4.8 Hereditary Non-Polyposis Colorectal Cancer (HNPCC) 47
References 47

4.1 Introduction

The word "polyp" (derived from the Greek for "multiple feet" or "little nipple") is used to describe a mucosal protrusion which is more or less circumscribed and discrete from surrounding mucosa. As such it is a descriptive term and not a histological diagnosis. Macroscopically polyps may be pedunculated (possess a stalk) or sessile (have a broad base). They vary enormously in shape and size, some being only 1–2 mm in diameter while others measure several centimetres across. Most are due to mucosal pathology but a significant minority originate in the submucosa and stretch or ulcerate the overlying large bowel epithelium. Polyps are not uncommonly multiple, usually numbering between two and five in total. However, a group of polyposis syndromes exist where tens, hundreds and literally thousands of polyps carpet the colonic mucosa. These polyposis syndromes are described at the end of this chapter and constitute a heterogenous group of disorders. Some are inherited, others are sporadic and they are enormously variable in the number and type of polyps encountered.

Polyps are best classified histologically as this gives precise information about their histogenesis (tissue of origin), pathogenesis, likelihood of recurrence, risk of malignant change and possibility of any associated pathology (e.g. polyposis syndromes; MEN syndrome; neurofibromatosis, etc.). This means of course that biopsy of the polyp, or preferably polypectomy, is necessary for the correct management of the patient. Table 4.1 outlines the histological classification used

N. SCOTT, MD, MRC Path
Consultant Pathologist, St. James's University Hospital, Bekett Street, Leeds, West Yorkshire LS9 7TF, UK
A. H. CHAPMAN, MD, FRCP, FRCR
Clinical Director of Radiology, Department of Clinical Radiology, Leeds Teaching Hospitals Trust, St. James's University Hospital, Bekett Street, Leeds, West Yorkshire LS9 7TF, UK

Table 4.1. Histological classification of large bowel polyps

Neoplastic Polyps
- Benign
  Adenoma
  Polypoid dysplasia in UC
  Lipoma
  Leiomyoma
  Schwannoma
  Ganglioneuroma
  Haemangioma
- Malignant
  Polypoid carcinoma
  Carcinoid
  GIST
  Leiomyosarcoma
  Lymphoma
  Metastatic tumours

Non-Neoplastic Polyps
- Hamartomas
  Peutz-Jeghers polyps
  Juvenile polyps
- Metaplastic (hyperplastic) polyps
- Benign lymphoid polyps
- Inflammatory polyps
- Polyps related to mucosal prolapse
- Inflammatory fibroid polyps

in this chapter and is based on a simple subdivision into neoplastic versus non-neoplastic, benign versus malignant and epithelial versus mesenchymal polyps.

Many common polyps, e.g. adenomas, are neoplastic. A neoplasm (Latin: new growth) is a mass of abnormal tissue that grows in a progressive and autonomous fashion. It is usually derived from a single cell, i.e. demonstrates monoclonality. A malignant neoplasm is one that is invasive and can spread from its site of origin.

4.2
Neoplastic Polyps

4.2.1
Benign Neoplastic Polyps

4.2.1.1
Adenomas

Adenomas are benign glandular epithelial neoplasms. They are probably the commonest type of polyp in the large bowel, being slightly more frequent than metaplastic polyps. In a prospective study of resected polyps at colonoscopy 62% were found to be adenomas and 29% metaplastic polyps. Autopsy series from Western European and North American populations show that prevalence increases with age and is greater in men than women (WILLIAMS et al. 1982). Adenomas are rare before 30 years of age but occur in 30%–50% of the population after 50. Colonoscopic screening studies of "average risk" asymptomatic adults 50–75 years of age report similar frequencies to those determined at post mortem (LIEBERMAN et al. 2000). Lower prevalences are seen in populations at low risk of large bowel cancer such as those of Africa and South-East Asia.

Overall adenomas are distributed fairly evenly around the colon; however, some studies suggest that caecal and ascending colon polyps become more prevalent in the older age groups (FIDE and STALSBERG 1978). A consistent finding is that adenomas located in the caecum, sigmoid colon and rectum tend to be larger than at other sites.

Multiple polyps are found in 20%–40% of individuals, a feature which is also related to age, male sex and co-existent metaplastic polyps (JASS et al. 1992).

Macroscopically adenomatous polyps may be pedunculated, sessile or "flat" (Fig. 4.1). Pedunculated polyps in which the adenoma sits on the end of a stalk, are most frequent in the rectum, sigmoid and descend-

ing colon. In contrast caecal and ascending colon polyps are predominantly sessile. The stalk in pedunculated polyps is often lined by normal mucosa and contains submucosal connective tissue and vessels. Flat adenomas are discussed in more detail below.

In autopsy series most adenomas are small and tubular; 85%–90% less than 10 mm; 60% less than 5 mm diameter (WILLIAMS et al. 1982). Micro-adenomas, which are invisible to the naked eye and consist of one or a few dysplastic crypts (unicrypt and oligocryptal adenomas), are the earliest lesion identifiable histologically (Fig. 4.2). They are very rarely seen in "average risk" populations but are well described in patients with familial adenomatous polyposis (FAP) (BRADBURN et al. 1991).

Histologically, adenomas are circumscribed, neoplastic epithelial tumours showing glandular differentiation. By definition they exhibit epithelial dysplasia which is an unequivocal neoplastic alteration to the crypt epithelial lining characterised by varying degrees of cytological and architectural atypia. This includes the morphological features of nuclear enlargement,

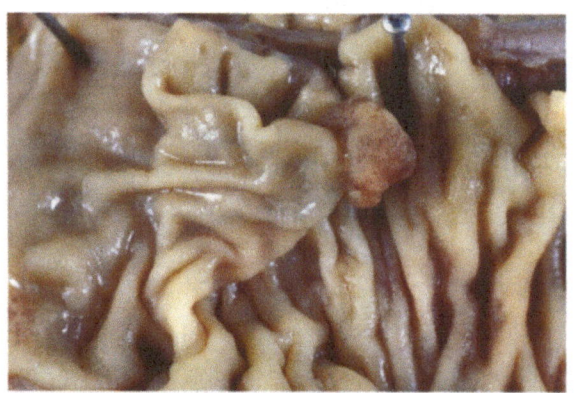

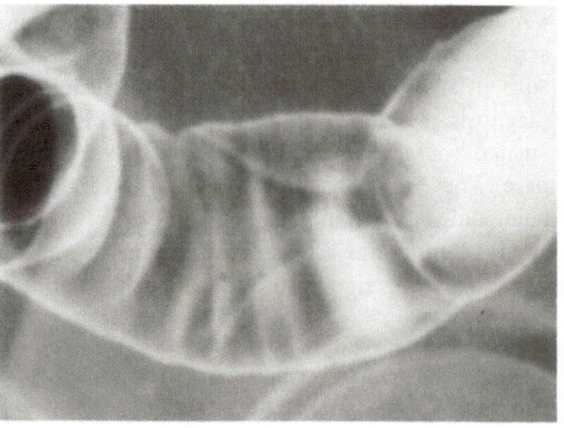

Fig. 4.1a,b. a Colectomy specimen showing a small tubular adenoma on the end of a broad triangle-shaped mucosal pedicle. **b** Barium enema

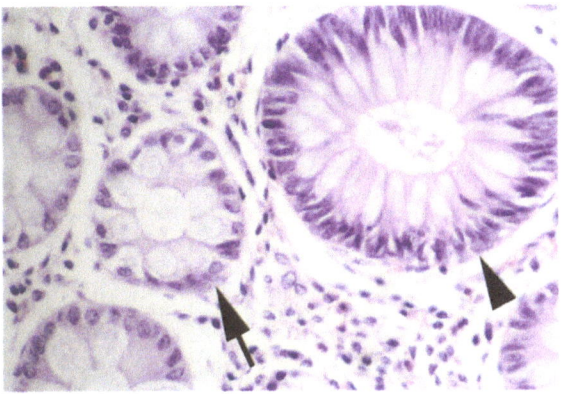

Fig. 4.2. Unicrypt (adenoma) adjacent to non-dysplastic colonic crypt in a patient with FAP. (H&E stain section magnification ×40). Dysplastic crypt (*arrowhead*), normal crypt (*arrow*)

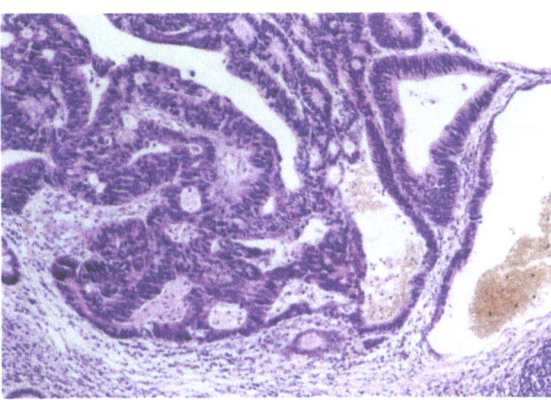

Fig. 4.3. Section showing severe dysplasia in an adenoma. (H&E stain, magnification ×20)

nuclear elongation, hyperchromasia and pseudostratification (layering of nuclei in adjacent cells); increased nuclear to cytoplasmic ratio; increased mitotic activity (which may include abnormal mitotic figures); reduced or absent cytoplasmic mucin production. These light microscopic abnormalities are paralleled by loss of ultrastructural and functional differentiation, as well as perturbations in the functional organisation of the crypt. In the normal colonic crypt, DNA synthesis is restricted to the basal half with progressive cellular maturation as colonocytes migrate up the crypt axis. In the adenomatous crypt, immature incompletely differentiated cells are seen at all levels from the base to the surface and the proliferative compartment is expanded to include dividing cells in the upper third and surface epithelium (JOHNSTON et al. 1989).

According to the severity of these architectural and cytological changes, adenomas can be classified as showing mild, moderate or severe dysplasia. Many polyps, especially large ones, contain areas showing different degrees of atypia. By convention, adenomas are graded according to the most severe dysplasia present rather than the predominant pattern (JASS and SOBIN 1989). Carcinoma in situ is a term most often employed in the United States to describe the most extreme examples of severe dysplasia (Fig. 4.3). Adenomas do not show invasion through the basement membrane of the colonic crypt. Intramucosal carcinoma, in which neoplastic epithelial cells infiltrate the mucosal connective tissue but not the submucosa, must occur at an early stage of tumour growth but is very rarely seen in routine diagnostic practice. Most pathologists diagnose adenocarcinoma only when malignant epithelial cells are seen invading through the muscularis mucosa into the submucosa or beyond (Fig. 4.4). Invasion through

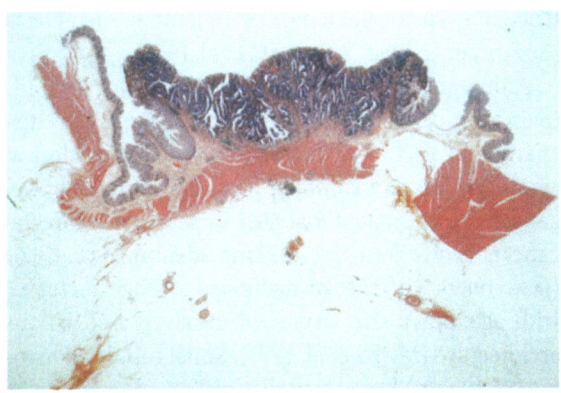

Fig. 4.4. Small flat adenocarcinoma showing early invasion into the sub-mucosa. (H&E stain, magnification ×10)

the muscularis mucosa gives access to submucosal lymphatics enabling tumours to metastasise.

In addition to degree of dysplasia, adenomas are classified according to their microscopic architecture. Most are composed of straight or branching tubules/crypts surrounded by a loose stroma containing fibroblasts, plasma cells, macrophages and connective tissue fibres similar to those in the normal lamina propria. A minority of adenomas contain villous or papillary structures. By convention where villi constitute less than 20% of the polyp, the adenoma is categorised as a tubular polyp (JASS and SOBIN 1989). Where over 80% of the polyp is villous in architecture, it is called a villous adenoma (Fig. 4.5). Tubulovillous polyps are those in which both tubules and villi are present in excess of 20% of the polyp volume. In most series tubulovillous and villous adenomas account for less than 10%–20% of all polyps. Villous elements are more common in large adenomas and are more often associated with severe dysplasia. Rarely adenomas

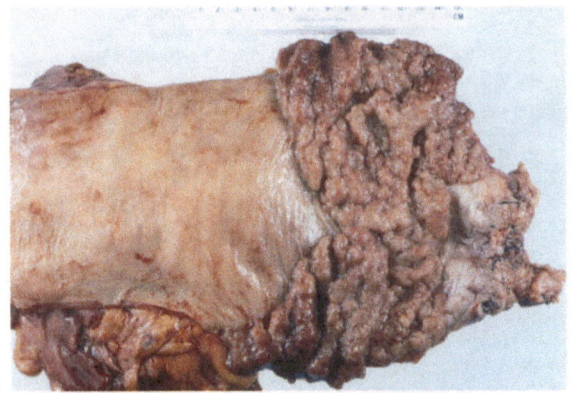 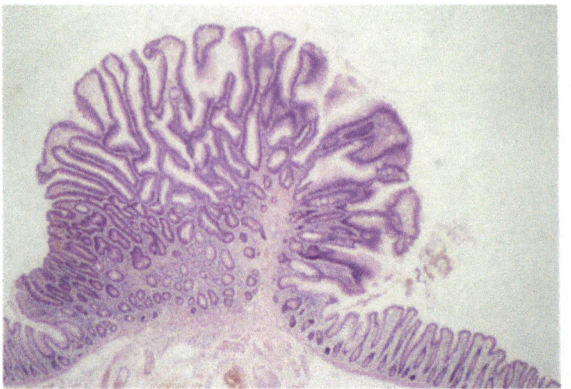

Fig. 4.5a,b. a Abdomino-perineal resection specimen containing a large sessile villous adenoma. **b** Polypoid villous adenoma exhibiting mild dysplasia. (H&E stain, magnification ×10)

may show clear cell change or squamous metaplasia (SUZUKI et al. 1998; WILLIAMS et al. 1979).

Although some large adenomas can cause morbidity in their own right from rectal bleeding, mucus discharge and electrolyte disturbances, their chief clinical significance is as a common precursor of large bowel cancer. It is estimated that 80% or more of colorectal cancers evolve from pre-existing adenomas (Fig. 4.6) (JASS 1989). The risk of malignant change increases with age, polyp size, degree of dysplasia and villous architecture (MUTO et al. 1975). Small tubular adenomas (<10 mm) have a very low risk of progression to cancer; many stay the same size or get smaller over time (HOFSTAD et al. 1996). However, a few will grow, become increasingly dysplastic and after 10–20 years become malignant. Several studies show that polypectomy reduces the incidence of colorectal cancer in patients with adenomas by as much as 76%–90% (WINAWER et al. 1993; CITARDA et al. 2001).

4.2.1.1.1
Flat Adenomas

While most adenomas in the large bowel are polypoid and protrude into the lumen, a minority may be only slightly elevated above the background mucosa. These plaque-like lesions are commonly referred to as "flat adenomas" (MUTO et al. 1985). Some have a central depression or dimple and these are called "depressed adenomas". Originally described by Japanese endoscopists, latterly they have been identified in colonoscopic studies from Sweden, the United Kingdom, Canada and the USA (TSUDA et al. 2002; REMBACKEN et al. 2000; SAITOH et al. 2001). As well as being flat in contour, they are typically small, usually less than 10 mm in diameter and some have a red or white surface (Fig. 4.7).

Using a dye spray technique and rigourous colonoscopic examination SAITOH et al. (2001)

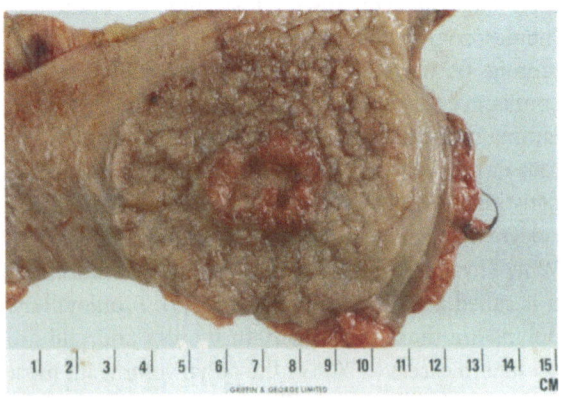 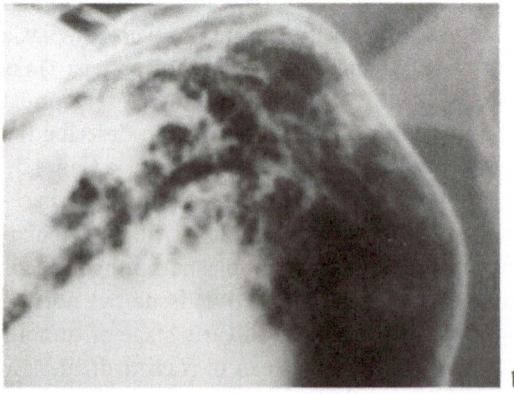

Fig. 4.6a,b. a Colectomy specimen showing ulcerated carcinoma arising in the middle of a large sessile villous adenoma. **b** Barium enema in a different patient. Large malignant villous adenoma of the rectum; a flat tumour with a reticular surface pattern caused by barium caught between the fronds of the tumour

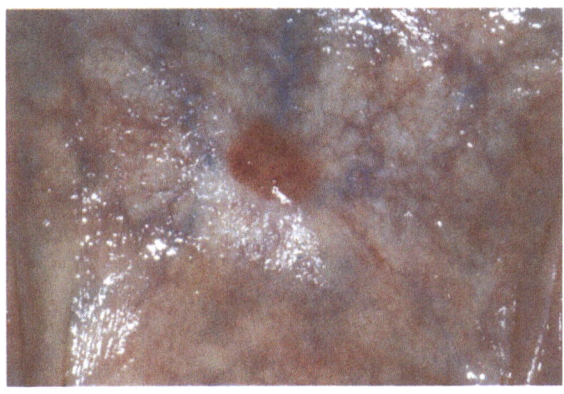

Fig. 4.7. Colectomy specimen. Erythematous flat well-defined mucosal lesion; a flat adenoma

found flat adenomas in 22.7% of adult American patients undergoing endoscopy for suspected large bowel neoplasia. In an unselected British series of 1000 patients (mean age 59 years) adenomas were found in 225 patients; 36% of these were flat and 0.6% were depressed (REMBACKEN et al. 2000).

Histologically, flat adenomas are mainly tubular in architecture although tubulovillous and villous types have been reported. By definition the dysplastic mucosa is less than twice the thickness of adjacent normal mucosa (Fig. 4.8). Japanese studies emphasise the much higher frequency of severe dysplasia/carcinoma in these tumours compared with polypoid adenomas of similar size (MUTO et al. 1985). While some Western series also describe a higher rate of severe dysplasia others have not been able to confirm this (REMBACKEN et al. 2000; SAITOH et al. 2001). However, most workers acknowledge the significance of a central depression which in all studies is associated with either severe dysplasia or invasive carcinoma. It is hypothesised that flat adenomas have an increased propensity to evolve into small, flat colorectal carcinomas.

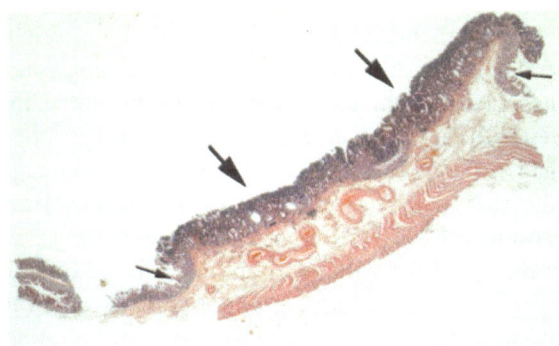

Fig. 4.8. Flat adenoma with dysplastic mucosa (*large arrows*). Adjacent normal mucosa (*small arrows*). (H&E stained section, magnification ×10)

4.2.1.1.2
Serrated Adenomas

Between 1% and 2% of adenomas have a serrated architecture reminiscent of a metaplastic (hyperplastic) polyp (Fig. 4.9) (JASS 2002). However, unlike metaplastic polyps they show distinct cytological atypia (nuclear enlargement, hyperchromasia, pseudostratification), as well as a greater degree of architectural complexity (glandular budding/branching, etc.). Because of this morphological overlap they have also been called "mixed hyperplastic-adenomatous" polyps. Portions of the polyp may have a pure metaplastic or conventional adenomatous morphology.

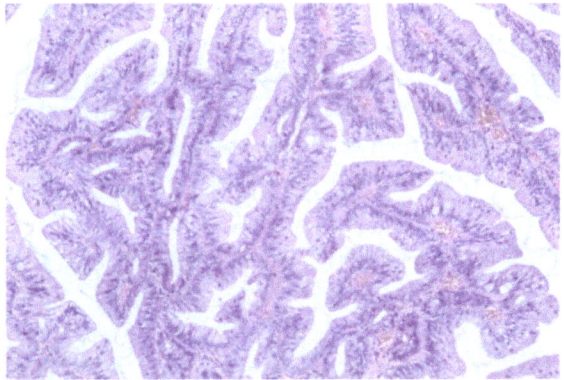

Fig. 4.9 Serrated adenoma showing saw-tooth configuration of crypts with dysplastic epithelium. (H&E stain section, magnification ×20)

Serrated adenomas are distributed throughout the bowel but are thought to be relatively common in the right colon (MAKINEN et al. 2001). Like other adenomas they may be flat, sessile or pedunculated. A proportion show severe dysplasia and transition to adenocarcinoma has been documented proving the existence of a serrated adenoma–carcinoma sequence. Interestingly some of the associated carcinomas also have a serrated morphology (YAO et al. 2000). It is hypothesised that serrated adenomas may evolve from pre-existing metaplastic polyps introducing for the first time the possibility of a metaplastic polyp–adenoma–carcinoma sequence.

4.2.1.2
Polypoid Dysplasia in Ulcerative Colitis

Chronic ulcerative colitis (UC) is associated with an increased risk of developing colorectal cancer which is preceded by epithelial dysplasia. While over 90% of pre-malignant dysplastic lesions occur in flat mucosa, approximately 5% occur in elevated or "polypoid" tumours (TYTGAT et al. 1995). This may take the form of discrete sessile nodules resembling sporadic adenomas; more diffuse irregular polypoidal lesions, or plaque-like tumours with a papillary or villous surface. Elevated dysplastic lesions in UC are known as DALMs (dysplasia associated lesion or mass) and are believed to carry a particularly high risk of malignant change (Fig. 4.10). In one study seven out of 12 patients (58%) with a DALM developed cancer (BLACKSTONE et al. 1981). Consequently their presence is generally taken as an indication for colectomy. However, more recently attention has focused on a subgroup of DALMs resembling sporadic adenoma (adenoma-like DALM; ALDs) (BERNSTEIN 1999). Macroscopically and histologically similar to an adenoma, molecular studies suggest these lesions are distinct from other UC related dysplasias and may be managed conservatively, i.e. by polypectomy (ODZE 1999). However, this is a decision which is taken only after considering the patient's duration of disease and excluding as far as possible co-existent flat dysplasia

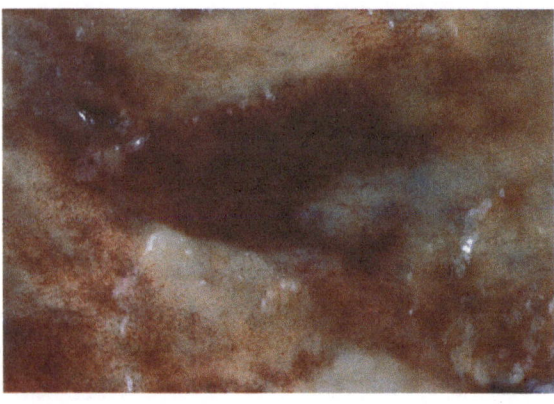

Fig. 4.10 Dysplasia associated lesion or mass (DALM). Erythematous plaque-like lesion in ulcerative colitis. Colectomy specimen

4.2.1.3
Lipomas

Lipomas, benign neoplasms of adipose tissue, are the commonest type of benign mesenchymal tumour in the colon. The vast majority are submucosal although occasional subserosal lesions are described. They are usually sessile but may be polypoid and sometimes adopt a particularly grotesque and irregular shape. Autopsy series suggest they are rare, being found in only 0.2% of the population (WEINBERG and FELDMAN 1955). Some studies suggest they are commoner in the right colon but others report a uniform distribution (TAYLOR and

WOLFF 1987). They are multiple in 10%–20% of cases and rare examples of lipomatous poliposis are documented in which hundreds of polyps cover the mucosal surface (SANTOS-BRIZ et al. 2001). These are invariably misdiagnosed as familial adenomatous polyposis. In most surgical series, lipomas are over 2 cm in diameter, largely reflecting the fact that tumours less than 2 cm in diameter are usually asymptomatic. Larger polyps may present with bleeding, abdominal pain, intestinal obstruction and intussusception. Histologically there is a proliferation of mature fat cells which expands the submucosa (Fig. 4.11). The overlying mucosa is usually intact and normal in appearance but may become ulcerated. Transformation to liposarcoma is not described.

Lipohyperplasia of the ileocaecal valve is often confused with a colonic lipoma but consists of a more diffuse, less circumscribed growth of fat in the submucosa of the ileocaecal valve. This causes the valve to appear thickened and protuberant. This condition is probably more frequent in obese individuals (Fig. 4.12).

4.2.1.4
Other Benign Mesenchymal Polyps

Other benign polypoid mesenchymal tumours of the colon and rectum include leiomyoma, schwannoma, ganglioneuroma, haemangioma and granular cell tumours. Leiomyomas (benign smooth muscle neoplasms) frequently arise from the muscularis mucosa (MIETTINEN et al. 2001a). They usually present as small sessile polyps, 10 mm or less in diameter. They are invariably asymptomatic, histologically well differentiated and composed of fascicles of spindle cells with eosinophilic cytoplasm and blunt ended, cigar shaped nuclei. Unlike GISTs (gastrointestinal stromal tumours) they are CD34 and C-kit negative, but strongly express immunohistochemical markers of smooth muscle differentiation, e.g. alpha smooth muscle actin and desmin. Colonic leiomyomas of the muscularis propria are rare.

Schwannomas and neurofibromas (benign peripheral nerve sheath tumours) are also exceedingly rare neoplasms in the colon and rectum. In one of the few series reported, colonic schwannomas often had a polypoid intraluminal component although the vast majority were transmural lesions (MIETTINEN et al. 2001b). None of the 20 cases in this series were associated with neurofibromatosis; however, it is well known that up to 25% of patients with Von Recklinghausen's disease will have gastrointestinal involvement (HOCHBERG et al. 1974).

Ganglioneuromas are spindle cell proliferations of neural origin with interspersed ganglion cells. In

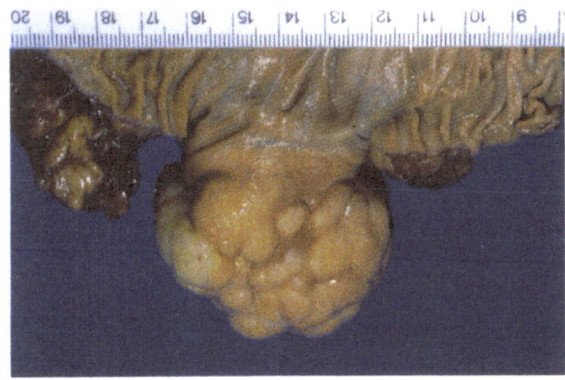
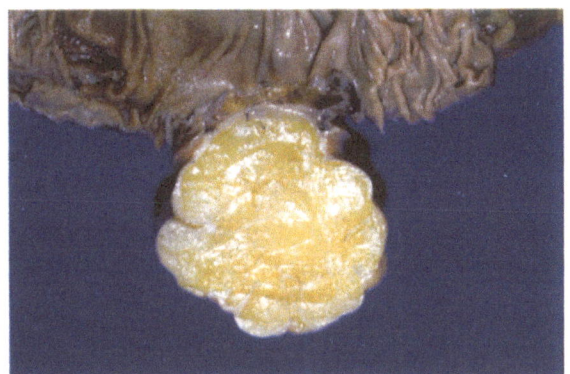

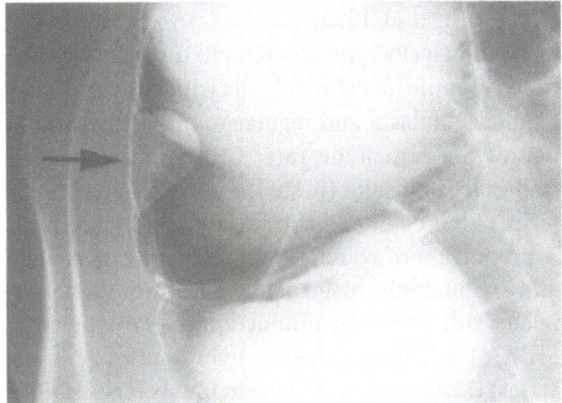

Fig. 4.11a–c. a Lipomatous polyp. Colectomy specimen. **b** Cut surface of the polyp. Note the uniform yellow appearance of the fat and that the overlying mucosa is intact. **c** Barium enema. A soft submucosal caecal tumour (*arrow*) that changed shape during the course of the examination

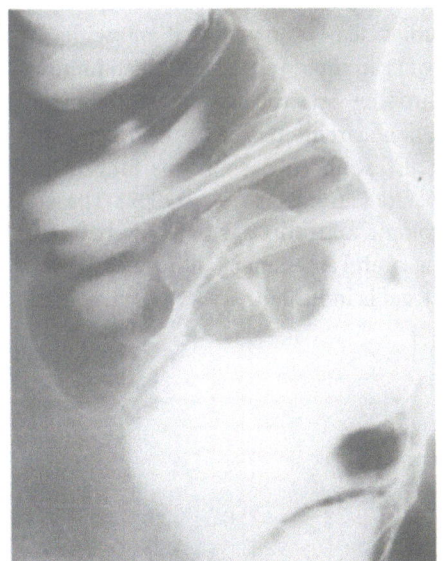
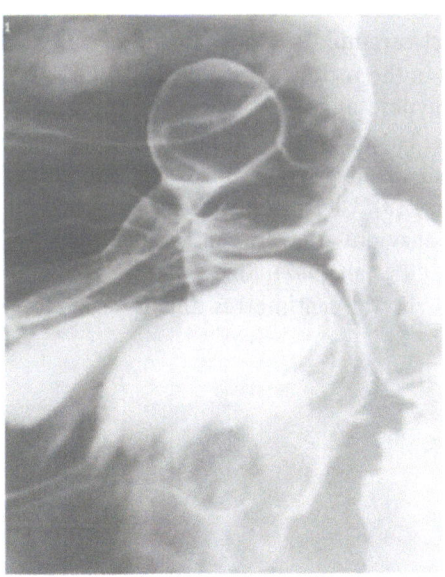

Fig. 4.12a,b. a Enlarged lipomatous ileocaecal valve. **b** Lipoma arising from the ileocaecal valve

the rectum and colon they present as small mucosal polyps. They may be sporadic or associated with multiple endocrine neoplasia syndrome type 2B (WEIDNER et al. 1984). Mucosal ganglioneuromas are also seen in patients with neurofibromatosis and in Cowdens/Bannayan-Reilly-Ruvalcaba syndrome (ERDMAN and BARNARD 2002).

Hemangiomas in the colon and rectum may be of capillary or cavernous type. Endoscopically they appear as circumscribed red sessile polypoid tumours covered by an intact mucosa. Histologically, they consist of a proliferation of small round blood vessels (capillary type) or large thin walled vascular channels (cavernous type). Acute thrombosis and organising thrombus are frequently seen in cavernous hemangiomas.

4.2.2
Malignant Neoplastic Polyps

4.2.2.1
Polypoid Carcinoma

While most adenocarcinomas of the large bowel have a stricturing, ulcerated or fungating exophytic appearance some may present as a polyp. Histology will show no evidence of any residual adenoma although it is assumed that most will have arisen in a pre-existing benign polyp. Polypoid carcinomas may be pedunculated, sessile or flat and many will be at an early stage of progression, i.e. confined to the bowel wall and lymph node negative.

4.2.2.2
Carcinoid

Carcinoids are low grade malignant epithelial tumours showing neuroendocrine differentiation (well differentiated neuroendocrine carcinomas). They are thought to arise via neoplastic transformation of endoderm derived endocrine cells in the colonic crypts. Most carcinoid tumours in the large bowel are located in the rectum and sigmoid. They are commonly polypoid and may have a distinct yellow appearance. The bulk of the tumour is usually submucosal and the overlying mucosa is smooth and intact (Fig. 4.13). Ulceration is associated with aggressive behaviour and an increased risk of metastasis (BURKE et al. 1987). Size ranges from less than 1 cm to several centimetres and is

an important prognostic factor. Carcinoids of the rectum less than 10 mm are invariably benign while tumours more than 20 mm diameter are associated with substantial mortality. Predicting the behaviour of tumours 10–20 mm in size is more problematic. Atypical histological features including invasion of the muscularis propria, identifies a group with a worse prognosis (KOURA et al. 1997). Occasionally intestinal carcinoids are associated with ischemic necrosis of the bowel wall due to mesenteric arterial occlusion (Fig. 4.13). Another rare association are numerous tiny granulation tissue polyps in the surrounding mucosa, the cause of which is unclear (ALLIBONE et al. 1993).

Histologically typical carcinoid tumours are composed of uniform cuboidal cells with granular eosinophilic cytoplasm and regular round nuclei. Mitotic figures are absent or rare. Cells are arranged in trabecular or insular (nested, island like) growth patterns, or less commonly form glands and solid sheets. A proportion of colonic carcinoids are argyrophilic and argentaffinic, histochemical features which correlate with serotonin production. However, urinary 5HIAA levels are rarely elevated (4 out of 22 in one series) (KOURA et al. 1997). Carcinoids may also produce a range of peptide hormones including pancreatic polypeptide, glucagon, gastrin and somatostatin although this is also rarely evident clinically.

Several studies clearly show that patients with small and large bowel carcinoid tumours have an increased risk of synchronous and metachronous malignancy, particularly adenocarcinomas of the colon and small intestine, but also stomach, oesophagus, lung, urinary tract and prostate (TICHANSKY et al. 2002). Therefore whenever a colonic, appendix or small bowel carcinoid is diagnosed a careful assessment of the rest of the gastrointestinal tract is indicated.

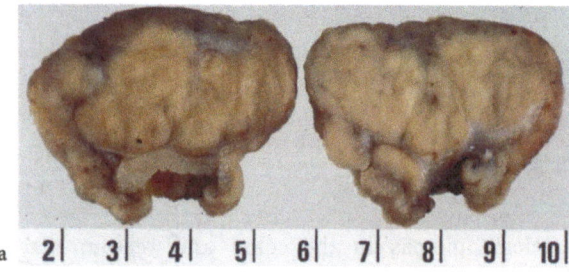

a

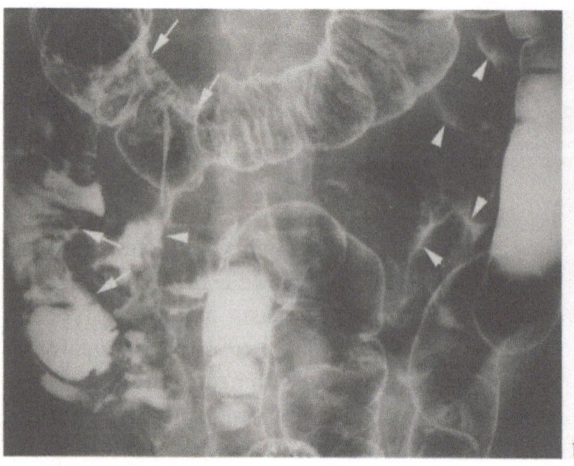

b

Fig. 4.13a,b. a Carcinoid tumour; note the pale yellow colour and the intact overlying mucosa. b Barium enema. Carcinoid tumour affecting caecum and hepatic flexure. Ischaemic necrosis has resulted in a perforation. Intraperitoneal barium between bowel loops (*arrowheads*)

4.2.2.3
Gastrointestinal Stromal Tumours

Gastrointestinal stromal tumours (GISTs) are mesenchymal neoplasms believed to originate from pacemaker cells in the bowel wall (interstitial cells of Cajal) (SIRCAR et al. 1999). In the past they have been confused with smooth muscle tumours (leiomyosarcoma and leiomyoma) but are now clearly defined by their morphology and unique immunohistochemical profile (CD34 positive, CD117 C-kit positive) (MIETTINEN et al. 1999). As a result it has become apparent that most malignant stromal tumours of the colon and rectum are GISTs rather than leiomyosarcomas. They show a range of malignant behaviour which is predicted best by size and mitotic activity, although it is well recognised that some small, mitotically inactive tumours can still behave in an aggressive fashion. GISTs are commoner in the rectum than the colon. Small tumours may present as submucosal polyps (Fig. 4.14), but most will form a large intramural mass which may ulcerate the overlying mucosa (MIETTINEN et al. 2001a).

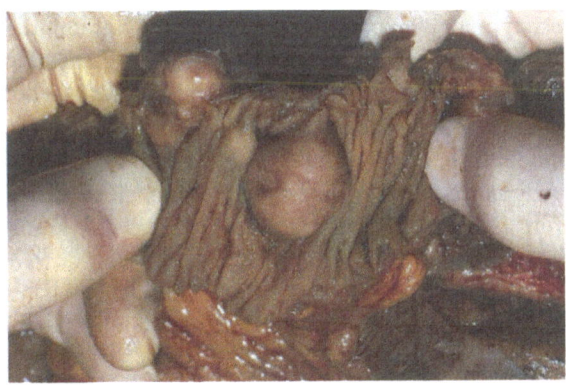

Fig. 4.14. Polypoid GIST with typical ulcer at apex

4.2.2.4
Malignant Lymphoma

Malignant lymphoma may occasionally affect the large bowel either as a primary gastrointestinal tumour or due to spread from nodal disease. This is dealt with further in the section on polyposis syndromes.

4.2.2.5
Metastatic Tumours

Tumours metastatic to the colon may occasionally produce polypoid lesions. Malignant melanoma is particularly likely to cause mucosal and submucosal nodules which can be mistaken for other types of colonic polyp (Fig. 4.15) (BLECKER et al. 1999).

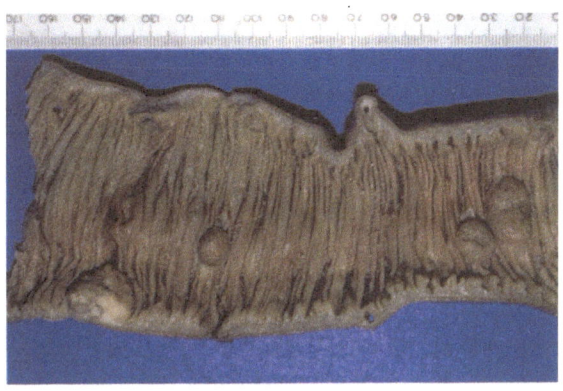

Fig. 4.15. Colectomy specimen showing sessile mucosal polyps due to metastatic malignant melanoma

4.3
Non-Neoplastic Polyps

4.3.1
Hamartomatous Polyps

Hamartomas are tumour like masses resulting from the disorganised growth of mature epithelium and stroma native to the organ in which they arise. This tissue may appear normal or hyperplastic but is not neoplastic. Originally thought to be congenital, most hamartomas are now known to be acquired. The two most common hamartomatous polyps in the colon are Peutz-Jeghers and juvenile polyps. The former usually occurs as part of a polyposis syndrome while most juvenile polyps are sporadic.

4.3.1.1
Peutz-Jeghers Polyps

Sporadic polyps similar to those seen in Peutz-Jeghers syndrome are extremely rare in the colon and have only been very occasionally described (NAKAYAMA et al. 1996). Like juvenile polyps, they are hamartomas and consist of an irregular branching core of smooth muscle fibres lined by histologically normal or hyperplastic mucosa. They may be sessile or pedunculated and can cause intestinal obstruction, often as a result of intussusception. Epithelial misplacement into the bowel wall is not uncommon in small bowel polyps and should not be mistaken for invasive carcinoma (SHEPHERD et al. 1987). However, this pseudo-malignant appearance has not been described in colonic tumours. A full description of Peutz-Jeghers syndrome can be found in Sect. 4.4.4. Peutz-Jeghers type polyps have also been found in patients with tuberous sclerosis.

4.3.1.2
Juvenile Polyps

Juvenile polyps, like Peutz-Jeghers polyps, are hamartomas and consist of a disorganised proliferation of mature epithelial and stromal elements. Most are smooth surfaced, spherical or ovoid polyps with a pedicle (Fig. 4.16). A minority are sessile. They range in size from less than 1 cm (27%) to over 4 cm (3%) (MAZIER et al. 1982), although most are 1–3 cm diameter. The surface may be ulcerated and cause

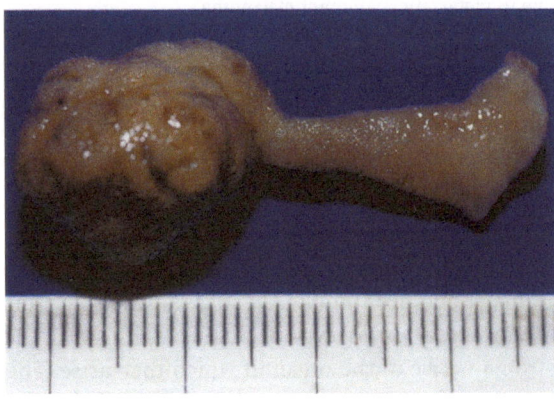

Fig. 4.16. Polypectomy specimen showing typical juvenile polyp with long pedicle and smooth surface

rectal bleeding which is the predominant mode of presentation. As the name suggests they are most often found in the paediatric population where they account for over 90% of all polyps (MESTRE 1986). In a large series of 144 juvenile polyps from Jordan, 68% occurred in children less than 10 years, 27% in the 10- to 19-year age group and 5% in adults (DAJANI and KAMAL 1984). Older studies describe a predominantly distal distribution with 60%–90% of polyps located in the rectum. However, a recent series reported from North America described 32% of polyps proximal to the splenic flexure, suggesting that this type of polyp might be more evenly distributed in the colon than previously thought (GUPTA et al. 2001). They are frequently multiple (23%–45%) and may rarely be part of an inherited polyposis syndrome (see Sect. 4.4.3) (JASS et al. 1988).

Histologically, there is a characteristic pattern of cystically dilated and distorted colonic crypts sepa-

rated by abundant oedematous stroma. The stroma contains inflammatory cells which may be numerous, variable numbers of smooth muscle fibres and granulation tissue in areas of ulceration. The epithelium lining the distended crypts is usually mature and mucin producing. In inflamed areas it may be mucin depleted and have a regenerative appearance. Epithelial dysplasia is uncommon in solitary juvenile polyps. Nevertheless, there are rare case reports of malignant change in these tumours indicating that a juvenile polyp–dysplasia–carcinoma sequence exists. However, this risk must be very small for sporadic polyps as a recent longitudinal study of 82 patients with solitary polyps followed over 25 years showed no increased risk of dying from large bowel cancer (NUGENT et al. 1993). In contrast, patients with juvenile polyposis have a substantial risk of developing gastrointestinal malignancy (JASS et al. 1988).

4.3.2
Metaplastic Polyps

Metaplastic polyps (synonym; hyperplastic polyp; serrated polyp) are probably the second commonest type of polyp in the large bowel. The majority are situated in the rectum and sigmoid with smaller numbers in the proximal colon and appendix. They are not seen in the small intestine. They are usually small, pale, sessile nodules with a smooth or slightly roughened surface, located on the apex of a mucosal fold (Fig. 4.17). In one large endoscopic series only 1% were over 10 mm in size and 83% were less than 5 mm in diameter (WILLIAMS et al. 1980). Larger polyps may be pedunculated and have a lobulated or villous surface. Studies suggest that the size of these lesions is significantly greater in the proximal colon

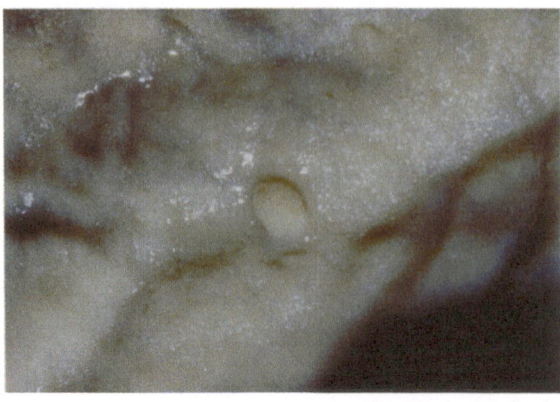

Fig. 4.17. Colectomy specimen showing small sessile metaplastic polyp with smooth pale surface

(TORLAKOVIC et al. 2003). They are commoner in men than women (ratio 4:1) and increase in number with age (FRANZIN et al. 1984). Clustering of metaplastic polyps may be seen around cancers and adenomas (CAPPELL and FORDE 1989).

Histologically metaplastic polyps are composed of colonic crypts which are elongated and mildly dilated. The crypt epithelium contains increased numbers of absorptive cells. A highly characteristic feature is the tufted, serrated outline of the crypt epithelium (Fig. 4.18). This is most pronounced in the superficial half of the crypt but occasionally may extend down into the crypt base. Unlike adenomatous polyps there is no evidence of nuclear or cytological atypia (dysplasia). Other findings include thickening of the subepithelial collagen plate, mild

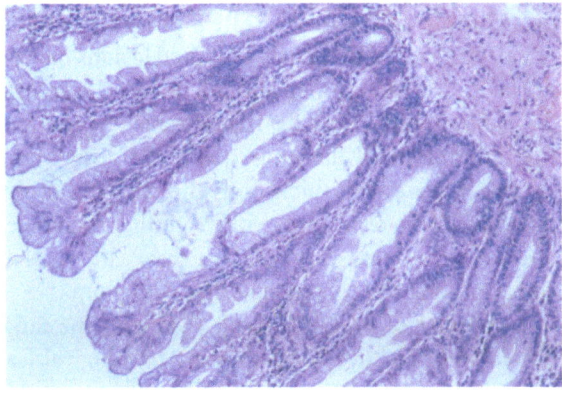

Fig. 4.18. Typical metaplastic polyp with serrated crypt outline. (H&E stain, magnification ×20)

chronic inflammation in the lamina propria and disorganisation of the muscularis mucosa with smooth muscle fibre extension into the polyp base. The latter two features have led some authors to suggest that either a reparative response to local inflammation or mucosal prolapse underlies the development of these polyps (ARTHUR 1968). Cell kinetic studies indicate that migration of colonocytes up the crypt towards the surface is delayed, leading to "hypermaturation" and cellular crowding. In contrast to adenomas, DNA synthesis is restricted to cells in the lower half of the crypt, a situation identical to that in the normal mucosa (LANE et al. 1971).

Traditionally metaplastic polyps have been viewed as biologically and clinically insignificant; however, in the past 5–10 years information has accrued that at least some, if not all serrated polyps may not be so innocent. It has been known for a long time that there is a strong epidemiological association between colorectal cancer, adenomas and metaplastic polyps

(CLARK et al. 1985). Metaplastic polyps are more frequent in populations with a high incidence of large bowel cancer. More recently a number of somatic mutations, e.g. k-ras mutation, chromosome 1p deletion and microsatellite instability have been identified in a proportion of metaplastic polyps indicating that they may be neoplastic (monoclonal) proliferations rather than reactive lesions (WILLIAMS 1997). Coupled with increasing recognition of polyps showing mixed features of hyperplastic and adenomatous polyps and the elevated cancer risk in hyperplastic polyposis, this has led to a growing belief that a subgroup of metaplastic polyps exist which may evolve into adenocarcinoma (JASS 2002; LEGGETT et al. 2001). Large right-sided metaplastic polyps appear to be particularly implicated in this pathway. Conversely the archetypal small sessile rectal and sigmoid polyp can probably still be regarded as having no significant malignant potential.

4.3.3
Benign Lymphoid Polyps

In a small number of individuals reactive hyperplasia of lymphoid tissue in the bowel wall can lead to a sessile or pedunculated polyp. Lymphoid polyps are most commonly seen in children and are invariably located in the rectum where they cause rectal bleeding, tenesmus and rectal prolapse (BYRNE et al. 1982). Size ranges from a few millimetres to 4 cm. They may be multiple. Histologically, the mucosa and submucosa are expanded by numerous lymphoid follicles with well developed germinal centres and a mantle of small lymphocytes. Rarely the whole bowel wall may be affected. The aetiology is unclear; it is postulated that a viral infection may trigger some to develop. Spontaneous regression is well described. Microscopic differentiation from other types of large bowel polyp, especially adenoma and lymphoma, is necessary. Excluding the latter may be particularly difficult in small biopsies.

4.3.4
Inflammatory Polyps

Inflammatory polyps (synonym: inflammatory pseudopolyps) are most often seen in patients with idiopathic inflammatory bowel disease but can also develop following ulceration in other conditions, e.g. amoebic colitis, schistosomiasis, ureterosigmoidostomy and blind ileal loops (GEBOES et al. 2002). They may be solitary but are usually multiple. They are more often sessile than pedunculated. Most are 2–10 mm in size; however, giant inflammatory polyps (greater than 15 mm) are well described and these may cause intestinal obstruction, intussusception and protein losing enteropathy as well as leading to diagnostic confusion with adenomas and carcinomas (ANDERSON et al. 1996; KELLY et al. 1986). Quite frequently inflammatory polyps assume a worm-like, filiform shape (Fig. 4.19), but can appear more bulbous or assume complex branching outlines. Sometimes mucosal bridges occur. Inflammatory polyps may be distributed diffusely around the colitic bowel or numerous polyps may be crowded in a relatively short segment with flat atrophic mucosa either side. Giant polyps are most often located in the transverse colon.

Inflammatory polyps have been reported in 10%–25% of patients with inflammatory bowel disease (TEAGUE and READ 1975). They are commoner in ulcerative colitis than Crohn's disease and are particularly associated with extensive severe colitis. Their pathogenesis is thought to involve severe ulceration which undermines adjacent mucosa causing it to become elevated above the surrounding denuded surface (KELLY and GABOS 1987). With healing the ulcer becomes re-epithelialized and this regenerated mucosa is flat and atrophic. In contrast the intervening elevated, polypoid mucosa either has a normal crypt architecture or shows crypt distortion and elongation. Some inflammatory polyps may develop cystically dilated glands and abundant, inflamed stroma very similar to juvenile polyps. Others consist entirely of granulation tissue. Dysplasia is not a common finding

in these polyps and there is no evidence that they are associated with an increased risk of colorectal cancer beyond that normally attributed to chronic UC (DE DOMBAL et al. 1966).

4.3.5
Polyps Related to Mucosal Prolapse

The solitary rectal ulcer syndrome (SRUS) may present endoscopically with an ulcer, localised hyperaemic and oedematous mucosa, a nodular mass or a polyp. In one of the largest series reported to date only 29% of patients had ulcerated lesions at diagnosis while 44% presented with polyps (TJANDRA et al. 1993). The majority of ulcers and polyps are located on the anterior wall (76%) anywhere from the dentate line to 15 cms from the anal verge. This variable macroscopic appearance of SRUS often leads to an erroneous clinical diagnosis. Polypoid lesions may be mistaken for carcinomas and adenomas. Histologically both polypoid and flat mucosa show typical features dominated by fibromuscular obliteration of the lamina propria with thickening and splaying of the muscularis mucosae. Regenerative epithelial changes are occasionally misdiagnosed as dysplastic further compounding the confusion with an adenoma.

A number of other polypoid lesions of the large bowel have been described showing histological features similar to those seen in SRUS. These include inflammatory cloacogenic polyp, inflammatory cap polyp, inflammatory myoglandular polyp, prolapsing mucosal polyp and polypoid prolapsing mucosal

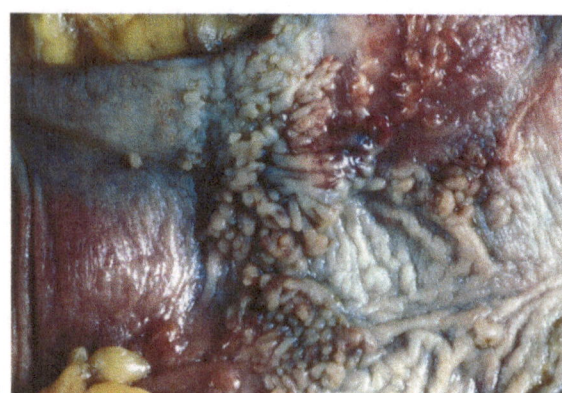
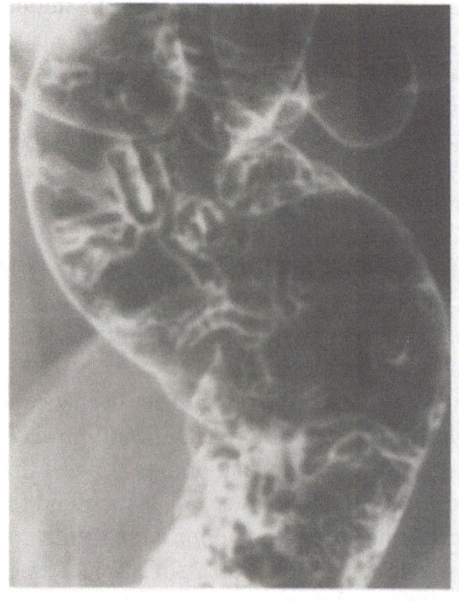

Fig. 4.19a,b. a Colectomy specimen. Filiform post-inflammatory polyps in ulcerative colitis. **b** Barium enema showing filiform polyps in a different patient

folds (SAUL 1987; WILLIAMS et al. 1985; NAKAMURA et al. 1992; TENDLER et al. 2002; KELLY 1991). They may be solitary or multiple, pedunculated or sessile. Apart from inflammatory cloacogenic polyps, which by definition are situated at the ano-rectal junction, these polyps are most commonly found in the sigmoid colon. Many though not all, are associated with redundant mucosal folds and diverticulosis (Fig. 4.20). Inflammatory cap polyps have also been described in prolapsing ileostomies and colostomies and in a prolapsed ileo-anal pouch (ATTANOOS et al. 1995).

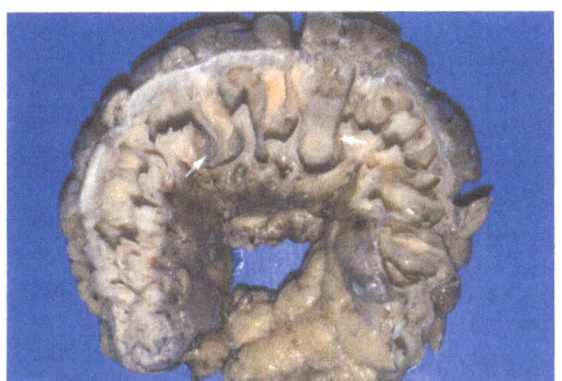

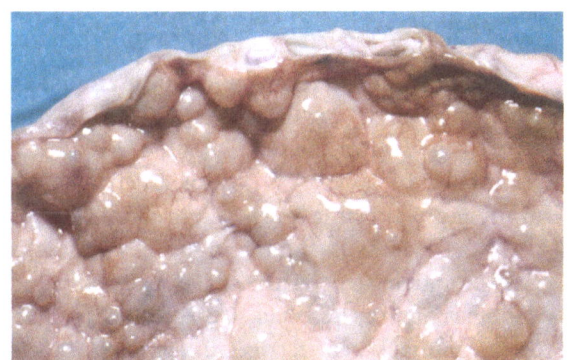

Fig. 4.20a,b. a Sigmoid colectomy specimen for diverticular disease. Note redundant, polypoid prolapsing mucosal folds (*arrows*). b Sigmoid colectomy specimen showing several polypoid prolapsing mucosal folds. Note pigmentation of the polyp mucosa due to mucosal haemorrhage

4.3.6
Inflammatory Fibroid Polyps

These are rare, non-neoplastic polyps more usually seen in the stomach and small bowel (KIM and KIM 1988). They may be pedunculated or sessile and are frequently ulcerated. Size ranges from 1.5 to 7 cms. Histologically the lesion is predominantly submucosal consisting of a proliferation of blood vessels and spindle cells, the latter characteristically arranged around vascular structures in a concentric, onion skin pattern. There is usually an accompanying diffuse infiltrate of lymphocytes, plasma cells and eosinophils. The spindle cells probably represent either fibroblasts or myofibroblasts. Once thought to be a localised form of eosinophilic gastroenteritis, inflammatory fibroid polyp is now considered to be an unusual fibrovascular reaction to trauma, ulceration or some other inflammatory stimulus (TRILLO and ROWDEN 1991).

4.3.7
Other Non-Neoplastic Polyps

A variety of other conditions can give rise to polyps or polypoid lesions. These include pneumatosis coli, endometriosis and heterotopic gastric mucosa (Fig. 4.21) (GALANDIUK and FAZIO 1986; YANTISS et al. 2001; CASTOLLANOS et al. 1984).

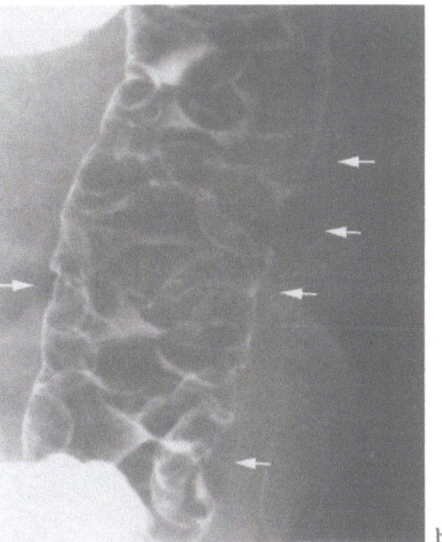

Fig. 4.21a,b. a Colectomy specimen. Diffuse polypoid appearance caused by multiple sub-mucosal gas bubbles. b Barium enema. Gas in bowel wall (*arrows*). Pneumatosis coli

4.4
Polyposis Syndromes

4.4.1
Familial Adenomatous Polyposis

Familial adenomatous polyposis (synonyms: FAP; adenomatous polyposis coli; familial polyposis coli) is undoubtedly the most well known and well described of the gastrointestinal polyposis syndromes. It is inherited as an autosomal dominant condition, is fully penetrant and if untreated leads to colorectal cancer in virtually 100% of gene carriers. Its incidence at birth is one in 8000–10,000 (CAMPBELL et al. 1994). A positive family history is not invariable as new mutations account for 20%–25% of cases (BISGAARD et al. 1994). The gene responsible (APC) is located on chromosome 5q and is a classical tumour suppressor gene, i.e. adenomas and carcinomas result from point mutations and chromosome deletions which cause loss of gene expression. In typical FAP multiple adenomatous polyps develop in the large bowel during adolescence and early adulthood. Distribution is relatively uniform around the rectum and colon. Polyps usually exceed 100 and are often present in thousands (Fig. 4.22); however, the number of polyps can vary dramatically both within and between families as a result of different APC gene mutations and the influence of modifier genes. An attenuated variant of FAP exists in which adenomas number less than 100 (LYNCH et al. 1995). Not uncommonly gene carriers may develop as few as 10–50 polyps. Other characteristics of this attenuated phenotype include a significantly later age at onset of adenoma/carcinoma (mean age at diagnosis greater than 40 years); more proximal location of polyps and over representation of flat adenomas.

Histologically adenomas in FAP are identical to their sporadic counterparts with the exception that microadenomas consisting of fewer than ten dysplastic crypts are also found in macroscopically normal mucosa. Rarely gene carriers may develop multiple benign lymphoid polyps in the small and large bowel which mimic adenomatous polyposis (GRUENBERG and MACKMAN 1972). This has led in the past to inappropriate surgery and highlights the importance of histological confirmation.

Extra colonic manifestations of FAP include gastric polyps and adenocarcinoma; duodenal adenomas and peri-ampullary carcinoma; hepatoblastoma; thyroid carcinoma; central nervous system tumours; osteomas and intra-abdominal fibromatosis (desmoid tumours). Some of these complications have previously gone under the name of Gardener's and Turcot's syndrome but are now recognised as part of the FAP phenotype (TURCOT et al. 1959).

4.4.2
Metaplastic Polyposis

A number of small series and case reports have described individuals and families in which multiple metaplastic (hyperplastic) polyps develop (JOR-

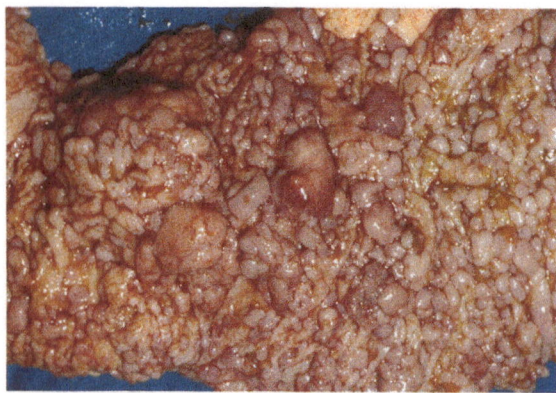

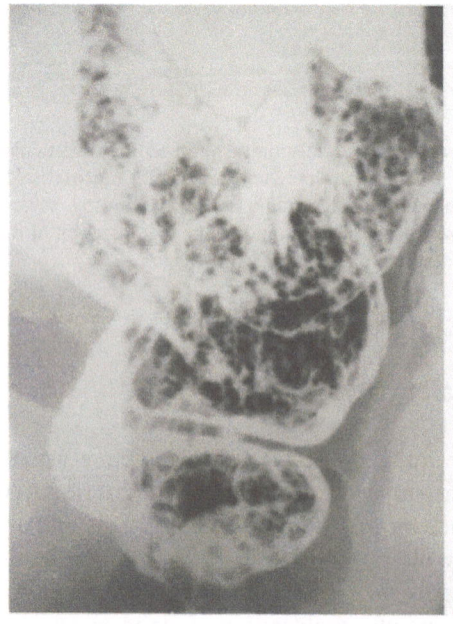

Fig. 4.22a,b. a Colectomy specimen. Familial adenomatous polyposis. A myriad of mucosal polyps of varying size **b** Barium enema

GENSEN et al. 1996; RASHID et al. 2000; JEEVARATNAM et al. 1996). In one family there appeared to be an autosomal dominant pattern of inheritance (JEEVARATNAM et al. 1996). These serrated polyps are distinctive in that they are usually larger and are more evenly distributed around the colon than sporadic metaplastic polyps, which are predominantly distal. The term "giant hyperplastic polyposis" has been used in some cases where polyps characteristically exceed 1–2 cm in size (JEEVARATNAM et al. 1996). The polyps in this syndrome are also unusual histologically. While many appear to be classical metaplastic polyps, there is invariably an admixture of mixed hyperplastic/adenomatous polyps, serrated adenomas and even typical tubular adenomas (RASHID et al. 2000). Recently JASS and BURT (2000) have proposed that hyperplastic polyposis be defined by:

- At least five histologically diagnosed hyperplastic polyps proximal to the sigmoid colon, of which two are greater than 10 mm in diameter, or
- Any number of hyperplastic polyps occurring proximal to the sigmoid colon in an individual who has a first-degree relative with hyperplastic polyposis, or
- Greater than 30 hyperplastic polyps of any size but distributed throughout the colon.

Like FAP, evidence is accruing that hyperplastic polyposis as defined above carries a significant risk of colorectal cancer. In a recent study seven out of 12 patients followed over 5 years at one institution developed large bowel adenocarcinoma (LEGGETT et al. 2001).

4.4.3
Juvenile Polyposis

Multiple juvenile polyps can affect the colorectum in two distinct clinical syndromes. In the first polyps are present from birth and infants present with diarrhoea, protein losing enteropathy, rectal prolapse and intussusception in the first year of life (SAHATELLO et al. 1974). This condition is non-familial and often fatal. In the second, patients present with polyps as adolescents and young adults (JASS et al. 1988). Tumours occur in the stomach, small bowel and colorectum where they may vary in number from less than ten to over 100. An autosomal dominant pattern of inheritance is described and recent genetic studies indicate inactivating mutations in SMAD4/DPC4 as the cause of at least some of these cases (HOWE et al.

1998). JASS et al. (1988) suggested the following definition of juvenile polyposis underlining its somewhat variable clinical phenotype:

- More than five juvenile polyps in the colorectum, or
- Juvenile polyps throughout the gastrointestinal tract, or
- Any number of juvenile polyps with a family history of juvenile polyposis.

Histologically most of the polyps are identical to a sporadic juvenile polyp; however, up to 20% show atypical morphology characterised by an unusual lobulated, villous or papillary configuration (GRIGIONI et al. 1981). Half of these atypical polyps show epithelial dysplasia similar to that seen in adenomas.

It is now recognised that juvenile polyposis carries a significant risk of colorectal and gastric cancer which may develop at a young age. In one series of 87 patients, including 18 with large bowel carcinoma, the mean age at diagnosis of malignancy was only 34 years (range 15–59 years) (JASS et al. 1988).

4.4.4
Peutz-Jeghers Polyposis

Multiple hamartomatous polyps affect the gastrointestinal tract in Peutz-Jeghers disease, an autosomal dominant inherited condition with an estimated prevalence of 1:120,000 (MCGARRITY et al. 2000). These polyps (described in Sect. 4.3.1.1) are most numerous in the small intestine, especially jejunum, but also affect the stomach and colon. In a series of 182 patients from the Mayo clinic, 27% had colonic polyps compared with small bowel polyps in 96% (BARTHOLOMEW et al. 1962). They are usually pedunculated and frequently grow to several centimetres in size when they cause intestinal obstruction, intussusception and gastrointestinal haemorrhage. Patients present clinically in their 20 s or 30 s. The syndrome, which is linked to mutation of a serine-threonine kinase gene on chromosome 19p, also includes mucocutaneous pigmentation (peri-oral, lips, buccal mucosa, fingers and toes) and an increased risk for both gastrointestinal and extra-intestinal malignancies (HEMMINKI et al. 1998). This includes oesophageal (relative risk 57×), gastric (relative risk 213×), small bowel (relative risk 520×) and large bowel malignancy (relative risk 84×), as well as cancers of the breast, pancreas, ovary and testis (GIARDIELLO et al. 2000). The relationship between the hamartomatous polyps and development of cancer in the intestine is not entirely clear as pre-malignant dysplasia is rarely seen in these tumours; however, at least some carcinomas appear to arise from neoplastic transformation of the polyp epithelium.

4.4.5
Cronkhite-Canada Syndrome

First described in 1955 by Cronkhite and Canada, this extremely rare condition is characterised by multiple gastrointestinal polyps, alopecia, nail dystrophy (onycholysis), hyperpigmentation, glossitis and cataracts (CRONKHITE and CANADA 1955). Most patients also develop a protein losing enteropathy and electrolyte imbalance. Multiple sessile, ill-defined polypoid thickenings occur in the mucosa of the stomach, small bowel, colon and rectum. The oesophagus is not involved. Polyps range in size from a few millimetres to a few centimetres. On microscopic examination these polyps resemble juvenile polyps (i.e. hamartomas). They are composed of oedematous and inflamed lamina propria in which is scattered cystically dilated colonic crypts. Dysplasia is not seen. However, unlike juvenile polyps the background non-polypoid mucosa in Cronkhite-Canada syndrome is also abnormal, and shows diffuse thickening due to oedema and chronic inflammation. This results in unusually prominent colonic mucosal folds. Cronkhite-Canada syndrome is not familial and presents clinically in later life (40–60 years). An association with colorectal cancer has been described (DANIEL et al. 1982).

4.4.6
Malignant Lymphomatous Polyposis

In 1961 Cornes described multiple polyps in the gastrointestinal tract due to lymphomatous involvement of the mucosa and submucosa (Fig. 4.23) (CORNES 1961). In the colon and ileocaecal region these sessile polyps range in size from a few millimetres to several centimetres. They are often associated with mesenteric node involvement (91%) and in one series 71% of patients had advanced disease at diagnosis (Ann Arbor stage 4) (FOUMESTRAUX et al. 1997). This clinical syndrome of multiple lymphomatous polyps is usually due to primary or secondary gastrointestinal involvement by mantle cell lymphoma and carries a poor prognosis. However, a minority of cases may be associated with follicular lymphoma or malt lymphoma (BRESLIN et al. 1999).

4.4.7
Other Polyposis Syndromes

Other polyposis syndromes include the development of multiple inflammatory fibroid polyps ("Devon polyposis syndrome"), lipomatous polyposis, Cowden's syndrome and Bannayan-Reilly-Ruvalcaba syndrome (ALLIBONE et al. 1992; SANTOS-BRIZ et al. 2001; ERDMAN and BARNARD 2002). The latter (CS and BRRS) are due to a germ-line mutation in the PTEN gene (WAITE and ENG 2002). In addition to gastrointestinal polyps, affected individuals exhibit multiple other abnormalities, e.g. macrocephaly, cutaneous pigmentation, skin tumours, thyroid goitre, thyroid and breast cancer. The intestinal polyps are usually hamartomas similar to sporadic juvenile polyps, but ganglioneuromas and adenomas may also occur. CS and BRRS are inherited as autosomal dominant conditions.

4.4.8
Hereditary Non-Polyposis Colorectal Cancer (HNPCC)

Approximately 1%–2% of all colorectal carcinomas develop in persons with HNPCC, an autosomal dominant inherited disorder. This disease is due to mutation in one of several genes involved in DNA mismatch repair, a process by which DNA coding errors incurred during DNA replication are corrected. HNPCC is defined clinically using the Amsterdam criteria (see Chap. 2, Sect. 2.2.1) (VASEN et al. 1999). Large bowel cancer occurs in up to 80% of affected

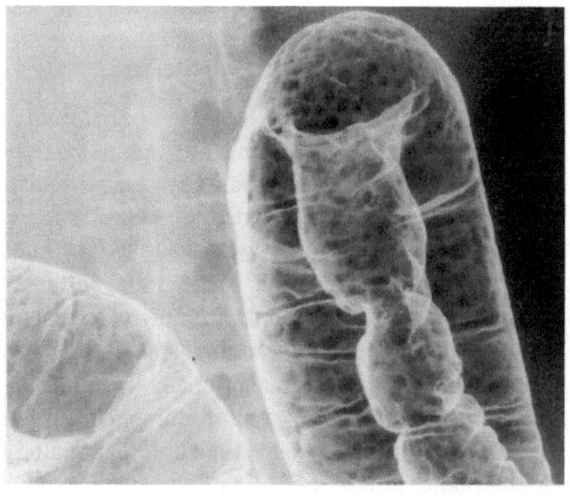

Fig. 4.23. Barium enema in a patient with lymphomatous polyposis. (Courtesy of T. Blakeborough, FRCR, Sheffield, UK)

individuals often at an earlier age than sporadic cancer (mean age of diagnosis 44 years) (VASEN et al. 1996). Tumours are commonly situated proximal to the splenic flexure (70%) and are more often multiple (45% rate of synchronous and metachronous cancer) (LYNCH and SMYRK 1996).This has important implications for diagnosis and surveillance since flexible sigmoidoscopy limited to the distal colon is not an adequate investigation.

A range of other cancers also occur in gene carriers including endometrial, ovarian, upper urinary tract, small bowel and gastric carcinomas.

While not by definition a polyposis syndrome, adenocarcinomas in HNPCC do appear to arise from adenomatous polyps. These adenomas are not thought to be any more prevalent in affected patients but have some unusual features (JASS and STEWART 1992). Like the cancers, they are more often located in the proximal colon and occur at a younger age. For any given size of polyp they are more frequently villous and show a greater degree of dysplasia, features which predict a higher risk of malignant change. Colonoscopic surveillance of patients with HNPCC suggests that the adenoma–carcinoma sequence is accelerated in this condition (AHLQUIST 1995). Polypectomy will reduce the incidence of carcinoma but surveillance intervals need to be short, probably of the order of 2 years.

References

Ahlquist DA (1995) Aggressive polyps in hereditary non-polyposis colorectal cancer: targets for screening. Gastroenterology 108:1590–1591

Allibone RO, Nanson JK, Anthony PP (1992) Multiple and recurrent inflammatory fibroid polyps in a Devon family ("Devon polyposis syndrome"): an update. Gut 33:1004–1005

Allibone RO, Hoffman J, Gosney JR et al (1993) Granulation tissue polyposis associated with carcinoid tumours of the small intestine. Histopathology 22:475–480

Anderson R, Kaariainen IT, Hanaver SB (1996) Protein losing enteropathy and massive pulmonary embolism in a patient with giant inflammatory polyposis. Am J Med 101:323–325

Arthur JF (1968) Sturcture and significance of metaplastic nodules in the rectal mucosa. J Clin Pathol 21:735–743

Attanoos R, Billings PJ, Hughes LE et al (1995) Ileostomy polyps, adenomas and adenocarcinomas. Gut 37:840–844

Bartholomew LG, Moore CE, Dahlion DC et al (1962) Intestinal polyposis with mucocutaneous pigmentation. Surg Gynecol Obstet 115:1–11

Bernstein CN (1999) ALMs versus DALMS in ulcerative colitis; polypectomy or colectomy? Gastroenterology 117:1488–1491

Bisgaard ML, Fenger K, Bulow S et al (1994) Familial adenomatous polyposis (FAP): frequency, penetrance and mutation rate. Hum Mut 3:121–125

Blackstone MO, Riddell RH, Gerald Rogers BH et al (1981) Dysplasia associated lesion or mass (DALM) detected by colonoscopy in long-standing ulcerative colitis; an indication for colectomy. Gastroenterology 80:366–374

Blecker D, Abraham S, Furth EE, Kochman ML et al (1999) Melanoma in the gastrointestinal tract. Am J Gastroenterol 94:3427–3433

Bradburn DM, Gunn A, Hastings A et al (1991) Histological detection of microadenomas in the diagnosis of familial adenomatous polyposis. Br J Surg 78:1394–1395

Breslin NP, Urbanski SJ, Shaffer EA (1999) Mucosa-associated lymphoid (MALT) lymphoma manifesting as multiple lymphomatous polyposis of the gastrointestinal tract. Am J Gastroenterol 94:2540–2545

Burke M, Shepherd N, Mann CV (1987) Carcinoid tumours of the rectum and anus. Br J Surg 74:358–361

Byrne WJ, Jimenez JF, Evler AR, Golladay ES et al (1982) Lymphoid polyps (focal lymphoid hyperplasia) of the colon in children. Pediatrics 69:598–600

Campbell WJ, Spence RA, Parks TG (1994) Familial adenomatous polyposis. Br J Surg 81:1722–1733

Cappell MS, Forde KA (1989) Spatial clustering of multiple hyperplastic, adenomatous and malignant colonic polyps in individual patients. Dis Colon Rectum 32:641–652

Castollanos D, Menchen P, Riva L et al (1984) Heterotopic gastric mucosa in the rectum. Endoscopy 16:197–199

Citarda F, Tomaselli G, Capocaccia R, Barcherini S, Crespi M et al. (2001) Efficacy in standard clinical practice of colonoscopic polypectomy in reducing colorectal cancer incidence. Gut 48:812–815

Clark JC, Callan Y, Eide TJ et al (1985) Prevalence of polyps in an autopsy series from areas with varying incidence of large bowel cancer. Int J Cancer 36:179–186

Cornes JS (1961) Multiple lymphomatous polyposis of the gastrointestinal tract. Cancer 14:249–256

Cronkhite LW, Canada WJ (1955) Generalized gastro-intestinal polyposis: an unusual syndrome of polyposis, pigmentation, alopecia and onychotrophia. NEJM 252:1011

Dajani YF, Kamal MF (1984) Colorectal juvenile polyps: an epidemiological and histopathological study of 114 cases in Jordanians. Histopathology 8:765–779

Daniel ES, Ludwig SL, Lewin KJ et al (1982) The Cronkhite-Canada syndrome. An analysis of clinical and pathologic features and therapy in 55 patients. Medicine 61:293–309

De Dombal FF, Watts J, Watkinson G et al (1966) Local complications of ulcerative colitis: stricture, pseudopolyposis and carcinoma of the colon and rectum. BMJ 1:1442–1447

Erdman SH, Barnard JA (2002) Gastrointestinal polyps and polyposis syndromes in children. Curr Opin Pediatr 14:576–582

Fide TJ, Stalsberg H (1978) Polyps of the large intestine in Northern Norway. Cancer 42:2839–2848

Foumestraux A, Delmer A, Lavergne A et al (1997) Multiple lymphomatous polyposis of the gastrointestinal tract: prospective clinicopathologic study of 31 cases. Gastroenterology 112:7–16

Franzin G, Dina R, Zamboni G et al (1984) Hyperplastic (metaplastic) polyps of the colon. Am J Surg Pathol 8:687–689

Galandiuk S, Fazio VW (1986) Pneumatosis cystoides intestinalis. Dis Colon Rectum 29:358–363

Geboes K, Shepherd N, Talbot I (2002) Polyps of the large intestine. Gastrointestinal polyps. GMM, Haboubi

Giardiello FM, Brensinger JD, Tersmette et al (2000) Very high risk of cancer in familial Peutz-Jeghers syndrome. Gastroenterology 119:1447–1453

Grigioni WF, Alampi G, Martinelli G et al (1981) Atypical juvenile polyposis. Histopathology 5:361–376

Gruenberg J, Mackman S (1972) Multiple lymphoid polyps in familial polyposis. Ann Surg 175:552–554

Gupta SK, Fitzgerald JF, Croffie JM et al (2001) Experience with juvenile polyps in North American children: the need for pancolonoscopy. Am J Gastroenterol 96:1695–1697

Hemminki A, Markie D, Tomlinson I et al (1998) A serine/threonine kinase gene defective in Peutz-Jeghers syndrome. Nature 391:184–187

Hochberg FH, DaSilva AB, Galdabini J (1974) Gastrointestinal involvement in von Reclinghausens neurofibromatosis. Neurology 24:1144–1151

Hofstad B, Vatn MH, Anderson SN et al (1996) Growth of colorectal polyps: redetection and evaluation of unresected polyps for a period of three years. Gut 39:449–456

Howe JR, Roth S, Ringold JC et al (1998) Mutations in the SMAD4/DPC4 gene in juvenile polyposis. Science 280:1086–1088

Jass JR (1989) Do all colorectal carcinomas arise in pre-existing adenoma? World J Surg 13:45–51

Jass JR (2002) Serrated adenoma of the colorectum. Curr Diag Pathol 8:42–49

Jass JR, Burt R (2000) Hyperplastic polyposis. In: Hamilton SR, Aaltonen LA (eds) WHO international classification of tumours, 3rd edn. Pathology and genetics of tumours of the digestive system. Springer, Berlin Heidelberg New York, pp 135–136

Jass JR, Sobin LH (eds) (1989) WHO international histological classification of tumours. Histological typing of intestinal tumours, 2nd edn. Springer, Berlin Heidelberg New York

Jass JR, Stewart SM (1992) Evolution of hereditary non-polyposis colorectal cancer. Gut 33:783–786

Jass JR, Williams CB, Bussey HJR et al (1988) Juvenile polyposis – a precancerous condition. Histopathology 13:619–630

Jass JR, Young PJ, Robinson EM (1992) Predictors of presence, multiplicity, size and dysplasia of colorectal adenomas. A necropsy study in New Zealand. Gut 33:1508–1514

Jeevaratnam P, Cottier DS, Browett PJ, Water NS, Pokos V, Jass JR et al (1996) Familial giant hyperplastic polyposis predisposing to colorectal cancer: a new hereditary bowel cancer syndrome. J Pathol 179:20–25

Johnston PG, O'Brien MJ, Dervan PA et al (1989) Immunohistochemical analysis of cell kinetic parameters in colonic adenocarcinomas, adenomas and normal mucosa. Hum Pathol 20:696–700

Jorgensen H, Mogensen A, Svendsen LB (1996) Hyperplastic polyposis of the large bowel. Scand J Gastroenterol 31:825–830

Kelly JK (1991) Polypoid prolapsing mucosal folds in diverticular disease. Am J Surg Pathol 15:871–878

Kelly JK, Gabos S (1987) The pathogenesis of inflammatory polyps. Dis Colon Rectum 30:251–254

Kelly JK, Lanevin JM, Price LM, Hershfield NB, Share S, Blustein P et al (1986) Giant and symptomatic inflammatory polyps of the colon in idiopathic inflammatory bowel disease. Am J Surg Pathol 10:420–428

Kim YI, Kim WH (1988) Inflammatory fibroid polyps of gastrointestinal tract. Am J Clin Pathol 89:721–727

Koura AN, Giacco GG, Curley SA et al (1997) Carcinoid tumours of the rectum. Cancer 79:1924–1298

Lane N, Kaplan H, Pascal RR (1971) Minute oedematous and hyperplastic polyps of the colon: divergent patterns of epithelial growth with specific associated mesenchymal changes. Gastroenterology 60:537–550

Leggett BA, Devereaux B, Biden K et al (2001) Hyperplastic polyposis: association with colorectal cancer. Am J Surg Pathol 25:177–184

Lieberman DA, Weiss DG, Bond JH et al (2000) Use of colonoscopy to screen asymptomatic adults for colorectal cancer. NEJM 343:162–168

Lynch HT, Smyrk T (1996) Hereditary non-polyposis colorectal cancer (Lynch syndrome): an updated review. Cancer 78:1149–1167

Lynch HT, Smyrk T, McGinn T et al (1995) Attenuated familial adenomatous polyposis (AFAP). Cancer 76:2427–2433

Makinen MJ, George SMC, Jernvall P (2001) Colorectal carcinoma associated with serrated adenoma – prevalence, histological features and prognosis. J Pathol 193:286–294

Mazier WP, MacKeigan JM, Billingham RP et al (1982) Dignan RD. Juvenile polyps of the colon and rectum. Surg Gynecol Obstet 154:829–832

McGarrity TJ, Kulin HE, Zaino RJ (2000) Peutz-Jeghers syndrome. Am J Gastroenterol 95:596–604

Mestre JR (1986) The changing pattern of juvenile polyps. Am J Gastroenterol 81:312–314

Miettinen M, Sarlomo-Rikala M, Lasota J (1999) Gastrointestinal stromal tumors: recent advances in understanding of their biology. Um Pathol 30:1213–1220

Miettinen M, Fulong M, Sarlomo-Rikala M (2001a) Gastrointestinal stromal tumors, intramural leiomyomas and leiomyosarcomas in the rectum and anus. Am J Surg Pathol 25:1121–1133

Miettinen M, Shekitha KM, Sobin LH (2001b) Schwannomas in the colon and rectum. Am J Surg Pathol 25:846–855

Muto T, Bussey HJR, Morson BC (1975) The evolution of cancer of the colon and rectum. Cancer 36:2251–2270

Muto T, Kamiya J, Sawada T et al (1985) Small "flat adenoma" of the large bowel with special reference to its clinicopathologic features. Dis Colon Rectum 28:847–851

Nakayama H, Fujii M, Kimura A (1996) A solitary Peutz-Jeghers type hamartomatous polyp of the rectum: report of a case. Jpn J Clin Oncol 26:273–276

Nakamura S, Kine I, Akagi T (1992) Inflammatory myoglandular polyps of the colon and rectum. Am J Surg Pathol 16:772–779

Nugent KP, Talbot IC, Hodgson SV et al (1993) Solitary juvenile polyps: not a marker for subsequent malignancy. Gastroenterology 105:698–700

Odze RD (1999) Adenomas and adenoma-like DALMS in chronic ulcerative colitis: a clinical, pathological and molecular review. Am J Gastroenterol 94:1746–1750

Rashid A, Houlihan PS, Booker S et al (2000) Phenotypic and molecular characteristics of hyperplastic polyposis. Gastroenterology 119:323–332

Rembacken BJ, Fujii T, Cairns A et al (2000) Flat and depressed colonic neoplasms: a prospective study of 1000 colonoscopies in the UK. Lancet 355:1211–1214

Sahatello CR, Hahn I, Carrington CB (1974) Juvenile gastrointestinal polyposis in a female infant: report of a case and review of the literature of a recently recognised syndrome. Surgery 75:107–114

Saitoh Y, Waxman I, West AB et al (2001) Prevalence and distinctive biologic features of flat colorectal adenomas in a North American population. Gastroenterology 120:1657–1665

Santos-Briz A, Garcia JP, Gonzalez C et al (2001) Lipomatous polyposis of the colon. Histopathology 38:81–83

Saul SH (1987) Inflammatory cloacogenic polyp. Hum Pathol 18:1120–1125

Shepherd NA, Bussey HJR, Jass JR (1987) Epithelial misplacement in Peutz-Jeghers polyps. A diagnostic pitfall. Am J Surg Pathol 11:743–749

Sircar K, Hewlett BR, Huizinga JD et al (1999) Interstitial cells of cajal as precursors of gastrointestinal stromal tumours. Am J Surg Pathol 23:377–389

Suzuki H, Ohta S, Tokuchi S et al (1998) Adenoma with clear cell change of the large intestine. J Surg Oncol 67:182–185

Taylor BA, Wolff BG (1987) Colonic lipomas; review of the Mayo clinic experience 1976–1985. Dis Colon Rectum 30:888–893

Tendler DA, Aboudola S, Zacks JF (2002) Prolapsing mucosal polyps: an under-recognized form of colonic polyp. Am J Gastroenterol 97:370–376

Teague RH, Read AE (1975) Polyposis in ulcerative colitis. Gut 16:792–795

Tichansky DS, Cagir B, Borrazzo et al (2002) Risk of second cancers in patients with colorectal carcinoids. Dis Colon Rectum 45:91–97

Tjandra JJ, Fazio VW, Petras RE et al (1993) Clinical and pathologic factors associated with delayed diagnosis in solitary rectal ulcer syndrome. Dis Colon Rectum 36:146–153

Torlakovic E, Skovlund E, Snover DC et al (2003) Morphologic reappraisal of serrated colorectal polyps. Am J Surg Pathol 27:65–81

Trillo AA, Rowden G (1991) The histogenesis of inflammatory fibroid polyps of the gastrointestinal tract. Histopathology 19:431–436

Tsuda S, Veress B, Toth E, Fork F-T (2002) Flat and depressed colorectal tumours in a Southern Swedish population. Gut 51:550–555

Turcot J, Despres JP, Pierre F (1959) Malignant tumours of the central nervous system associated with familial polyposis of the colon, report of two cases. Dis Colon Rectum 2:465–468

Tytgat GNJ, Dhir V, Gopinath N (1995) Endoscopic appearances of dysplasia and cancer in inflammatory bowel disease. Eur J Cancer 31:1174–1177

Vasen HFA, Wignen J, Menko FH et al (1996) Cancer risk in families with hereditary non-polyposis colorectal cancer diagnosed by mutation analysis. Gastroenterology 110:1020–1027

Vasen HFA, Watson P, Mecklin J et al (1999) New clinical criteria for hereditary non-polyposis colorectal cancer (HNPCC) proposed by the International Collaborative Group. Gastroenterology 116:1453–1456

Waite KA, Eng C (2002) Protean PTEN: form and function. Am J Hum Genet 70:829–844

Weidner N, Flanders DJ, Mitros FA (1984) Mucosal Ganglioneuromatosis associated with multiple colonic polyps. Am J Surg Pathol 8:779–786

Weinberg T, Feldman M (1955) Lipomas of the gastro-intestinal tract. Am J Clin Pathol 25:272–287

Williams AR, Balascoriya BAW, Day DW (1982) Polyps and cancer of the large bowel: a necropsy study in Liverpool. Gut 23:835–842

Williams GT (1997) Metaplastic (hyperplastic) polyps of the large bowel: benign neoplasms after all? Gut 40:691–692

Williams GT, Blackshaw AJ, Morson BC(1979) Squamous carcinoma of the colorectum and its genesis. J Pathol 129:139–147

Williams GT, Arthur JF, Bussey HJR et al (1980) Metaplastic polyps and polyposis of the colorectum. Histopatholoy 4:155–170

Williams GT, Bussey HJR, Morson BC (1985) Inflammatory cap polyps of the large intestine. Br J Surg 72:5133

Winawer SJ, Zauber AG, Nah Ho M et al (1993) Prevention of colorectal cancer by colonoscopic polypectomy. NEJM 329:1977–1981

Yantiss RK, Clement PB, Young RH (2001) Endometriosis of the intestinal tract. Am J Surg Pathol 25:445–454

Yao T, Nishiyama K, Oya M (2000) Multiple serrated adenocarcinomas of the colon with a cell lineage common to metaplastic polyp and serrated adenoma. J Pathol 190:444–449

5 An Introduction to Imaging Colonic Neoplasms

Alison Gillams

CONTENTS

5.1   Defining the Problem –
        What Do We Need to Detect? *51*
5.2   The Role of Imaging Compared to Colonoscopy *51*
5.2.1   Barium Enema *51*
5.2.1.1 Accuracy *52*
5.2.1.2 Safety *53*
5.2.1.3 Completeness *53*
5.2.2   CT Colonography *53*
5.2.2.1 Accuracy *53*
5.2.2.2 Safety *54*
5.2.2.3 Completeness *54*
5.2.3   MR Colonography *54*
5.3   Imaging the Frail/Elderly *55*
5.4   Imaging Following Incomplete Colonoscopy *56*
5.5   Screening *57*
5.6   Imaging Strategy *57*
        References *58*

5.1
Defining the Problem – What Do We Need to Detect?

There has been a great deal of discussion as to the importance of detecting small polyps. The incidence of malignancy in polyps less than 1 cm is 1%, this increases to 10%–20% for polyps with diameters between 1 and 2 cm. For polyps larger than 2 cm the incidence of malignancy is 46% (MUTO 1975). Not only is the incidence of malignancy low in small polyps, but also polyps usually grow very slowly. The estimated time for a pre-cancerous polyp to progress to a carcinoma is 10 years (MORSON 1984). This is supported by more recent, 5-year colonoscopic surveillance data. In one group, 41 patients from a total of 368 studied developed a small (less than 1 cm) adenoma but only one had developed a polyp with a diameter greater than 1 cm and there were no cancers (REX et al. 1996). Given these facts, the detection of

small polyps should not be the focus of this debate. Instead the aim should be to detect lesions larger than 1 cm. For the purposes of this chapter a small polyp is one that measures less than 1 cm in maximum diameter and a large polyp is one with a diameter of more than 1 cm. Some authors use a third category dividing small polyps into those of more or less than 5 mm. However, polyp measurement is inaccurate on both barium studies, due to magnification and the orientation of the polyp, and on colonoscopy, where sizes are usually estimated. Therefore this third category has not been included. Another area of controversy surrounds the importance of the flat polyp. There is a wide range of reported overall incidence and a variable reported incidence of dysplasia. Depending on the series quoted, flat polyps are either common with low levels of dysplasia or rare with high levels of dysplasia (REMBACKEN et al. 2000). This may be due to racial differences.

5.2
The Role of Imaging Compared to Colonoscopy

In this section the relative merits of barium enema and CT colonography are discussed under the broad headings of accuracy, safety and completeness. A brief discussion of the newer technique of MR colonography follows. A summary is provided in Tables 5.1–5.3.

5.2.1
Barium Enema

The literature is full of conflicting reports of the relative merits of barium enema (BE) and colonoscopy. Multiple variables account for these disparities. The patient population, the skill, the experience and the techniques used by endoscopists and radiologists, the inadequacy of the gold standard,

A. GILLAMS, MD
Department of Medical Imaging, The Middlesex Hospital, Mortimer Street, London, W1T 3AA, UK

Table 5.1. Accuracy

Lesion	DCBE	Colonoscopy	Prepared CT colonography
Cancer	90.2%	95%	98%
>1 cm polyps	82.7%	89.9%	91%

Table 5.2. Safety

	SCBE	DCBE	Colono-scopy	Normal dose CT: symptomatic patients	Faecal tagging CT	Screening low dose CT	MR	Faecal tagging MR
Complications	+	+	++	+/-	+/-	+/-	+/-	+/-
Radiation dose (mGy) (male:female)	3.4:6.4	3.4:6.4	0	7.5:11.4	Either normal dose/screening dose depending on population	3.9:5.7	0	0
Need for bowel cleansing	+	+++	+++	++	0	++	++	0

Table 5.3. Completeness

Factor	SCBE	DCBE	Colonoscopy	Prepared CT	Faecal tagging CT	MR Colonography	Faecal tagging MR
Collapse/Spasm/Diverticular disease	+/-	+/-	0	+	++	+	+
Importance of bowel cleansing	+	+++	+++	++	0	++	0
Extra-luminal information	0	0	0	+++	+++	++	++
Impact of an obstructing distal lesion	Usually successful	Usually successful	Incomplete study	Does not impact	Does not impact	Does not impact	Does not impact
% studies complete	90-98%	90-98%	65-90%	95%	95%	Not known	Not known

usually colonoscopy, and the difficulty of accurately localising lesions on colonoscopy. Results will inevitably differ depending on the prevalence of polyps and cancers in the patient population studied. Both techniques require training, skill and experience. One indicator of the importance of the operator is the percentage of complete colonoscopies. A caecal intubation rate of 90% is considered desirable but when the results from multiple centres are analysed the complete colonoscopy rate falls to as low as 65%–75% (DAFNIS et al. 2001).

Another problem in deciphering the literature is that colonoscopy has been accepted as the gold standard in comparisons with barium studies. Yet back-to-back colonoscopies show a not insubstantial miss rate and there are several reports of cancers missed on apparently complete colonoscopies. Colonoscopy has a false positive rate, particularly for small polyps; histological analysis reveals normal mucosa with no evidence of hyperplasia in a number of colonoscopi-cally identified small polyps. Finally, localisation is problematic. Some colonoscopists use fluoroscopy to check the location of the endoscope. Without this the colonoscopist has difficulty accurately locating lesions, particularly in older patients with long loops of redundant colon. In one study 19% of lesions were incorrectly sited (LAM et al. 1998). This mis-location can be such that a change in surgical management is required in as many as 7% (HANCOCK and TALBOT 1995).

5.2.1.1
Accuracy

In experienced hands, the detection of cancer using DCBE techniques in symptomatic patients shows a high sensitivity of 90.2% with a specificity of 99.5% (CONNOLLY et al. 2002) (Fig. 5.1). Large polyp detection is also good with a sensitivity of 82.7% compared to colonoscopy which has detection rates of 89.9% (OTT 2000) (Fig. 5.2). However, small polyp

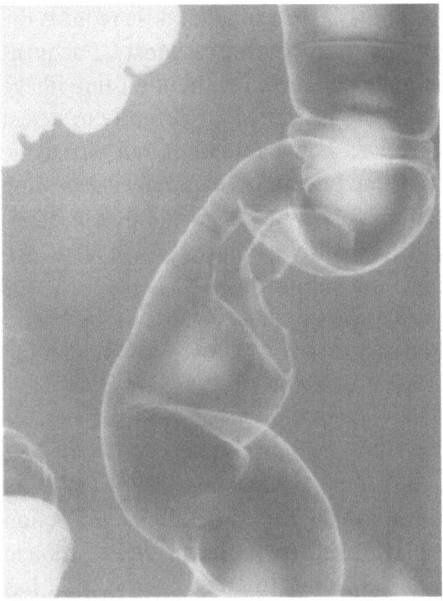

Fig. 5.1. Double contrast barium enema showing a cancer of the descending colon

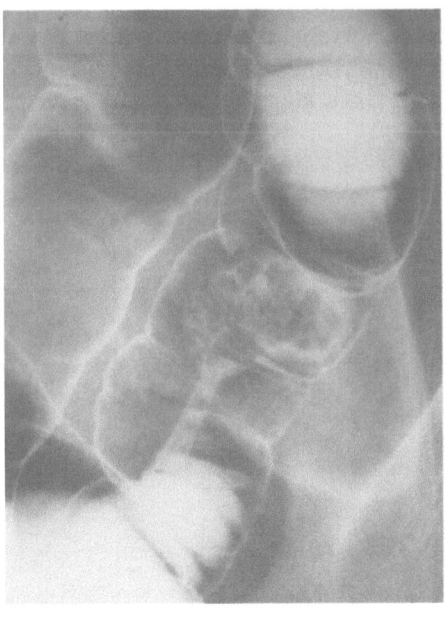

Fig. 5.2. Double contrast barium enema showing a polyp on a long stalk

detection is poor, whereas colonoscopy will detect 76%–85% of small polyps (HIXSON et al. 1990; REX et al. 1997).

5.2.1.2
Safety

Colonoscopy is the more invasive procedure. It carries a small risk of haemorrhage, less than 0.1%–0.8% and a mortality of 1–3/10,000 procedures (JENTSCHURA et al. 1994; HUANG and MARKS 2001). Most colonoscopists use sedation and there is a small incidence of aspiration- and sedation-related complications. The radiation dose from barium enema varies with the experience of the operator and the degree of tortuosity of the colon. The average figure for 5 min screening and six images is 3.43 mGy for men and 6.38 mGy for women (HARA 1997). The risk of perforation from barium enema is very small at 1/25,000 procedures (BLAKEBOROUGH et al. 1997).

5.2.1.3
Completeness

Both techniques require good bowel preparation. Both techniques are hampered by the presence of diverticular disease: barium studies because it is harder to detect polyps or cancers in the presence of diverticular disease, and colonoscopy because it may be impossible to safely negotiate the diverticular segment. Finally barium studies are harder in the patient who is unable to retain air or barium when it may be necessary to resort to a single contrast barium enema (SCBE) technique.

5.2.2
CT Colonography

CT technology has changed rapidly through the 1990s with a series of dramatic improvements, many of which facilitate CT colonography. Currently CT colonography involves interrogation of the prepared, cleansed and distended colon. The post-processing techniques have changed in speed and automation but routinely a combination of multi-planar and 3D techniques are used. IV contrast is used in symptomatic patients with suspected carcinoma but not routinely for screening.

5.2.2.1
Accuracy

Multiple studies comparing CT colonography and colonoscopy have shown a sensitivity for the detection of cancers and large polyps of at least 90% (FENLON et al. 1999). The detection of small polyps can be as high as 55% but at the expense of a higher false positive rate (FENLON et al. 1999). The most difficult lesions to detect are the so-called flat lesions that proffer minimal profile to the bowel wall (FIDLER et al. 2002). False positive diagnoses are particularly a problem for CT colonography in the presence of residue. The presence of heterogeneous attenuation on the multi-planar images, a change in location between the supine and prone imaging or the lack of enhancement following IV contrast aids differentiation. If CT is used for screening, attempts at the diagnosis of small polyps will result in high false positive rates which in turn will commit a number of patients to an unnecessary endoscopic procedure.

5.2.2.2
Safety

The risks of IV iodinated contrast media are small. In a large-scale study of more than 335,000 cases, the overall incidence of a reaction to non-ionic contrast was 3% with a less than 0.05% incidence of a severe reaction (KATAYAMA et al. 1990). The average radiation dose of a single supine acquisition at routine mA (120mA) is 7.48 mGy for males and 11.4 mGy for females. For a full prone and supine, non-contrast enhanced study at a reduced mA (70 mA) the dose is 3.8 mGy for males and 5.7 mGy for females (HARA 1997). Some centres are working on reducing the radiation dose further (50 mA) with a view to using CT for screening. Until improvements in MR make MR colonography competitive, low dose CT techniques will be the imaging alternative to double contrast barium enema (DCBE) for screening. Dosimetry depends on collimation, the need for two acquisitions, i.e. prone and supine imaging, and the use of IV contrast. Several authors have looked at the importance of spatial resolution and standard mA dosimetry. For example there is very little difference in detection rates at collimations of less than 2.5 mm, although there are important differences between 3 and 5 mm. Therefore, the radiation burden can be reduced by using a 2.5–3 mm collimation. Lowering the mA reduces the usefulness of IV contrast and in the presence of residue will mandate both supine and prone imaging. Despite this, radical reductions in mA have been shown not to reduce the diagnostic efficacy despite poor signal-to-noise ratios and aesthetically displeasing images.

5.2.2.3
Completeness

Whereas with barium studies a collapsed segment of bowel can be re-interrogated, an area of spasm can be shown to relax, CT is often a single shot or at most two-acquisition technique. The radiation dose reduces the desirability of repeated acquisitions. Most CT acquisitions are currently completed without on-line image evaluation and there is limited opportunity to detect an area of collapsed bowel or spasm and repeat the acquisition. This can be avoided in part by performing a scout view immediately prior to the data acquisition. More rapid reconstruction times will allow on-line evaluation and limited repeat acquisitions. CT is less vulnerable to poor bowel preparation. Faecal residue often demonstrates heterogenous attenuation on cross-sectional imaging. If IV contrast is used, then enhancing polyps and cancers are detectable within fluid residue (MORRIN et al. 2000) (Fig. 5.3). Overlapping bowel loops that interfere with lesion detection in traditional two-dimensional projection imaging (i.e. barium enema studies) is not a problem in cross-sectional imaging. Contrast enhanced CT has the additional benefit of assessing the remainder of the abdomen and pelvis in symptomatic patients. The incidence of other significant management-changing extra-colonic pathology (e.g. pancreatic or renal cancer) is of the order of 11% (HARA et al. 2000). Contrast-enhanced CT can provide staging information with an overall accuracy of 79% (HARVEY et al. 1998) (Fig. 5.4) and a 94% accuracy for the detection of liver metastases larger than 1 cm (SCOTT et al. 2001).

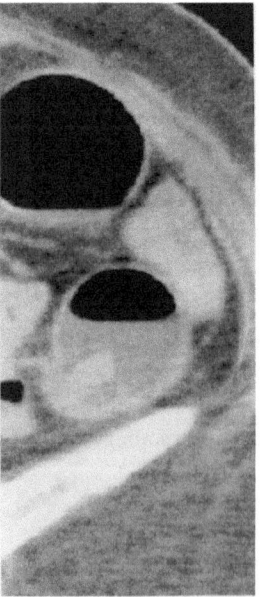

Fig. 5.3. CT colonography showing an enhancing polyp surrounded by fluid residue. The use of intravenous contrast permits polyp detection despite the polyp being completely immersed in fluid

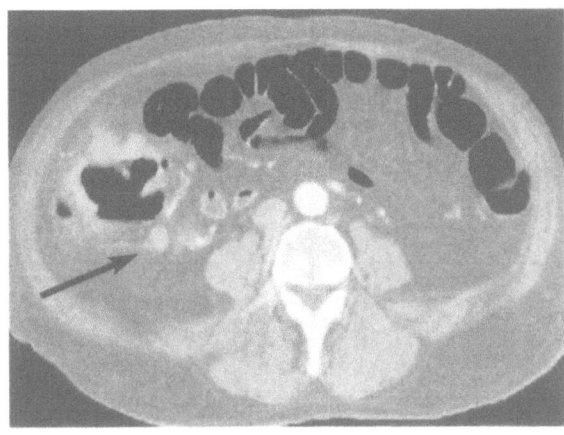

Fig. 5.4. CT colonography showing a Dukes' C caecal carcinoma with an enhancing enlarged pericolic node (*arrow*)

5.2.3
MR Colonography

MR colonography is a relatively new technique with only a few studies published to date. In the largest series MR colonography detected 19 out of a total of 31 polyps of 6–10 mm size and 26 of 27 polyps larger than 1 cm (LUBOLDT et al. 2000). The great advantages of MR, i.e. multi-plantar capability and superb soft tissue contrast, can also be achieved using CT in this context. Multi-slice CT provides volumetric data and in CT colonography there is inherent superb contrast between the air filled bowel and brightly enhancing polyps and cancer. Whereas historically MR has not been able to provide the necessary spatial and temporal resolution now for the first time MR is able to deliver. Using 3D T1 weighted acquisitions, 2–3 mm slice thickness with an in-plane resolution of 1–3 mm can be obtained in a breath-hold. MR is not widely available, it is time consuming (imaging time of 20 min) and it is vulnerable to a range of artefacts e.g. magnetic susceptibility artefact from hip replacements and breathing artefact. If MR overcomes these difficulties, then the ultimate advantage of absence of radiation will make MR the more attractive imaging technique, particularly where radiation considerations are paramount. Faecal tagging to obviate the need for bowel preparation can be used in MR as well as CT. A small prospective trial of faecal tagging and MR colonography, following water enema and IV gadolinium enhancement, in symptomatic patients detected 15 out of 18 polyps (5 – 20 mm) and all 10 cancers (LAUENSTEIN et al. 2002).

5.3
Imaging the Frail/Elderly

Single contrast enema, unprepared CT colonography or prepared CT.

The advantage of prepared CT over barium enema examination is that less is required of the patient to achieve a complete diagnostic study (Fig. 5.5). A supine and possibly a prone examination, with two breath-hold acquisitions of 20 s, is much easier to tolerate than the multiple positions and repeat views of the DCBE or even the SCBE. SCBE has a reduced sensitivity for small polyps (72% vs. 91% in one study) but a comparable sensitivity for large polyps (94% vs. 96%) and therefore is considered a reasonable alternative in

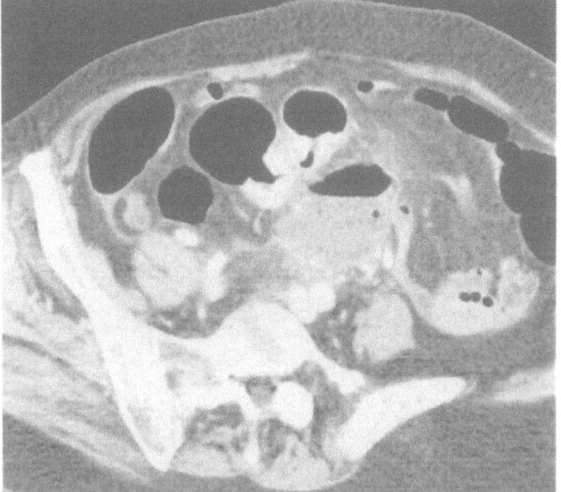

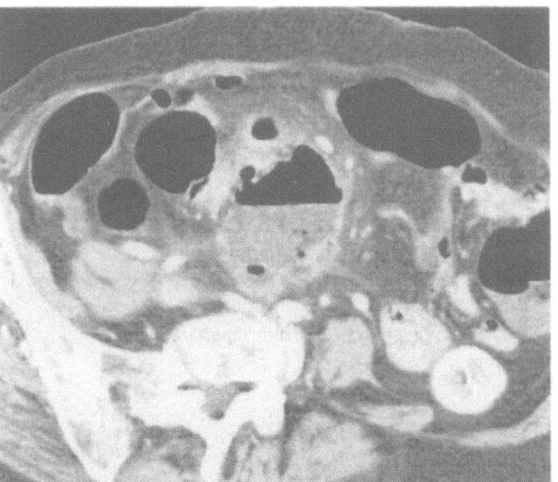

Fig. 5.5a,b. a Perforated cancer with an associated abscess. The stenosing sigmoid carcinoma is seen as an enhancing mass with an adjacent air fluid collection. **b** Part of the track from the bowel to the abscess is seen on the lower image

elderly patients (OTT et al. 1986) (Fig. 5.6). Yet studies looking at patient acceptability and comparing colonoscopy and CT colonography have highlighted that the most unpleasant part of the experience is the bowel preparation. Bowel preparation results in fluid depletion and electrolyte disturbance, particularly hypokalaemia ,and is particularly hazardous in the elderly whose postural hypotension can be exacerbated by dehydration (BARKER et al. 1992; DOWNING et al. 1983). Faecal tagging techniques have been developed to circumvent the need for bowel preparation (CALLSTROM et al. 2001). Faecal tagging is achieved by the ingestion of dilute positive contrast agents in the days prior to the examination. The contrast agents become intermixed with stool and this permits differentiation of neoplastic lesions from stool residue (Figs. 5.7, 5.8). Using a regime of multiple doses of dilute barium over 48 h, polyp sensitivity of 80%–100% has been achieved for large polyps (CALLSTROM et al. 2001). Some groups combine faecal tagging with milder cathartic agents. This combination technique has shown similar sensitivities for polyp detection when compared to standard bowel preparation techniques (LEFERE et al. 2002).

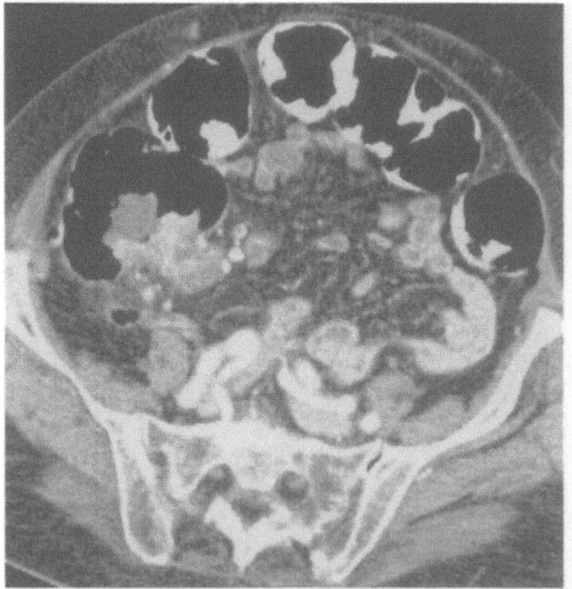

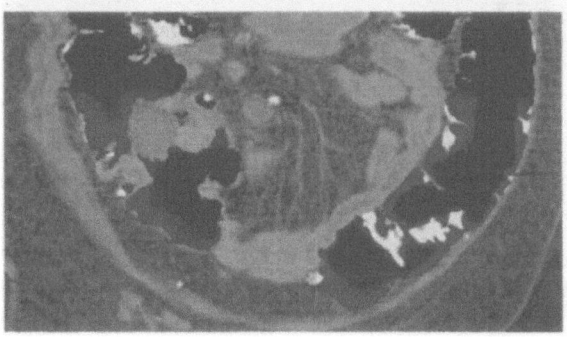

Fig. 5.7a,b. CT faecal tagging: axial (a) and coronal (b) reformatted CT images showing an enhancing mass at the ileocaecal valve. This was histologically proven adenocarcinoma. The untagged material immediately adjacent to the cancer was blood clot

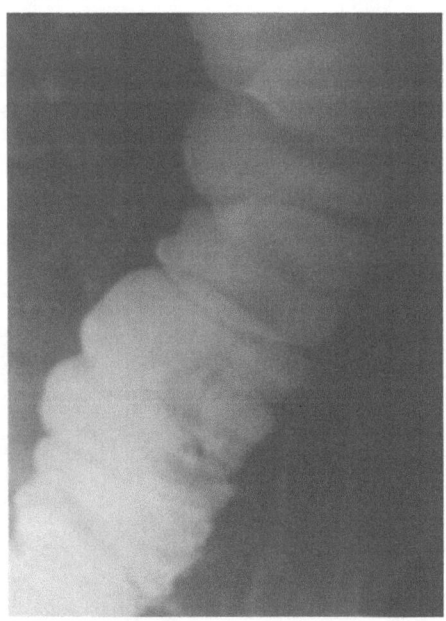

Fig. 5.6. Single contrast barium enema showing a polyp on a stalk

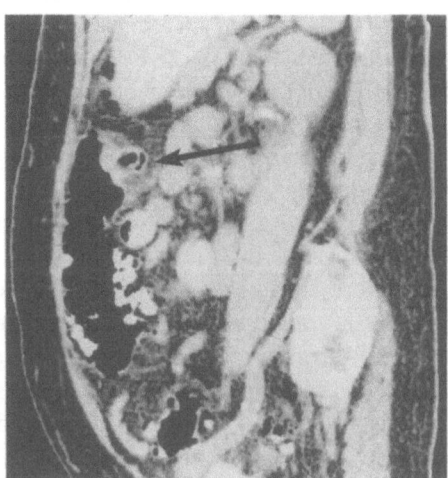

Fig. 5.8. CT faecal tagging: multiplanar reformat showing an inflamed diverticulum (*arrow*)

5.4
Imaging Following Incomplete Colonoscopy

Even experienced colonoscopists fail to reach the caecum in 6%–26% of examinations and repeat colonoscopy has a subsequent completion rate of only 50% (MARSHALL and BARTHEL 1993). Women with a history of abdominal hysterectomy are particularly likely to have an incomplete colonoscopy usually due to an impassable sigmoid (CIROCCO and RUSIN 1995). In a group of 103 patients who underwent DCBE immediately after failed colonoscopy, complete examination was achieved in 97 (94%) and significant additional information was provided in 14 (BROWN et al. 2001). Immediate CT colonography is the ideal solution to failed colonoscopy, although rectal intubation and the addition of some air is required in most patients; 21 out of 23 in one study. However, following polypectomy there is a risk of perforation (BRITTON et al. 2001; NERI et al. 2002; CHONG et al. 2002).

5.5
Screening

The need for colorectal screening is no longer disputed, but the choice of optimal screening programme will be the subject of much debate for some time to come. There are many factors to be considered in choosing the optimal screening protocol. The ideal non-invasive test with no radiation dose, and in the future no bowel cleansing, will be MR colonography. However, it is likely that machine availability and cost will prevent this screening strategy. In the interim the debate will revolve around flexible sigmoidoscopy with or without DCBE or CT colonography. One worrying feature of existing screening programmes is the very poor take-up; finding a technique that is acceptable to patients is going to be one of the deciding factors (MCMAHON and GAZELLE 2002).

5.6
Imaging Strategy

The current situation is shown in Fig. 5.9. Resource issues continue to have a major impact. Whilst the lack of adequate numbers of skilled personnel has partly been circumvented by training radiographers to perform barium enemas and by training nurse endoscopists to perform flexible sigmoidoscopy and colonoscopy, manpower and machine shortages will always be a factor in the investigation strategy adopted. An idealised, optimal strategy for the future is shown in Fig. 5.10.

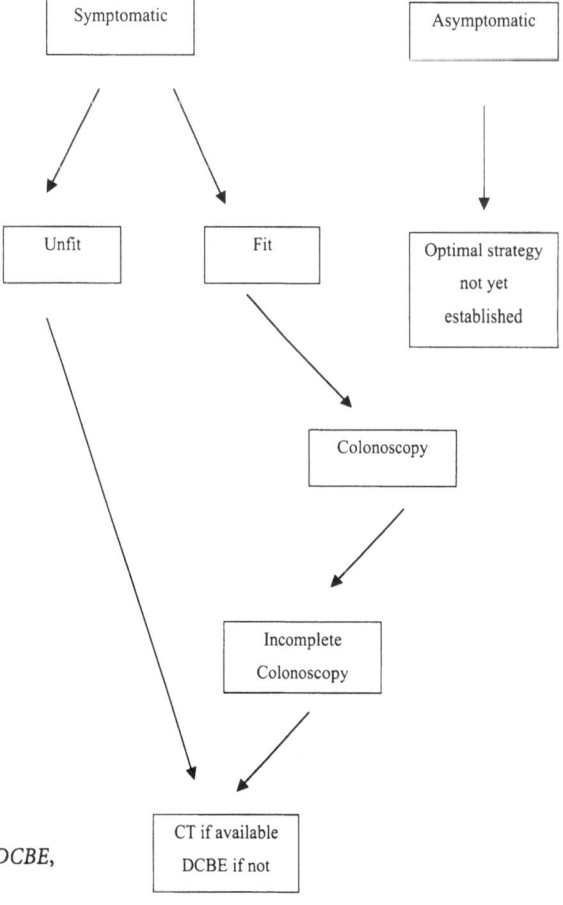

Fig. 5.9. Current investigation strategy. *DCBE*, double contrast barium enema

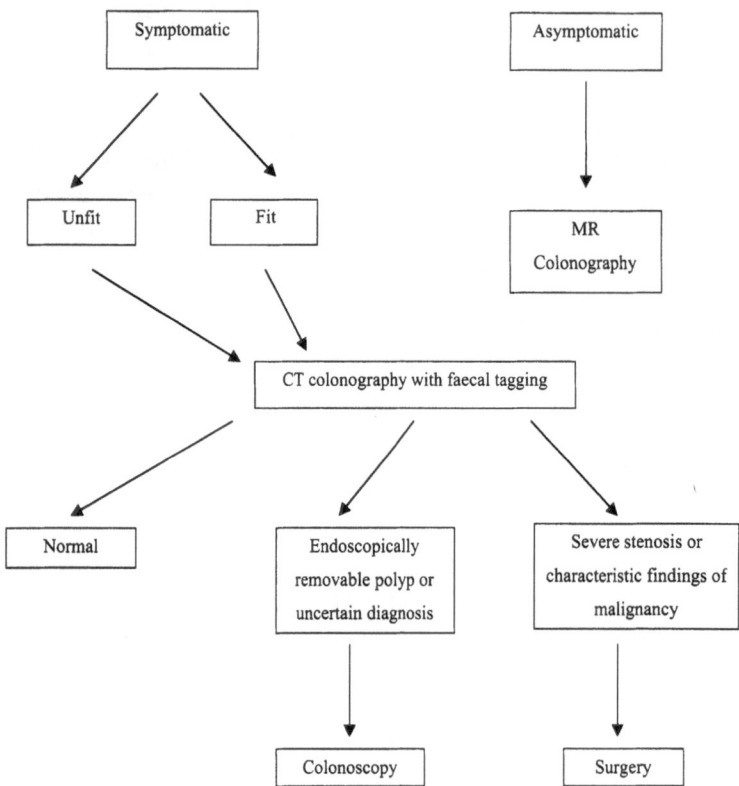

Fig. 5.10. An idealistic futuristic imaging strategy

References

Barker P, Hanning C, Trotter T (1992) A study of the effect of Picolax on body weight, cardiovascular variables and haemoglobin concentration. Ann R Coll Surg England 74: 318–319

Blakeborough A, Sheridan M, Chapman A (1997) Complications of barium enema examinations: a survey of UK consultant radiologists 1992–1994. Clin Radiol 52:142–148

Britton I, Dover S, Vallance R (2001) Immediate CT pneumocolon for failed colonoscopy; comparison with routine pneumocolon. Clin Radiol 56:89–93

Brown A, Skehan S, Greaney T et al (2001) Value of double-contrast barium enema performed immediately after incomplete colonoscopy. AJR Am J Roentgenol 176:943–945

Callstrom M , Johnson C, Fletcher J et al (2001) CT colonography without cathartic preparation: feasibility study. Radiology 219:693–698

Chong A, Shah J, Levine M et al (2002) Diagnostic yield of barium enema examination after incomplete colonoscopy. Radiology 223:620–624

Cirocco WC, Rusin LC (1995) Factors that predict incomplete colonoscopy. Dis Colon Rectum 38:964–968

Connolly D, Traill Z, Reid H et al (2002) The double contrast barium enema: a retrospective single centre audit of the detection of colorectal carcinomas. Clin Radiol 57:29–32

Dafnis G, Granath F, Pahlman L et al (2001) The impact of endoscopists' experience and learning curves and inter-endoscopist variation on colonoscopy completion rates. Endoscopy 33:511–517

Downing T, Bennion R, Sadeghi A (1983) Effect of pre-operative colon preparation on serum potassium. Am Surg 49: 414–416

Fenlon H, Nunes D, Schroy P et al (1999) A comparison of virtual and conventional colonoscopy for the detection of colorectal polyps. N Engl J Med 341:1496–1503

Fidler JL, Johnson C, MacCarty R et al (2002) Detection of flat lesions in the colon with CT colonography. Abdom Imaging 27:292–300

Hancock J, Talbot R (1995) Accuracy of colonoscopy in localisation of colorectal cancer. Int J Colorectal Dis 10: 140–141

Hara AK (1997) Reducing data size and radiation dose for CT colongraphy. AJR Am J Roentgenol 168:1181–1184

Hara A, Johnson C, MacCarty R et al (2000) Incidental extracolonic findings at CT colongraphy. Radiology 215:353–357

Harvey CJ, Amin Z, Hare CMB et al (1998) Helical CT pneumocolon to assess colonic tumours: radiologic-pathologic correlation. AJR Am J Roentgenol 170:1439–1443

Hixson L, Fennery M, Sampliner R et al (1990) Prospective study of the frequency and size distribution of polyps missed by colonoscopy. J Natl Cancer Inst 82:1769–1772

Huang E, Marks J (2001) The diagnostic and therapeutic roles of colonoscopy; a review. Surg Endosc 15:1373–1380

Jentschura D, Raute M Winter J et al (1994) Complications in endoscopy of the lower gastrointestinal tract: Therapy and prognosis. Surg Endosc 8:672–676

Katayama H, Yamaguchi K, Kozuka T et al (1990) Adverse reactions to ionic and non-ionic contrast media. A report from the Japanese Committee on the Safety of Contrast Media. Radiology 175:621–628

Lam DT, Kwong K, Lam C et al (1998) How useful is colonoscopy in locating colorectal lesions? Surg Endosc 12: 839–841

Lauenstein T, Goehde S, Ruehme S et al (2002) MR colonography with barium-based fecal tagging: initial clinical experience. Radiology 223:248–254

Lefere P, Gryspeerdt S, Dewyspelaere J et al (2002) Dietary fecal tagging as a cleansing method before CT colongraphy: initial results polyp detection and patient acceptance. Radiology 224:393–403

Luboldt W, Bauerfeind P, Wildermuth S et al (2000) Colonic masses: detection with MR colonography. Radiology 216: 383–388

Marshall JB, Barthel JS (1993) The frequency of total colonoscopy and terminal ileal intubation in the 1990s. Gastrointest Endosc 39:518–520

McMahon P, Gazelle S (2002) Colorectal cancer screening issues: a role for CT colonography? Abdom Imaging 27: 235–243

Morrin M, Farrell R, Kruskal J et al (2000) Utility of intravenously administered contrast material at CT colonography. Radiology 217:765–771

Morson B (1984) The evolution of colorectal carcinoma. Clin Radiol 35:425–431

Muto T, Bussey H, Morson B (1975) The evolution of cancer of the colon and rectum. Cancer 36:2251–2270

Neri E, Giusti P, Battolla L et al (2002) Colorectal cancer: role of CT colonography in preoperative evaluation after incomplete colonoscopy. Radiology 223:615–619

Ott D (2000) Accuracy of double-contrast barium enema in diagnosing colorectal polyps and cancer. Semin Roentgenol 35:333–341

Ott D, Chen Y, Gelfand D et al (1986) Single-contrast vs. double-contrast barium enema in the detection of colonic polyps. AJR Am J Roentgenol 146:993–996

Rembacken B, Fujii T, Cairns A et al (2000) Flat and depressed colonic neoplasms: a prospective study of 1000 colonoscopies in the UK. Lancet 355:1211–1214

Rex D, Cummings O, Helper D et al (1996) 5-year incidence of adenomas after negative colonoscopy in asymptomatic average-risk persons. Gastroenterology 111:1178–1181

Rex D, Cutler C, Lemmel G et al (1997) Colonoscopic miss rates of adenomas determined by back-to-back colonoscopies Gastroenterology 112:24–28

Scott DJ, Guthrie J, Arnold P et al (2001) Dual phase helical CT versus portal venous phase CT for the detection of colorectal liver metastases: correlation with intra-operative sonography, surgical and pathological findings. Clin Radiol 56:235–242

6 Virtual Colonography

John Bruzzi and Helen Fenlon

CONTENTS

6.1 Introduction 61
6.2 Technique 61
6.2.1 Bowel preparation 61
6.2.2 Colonic distension 62
6.2.3 Scanning Parameters 62
6.2.4 IV Contrast 63
6.3 Image Display 63
6.3.1 2D Axial and Multiplanar Images 63
6.3.2 3D Endoluminal Images 64
6.3.3 Other Display Methods 64
6.4 Image Interpretation 64
6.4.1 General Considerations 64
6.4.2 Normal Findings 64
6.4.3 Abnormal Findings 65
6.5 Diagnostic Accuracy of CT Colonography 66
6.5.1 Diagnostic Performance in High Risk Populations 66
6.5.2 CT Colonography in Pre-operative Assessment 67
6.5.3 CT Colonography and Screening 68
References 68

6.1 Introduction

Colon cancer is the second leading cause of death in the United States and the commonest cause among non-smokers. Early detection can lead to curative surgery and prolonged survival (WINAWER et al. 1997). Traditional non-invasive tests such as faecal occult blood testing have been criticised for their poor sensitivity and specificity, while conventional colonoscopy, the gold standard method of examining the colon, is an uncomfortable procedure that carries a definite mortality rate and may miss up to 24% of polyps (REX et al. 1997).

The introduction in 1994 of a genuinely novel, safe and accurate means of evaluating the colon has been credited to VINING and GELFAND (1994). 'Virtual colonoscopy' relies entirely on information acquired at CT scanning to produce two-dimensional (2D) multi-

J. BRUZZI FFRRCSI, FRCR; H. FENLON, FFRRCSI, FRCR
Department of Radiology, Mater Misericordiae Hospital, Eccles Street, Dublin 7, Ireland

planar views of the air-filled colon, in addition to creating reconstructed three-dimensional (3D) images of the inside of the colon that simulate appearances seen at endoscopy. Reported diagnostic accuracy for polyps >5 mm exceeds that of barium enema and approaches that of conventional colonoscopy. The widespread excitement stimulated by this innovation has led to rapid development and refinement of the technique, and fostered intense debate over the nature of colorectal neoplasia and how it should be diagnosed.

In 1999, it was proposed that the term 'virtual colonoscopy' be replaced by the term 'CT colonography', and it is by this name that the technique is now generally known.

6.2 Technique

Although centres vary somewhat in certain aspects of the performance of CT colonography, the basic principles remain the same. Studies are performed by scanning the abdomen and pelvis using helical or multislice CT and reconstructing the data to produce multiplanar 2D and/or 3D images of the colonic lumen. Images can be read at remote computer workstations that facilitate rapid review and ease of interpretation.

6.2.1 Bowel preparation

As retained faecal material can simulate endoluminal masses, the patient must first undergo thorough bowel cleansing prior to scanning. Low residue diets and phospho-soda preparations such as Picolax (Ferring Pharmaceuticals, Berkshire, UK) and FleetPrep (De Witt International, David Mayers Ltd, Dublin, Ireland) that are commonly employed prior to barium enema are ideal for CT colonography, as they produce a thoroughly cleansed, dry bowel mucosa. Polyethylene glycol solutions (Klean-prep, Helsinki Birex Pharmaceuticals, Dublin, Ireland) are preferred by endoscopists because they cause less internal fluid shifts and result in a wet mucosa that facilitates easier colonoscopy. However, they tend to leave a significant amount of retained fluid that can hide submerged polyps and hinder adequate colonic evaluation.

Bowel preparation is generally the source of greatest inconvenience and discomfort for the patient and an important potential cause of non-compliance with the test. Recent published studies on the viability of limited bowel catharsis using faecal-labelling techniques have been encouraging, with improved patient tolerance and diagnostic accuracy comparable to results using total bowel cleansing (CALLSTROM et al. 2001; LEFERE et al. 2002). Faecal-labelling involves administering small doses of oral contrast medium such as dilute barium sulphate in conjunction with low residue diets, leading to a partially-cleansed bowel in which faecal material can be readily identified due to the admixed high-density contrast medium. Alternatively, labelled material can be 'digitally subtracted' to leave an artificially clean colon (ZALIS and HAHN 2001). The optimal dosage regimen of oral contrast medium has yet to be agreed upon, but results indicate that small frequent doses over a 48-h period may be the most satisfactory.

6.2.2
Colonic distension

The basis of polyp detection in CT colonography depends on the high contrast resolution between colonic mucosa and endoluminal gas. In order to optimise this contrast difference, the colon must be adequately distended with gas so that mucosal excrescences can be seen in profile.

Several methods exist for achieving satisfactory colonic distension. With the patient in the decubitus position on the scanning table, a soft-tipped enema tube is inserted into the rectum. The colon can then be insufflated with room air using a hand pump up to maximum patient tolerance (approximately 40 puffs). Some workers advocate the use of carbon dioxide instead of room air (ROGALLA et al. 1999). Carbon dioxide is absorbed by the mucosa more quickly than room air and theoretically may cause less patient discomfort. However, the use of gas cylinders is inconvenient and, in practise, it may be easier to administer room air via a hand pump. The adequacy of colonic distension can be assessed on the CT scout images and further gas insufflated if necessary.

The additional use of IV muscle relaxants such as glucagon (Eli Lilly, Indianapolis, Indiana, USA) and hyoscine n-butylbromide (Buscopan, Boehringer Ingelheim, Berkshire, UK) derives from their traditional use in barium enema studies, where they have been shown to reduce colonic wall spasm, particularly in patients with diverticulosis (MURRAY 1966). They also decrease peristalsis, thereby limiting motion artefact. However, studies on the efficacy of IV glucagon in CT colonography have failed to demonstrate any significant benefit, either in terms of colonic distension or of polyp detection (YEE et al. 1999; MORRIN et al. 2002). It is possible that Buscopan may have a greater effect and is under current investigation.

6.2.3
Scanning Parameters

Following gas insufflation into the colon, the patient then undergoes abdominal CT scanning in both the supine and prone positions. The value of additional prone scanning is that it leads to a redistribution of gas and intraluminal contents and the dilatation of previously collapsed colonic segments. This has been emphasised by numerous workers to be the most useful technique in ensuring optimal colonic visualisation (CHEN et al. 1999; FLETCHER et al. 2000). Bowel distension is enhanced compared to scanning in a single position, leading to greater polyp detection and a reduction in perceptual errors.

Colonic distension has consistently been shown to be better in the prone position than in the supine position, and where scanning has to be limited to a single position because of poor patient mobility, should probably be chosen in favour of supine scanning.

Scanning can be performed using single slice helical CT or multidetector CT. The following parameters have been described for single slice helical CT: 70–100 mA, 110 kVp, 5 mm collimation with a table speed of 6.25 mm/sec (pitch of 1.25), 2 mm reformatting index and smallest field of view (FOV) to fit. Scanning takes approximately 50 s and can be performed with a single breath hold for the upper cuts and slow exhalation thereafter, or with multiple scans over several breath holds.

The primary advantage of multidetector CT scanning is that it only takes 15 s and can be performed with a single breath hold, thereby minimising respiratory misregistration artefact. Standard protocols use parameters of 70–100 mA, 120 kVp, pitch of 2.5×4 mm and slice width reconstructions of 3 mm.

Radiation dose to the patient can be minimised by reducing the mA – or by increasing the pitch and using a narrower collimation – without significantly impairing image quality. Because of the high inherent contrast difference between soft tissue and gas, the mA can be lowered to as far as 50 mA, and still result in a diagnostic study. In this way, radiation dosage to the patient can be kept to a level lower than that incurred from a standard double contrast barium enema (HARA et al. 1997; MACARI et al. 2002).

6.2.4
IV Contrast

The high contrast resolution between endoluminal gas and the colonic mucosa means that the administration of IV contrast agent is not necessary. The attractions of a non contrast-enhanced study, particularly as a potential screening tool, are its greater patient acceptability and its lower cost.

However, in patients with known or at high risk of colon cancer, IV contrast may confer additional important information. IV contrast administration increases bowel wall conspicuity, allowing differentiation of mucosal abnormalities from retained fluid and faecal material and leading to greater reader confidence (MORRIN et al. 2000a). Pericolic infiltration with tumour can be evaluated, and metastatic disease to local lymph nodes and to distant sites may be identified. The potential exists, therefore, for an all-in-one test that can diagnose and stage colonic tumours, obviating the need for further scanning. Such an approach may be particularly useful in patients with a high suspicion of colorectal cancer and in patients undergoing surveillance following resection of a tumour. The low milliamperage that is normally employed in CT colonography means that tissue characterisation in organs such as the liver is not optimal, and if IV contrast is used for combined diagnosis and staging purposes, scanning should be performed at a higher milliamperage. NERI et al. (2000) have described how triphasic scanning can be performed in CT colonography to take into account the hepatic arterial and portal venous phases of liver imaging.

It is important, therefore, to define two separate roles for CT colonography, which involve different technical considerations. As a potential screening tool in asymptomatic patients, where disease prevalence would be relatively low, CT colonography could be routinely performed at low mA settings and without the use of IV contrast. As a diagnostic test in symptomatic patients where there is a high risk

of colorectal neoplasia, IV contrast and higher mAs could be employed to optimise diagnostic yield.

Another argument for the employment of IV contrast involves the high detection rate of unsuspected extracolonic abnormalities. The poor tissue characterisation of routine non contrast-enhanced CT colonography means that incidental findings such as simple liver and renal cysts cannot be adequately evaluated, often necessitating further radiological work-up and incurring unexpected expense (HARA et al. 2000). The detection of such extracolonic findings at CT colonography will have important implications when defining its role in any colorectal cancer screening programme.

6.3
Image Display

Volumetric data sets of the abdomen acquired by CT scanning are reconstructed into multiplanar 2D and/or 3D image sets, and studies are read at remote computer workstations. Various software applications exist to facilitate speed and ease of interpretation. While most workers agree on the need to examine the colon using a variety of views (2D and/or 3D), centres differ in their individual reading techniques.

6.3.1
2D Axial and Multiplanar Images

2D axial images are the primary means of reading CT colonography studies, as the image display is familiar to radiologists and requires minimal manipulation of the data. A method known as 'colon tracking' is used to trace the colon from the rectum to the caecum, following the colonic lumen from slice to slice in order to comprehensively assess each loop and avoid skipping segments. At lung window settings, there is high contrast resolution between soft tissue and luminal gas, and polyps are identified in profile as polypoid elevations from the mucosal surface. At soft tissue window settings, more information is provided regarding the nature of endoluminal masses, the colonic wall, and extracolonic tissue. Retained faecal material can be distinguished from polyps by the presence of admixed gas. Mucosal lipomas and inverted diverticula can be identified by their fatty constituency. For these reasons, 2D axial image sets should always be reviewed at both lung and soft tissue window settings.

2D multiplanar reconstructions in the relevant coronal and sagittal planes can be displayed concurrently with axial images, and can be referred to for further characterisation and localisation of abnormalities.

6.3.2
3D Endoluminal Images

Published series have demonstrated that use of both 2D and reconstructed 3D images of the colonic lumen provides more information than either data set alone, leading to greater interpreter confidence and higher diagnostic accuracy (HARA et al. 1996; ROYSTER et al. 1997; DACHMAN et al. 1998). 3D images can be displayed using either information about the surface topology of structures, called surface rendering, or, additionally, by incorporating information about the soft tissue density of structures, called volume rendering. The latter modality provides more information about the nature of structures but requires greater computer power and time to generate the images. With the additional use of perspective rendering, which causes blurring of structures in the far field and sharpening of objects close up, 3D images simulate appearances at conventional colonoscopy.

Some workers like to examine the entire colon with 3D images, navigating from rectum to caecum in the form of a simulated colonoscopy, hence the term 'virtual colonoscopy'. However, performing complete virtual colonoscopic 'fly-throughs' of the large bowel markedly increases interpretation times. Most workers prefer to reserve 3D images for problem-solving of abnormalities seen on 2D axial slices (MACARI et al. 2000). This approach adds little to interpretation times and does not detract from diagnostic performance. The relevant three-dimensional endoluminal images can be generated concurrently with the axial views, allowing ready characterisation of findings of interest. With experience and increased familiarity with the 2D appearance of both polyps and normal variants at CT colonography, less referral to 3D images is necessary. Since interpretation times can range from as short as 10 min using axial images alone to 50 min with endoluminal navigation of the entire colon, the choice of an optimal display modality will become an important issue when considering CT colonography in the context of population screening.

6.3.3
Other Display Methods

Attention has also focussed on manipulating and displaying CT colonography data in ways other than traditional 2D axial and 3D virtual colonoscopic modes. Automatic segmentation of the colon can be performed, facilitating quicker reading and allowing instant localisation of abnormalities. Ways of laying out the mucosa in the form of a Mercator map projection have been developed, ensuring a more complete visualisation of the entire colon than can be achieved with conventional 3D endoluminal images (PAIK et al. 2000a). Early studies have also been published on computer-aided detection of abnormalities, promising greater test sensitivities and shorter reading times in the future (YOSHIDA et al. 2002; PAIK et al. 2000b). These techniques are still undergoing active investigation and development and have not yet been routinely employed in a clinical setting.

6.4
Image Interpretation

6.4.1
General Considerations

The accuracy of interpretation of CT colonography images is greatly dependent on observer experience with the technique, as described by MCFARLAND et al. (2001) and by GLUECKER et al. (2002). Double reading increases observer confidence, at least in the early stages, and we recommend that radiologists should attempt to report CT colonography studies only after an initial training period (approximately 50 cases). Results from study series where readers have been relatively inexperienced at interpreting CT colonography have reflected unacceptably poor diagnostic accuracy. It should be borne in mind that patients with positive findings at CT colonography will need to proceed to conventional colonoscopy and biopsy. The purpose of CT colonography should be the accurate detection of polyps that need to be removed, minimising false positive errors that will lead to unnecessary further examination and high costs.

6.4.2
Normal Findings

The normal colonic mucosa should be visualised on both 2D axial and 3D images as a smooth surface without discontinuous elevation. Haustral folds can be recognised by their smooth concave edges as they run from one wall to another. Orientation on 3D endoluminal images can be accomplished by recognising the tortuous nature of the sigmoid colon, the relatively straight tubular course of the descending colon and the triangular configuration of the transverse colon, cues that have traditionally been appreciated by endoscopists. Orientation can also be achieved by referral to 2D multiplanar images.

The ileocaecal valve is a troublesome area that can vary tremendously in appearance (Figs. 6.1a,b, 6.2). Its morphology can be lobular and may even simulate a caecal mass. Confident identification of the valve improves with reader experience and depends on recognition of its various appearances, its relationship to the terminal ileum, and its fatty texture.

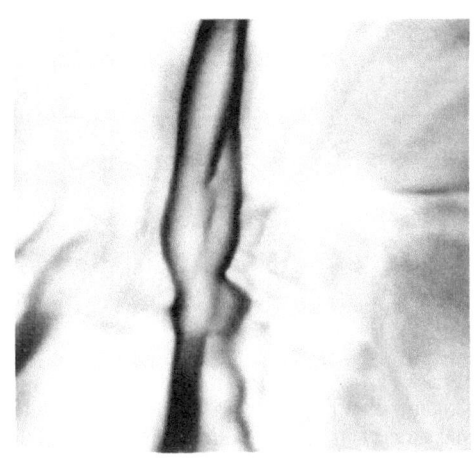

Fig. 6.2. Endoluminal 3D view of the normal ileocaecal valve, demonstrating its lobulated free edge. The ileocaecal valve can have a wide range of appearances which should not be mistaken for neoplastic disease

Extrinsic impressions on the colonic wall from normal abdominal organs such as the spleen and kidneys can often simulate neoplastic masses on 3D endoluminal views. Definitive identification can be made by referral to 2D multiplanar images (FENLON et al. 1998).

6.4.3
Abnormal Findings

Colonic polyps are identified on 2D axial images as focal rounded elevations with attenuation values on soft tissue windows equivalent to that of colonic mucosa. They can be differentiated from haustral folds by their polypoid morphology and by the tendency of haustral folds to be traceable from one wall to the next. Difficulties arise at sharp turns and at the flexures where haustral folds converge and may have a bulbous appearance, simulating polyps (Fig. 6.3). It can also be troublesome to detect small polyps located on or adjacent to mucosal folds. With experience, such pitfalls can be overcome.

On 3D images, polyps are readily identified as rounded protuberances on the mucosal surface (Figs. 6.4, 6.5). However, particularly with surface-rendered images, it may be impossible to differentiate polyps from residual faecal material, inverted diverticula, mucosal lipomas and extrinsic impressions. Errors can be avoided by referring to corresponding 2D images (FLETCHER et al. 1999).

Diagnostic accuracy can also be severely limited where there are significant amounts of retained stool

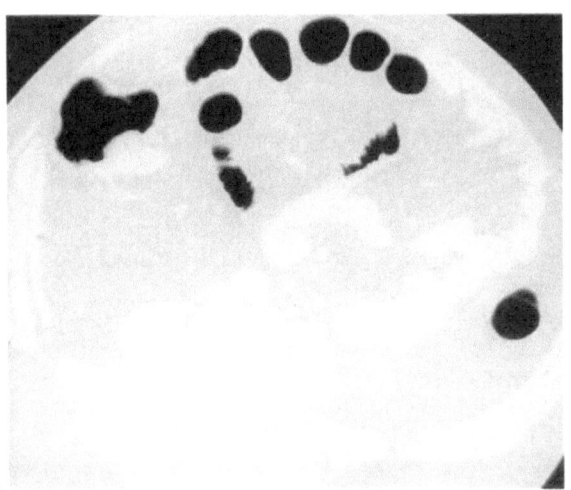

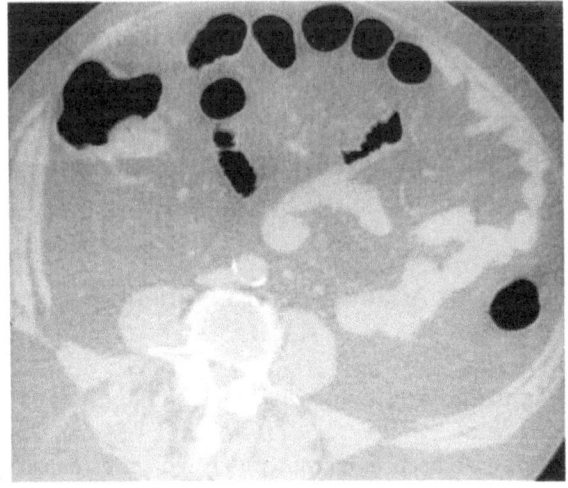

Fig. 6.1 a,b. a Apparent flat polyp in the caecum, demonstrated at lung window settings on a 2D axial slice. **b** On soft tissue window settings, the same polypoid mass is more clearly identified at the junction of terminal ileum and caecum and is of fatty tissue attenuation, thereby confirming it as the ileocaecal valve. Accurate determination of the relationship of the ileocaecal valve to the terminal ileum and recognition of its attenuation values can be helpful in establishing the benign nature of this normal structure

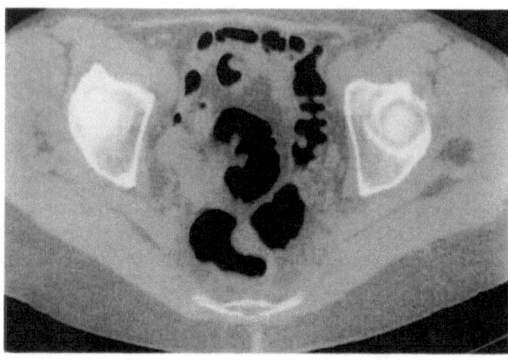

Fig. 6.3. Demonstration of prominent bulbous haustral folds on a 2D axial slice at soft tissue settings. Familiarity with the range of appearances of the normal colonic anatomy can avoid confusion with polyps and masses

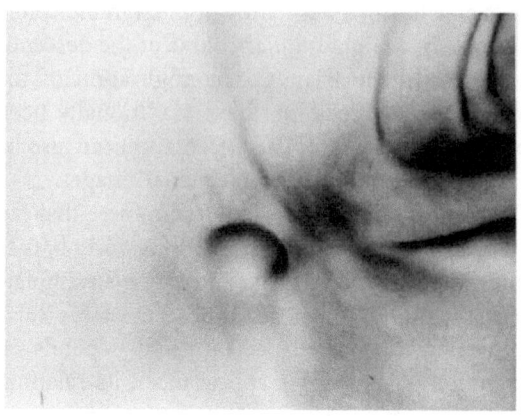

Fig. 6.4. Endoluminal 3D view of 3 mm polyp in transverse colon

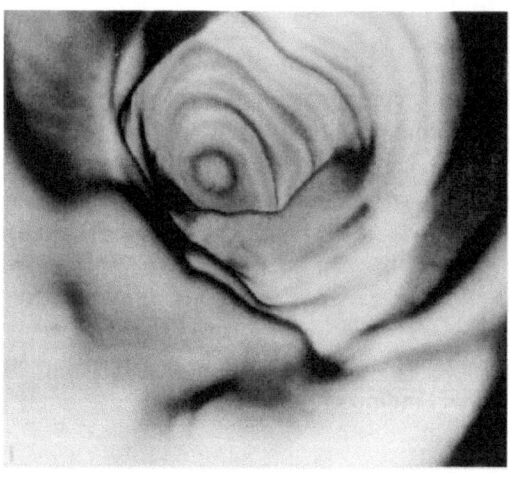

Fig. 6.5. Endoluminal 3D view of a polypoid carcinoma in the ascending colon

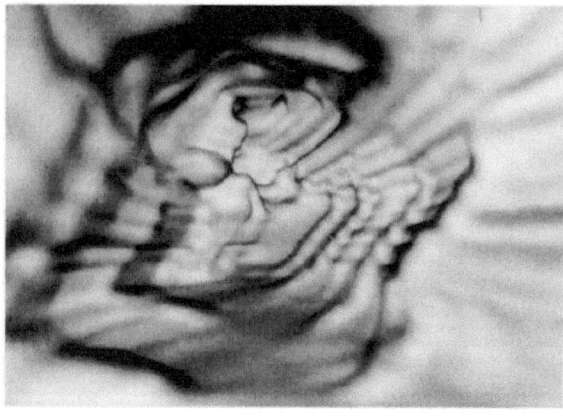

Fig. 6.6. Endoluminal 3D view of an annular carcinoma causing almost complete colonic obstruction. Examination of the proximal bowel in such cases can often be impossible by conventional colonscopy, whereas the passage of sufficient air to enable evaluation by CT colonography can usually be achieved

and fluid. In such cases, the change in position of loose material within the lumen on prone scanning may be the only method of differentiating polyps from such luminal contents. However, pedunculated polyps with a long stalk may be relatively mobile and can be mistaken for stool in this manner (FENLON et al. 1999a). Reports of such incidents emphasise the importance of adequate bowel cleansing or stool labelling.

Specificity is reduced in patients with severe diverticular disease, where segments of narrowed and thick-walled colon may simulate strictures and constricting annular carcinomas (Fig. 6.6). Reliable differentiation between the two may not be possible at CT colonography alone.

6.5
Diagnostic Accuracy of CT Colonography

6.5.1
Diagnostic Performance in High Risk Populations

There have been numerous published series on the performance of CT colonography in moderate to high risk populations. The results of some of the largest of these studies are listed in Table 6.1. Sensitivities for polyps >1 cm range from 70%–100%; for polyps between 6 mm and 9 mm, from 47%–82%; and for polyps <6 mm, 26%–59%. Respective specificities are 90%–96%, 63%–96% and 80%–92% (Table 6.2). Although there have been no direct comparisons

Table 6.1. Sensitivity of CT colonography in published series

Investigators	Patients (n)	Sensitivity (%) per polyp			Sensitivity (%) per patient		
		>10mm	6–9mm	<6mm	>10mm	6–9mm	<6mm
HARA et al. (1997)	70	70	63	26	75	66	42
FENLON et al. (1999a)	100	91	82	55	96	92	N/A
MORRIN et al. (2000b)	200	100	65	33	100	73	57
FLETCHER et al. (2000)	180	75	47	N/A	85	88	N/A
YEE et al. (2001)	300	90	80	59	100	93	82
LAGHI et al. (2002)	165	92	82	50	N/A	N/A	N/A
MACARI et al. (2002)	105	93	70	12	N/A	N/A	N/A

Table 6.2. Per-patient specificity of CT colonography in published series

Investigators	Patients (n)	>10mm	6-9mm	<6mm
HARA et al. (1997)	70	90%	63%	80%
FENLON et al. (1999b)	100	96%	92%	N/A
MORRIN et al. (2000a)	200	90%	96%	92%
FLETCHER et al. (2000)	180	93%	72%	N/A

made between CT colonography and barium enema, the diagnostic accuracy of CT colonography for polyps larger than 5 mm would appear to exceed that of barium enema, and certainly approaches that of conventional colonoscopy. Results are somewhat better on a per-patient basis, reflecting the reliability of the test in identifying those patients who need to proceed to colonoscopy and biopsy.

Causes for false positive and negative exams include technical errors and perceptual errors. Technical errors include poor bowel cleansing, excess residual fluid, under-inflation of the colon and artefacts related to the scanning process itself, such as respiratory mis-registration, motion artefact and the limited resolution capability for discrimination of small lesions. Most of these problems are overcome with careful patient preparation and performance of high-quality exams on multi-detector CT scanners.

Perceptual errors refer to the failure to recognise pathology that can be identified in retrospect, usually due to lesion morphology or location. Such errors can be minimised by adequate interpreter training and by optimal colonic distension, which will increase the conspicuity of lesions in most cases. Adequate distension can be difficult to achieve where there is pronounced bowel wall thickening and spasm, such as in segments of colon affected by diverticulosis, and confident reading of such segments may be limited (FLETCHER et al. 2000).

6.5.2
CT Colonography in Pre-operative Assessment

One of the proven situations in which CT colonography may be the diagnostic test of choice is in the pre-operative assessment of patients with obstructing carcinomas. Synchronous cancers can be present in as many as 9% of such patients, and may influence the surgical plan. Complete colonoscopy in these cases may not be possible due to the obstructing nature of the lesions, and traditionally these patients have undergone either pre-operative barium enema or colonic palpation at the time of surgery. Recent studies have shown how CT colonography is superior to any of these other diagnostic options, successfully evaluating the entire colon in almost all cases and detecting previously unsuspected synchronous adenomas and carcinomas (FENLON et al. 1999b; MACARI et al. 1999; MORRIN et al. 2000b). Other workers have found that enhancement of pre-operative CT colonography scans with IV contrast can also satisfactorily assess extra-colonic structures, enabling complete pre-operative abdominal assessment with a single procedure (NERI et al. 2002).

6.5.3
CT Colonography and Screening

To date, there have been no large published series on the diagnostic performance of CT colonography in an average-risk screening population. For CT colonography to become a viable screening tool, it must be shown to be accurate, safe, acceptable to patients and cost-effective.

Data from the performance of CT colonography in high-risk patients would suggest that it is more accurate than barium enema, with sensitivities and specificities for polyps >1 cm approaching those of conventional colonoscopy. These results need to be validated in average-risk population groups. Although there is some criticism of the technique for its poor detection of small polyps, debate continues as to the clinical relevance of such small polyps. Most polyps smaller than 5 mm are hyperplastic lesions with no neoplastic potential. The risk of malignancy in polyps under 1 cm is only 0.1%, with a probability of malignant transformation within 1 year of less than 5% (CHANTEREAU et al. 1992; WAYE et al. 1998). While it is true that, at the moment, CT colonography cannot reliably exclude the presence of small polyps under 5 mm, its value may lie in its ability to detect larger polyps (larger than 1 cm), correctly identify patients who need to proceed to colonoscopy, and obviate the need for further tests for in patients without symptomatic polyps. It may be neither clinically necessary nor economically justifiable to attempt to identify or remove all smaller polyps. The size of the 'significant polyp' is hotly debated, and it may be that a size of >5 mm will be widely acceptable as a realistic diagnostic target.

SONNENBERG et al. (1999) have calculated that for CT colonography to become a cost-effective screening tool, it must attain patient compliance rates of 15–20% greater, or procedural costs 54% less, than conventional colonoscopy, assuming test sensitivity rates of 80%. Patient compliance is likely to be favourable as this is a non-invasive screening test that can be performed without the use of sedation, allowing a return to work on the same day. Similarly, the popularity of the test will be heavily influenced by the successful development of more convenient and comfortable bowel preparation techniques. As CT colonography becomes more firmly established as the radiological test of choice for examining the colon and competition for development of efficient software escalates, procedural costs will surely fall. In the future, these factors may combine to make CT colonography a competitive screening option.

References

Callstrom MR, Johnson CD, Fletcher JG, Reed JE, Ahlquist DA, Harmsen WS, Tait K, Wilson LA, Corcoran KE (2001) CT colonography without cathartic preparations: feasibility study. Radiology 219:693–699

Chantereau MJ, Faivre J, Boutron MC, Piard F, Arveux P, Bedenne L, Hillon P (1992) Epidemiology, management and prognosis of malignant large bowel polyps within a defined population. Gut 33:259–263

Chen S, Lu DS, Hecht JR, Kadell BM (1999) CT colonography: value of scanning in both the supine and prone positions. AJR Am J Roentgenol 172:595–599

Dachman AH, Kuniyoshi JK, Boyle CM, Samara Y, Hoffmann KR, Rubin DT, Hanan I (1998) CT colonography with three-dimensional problem solving for detection of colonic polyps. AJR Am J Roentgenol 171:989–995

Fenlon HM, Clarke PD, Ferrucci JT (1998) Virtual colonoscopy: imaging features with colonoscopic correlation. AJR Am J Roentgenol 170:1303–1309

Fenlon HM, McAnaeny DB, Nunes DP (1999a) Occlusive colon carcinoma: virtual colonoscopy in the preoperative evaluation of the proximal colon. Radiology 210:423–428

Fenlon HM, Nunes DP, Schroy PC III, Barish MA, Clarke PD, Ferrucci JT (1999b) A comparison of virtual and conventional colonoscopy for the detection of colorectal polyps. N Engl J Med 341:1496–1503

Fletcher JG, Johnson CD, MacCarty RL, Welch TJ, Reed JE, Hara AK (1999) CT colonography: potential pitfalls and problem-solving techniques. AJR Am J Roentgenol 172:1271–1278

Fletcher JG, Johnson CD, Welch TJ, MacCarty RL, Ahlquist DA, Reed JE, Harmsen WS, Wilson LA (2000) Optimization of CT colonography technique: prospective trial in 180 patients. Radiology 216:704–711

Gluecker T, Meuwly J-Y, Pescatore P, Schnyder P, Delarive J, Jornod P, Meuli R, Dorta G (2002) Effect of investigator experience in CT colonography. Eur Radiol 12:1405–1409

Hara AK, Johnson CD, Reed JE, Ehman RL, Ilstrup DM (1996) Colorectal polyp detection with CT colography: two-versus three-dimensional techniques. Radiology 200:49–54

Hara AK, Johnson CD, Reed JE, Ahlquist DA, Nelson H, Ehman RL, Harmsen WS (1997) Reducing data size and radiation dose for CT colonography. AJR Am J Roentgenol 168:1181–1184

Hara AK, Johnson CD, MacCarty RL, Welch TJ (2000) Incidental extracolonic findings at CT colonography. Radiology 215:353–357

Laghi A, Iannaccone R, Carbone I, Catalano C, Di Giulio E, Schillaci A, Passariello R (2002) Detection of colorectal lesions with virtual computed tomographic colonography. Am J Surg 183:124–31

Lefere PP, Gryspeerdt SS, Dewyspelaere JK, Baekelandt MS, van Holsbeeck BG (2002) Dietary fecal tagging as a cleansing method before CT colonography: initial results polyp detection and patient acceptance. Radiology 224:393–403

Macari M, Megibow AJ, Barman P, Milano A, Dicker M (1999) CT colography in patients with failed colonoscopy. AJR Am J Roentgenol 173:561–564

Macari M, Milano A, Lavelle M, Berman P, Megibow AJ (2000) Comparison of time-efficient CT colonography with two- and three-dimensional colonic evaluation for detecting colorectal polyps. AJR Am J Roentgenol 174:1543–1549

Macari M, Bini EJ, Xue X, Milano A, Katz SS, Resnick D, Chandarana H, Krinsky G, Klingenbeck K, Marshall CH, Megibow AJ (2002) Colorectal neoplasms: prospective comparison of thin-section low-dose multi-detector row CT colonography and conventional colonoscopy for detection. Radiology 224:383–392

McFarland EG, Brink JA, Pilgram TK, Heiken JP, Balfe DM, Hirseli DA, Weinstock L, Littenberg B (2001) Spiral CT colonography: reader agreement and diagnostic performance with two- and three-dimensional image display techniques. Radiology 218:375–383

Morrin MM, Farrell RJ, Kruskal JB, Reynolds K, McGee JB,

Raptopoulos V (2000a) Utility of intravenously administered contrast material at CT colonography. Radiology 217:765–771

Morrin MM, Farrell RJ, Raptopoulos V, McGee JB, Bleday R, Kruskal JB (2000b) Role of virtual computed tomographic colonography in patients with colorectal cancers and obstructing colorectal lesions. Dis Colon Rectum 43:303–311

Morrin MM, Farrel RJ, Keogan MT, Kruskal JB, Yam CS, Raptopoulos V (2002) CT colonography: colonic distention improved by dual positioning but not intravenous glucagon. Eur Radiol 12:525–530

Murray JP (1996). Buscopan in diagnostic radiology of the alimentary tract. Br J Radiol 93:102–111

Neri E, Giusti P, Battolla L, Vagli P, Boraschi P, Lencioini R, Caramella D, Bartolozzi C (2002) Colorectal cancer: role of CT colonography in preoperative evaluation after incomplete colonoscopy. Radiology 223:615–619

Paik DS, Beaulieu CF, Jeffrey RB Jr, Karadi CA, Napel S (2000a) Visualization modes for CT colonography using cylindrical and planar map projections. J Comput Assist Tomogr 20:179–188

Paik DS, Beaulieu CF, Jeffrey RB, Yee J, Steinauer-Gebauer AM, Napel S (2000b) Computer-aided detection of polyps in CT colonography: method and free-response ROC evaluation of performance. Presented at the 86th scientific assembly and annual meeting of the RSNA, 2000. Radiology 217:370

Rex DK, Cutler CS, Lemmel GT, Rahmani EY, Clark DW, Helper DJ, Lehman GA, Mark DG (1997) Colonoscopic miss rates of adeonomas determined by back-to-back colonoscopies. Gastroenterology 112:24–28

Rogalla P, Schmidt E, Korvea M, Hamm BK III (1999) Optimal colon distension for virtual colonoscopy: room air versus CO2 insufflation. (Presented at the 86th scientific assembly and annual meeting of the RSNA, 1999.) Radiology 213:341

Royster AP, Fenlon HM, Clarke PD, Nunes DP, Ferrucci JT (1997) CT colonoscopy of colorectal neooplasms: two-dimensional and three-dimensional virtual-reality techniques with colonoscopic correlation. AJR Am J Roentgenol 169:1237–1242

Sonnenberg A, Delco F, Bauerfeind P (1999) Is virtual colonoscopy a cost-effective option to screen for colorectal cancer? Am J Gastroenterol 94:2268–2274

Vining DJ, Gelfand DW (1994) Noninvasive colonoscopy using helical CT scanning, 3D reconstruction, and virtual reality. Paper presented at the annual meeting of the Society of Gastrointestinal Radiologists. 13–18 Febr 1994, Maui, HI

Waye JD, Lewis BS, Frankel A, Geller SA (1998) Small colon polyps. Am J Gastroenterol 83:120–122

Winawer SJ, Fletcher RH, Miller L, Godlee F, Stolar MH, Mulrow CD, Woolf SH, Glick SN, Ganiats TG, Bond JH, Rosen L, Zapka JG, Olsen SJ, Giardiello FM, Sisk JE, van Antwerp R, Brown-Davis C, Marciniak DA, Mayer RJ (1997) Colorectal cancer screening: clinical guidelines and rationale. Gastroenterology 112:594–642

Yee J, Hung RK, Akerar GA, Wall SD (1999) The usefulness of glucagon hydrochloride for colonic distension in CT colonography. AJR Am J Roentgenol 173:169–172

Yee J, Akerbar GA, Hung RK, Steinauer-Gebauer AM, Wall SD, McQuaid KR (2001) Characteristics of CT colonography for the detection of colorectal neoplasia in 300 patients. Radiology 219:685–692

Yoshida H, Masutani Y, MacEneaney P, Rubin DT, Dachman AH (2002) Computerized detection of colonic polyps at CT colonography on the basis of volumetric features: pilot study. Radiology 222:327–336

Zalis ME, Hahn PF (2001) Digital subtraction bowel cleansing in CT colonography. AJR Am J Roentgenol 176:646–648

7 Dietary Faecal Tagging

Philippe Lefere and Stefan Gryspeerdt

CONTENTS

7.1 Definition 71
7.2 History 71
7.3 Background 71
7.3.1 Conventional Colonoscopy and Barium Enema 71
7.3.2 CT Colonography 72
7.3.2.1 Fluid Residue 72
7.3.2.2 Faecal Residue 73
7.3.2.3 The Solution 73
7.4 Techniques 74
7.4.1 Faecal Tagging with Cathartic Colon Cleansing 74
7.4.1.1 Faecal Tagging with Barium 74
7.4.1.2 Faecal Tagging with Iodinated Contrast Media 75
7.4.2 Faecal Tagging without Cathartic Colon Cleansing 75
7.4.2.1 Without Stool Subtraction 75
7.4.2.2 With Stool Subtraction 76
7.5. Imaging Features 76
7.5.1 Residual Stool 77
7.5.2 Residual Fluid 77
7.6 Conclusion 77
References 78

7.1
Definition

In Webster's dictionary the verb "to tag" is defined as: to fasten a label of paper, plastic, metal etc. to something to show information about it or for its identification. In the same way in dietary faecal tagging, the faecal residue is labelled with a contrast agent so as to be recognised. "Dietary" refers to the manner of administration of the contrast agent: it is ingested with meals, during the preparation for CT colonography. The technique is based on the ability of an orally administered contrast agent to mix with colonic contents. As faecal residue can consist of both residual fluid and stool, the contrast agent has to label both components. Stool tagging refers to the ability to impregnate or label residual stool with the contrast agent (Fig. 7.1). Fluid tagging refers to the ability to increase the attenuation of residual fluid (Fig. 7.2) (FLETCHER 2002).

P. LEFERE, MD; S. GRYSPEERDT, MD
Stedelijk Ziekenhuis, Bruggesteenweg 90, B-8800 Roeselare, Belgium

7.2
History

The first experience of impregnating stool in the colon with barium goes back to the seventies. MILLER (1977) suggested performing the upper GI series prior to the barium enema when both examinations were requested. This allowed residual stool in the colon to be easily identified because of admixed barium. This idea was further developed by SHORT (1980) who administered a tracer dose of barium orally, at the start of the barium enema preparation, in order for the barium to mix with residual stool in the colon. The advantages of labelling residual stool prior to a barium enema were that colon cleansing was easily assessed, reducing the need for additional cleansing enemas immediately before the examination, and it was possible to differentiate residual stool from polypoid lesions. Ease of recognition of residual stool was confirmed by POCHACZEVSKY (1987, 2002).

7.3
Background

7.3.1
Conventional Colonoscopy and Barium Enema

A full structural examination of the colon involves intensive cathartic cleansing, as both conventional colonoscopy and double contrast barium enema need an entirely clean colon for the best diagnostic results (REEDERS and ROSENBUSCH 1994). However, a taxing bowel preparation threatens patient compliance and is a significant burden for asymptomatic patients requiring colon cancer screening (MORRIN 1999). Clinical research using different cathartic agents has been performed to decide on the best compromise between patient compliance and a clean colon. This research has never reached a consensus as to how best to prepare the colon and so methods frequently differ from hospital to hospital (FORDHAM 1979).

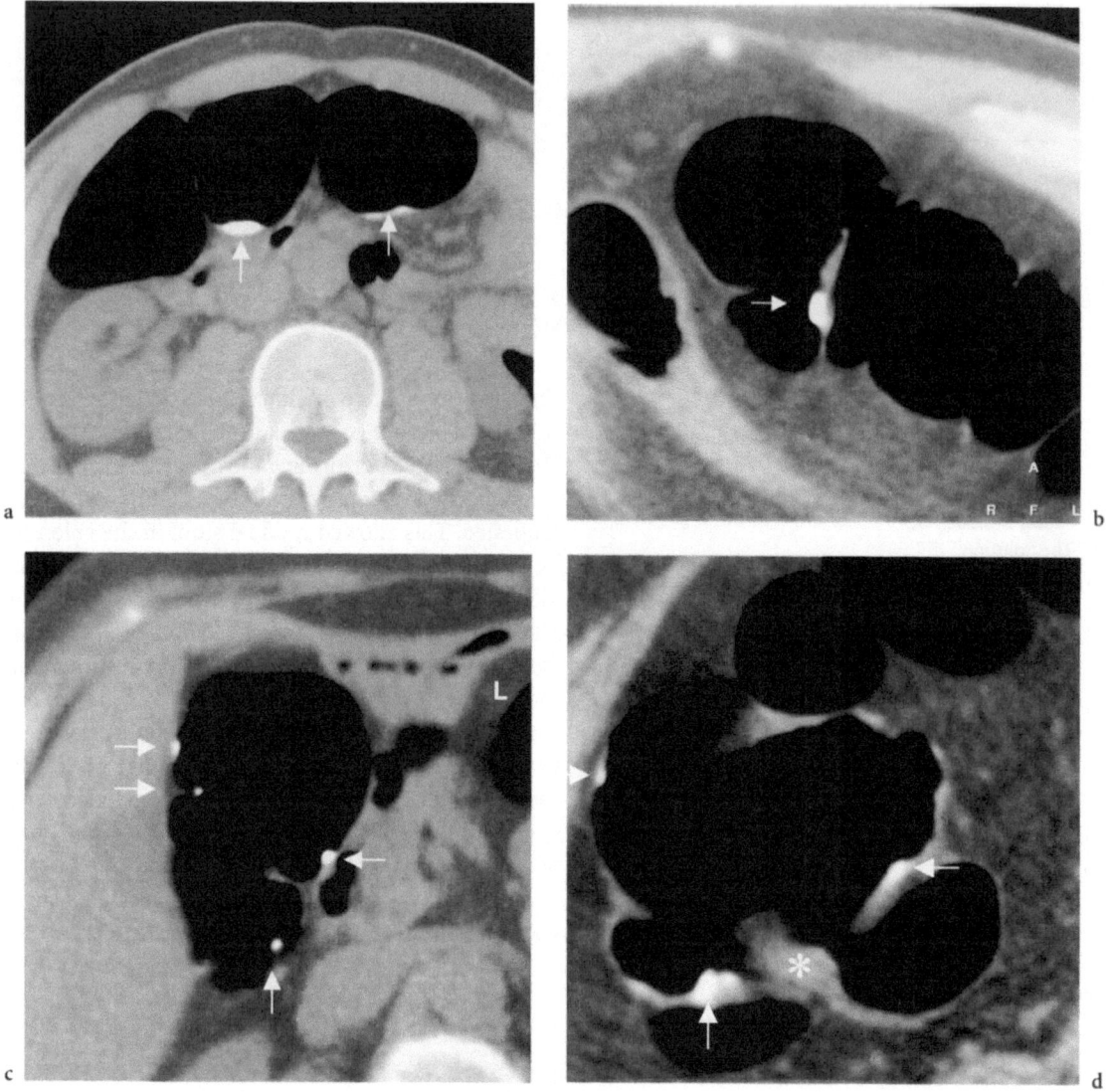

Fig. 7.1a-d. Tagged residual stool (*white arrows*) at different locations (**a,b** transverse colon; **c**, ascending colon; **d**, caecum). The tagged residual stool is easily differentiated from a polypoid lesion. *Asterisk* in (**d**), ileocecal valve

7.3.2
CT Colonography

CT colonography is a more comfortable and less invasive examination than conventional colonoscopy and double contrast barium enema but still requires a clean colon to ensure diagnostic accuracy (VINING 1996; FENLON and FERRUCCI 1997). Even after cathartic cleansing and dietary privation there is frequently residual stool and fluid in the colon leaving the radiologist with diagnosic difficulties (JOHNSON and DACHMAN 2000). In view of this, intensive bowel preparation based on cathartic colon cleansing is felt to be essential for CT colonography (FERRUCCI 2001;

BRUZZI et al. 2001; LUBOLDT et al. 2002) and this is a critical issue that needs to be solved if this technique is to further develop (JOHNSON 2002).

7.3.2.1
Fluid Residue

Although not compromising sensitivity (FLETCHER et al. 2000), residual fluid produces drowned segments and this is a particular problem associated with the use of polyethylene glycol for colon cleansing. Changing the distribution of fluid within the colon by prone-supine scanning (dual scanning) can overcome this problem (FLETCHER 2002) or the

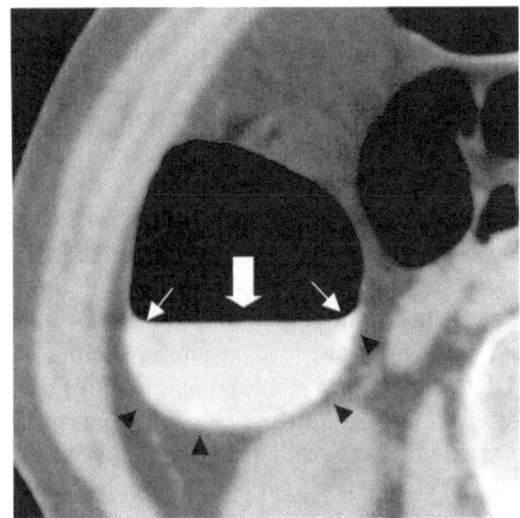

Fig. 7.2. A fluid level homogeneously tagged with barium in the ascending colon (*large white arrow*). A meniscus (*small white arrows*) is seen at its junction with the colonic wall. Small marginal white densities in the fluid (*black arrowheads*) result from tagged stool

problem of the "wet prep" can be avoided by replacing polyethylene glycol by phosphosoda or magnesium citrate (MACARI et al. 2001).

7.3.2.2
Faecal Residue

Faecal residue sometimes mimics tumour and so can result in a false positive diagnosis (MACARI and MEGIBOW 2001; FENLON 2002). This problem can also be overcome by dual scanning (FLETCHER et al. 2000; FENLON 2002) which although increasing interpretation time does allow residual stool to be recognised as it moves to remain in a dependent position. Residual stool can also be recognised if it presents as a round lesion without clear attachment to the colon wall or if it shows the presence of air inclusions (FLETCHER et al. 1999). However these characteristics are inconstant and diagnostic problems can arise as stool can stick to the colon wall and so by not changing position can mimic a polyp, or a polyp with a long stalk can mimic faecal residue if it is seen to change position with dual scanning.

7.3.2.3
The Solution

False positive and negative findings caused by residual stool and fluid have been reported in all major studies (FENLON et al. 1999) and faecal tagging or labelling has been conceived to overcome the problem. An orally administered contrast agent impregnates residual stool (stool tagging) (Fig. 7.1) and mixes with fluid (fluid tagging) (Fig. 7.2). Only a small amount of contrast agent is needed to mix with stool to produce a hyperdense lesion on CT and in the presence of labelled residual fluid, a tumoral lesion can be recognised as a filling defect (Fig. 7.3).

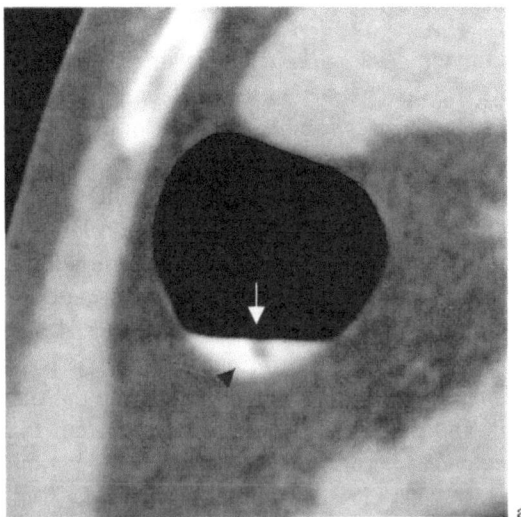

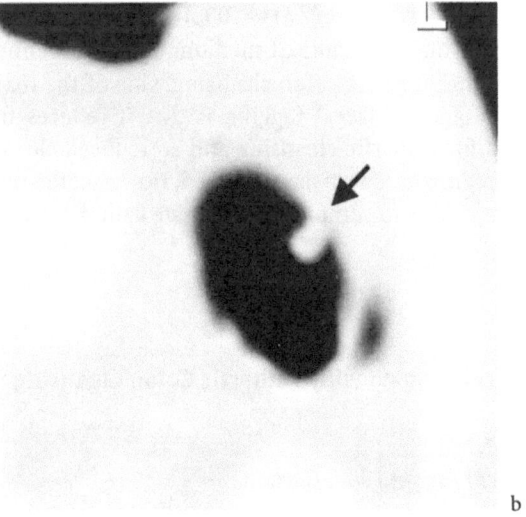

Fig. 7.3a,b. **a** Prone view of a small fluid level with a rounded filling defect in the descending colon (*white arrow*). Some denser material is adjacent to it (*black arrowhead*). There was uncertainty as to whether this represented non-tagged stool or a polyp. **b** The supine view of the same colonic segment shows that the lesion (*black arrow*) has not moved with gravity. The presence of a polyp was confirmed at conventional colonoscopy

Because of this ability to recognise stool and fluid in the colon, it should be possible to diminish the intensity of the colon cleansing regime (McFarland and Brink 1999; Fletcher and Johnson 2000) and still achieve the same diagnostic accuracy.

To summarise, faecal tagging has two purposes, to diminish false positive and false negative findings and to reduce the patient preparation and so improve patient compliance.

7.4
Techniques

Barium, iodinated contrast media, or a combination of the two, have all been used for faecal tagging but so far no study has compared the use of these different faecal tagging agents. Barium offers the advantage of being cheap and inert, so there is minimal bowel absorption. The taste of both barium and iodinated contrast agents can be improved by the addition of flavours. Adverse reactions have been described with both, but are exceptional (Jobling et al. 1999; Skucas 2000). The high osmolality of ionic water-soluble contrast agents attracts water into the small bowel and can occasionally cause dehydration, diarrhoea and hyperperistalsis with abdominal cramps (Skucas 2000). It is for this reason that the use of the more expensive non-ionic water-soluble agents has been advocated (Zalis 2002).

The intake of contrast medium can be combined with the cathartic colon cleansing. One of the main advantages of faecal tagging is that it reduces the need for cathartic cleansing and so reduced cleansing regimens have been proposed. However, the ultimate goal is to completely eliminate cathartic bowel preparation.

7.4.1
Faecal Tagging with Cathartic Colon Cleansing

7.4.1.1
Faecal Tagging with Barium

The use of barium as the sole faecal tagging agent in combination with a milder colon cleansing regime has been described (Lefere et al. 2002b). Two groups of 50 patients undergoing CT colonography were compared. The first group was prepared with a combination of a classic low residue diet combined with polyethylene glycol and bisacodyl as cathartic

agents the day prior to CT colonography, but with no faecal tagging. The second group was prepared using a nutritional kit providing a low residue diet consisting of meals and beverages for breakfast, lunch and dinner the day prior to the examination, and with each meal 250 ml of 2.1% barium suspension was taken for faecal tagging. Cathartic cleansing was performed with magnesium citrate and bisacodyl.

Conventional colonoscopy was performed and both patient groups were interviewed to determine the convenience of the preparation.

Both groups had nearly identical sensitivities for polyp detection (88% faecal tagging; 85% polyethylene glycol) equalling those of previous reports using polyethylene glycol as a cathartic agent (Fenlon et al. 1999; Yee et al. 2001). The specificity for polyp detection at CT colonography improved in the group with faecal tagging as compared to polyethylene group (88% v 77%) and there was less discomfort and sleep disturbance in the faecal tagged group.

Magnesium citrate produced a less intense cleansing of the colon and so there was more faecal residue than in the patients prepared with polyethylene glycol (Regev et al. 1998; Frommer 1997). However, this problem was overcome as stool labelled with barium was hyperdense on CT. Improved detection of residual stool improved specificity without influencing sensitivity. The reduced intensity of the bowel cleansing reduced patient discomfort and yet accuracy of diagnosis was improved.

In the same study the efficacy of the faecal tagging with barium was evaluated. All faecal residue ≥ 6 mm, except for one residue measuring 13 mm, was sufficiently tagged to be recognised as stool. For stool ≤ 5 mm there was a visual labelling score ranging between 77% and 87% depending on the colonic segment. In a review of 100 patients undergoing the same preparation with faecal tagging, the efficacy of tagging both fluid and residual stool was evaluated. Of a total of 600 colonic segments, five showed non-tagged stool ranging between 6 and 9 mm and two showed non-tagged stool ≥ 1 cm. The tagging of the residual fluid was less efficient with non-tagged fluid in 25% of the segments containing residual fluid (Lefere et al. 2002a).

7.4.1.2
Faecal Tagging with Iodinated Contrast Media

Iodinated contrast agents, given shortly before CT colonography, have been used to tag residual fluid. The aim is to uniformly and densely opacify colonic contents, especially in the caecum (Fletcher et al. 2000).

VINING (1998) combined iodinated contrast medium with oral sodium phosphate lavage for fluid tagging in 35 patients. A small amount of contrast medium was administered 1-2 h prior to the examination. They concluded that this method improved sensitivity and specificity for the detection of lesions ≥5 mm.

FLETCHER et al. (2000) failed to confirm an improvement in sensitivity when using an iodinated contrast medium to tag residual fluid. They combined polyethylene glycol with 120 ml of ionic contrast medium the night before CT colonography in 89 patients.

However, in a more recent and larger study involving 250 patients, VINING et al. (2001) were able to confirm their preliminary promising results. None of these reports provided any data on the efficacy of residual stool tagging.

7.4.2
Faecal Tagging without Cathartic Colon Cleansing

The ultimate goal of faecal tagging is to eliminate cathartic cleansing and provide a screening test for colorectal cancer that is minimally invasive and so acceptable to patients (WINAWER et al. 1995; REX 2000; BAUERFEIND 2001; HAWES 2002).

There are two techniques for faecal tagging of the unprepared colon. The first, without stool subtraction (CALLSTROM et al. 2001; LEFERE et al. 2002a), involves minimal software manipulation and so can be performed on any workstation, but does not allow 3D images to be adequately read if the colon is covered with faecal residue. The second (ZALIS and HAHN 2001) involves stool subtraction. Residual stool and fluid are removed electronically by means of software manipulation. This technique offers 3D imaging which is generally accepted as being an essential problem-solving requirement for the interpretation of CT colonography (DACHMAN et al. 1998).

7.4.2.1
Without Stool Subtraction

7.4.2.1.1
A Combination of Barium and Iodinated Contrast

CALLSTROM et al. (2001) performed CT colonography without cathartic cleansing using a combination of several doses of barium with and without the addition of a final dose of ionic iodinated contrast medium. They tried several regimes spread over 1 or 2 days. They obtained the best results by administering 6 doses of 225 ml of a 1.2% barium suspension over 2 days and a single dose of 225 ml dilute diatrizoate meglumine and diatrizoate sodium 30 min before CT colonography. To assess the efficacy of tagging and to recognise stool, they electronically labelled colonic contents having a density ≥150 H.U. The studies were interpreted by two reviewers and resulted in an 80%-100% detection rate for polyps ≥1 cm; comparable to results obtained with a fully cleansed colon (Fig. 7.4).

7.4.2.1.2
Barium

Using a low residue diet, a hydration regime and barium as the sole faecal tagging agent, we performed CT colonography without cathartic colon cleansing. The hydration regime, allowing a maximum fluid

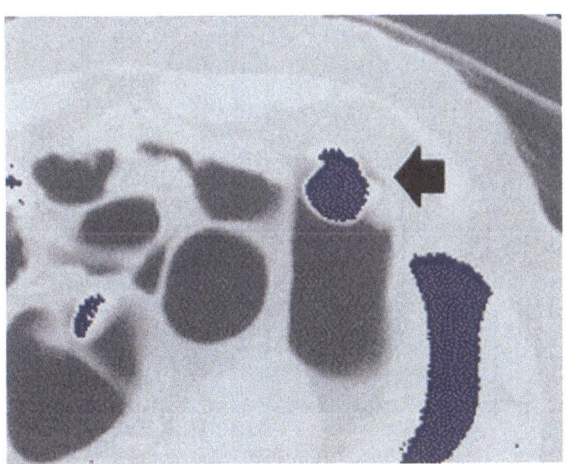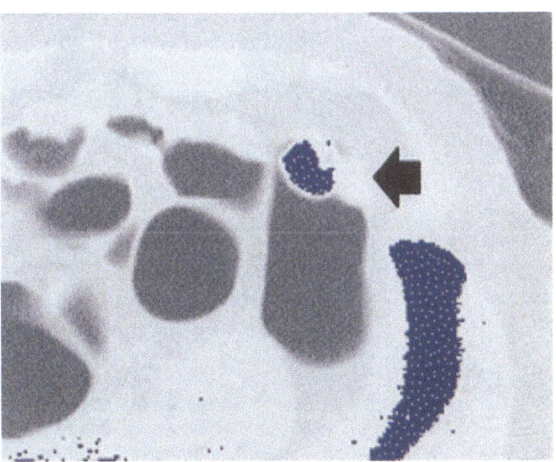

Fig. 7.4a,b. Two images (a,b) at the level of the junction of the descending and sigmoid colon. The stool is electronically labelled. A polyp approximately 1 cm in diameter is identified (*black arrow*). (Courtesy of Drs C.D. Johnson and M.R. Callstrom)

intake of 2 l the day before, was conceived to obtain a balance between the fluid ingested and absorbed in the human body. This resulted in a dry colon with efficient, dense and homogeneous stool labelling. We didn't however look into the accuracy of polyp detection (LEFERE et al. 2002a).

7.4.2.2
With Stool Subtraction

7.4.2.2.1
A Combination of Barium and Iodinated Contrast

After previous research (WAX et al. 1998; WAX 2000; CHEN et al. 2000) involving combining faecal tagging with cathartic colon cleansing, CHEN et al. (2002) performed electronic cleansing (stool subtraction) in 18 healthy volunteers without cathartic cleansing. They used a combination of barium and hyperosmolar iodinated contrast medium and obtained homogeneous tagging with good electronic cleansing in 71% of cases.

7.4.2.2.2
Barium

SHEPPARD et al. (1999) were the first to report stool subtraction in an animal model with simulated polyps. They used a mixture of barium and peanut butter to mimic tagged stool and achieved an acceptable sensitivity for polyp detection of 94%.

7.4.2.2.3
Low Osmolar Iodinated Contrast

ZALIS and HAHN (2001) were the first to report stool subtraction in humans. They initially used 6-7 doses of 5 ml dilute barium or hyperosmolar ionic contrast over the 48 h prior to CT colonography (barium: 2.1% w/v; iodine: 1/40 dilution of diatrizoate meglumine and diatrizoate sodium). A final large dose of 800 ml of barium or iodine at the same concentration was administered 3 h before the examination. Neither cathartic cleansing, nor diet was used. They succeeded in removing the opacified bowel contents without affecting the surrounding colonic soft tissue structures (Fig. 7.5). In a more recent study they preferred to use low-osmolar iodinated contrast media over 48 hours because of the improved homogeneity of the tagging (ZALIS 2002).

7.5.
Imaging Features

To date in the literature, little attention has been given to the imaging features of tagged residue.

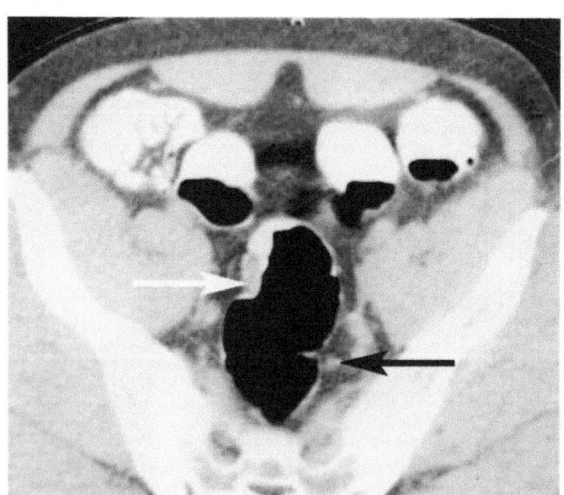 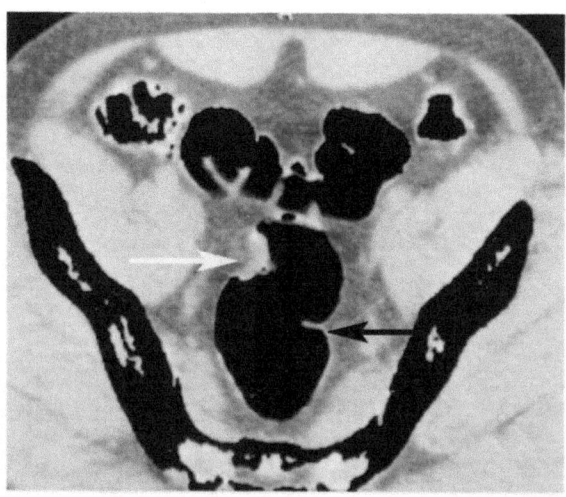

Fig. 7.5a,b. a A 40-year old male with colonoscopy-confirmed rectal mass. Image obtained before digital processing shows a mass partially obscured by opacified bowel contents (*white arrow*). A haustral fold is indicated (*black arrow*). [Courtesy of ZALIS and HAHN (2001), reprinted with permission]. **b** The same image obtained after digital processing. The opacified bowel contents has been subtracted, whereas the mass (*white arrow*) and the fold (*black arrow*) are left unaffected

7.5.1
Residual Stool

In two series of patients prepared with faecal tagging and cathartic cleansing we found that tagged stool had a variety of appearances (LEFERE et al. 2002a). There were wide inter- and intra-patient differences with densities ranging from 50 to 2900 HU. The stool varied in homogeneity so special care has to be taken not to misinterpret a polyp surrounded by tagged stool as non-tagged stool (Fig. 7.6); dual scanning helped in such cases. Residual stool varied in size from large, easy to recognise balls to particulate matter, sometimes too small to appreciate the tagging.

7.5.2
Residual Fluid

In the same study of 100 patients we found varying amounts of fluid to be present in 82 (LEFERE et al. 2002a) (Fig. 7.7). A fluid level with a meniscus where it meets the colon wall may be seen, or a thin layer or film of barium may coat the dependent and non-dependent walls of the colon (Fig. 7.8). Inter- and intra-patient variation in density of the fluid was also noted (Fig. 7.9).

7.6
Conclusion

As yet there is no consensus as to the best method of fluid/faecal tagging and large clinical studies are necessary to confirm the results of the small studies performed so far. Cathartic cleansing, preferably using phosphosoda and bisacodyl is still an essential requirement for CT colonography (FERRUCCI 2001). However, colorectal cancer screening of asymptomatic individuals needs a test that has high patient compliance (JOHNSON 2002), as patient attendance is a problem with the methods of testing that are currently available. A screening test should only interrupt a patient's daily activities for the duration of the examination, be minimally invasive and have a short examination time. Minimal bowel preparation by using faecal tagging shows promise and could become the preparation of choice for CT colonography.

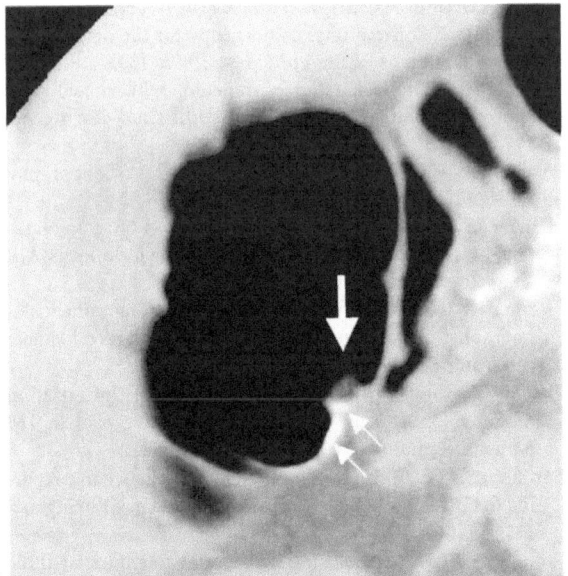
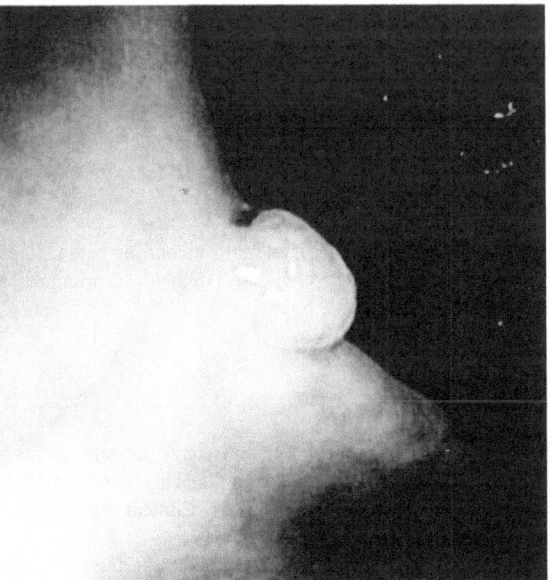

a   b

Fig. 7.6a,b. a A thin barium film (*small white arrows*) surrounds an 8-mm lesion in the ascending colon. Image suggests a polypoid lesion. **b** Conventional colonoscopy confirms the presence of an 8-mm sessile polyp

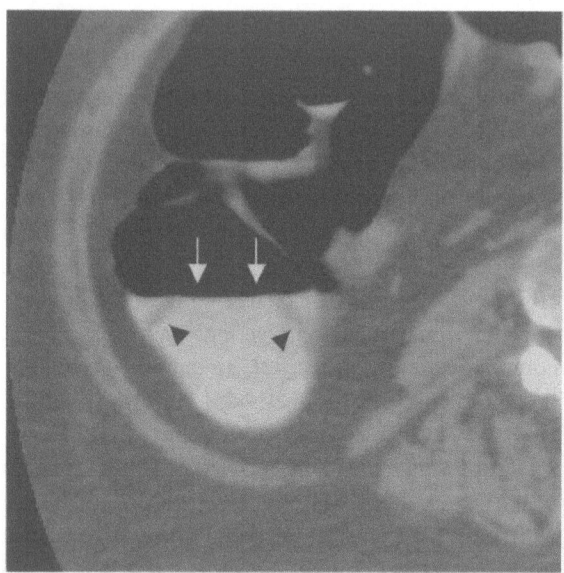

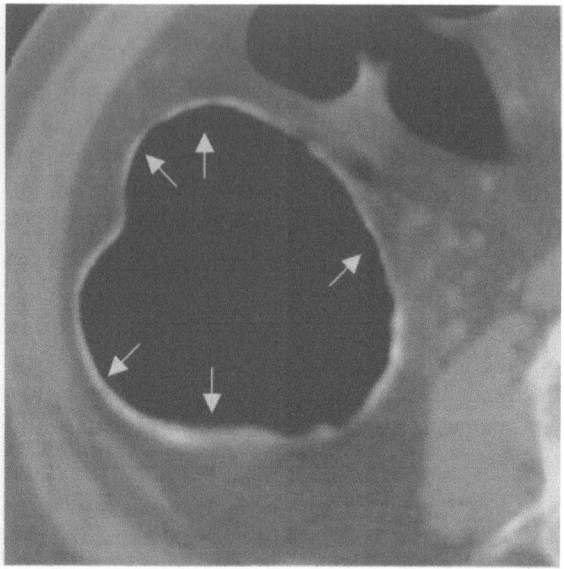

Fig. 7.7. A homogeneously tagged fluid level with barium (*white arrows*), surrounding normal semi-circular folds (*black arrowheads*)

Fig. 7.8. An example of a thin barium film covering the ascending colon on both the dependent and non-dependent side (*white arrows*)

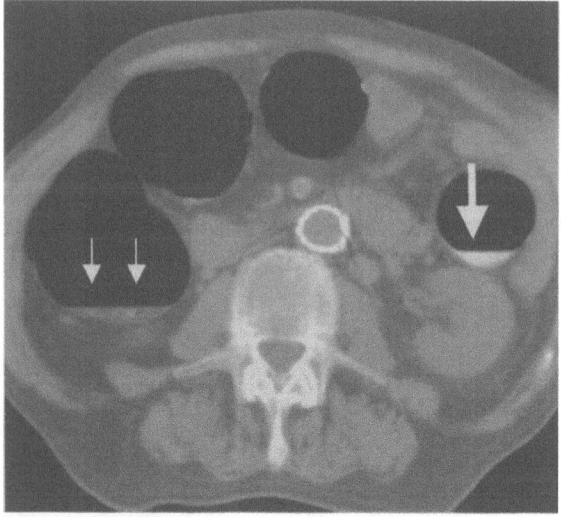

Fig. 7.9. A non-tagged fluid level in the ascending colon (*small white arrows*) and a tagged fluid level in the descending colon (*large white arrow*)

References

Bauerfeind P (2001) Virtual colonoscopy: the endoscopist's point of view. Semin Ultrasound CT MR 22:403–404

Bruzzi JF, Moss AC, Fenlon HM (2001) Clinical results by CT colonoscopy. Eur Radiol 11:2188–2194

Callstrom MR, Johnson CD, Fletcher JG et al (2001) CT colonography without cathartic preparation: feasibility study. Radiology 219:693–698

Chen D, Liang Z, Wax MR et al (2000) A novel approach to extract colon lumen from CT images for virtual colonoscopy. IEEE Trans Med Imaging 19:1220–1226

Chen D, Lakare S, Li L et al (2002) Laxative free virtual colonoscopy: feasibility study. Proceedings of the third international symposium on virtual colonoscopy in Boston, p 138

Dachman AH, Kunyoshi JK, Boyle CM et al (1998) CT colonography with three-dimensional problem solving for detection of colonic polyps. AJR Am J Roentgenol 171:989–995

Fenlon HM (2002) CT colonography: pitfalls and interpretation. Abdom Imaging 27:284–291

Fenlon HM, Ferrucci JT (1997) Virtual colonoscopy: what will the issues be? AJR Am J Roentgenol 169:453–458

Fenlon HM, Nunes DP, Schroy PC et al (1999) A comparison of virtual and conventional colonoscopy for the detection of colorectal polyps. N Engl J Med 341:1496–1503

Ferrucci JT (2001) Colon cancer screening with virtual colonoscopy: promise, polyps, politics. AJR Am J Roentgenol 177:975–988

Fletcher JG (2002) Future directions in CT colonography. Abdom Imaging 27:301–308

Fletcher JG, Johnson CD, MacCarty RL (1999) CT colonography: potential pitfalls and problem-solving techniques. AJR Am J Roentgenol 172:1271–1278

Fletcher JG, Johnson CD (2000) Computed tomographic colonography: current and future status for colorectal cancer screening. Semin Roentgenol 35:385–393

Fletcher JG, Johnson CD, Welch TJ et al (2000) Optimization of CT colonography technique: prospective trial in 180 patients. Radiology 216:704–711

Fordham SD (1979) Increasing patient compliance in preparing for barium enema examination. AJR Am J Roentgenol 133:913–915

Frommer D (1997) Cleansing ability and tolerance of three bowel preparations for colonoscopy. Dis Colon Rectum 40:100–104

Hawes RH (2002) Does virtual colonoscopy have a major role in population-based screening? Gastrointest Endosc Clin North Am 12:85–91

Jobling C, Halligan S, Bartram C (1999) The use of non-ionic water-soluble contrast agents for small bowel follow-through examination. Eur Radiol 9:706–710

Johnson CD (2002) CT colonography: an overview. Abdom Imaging 27:232–234

Johnson CD, Dachman AH (2000) CT colonography: the next colon screening examination? Radiology 216:331–341

Lefere PA, Gryspeerdt SS, van Holsbeeck BG et al (2002a) Prepless colonoscopy. Proceedings of the third international symposium on virtual colonoscopy in Boston, pp 31–37

Lefere PA, Gryspeerdt SS, Dewyspelaere J et al (2002b) Dietary fecal tagging as a cleansing method before CT colonography: initial results – polyp detection and patient compliance. Radiology 224:393–403

Luboldt W, Fletcher JG, Vogl TJ (2002) Colonography: current status, research directions and challenges. Update 2002. Eur Radiol 12:502–524

Macari M, Megibow AJ (2001) Pitfalls of using three-dimensional CT colonography with two-dimensional imaging correlation. AJR Am J Roentgenol 176:137–143

Macari M, Lavelle M, Pedrosa I et al (2001) Effect of different bowel preparations on residual fluid at CT colonography. Radiology 218:274–277

McFarland EG, Brink JA (1999) Helical CT colonography (virtual colonoscopy): the challenge that exists between advancing technology and generalizability. AJR Am J Roentgenol 173:549–559

Miller RE (1977) Order of preference of roentgenographic examinations. JAMA 237:63–64

Morrin M (1999) Virtual colonoscopy: a kinder gentler colorectal cancer screening test. Lancet 354:1048–1049

Pochaczevsky R (1987) The barium enema scout film: cost effectiveness and clinical efficacy. Radiology 162:581–582

Pochaczevsky R (2002) Digital subtraction bowel cleansing in CT colonography. AJR Am J Roentgenol 178:241

Reeders JWAJ, Rosenbusch G (1994) Methods and techniques of the radiologic examination of the colon. In: Reeders JWAJ, Rosenbusch G (eds) Clinical radiology and endoscopy of the colon. Thieme, Stuttgart, pp 24–63

Regev A, Fraser G, Delpre G et al (1998) Comparison of two bowel preparations for colonoscopy: sodium picosulphate with magnesium citrate versus sulphate-free polyethylene glycol lavage solution. Am J Gastroenterol 93:1478–1482

Rex DK (2000) Virtual colonoscopy: time for some tough questions for radiologists and gastroenterologists. Endoscopy 32:260–263

Sheppard DG, Iyer RB, Herron D et al (1999) Subtraction CT colonography: feasibility in an animal model. Clin Radiol 54:126–132

Short WF (1980) Use of a tracer dose of barium for evaluating bowel preparation. Gastrointest Radiol 5:67–68

Skucas J (2000) Contrast media. In: Gore RM, Levine MS (eds) Textbook of gastrointestinal radiology, 2nd edn. Saunders, Philadelphia

Vining DJ (1996) Virtual endoscopy: is it reality? Radiology 200:30–31

Vining DJ (1998) Optimizing bowel preparation. Proceedings of the first symposium on virtual colonoscopy in Boston, pp 79–80

Vining DJ, Pineau B, Black T (2001) Accuracy of virtual colonoscopy using an oral contrast preparation and controlled gas distension. Radiology 221:578

Wax MR (2000) Virtual colonoscopy – CT contrast agents. Proceedings of the second symposium on virtual colonoscopy in Boston, pp 66–69

Wax MR, Liang Z, Chiou R et al (1998) Electronic cleansing for virtual colonoscopy. Proceedings of the first symposium on virtual colonoscopy in Boston, p 94

Winawer SJ, St John DJ, Bond JH et al (1995) Prevention on colorectal cancer. Guidelines based on new data. Bull World Health Organ 73:7–10

Yee J, Akerkar GA, Hung RK et al (2001) Colorectal neoplasia: performance characteristics of CT colonography for detection in 300 patients. Radiology 219:685–692

Zalis ME (2002) Electronic prep. Proceedings of the third symposium on virtual colonoscopy in Boston, pp 38–39

Zalis ME, Hahn PF (2001) Digital subtraction bowel cleansing in CT colonography AJR Am J Roentgenol 176:646–648

8 MR Colonography

Andrea Laghi, Isabella Baeli, Pasquale Paolantonio, Franco Iafrate,
Daniele Marin, Carlo Miglio, Roberto Passariello

CONTENTS

8.1 Introduction *81*
8.2 Technique *81*
8.2.1 Technical Requirements *81*
8.2.2 Bowel Preparation *82*
8.2.3 Colonic Distension *82*
8.2.4 Data Acquisition *83*
8.2.5 Data Elaboration and Viewing *83*
8.3 Clinical Results *84*
8.4 MR versus CT Colonography *85*
8.5 Future Developments *86*
8.6 Conclusion *87*
References *87*

8.1
Introduction

Virtual colonoscopy (VC) is an imaging modality that provides an excellent evaluation of the inner surface of the colon and is based on the acquisition of high spatial resolution three-dimensional data sets extracted either from CT or MR scans.

VC was first used in 1994 as a CT-based imaging modality (Vining 1996), but since 1997 MR colonography has developed as an alternative (Debatin et al. 1997).

VC has unique advantages over existing imaging modalities in that it is quick, non-invasive, acceptable to the patient, provides a full structural colonic examination together with axial images, which also allow the detection of extra-colonic pathology. Moreover, it has the potential to be accurate and reproducible.

VC is indicated when colonoscopy is incomplete (Morrin et al. 1999; Fenlon et al. 1999; Macari et

A. Laghi, MD; I. Baeli, MD; P. Paolantonio, MD;
F. Iafrate, MD; D. Marin, MD; C. Miglio, MD
Department of Radiology, University of Rome "La Sapienza",
Policlinico Umberto I, Viale Regina Elena 324, 00161 Rome,
Italy
R. Passariello, MD
Professor and Director of Department of Radiology, University of Rome "La Sapienza", Policlinico Umberto I, Viale
Regina Elena 324, 00161 Rome, Italy

al. 1999), when it can be performed on the same day, and when no additional bowel preparation is necessary, in order to provide a complete evaluation of the colon and to identify the cause of endoscopic failure (Morrin et al. 1999). In cases of occlusive colorectal carcinoma, virtual endoscopy is able to detect synchronous carcinomas (Morrin et al. 1999; Fenlon et al. 1999) occurring in 4.9% of cases (Arenas et al. 1997). It can also provide a complete staging examination as combining the administration of intravenous contrast medium with axial and endoscopic images delineates the primary pathology and shows how far the disease has extended to adjacent or distant organs (Harvey et al. 1998).

High performance gradient systems together with fast MRI scanning techniques allows the acquisition of complex 3D data sets within a comfortable breathhold. The major advantages of MRI are optimal soft-tissue contrast and the lack of radiation exposure. Compared to CT, this technique is still under development, but promises to improve the accuracy of VC.

8.2
Technique

Five aspects of the technique need to be considered: technical requirements, bowel preparation, colonic distension and data acquisition and elaboration.

8.2.1
Technical Requirements

MR colonography requires a high field strength magnet that can generate powerful gradients and fast sequences and a body, or optimally, a phased array multi-coil. The rather low intrinsic signal to noise (S/N) ratio of 3D gradient echo sequences, requires powerful gradients to implement short TR and TE values. To increase the S/N ratio a phased-array multi-coil is preferred; however, one limitation of this coil is the limited field-of-view with occasional incomplete coverage of the colon in some patients and signal loss in the more cephalic and caudal sections. The sequence used is a T1 weighted 3D spoiled gradient echo, with short TR and TE, so as to reduce acquisition time and susceptibility artefacts. To further reduce acquisition time without a significant decrease in spatial resolution this kind of sequence benefits from a partial Fourier acquisition technique. In this way it is possible to acquire a volume that covers the entire abdomen within 20 s, an acquisition time compatible with a single breath-hold.

8.2.2
Bowel Preparation

For optimal imaging of the bowel lumen the colon should be free of stool and other residues. The requirements for colon cleansing are the same as for CT; it should be simple, safe, acceptable to patients, cause minimal discomfort, reliably empty the colon of all formed faecal matter and most liquid material, and should not lead to electrolyte or fluid imbalance. At present no ideal bowel preparation is available and the choice is between polyethylene glycol solution and sodium phosphate. Polyethylene glycol solution is safe and effective and does not cause electrolyte imbalance, but 4 l of an unpalatable solution needs to be taken and around 20% of patients are unable to complete the preparation program (GOLUB et al. 1995). Sodium phosphate involves the ingestion of a smaller amount of fluid, but is contraindicated in patients with renal or cardiac disease (SCHILLER 2002). More recently, low sodium preparations (SCHILLER 2002) have been developed overcoming the problems of sodium phosphate. However, as sodium phosphate results in less residual fluid it is often the preferred preparation for CT colonography where air or CO_2 are used to distend the colon, but this is less important for MR colonography when a water enema is used for colonic distension.

8.2.3
Colonic Distension

With the patient in a prone position, a disposable enema tube is introduced into the rectum. To minimise peristalsis and alleviate colon spasm, 20 mg of scopolamine butylbromide (Buscopan; Boehringer Ingelheim, Florence, Italy) is injected intramuscularly or intravenously. Subsequently, 2–3 l of a watery solution of 0.5 mol/l gadolinium chelate (1:100) is administered as an enema via the rectal tube, completely filling the colon to the caecum. The rationale for using a water enema spiked with gadolinium chelate is to have a high signal intensity colonic lumen on T1 weighted images (Fig. 8.1). To ensure safe and optimal filling of the colon, with no reflux through the ileocecal valve, the filling process is monitored with a non-section-selective MR sequence (temporal resolution – one image per second) (Fig. 8.2). The minimum effective concentration of gadolinium is used in the enema solution to minimise cost. By exploiting the synergistic effect between iron glycerophosphate and gadolinium, the gadolinium concentration in the contrast enema can be significantly reduced (LUBOLDT et al. 1999), decreasing the cost of the procedure. An alternative to the positive contrast enema usually employed in MR colonography is to use a negative contrast agent, such as water or air to distend the colon (LOMAS et al. 2001; MORRIN et al. 2001; LAUENSTEIN et al. 2002a,b) (Fig. 8.3). Negative contrast has the advantage of better delineating the enhancement of the colonic wall when intravenous contrast is given. Whether water or air should be used for negative contrast depends on the signal characteristics of colorectal masses on T2-weighted images. The bright signal of water on two-dimensional single-shot fast spin echo (HASTE/SSFSE) imaging appears favourable because most carcino-

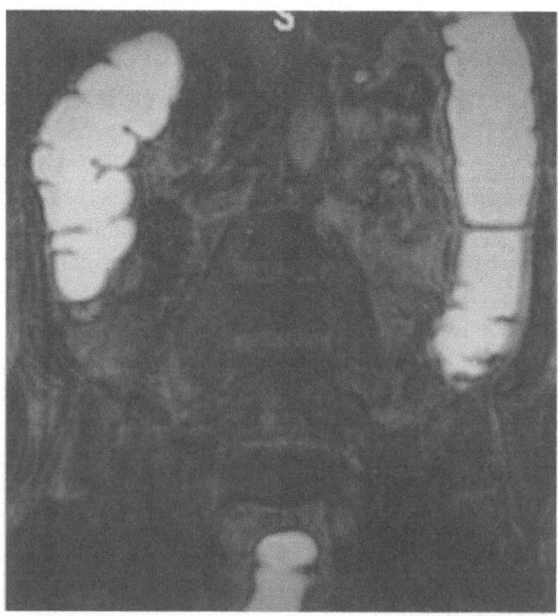

Fig. 8.1. An enema of water and gadolinium providing high signal intensity to the colonic lumen in this single slice of a 3D spoiled gradient echo sequence.

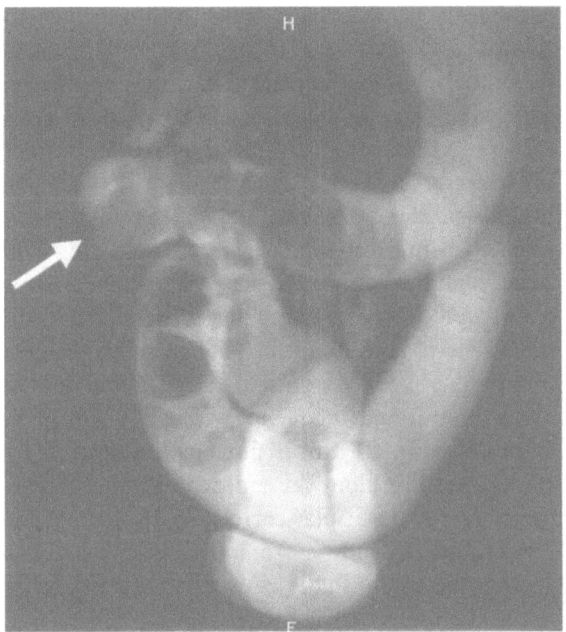

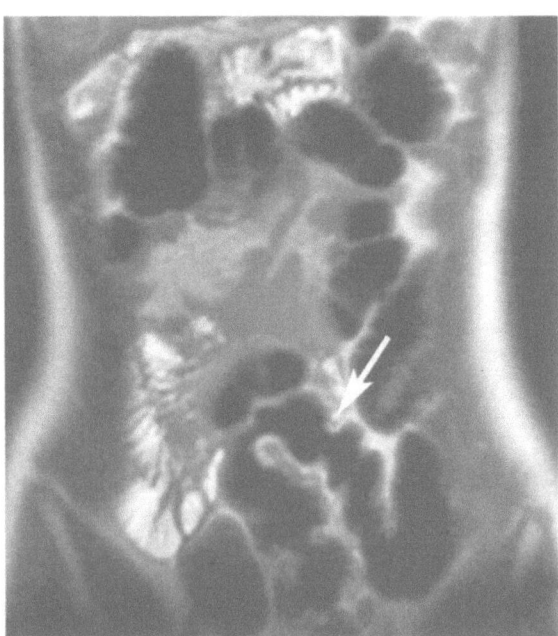

Fig. 8.2. Single-shot non slice selective turbo spin echo sequence used for monitoring the progression of the enema through the colon shows partial filling of the colonic lumen, with the enema reaching the hepatic flexure (*arrow*).

Fig. 8.3. Air-distended colon imaged with a single-shot turbo spin echo sequence. Air provides complete signal void of the visceral lumen, with the wall showing a relatively hyperintense signal; haustral folds (*arrow*) are clearly seen.

mas appear relatively dark on HASTE/SSFSE images and therefore are optimally depicted between the bright signal of the intraluminal water and the pericolonic fat. However, in small sample sized studies, it has been found that most polyps larger than 10 mm show a bright signal on the HASTE/SSFSE images (LAUENSTEIN et al. 2002; LUBOLDT et al. 2000). Thus, the signal characteristics of colorectal masses need to be further investigated to determine which endoluminal signal provides the optimal lumen-to-mass contrast on T2-weighted imaging.

8.2.4
Data Acquisition

Once complete filling and adequate distension of the entire colon is obtained, a 3D spoiled gradient echo (3.8/2.5, 40° flip angle) sequence is acquired with the patient in a prone and then supine position. Each imaging sequence is performed in the coronal plane within a single breath-hold of less than 30 s. The imaging protocol also includes 2D single-shot fast spin echo (SS-FSE or HASTE) (∞/64–90 ms [effective], 150° flip angle) pulse sequence and a contrast-enhanced 2D spoiled gradient echo (177ms/4.1ms, 80° flip angle) sequence to evaluate extra-colonic

findings (i.e. liver metastases, lymphadenopathy). These sequences are also preferably acquired in the coronal plane.

8.2.5
Data Elaboration and Viewing

Once 3D data sets are acquired they are downloaded to a dedicated off-line workstation to generate 3D reconstructions. 3D data sets can be examined using different 2D and 3D reconstruction techniques, starting with multiplanar reformations along three orthogonal axes and oblique planes. 3D reconstructions can be obtained by using either maximum intensity projection (MIP), or surface rendering or volume rendering algorithms. MIP is the easiest, fastest and most widely available reconstruction algorithm providing an overall 2D image of the colon projected in a bi-dimensional plane (Fig. 8.4). MIP post-processing may provide different projections of the colon from the original dataset. Shaded surface display (SSD) generates a 3D image of the colonic surface, mimicking a single contrast barium examination (Fig. 8.5). An adequate threshold value needs to be chosen with SSD and all pixels other than those of this value are automatically removed. Contiguous

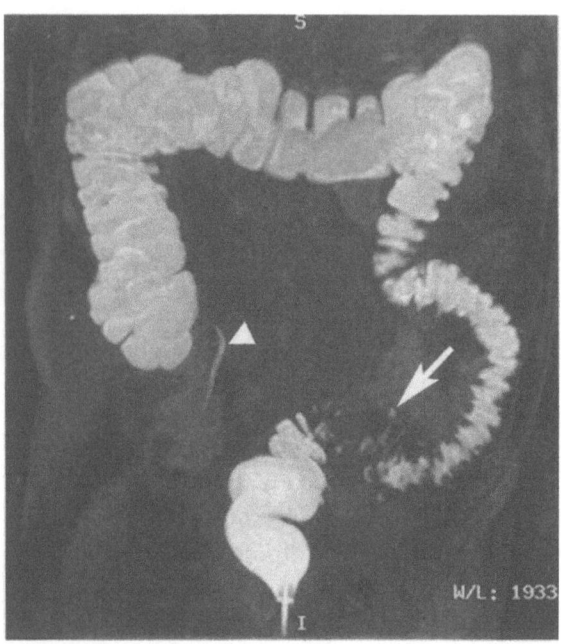

Fig. 8.4. Maximum intensity projection (MIP) reconstruction giving a single contrast depiction of the colon. There is sigmoid diverticulosis (*arrow*) and the appendix is clearly seen (*arrowhead*).

With volume rendering, more flexible management of the 3D data set is possible, with the generation of surface views (similar to surface rendering), 3D models, and tissue transition projection images, which look like a "double contrast" barium study (Fig. 8.6). The major advantage of volume rendering is that the entire data set is preserved, with little or no data segmentation, and tissue is reconstructed using different opacity levels. Using both surface and volume rendering algorithms, virtual endoscopic images resembling conventional endoscopic views are obtained. Colour can be assigned to simulate expected normal tissue colour in vivo and a "fly through" sequence within the lumen can be produced by creating a "flight path" (Fig. 8.7). The camera position along the endoscopic path is defined by an interactive display correlating 2D and 3D data sets in a multi-window format. This helps the virtual endoscopist establish the camera position in relation to the anatomy of the colon.

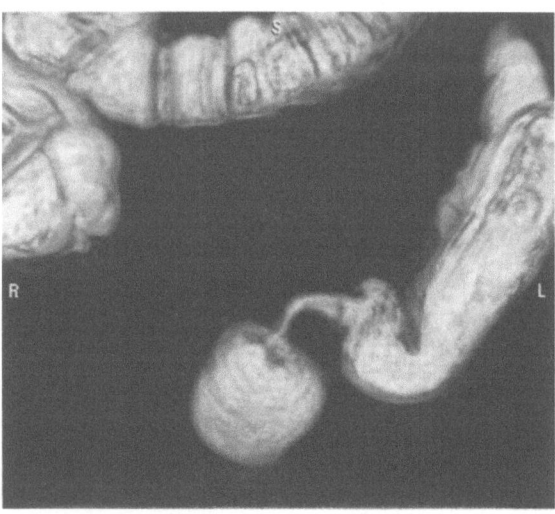

Fig. 8.5. Surface-rendered reconstruction showing a sigmoid carcinoma, with the typical apple-core appearance.

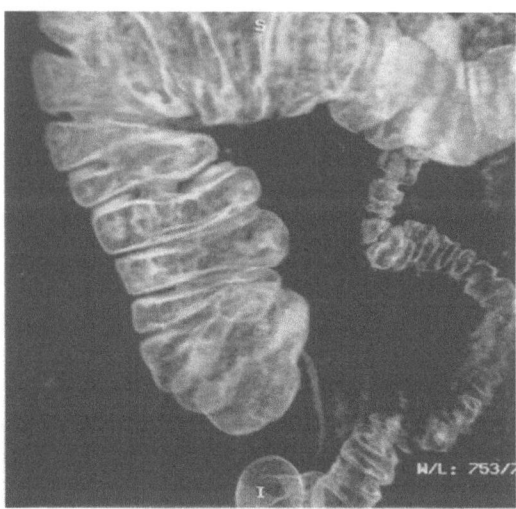

Fig. 8.6. View of the caecum and ascending colon with a virtual "double-contrast" enema effect obtained by using volume-rendering algorithm.

8.3
Clinical Results

pixels at the boundary of the predefined threshold value are modelled as surfaces. In SSD, the first voxel encountered along the projection ray that is above the user-defined threshold is selected as an inner surface of the colonic lumen. Computer-generated imaginary sources of illumination depict surface reflections and are encoded in the image gray scale.

In contrast to CT colonography, there is little data available on the performance of MR for the detection of colorectal lesions.

LUBOLDT et al. (2000) evaluated 132 patients, using conventional colonoscopy as the reference standard. The mean age in the study population was 60 years (±14 years), with a prevalence for mass

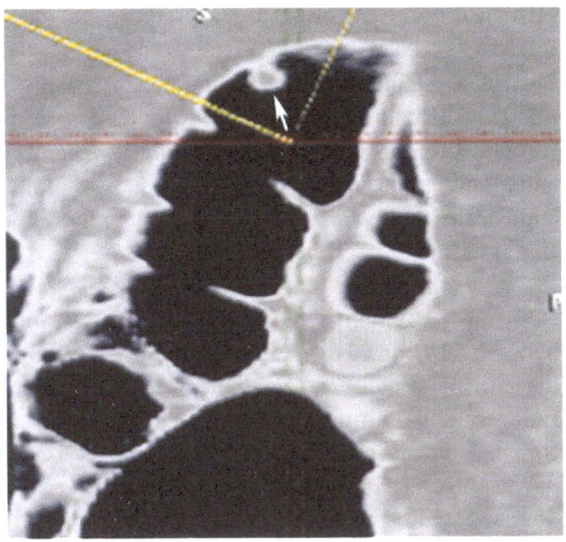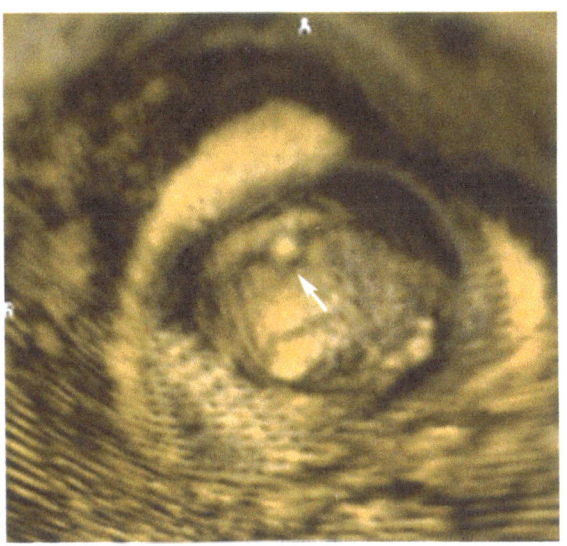

Fig. 8.7a,b. 10 mm polyp at the splenic flexure. **a** Sagittal reconstruction from the 3D dataset, showing the polyp (*arrow*) and the positioning of the virtual camera (field of view defined by yellow lines). **b** Volume-rendered endoluminal view of the same polyp (*arrow*).

lesions larger than 10 mm of 12%. Diagnostic images were obtained in 96% of patients. Most mass lesions smaller than 5 mm in size were not visualised but MR colonography correctly identified 19 of 31 (61%) lesions ranging in size from 6 to 10 mm, and 26 of 27 (96%) lesions exceeding 10 mm in size. In the detection of patients with polyps equal to or larger than 10 mm, MR colonography had a sensitivity of 93%, a specificity of 99%, a positive predictive value of 92% and a negative predictive value of 98%.

PAPPALARDO et al. (2000) evaluated 70 consecutive patients referred for conventional colonoscopy with MR colonography. The detection of colonic endoluminal lesions was compared with that of colonoscopy, and related to histological findings. All lesions exceeding 10 mm in size were correctly identified, the sensitivity was 96% (29 of 30) for lesions between 6 and 9 mm and 33% for lesions smaller than 5 mm.

Overall MR colonography was shown to have a diagnostic accuracy similar to colonoscopy, with a sensitivity of 96%, a specificity of 93%, a positive predictive value of 98% and a negative predictive value of 87.5%.

MEIER and WILDERMUTH (2002) evaluated 23 patients with proven colorectal cancer to establish MR colonography performance in tumour detection and staging. No lesions larger or equal to 8 mm was missed and all 23 carcinomas were detected. In addition one synchronous carcinoma was newly diagnosed, a lesion missed at colonoscopy as a more distal tumour was impassable.

8.4
MR versus CT Colonography

Further debate as to whether CT or MRI is superior for colorectal cancer detection and screening is to be expected (Table 8.1). Advantages of CT over MRI include fewer contraindications, shorter examination time, fewer imaging artefacts and higher voxel resolution. MRI has absolute contraindications, such as the presence of implanted metallic devices (pacemaker, intracranial vascular clips, etc.), and it also requires sedation in patients with severe claustrophobia. When performed without intravenous contrast media, however, CT colonography has virtually no contraindications.

Table 8.1. MR versus CT colonography

	MR	CT
Contraindications claustrophobia	Pace-maker,	None
Ionising radiations	No	Yes
Contrast medium	Gadolinium Air, barium	Air, CO_2
Artefacts	Metals, motion	Metals, motion
Spatial resolution	2.5×1.5×1.2 mm³	0.6×0.6×1(0.8)mm³ (multislice spiral CT)
Examination time	> 30 min	15 min
Extra-colonic findings	Yes	Yes

Shading indicates "advantage"

Compared to CT, MR colonography (MRC) involves a longer examination time. With multislice CT, a single breath-hold of approximately 20 s is necessary to acquire the entire data set, whereas a comprehensive MR study takes up to 10 min as different sequences have to be performed for a complete examination.

The longer examination time of MRC indirectly affects image quality as artefacts from colonic peristalsis increase as the effect of the antiperistaltic drug wears off. The higher voxel resolution inherent to CT results in a better quality endoluminal view. Thus, small polyps are better depicted with CT colonography (CTC), particularly when using narrow collimation with multidetector scanners. However, the impact of the higher spatial resolution on the detection of clinically relevant larger lesions is still unclear.

It is generally accepted that 80%–85% of colorectal cancers have an adenoma as a precursor (WINAWER et al. 1993; TORIBARA and SLEISENGER 1995) and that progression from adenoma to carcinoma takes 10 years or more (EIDE 1991). Thus, removal of adenomas at appropriate intervals constitutes simple and effective cancer prophylaxis.

Histology and size are regarded as criteria for increased risk for malignant transformation. The use of size as a criterion may trigger unnecessary polypectomies. Supporting the use of 10 mm as a cut-off value for colorectal cancer is that most malignant polyps are larger than 20 mm, most polyps (70%) are smaller than 10 mm, and more than 99% of such polyps are benign.

The advantages of MR over CT include lack of ionising radiation, possible better distension of the colon with liquid filling, selective imaging of the colon without superposition of the small bowel, T2-weighted contrast, and the sensitivity to intravenous contrast, when dynamic gradient echo imaging is used.

Air is cheaper than a liquid enema but may require a higher pressure than that required for a liquid enema in order to achieve and maintain colonic distension and so may cause more patient discomfort.

Currently, multislice CT appears to be more suitable for colorectal cancer screening than MR, given the speed of performing the examination, the increased spatial resolution and the robustness of the image quality.

MRC avoids ionising radiation but currently fails to demonstrate the colonic wall in a spatial resolution comparable to that of multislice CT. However, MRC is in its infancy, and has greater contrast potential than CTC.

8.5
Future Developments

MRC is a reliable imaging technique for the identification of colonic polyps and compared to conventional colonoscopy is considerably less painful. Patient acceptance is essential for the success of any large-scale colorectal cancer screening programme (LIEBERMAN 1995).

Today, the major limitation of MRC is bowel cleansing. BAUERFEIND (2001) in a comparative study between MRI and conventional colonoscopy found that the major concern of patients was bowel preparation rather than the pain related to conventional colonoscopy, although it should be remembered that most centres use sedation for colonoscopy. In a randomised trial comparing flexible sigmoidoscopy and colonoscopy, 75% of subjects who underwent colonoscopy complained of symptoms related to the bowel preparation; these ranged from "feeling unwell" to "inability to sleep" (LAUENSTEIN et al. 2002).

Consequently efforts have been directed at avoiding bowel preparation. This is the concept of "faecal tagging", where bowel cleansing can be eliminated if the signal intensity of faecal material is rendered similar to that of the contrast agent used to distend the colon. The principle of faecal tagging is to brightly tag stool, in order to render its signal intensity different from polyps but identical to the high signal enema used to fill and distend the colon (LAUENSTEIN et al. 2002). This effect can be obtained by means of an orally administered paramagnetic contrast agent mixed with regular meals. WEISHAUPT et al. (1999) optimised a technique which involved patients ingesting 10 ml of Gd-chelate (GD-DOTA, Guerbet, France) with meals for 2 days prior the colonic examination, together with lactulose (700 mg/ml) as an osmotic agent to soften stool and 10 mg/ml of Symeticon to reduce residual air. Despite promising results the cost of the technique has to date limited its widespread use in clinical practice.

More recently, LAUENSTEIN et al. (2002a,b) used a different technique rendering the colonic lumen dark by means of a rectal enema of water and stool dark by the oral ingestion of barium sulphate with meals prior to the MR examination (Fig. 8.8). The presence of air, which shows no MR signal, does not impair colonic lumen evaluation since the low signal is comparable to the low intensity of the barium and water enema; this is a further advantage of using barium sulphate as a tagging agent, as there is no need to acquire both prone and supine images. This approach differs from previous methods of "faecal tagging" where the lumen

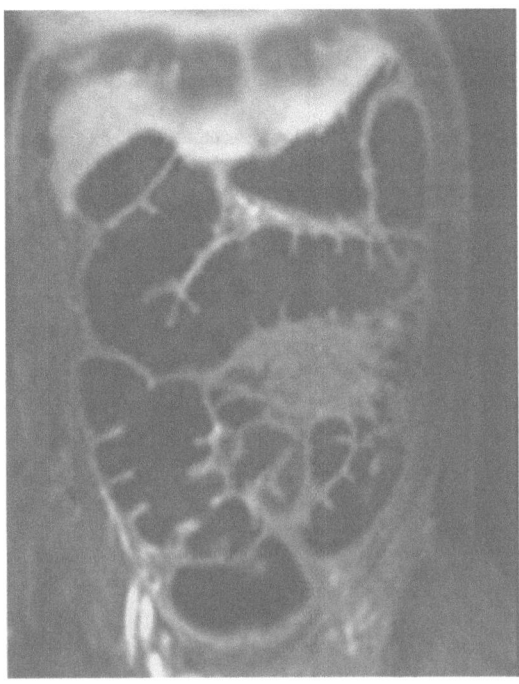

Fig. 8.8. Colonic distension using water enema and barium tagged stools; stools although present within the colon lumen are indistinguishable from the water due to the low signal intensity generated by the barium tagging (From LAUENSTEIN et al. 2002b with permission).

is bright and lesions are identified as filling defects. With barium the identification of the colonic wall as well as polypoid lesions is based on the enhancement following intravenous injection of gadolinium chelate. Further advantages of barium sulphate are its low cost, its palatability when flavoured, and the rarity of anaphylactoid reactions. About 200 ml of barium sulphate are ingested with each meal, starting 36 hours prior to the examination and care is taken to avoid foods rich in fibre and fruits which contain manganese and might shorten T1 relaxation time, thus increasing the signal intensity of stool. Faecal tagging obviates bowel cleansing and therefore should enhance patient acceptance of MRC. Although the feasibility of faecal tagging has been demonstrated, further refinements of the technique in terms of the length of the period of contrast administration are to be expected (CALLSTROM et al. 2001).

8.6
Conclusion

In conclusion, MRC is a reliable imaging technique for the evaluation of colorectal tumours, with an overall accuracy close to 90%. It provides an assessment of both the colon and extra-colonic structures and a future development is faecal tagging which may avoid bowel cleansing prior to the examination.

References

Arenas RB, Fichera A, Mhoon D et al (1997) Incidence and therapeutic implications of synchronous colonic pathology in colorectal adenocarcinoma. Surgery 2:706–709

Bauerfeind P (2001) Virtual colonoscopy: the endoscopist's point of view. Semin Ultrasound CT MR 22:403–404

Callstrom MR, Johnson CD, Fletcher JG et al (2001) CT colonography without cathartic preparation: feasibility study. Radiology 219:693–698

Debatin JF, Schoenenberger AW, Luboldt W et al (1997) In vivo exoscopic and endoscopic MR imaging of the colon. Am J Roentgenol 69:1085–1088

Eide TJ (1991) Natural history of adenomas. World J Surg 15: 3–6

Fenlon HM, McAneny DB, Nunes DP et al (1999) Occlusive colon carcinoma: virtual colonoscopy in the preoperative evaluation of the proximal colon. Radiology 210:423–428

Golub RW, Kerner BA, Wise WE Jr, Meesig DM, Hartmann RF, Khanduja KS, Aguilar PS (1995) Colonoscopic bowel preparations--which one? A blinded, prospective, randomized trial. Dis Colon Rectum 38:594–599

Harvey CJ, Amin Z, Hare CM (1998) Helical CT pneumocolon to assess colonic tumors: radiologic-pathologic correlation. Am J Roentgenol 170:1439–1443

Lauenstein TC Goehde SC, Ruehm SG, Holtmann G, Debatin JF (2002a) MR colonography with barium-based fecal tagging: initial clinical experience. Radiology 223:248–254

Lauenstein TC, Goehde SC, Debatin JF (2002b) Fecal tagging: MR colonography without colonic cleansing. Abdom Imaging 27:410–417

Lieberman DA (1995) Cost-effectiveness model for colon cancer screening. Gastroenterology 109:1781–1790

Lomas DJ, Sood RR, Graves MJ, Miller R, Hall NR, Dixon AK (2001) Colon carcinoma: MR imaging with CO2 enema – pilot study. Radiology 219:558–562

Luboldt W, Frohlich JM, Schneider N, Weishaupt D, Landolt F, Debatin JF (1999) MR Colonography: optimized enema composition. Radiology 212:265–269

Luboldt W, Bauerfeind P, Wildermuth S et al (2000) Colonic masses: detection with MR colonography. Radiology 216: 383–388

Macari M, Berman P, Dicker M (1999) Usefulness of CT colonography in patients with incomplete colonoscopy. Am J Roentgenol 173:561–564

Meier C, Wildermuth S (2002) Feasibility and potential of MR-Colonography for evaluating colorectal cancer. Swiss Surg 8:21–24

Morrin MM, Kruskal JB, Farrell RJ (1999) Endoluminal CT colonography after an incomplete endoscopic colonoscopy. Am J Roentgenol 172:913–918

Morrin MM, Hochman MG, Farrell RJ, Marquesuzaa H, Rosenberg S, Edelman RR (2001) MR colonography using colonic distension with air as the contrast material: work in progress. Am J Roentgenol 176:144–146

Pappalardo G, Polettini E, Frattaroli FM et al (2000) Magnetic resonance colonography versus conventional colonoscopy for the detection of colonic endoluminal lesions. Gastroenterology 119:300–304

Schiller LR (2002) Low-volume oral colonoscopy bowel preparation: sodium phosphate and magnesium citrate. Curr Gastroenterol Rep 4:401–403

Toribara NW, Sleisenger MH (1995) Screening for colorectal cancer. N Engl J Med 332:861–867

Vining DJ (1996) Virtual endoscopy: is it reality? Radiology 200:30–31

Weishaupt D, Patak MA, Froehlich J et al (1999) Faecal tagging to avoid colonic cleansing before MRI colonography. Lancet 354:835–836

Winawer SJ, Zauber AG, Ho MN, et al (1993) Prevention of colorectal cancer by colonoscopic polypectomy. The National Polyp Study Workgroup. N Engl J Med 329: 1977–1816

9 Self-Expanding Metal Colonic Stents

Stephen Halligan

CONTENTS

9.1   Introduction   89
9.2   Self-Expanding Metal Colorectal Stents   90
9.2.1 Patient Selection   90
9.2.2 The Team   91
9.2.3 Deployment Technique   91
9.3   Aftercare and Complications   94
9.4   Literature Review   94
9.5   Conclusion   95
       References   95

9.1
Introduction

The treatment of large bowel obstruction using self-expanding metal stents is now well established and widely disseminated. Stenting may be used either as a 'bridge to surgery' to buy time to prepare those patients in whom curative resection is possible or for definitive palliation in those with incurable disease, thereby avoiding an operation and stoma. Deployment is relatively straightforward and can be accomplished by most radiologists familiar with catheter and guide wire manipulation techniques. This chapter details the rationale for deployment, the stents and techniques used, and a literature review.

Large bowel obstruction is a common surgical emergency and in the developed world the commonest underlying cause is an occluding colorectal cancer. Unfortunately, emergency surgery for malignant large bowel obstruction is particularly badly tolerated by patients; mortality may be as high as 40% as opposed to less than 5% for elective cases (McIntyre et al. 1997). A review of 272 patients presenting as an emergency with colorectal cancer found that they were more likely to have a stoma fashioned, took longer to become fully ambulatory after their operation, and spent longer in hospital when compared to those undergoing elective treatment (Scott et al. 1995).

S. Halligan, MD, MRCP, FRCR
Intestinal Imaging Centre, St. Mark's Hospital, Northwick Park, Watford Road, Harrow, Middlesex HA1 3UJ, London, UK

Furthermore, patients were more likely to die on that admission and had reduced 5-year survival (Scott et al. 1995). The reasons for this are seemingly obvious; tumours that present with obstruction tend to be of a higher stage and only 50% are candidates for a cure. However, whilst this is true, it is not the whole story because stage-for-stage survival is also reduced (Runkel et al. 1991). Instead, morbidity and mortality is increased in this group because of the considerable systemic disturbance that accompanies malignant large bowel obstruction, with the result that their general condition is poor by the time they present to hospital. Emphasising this point, patients presenting acutely have twice the frequency of wound infection, 11 times the frequency of renal failure, and 25 times the rate of respiratory complications compared to patients who are operated on electively (Runkel et al. 1991). It is now well established that poor general condition is the major cause of mortality in patients presenting with malignant large bowel obstruction and outweighs local factors related to the primary tumour.

The site of the primary tumour influences whether it is likely to cause obstruction or not, a feature that is again relatively independent of stage (Aldridge et al. 1986). In all, 70% of obstructing cancers are left sided, which itself adds a degree of surgical uncertainty. Curative surgery for obstructing right-sided tumours is uncontroversial (right hemicolectomy and primary anastomosis) and these patients tend to do well as a group. However, surgery for left-sided obstruction is less clear-cut and a variety of approaches are possible. Some surgeons advocate a three-stage procedure, with initial relieving colostomy followed by resection and then finally closure. However, 40% of these patients never have intestinal continuity restored. Others advocate a two-stage procedure with primary resection and either a Hartman's (i.e. formation of a blind rectal stump) or mucous fistula. A more recent approach is a single stage resection with on-table colonic lavage.

All of this is complicated by the possibility that the disease is incurable. The median survival for patients with disseminated colorectal cancer is only 7 months and surgery should generally be avoided in this group if at all possible so that quality of remaining life is not compromised. However, adequate staging of the disease is frequently not possible when patients present as a surgical emergency and, moreover, no patient should be allowed to die from large bowel obstruction. The result is that many patients who are incurable are unavoidably subjected to major surgery in what will prove to be the last few months of their life.

The Holy Grail of surgery for obstructing colorectal cancer would therefore be a relatively non-invasive procedure that could be applied to left-sided tumours. This would also allow time for the patient's general condition to be stabilised so that the risk of any subsequent curative surgery would equal that of elective procedures for similar stage tumours. Furthermore, such a procedure would also buy time for adequate staging of the disease. If the patient were found to have incurable disease in the interim, then the procedure could potentially offer definitive palliation whilst avoiding the need for a stoma. Self-expanding metal colorectal stents can potentially fulfil these requirements.

9.2
Self-Expanding Metal Colorectal Stents

Self-expanding metal stents are well established in palliation of oesophageal malignancy and the rationale for their use in the colon is clear from the previous discussion; the left colon is potentially accessible to metal stents, which can be placed to relieve obstruction with minimal intrusion, buying time to stabilise and improve the patient's general condition and allowing time for staging of the disease. If the patient is found not to be a candidate for cure, either because of disseminated disease or because of frailty and associated operative risk, the stent can be left in situ for definitive palliation, thus avoiding the need for surgery and possibly also a stoma. It has also become evident that stent deployment is possibly beneficial in some patients suffering from malignant colonic obstruction due to causes other than primary colorectal carcinoma and there may also be a role in benign disease where surgery is not an easy option.

9.2.1
Patient Selection

Firstly, in any scenario where stent placement is being considered, it is important to establish both the diagnosis of obstruction and its underlying cause. Furthermore, for stent deployment to be practicable, obstruction should be confined to a single, well-defined area of colon. Referrals will generally fall into one of two groups; those presenting acutely as an emergency and those with more indolent disease, who are thought likely to obstruct in the very near future. The latter group will usually have a well-established diagnosis and may include those with a known colorectal cancer or alternatively patients with other disseminated malignancies, where colonic obstruction is a clinically evident complication of their underlying disease, for example ovarian carcinoma. In this (or indeed any) scenario it is important that the stenting radiologist directly inspects any accompanying imaging, rather than accept the clinician's story. In the author's experience, the clinical diagnosis of obstruction is frequently unconfirmed on contemporaneous imaging. Also, radiological scrutiny may reveal that obstruction is either at several separate locations or extends over a long length of colon, which may mean deployment is impracticable (or that more than one stent is necessary for colonic decompression). Thorough assessment of the clinical situation will prevent the stenting team being pointlessly assembled (Fig. 9.1). Colonic stenting does not suit everyone with large bowel obstruction and careful patient selection is the key to success, both technical and clinical.

Similarly, patients presenting as acute emergencies will again tend to fall into one of two groups; subjects with an established diagnosis of colorectal cancer (usually awaiting elective surgery scheduled for the near future) and those with no known diagnosis. In the latter case it is again especially important to establish the underlying diagnosis before contemplating a stent. This point cannot be stressed enough. At the very least, the diagnosis of acute large bowel obstruction should be made by abdominal radiographs that have been seen by a radiologist; in the author's experience, junior surgeons and physicians are increasingly unable to make this diagnosis with certainty. If obstruction is present, water-soluble enema is perhaps the easiest way to establish the underlying cause although computed tomography is an increasingly useful alternative, especially when patients are frail or in extremis. Computed tomography also allows distant staging where the underlying cause is a carcinoma. Inevitably, in some cases it will be difficult to establish the cause using imaging alone and in such instances the threshold to employ endoscopy should be low.

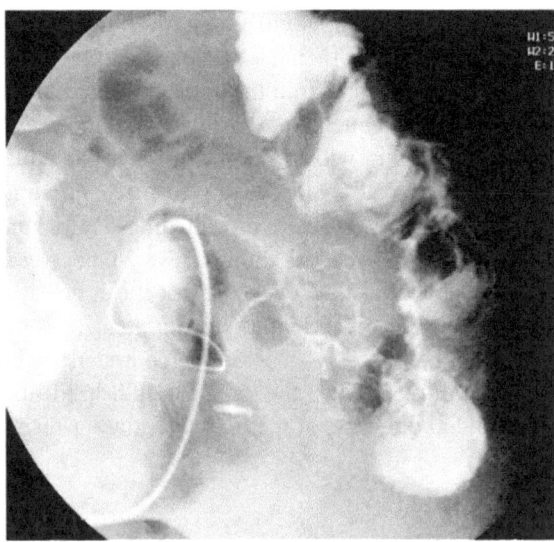

Fig. 9.1. A stricture at the descending-sigmoid junction has been reached by an angiographic catheter and guide-wire. Contrast injection reveals extensive proximal extrinsic disease in this patient with peritoneal metastases. There is not a dominant stricture

9.2.2
The Team

Once the diagnosis of colonic obstruction and its cause have been established, and a stent considered the best option, then the team can be assembled. There are essentially three philosophical approaches to colonic stenting: radiologist alone, endoscopist alone, or a combined procedure. The approach chosen will depend on local circumstances such as staff and room availability (e.g. endoscopy suite or fluoroscopy/interventional room), clinician willingness to develop the procedure, and perceived 'turf-battles'. However, there can be no doubt that the skills possessed by radiologists and endoscopists are complimentary in this scenario so the best approach would seem to be 'combined'. Generally, for obvious reasons, tumour cannulation is easiest under direct vision using an endoscope. This is especially true when the ostium is narrow or when the tumour has bulky, rolled margins. In contrast, endoscopists tend to lack the catheter and guide-wire manipulation skills possessed by trained radiologists. Furthermore, in some instances it is impossible to deploy the stent through the colonoscope (perhaps because fixity due to adjacent disease prevents scope angulation) whereas in others this may be the only option (especially for very proximal colonic tumours). The author prefers a combined approach, which undoubtedly accelerates the procedure.

9.2.3
Deployment Technique

Once the patient has been consented for the procedure, light conscious sedation and analgesia is administered intravenously with appropriate monitoring facilities in place. With the patient in the left-lateral position on a fluoroscopy couch, the endoscope (colonoscope or sigmoidoscope) is introduced to the level of the known occlusion, which is then directly inspected. Occasionally, the endoscope can easily traverse the stricture, in which case the team should reconsider the rationale of placing a stent at that time. The author has found it very helpful to place a small metal mucosal clip at the distal tumour margin because this helps identify this site during subsequent stricture imaging and stent deployment. The tumour ostium can then be cannulated using a thin ERCP type catheter passed through the scope channel and contrast injected to define the stricture length and general morphology. In most circumstances, the author has found stent deployment easiest when performed in isolation rather than through the endoscope. To achieve this when using endoscopic cannulation, the scope must be withdrawn whilst leaving the catheter placed across the stricture, a tricky procedure at the best of times! Ideally, the scope is carefully withdrawn whilst the catheter position is monitored using fluoroscopy. Once the tip of the scope is free of the anus, the catheter can be cut (allowing the endoscope to be completely removed) and a guide wire then inserted through the catheter to cross the stricture. In order to facilitate this manoeuvre, as much catheter as possible should be deployed above the stricture and a short scope (i.e. sigmoidoscope or paediatric colonoscope) used where possible. If catheter dislodgement is likely then an ERCP guidewire or alternative can be passed through the catheter and is usually a little easier to manoeuvre proximal to the occlusion because it is stiffer.

If the exchange cannot be performed then there are two options; either the stent is deployed through the endoscope or deployment is attempted solely using radiology. The approach used will depend on the site and morphology of the stricture but the author would usually attempt radiological cannulation first. The stricture must be reached using a catheter; the author favours a 6.5-F biliary manipulation catheter for recto-sigmoid lesions or a longer angiographic catheter for more proximal occlusions. However, like angiographic practice, the site and type of stricture encountered will usually determine the final catheter configuration chosen. A combination of guide wire probing followed by catheter advance will usually be needed to reach the stricture if this is proximal to the rectosigmoid junction; more distal strictures are easily reached merely by inserting the catheter directly (Fig. 9.2). Contrast should also be used liberally to reveal the bowel lumen and required direction for probing. Gas insufflation is also vital to open out and distend the bowel lumen. Like endoscopic cannulation, changes in patient position may be necessary to achieve catheter advance. For more proximal strictures it is frequently necessary to continually alternate between a hydrophilic wire and a stiffer type since the characteristics of the latter help prevent catheter looping within mobile bowel. If hand movements do not seem to be effectively transmitted to the catheter or wire tip, then it is worth screening distally to look for looping within the lumen or of the bowel loop itself (a frequent cause of failed colonoscopy). Catheter looping within the rectum is a particular problem, especially when trying to reach proximal strictures, and some sort of stiffening device may need to be employed; the author uses a 9-F peel-away sheath, which has the advantage that it can be easily removed when it is time to deploy the stent.

Once the stricture is encountered water-soluble contrast injected down the catheter will help identify the general direction of the tumour ostium, which is

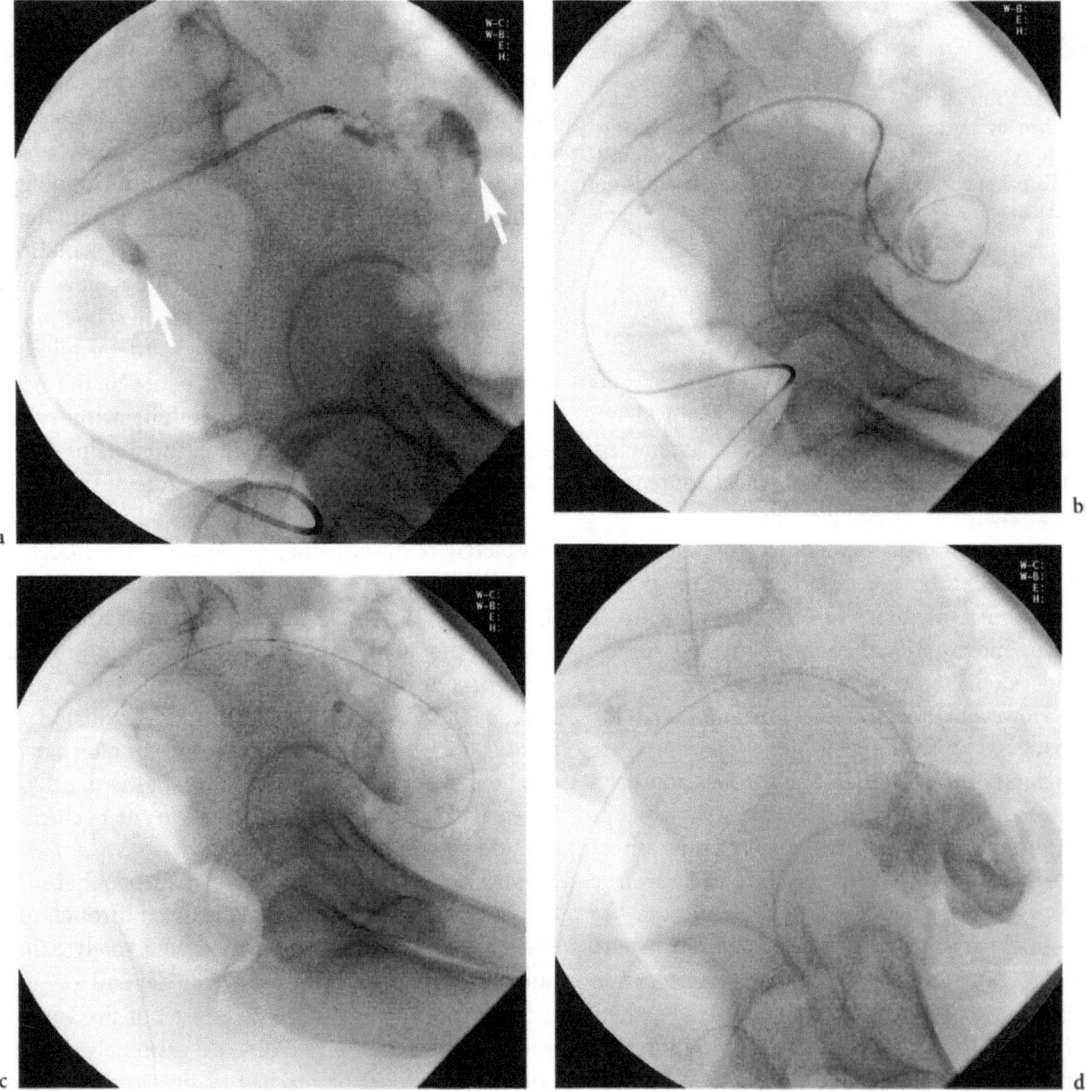

Fig. 9.2a–d. a The distal end of a rectosigmoid tumour has been entered with a biliary manipulation catheter. Water-soluble contrast injection reveals the extent of disease (*between arrows*). **b** The stricture is crossed by the catheter using a combination of probing with a hydrophilic wire and catheter advance. **c** The hydrophilic wire is exchanged for a stiff wire over which the stent can be deployed. **d** The stent is deployed and pulled back into the proximal stricture using gentle manual traction

cannulated using torque to direct the catheter tip in combination with probing using a hydrophilic guide-wire passed through the catheter (Fig. 9.2). Again, patient positional change may be necessary to observe the direction of the ostium and facilitate cannulation. Tumours with shouldered margins and tight ostia may take a considerable time to cannulate but this is usually possible if the catheter can reach the tumour. Once the guide-wire has passed the stricture the catheter is advanced over it, the wire withdrawn, and contrast injected to define stricture length and morphology.

At this time, the type of stent used should be chosen. The author has experience of two types, the Memotherm (Bard) and the Wallstent (Boston Scientific), although the Ultraflex (Boston Scientific) knitted nitinol type is also available, which is polyurethane coated and has a proximal flange (a type extensively used for oesophageal stenting). A variety of lengths and diameters are available. Generally, the most useful is the largest, which is 10 cm×3 cm at the time of writing. The stent is deployed over a stiff guide wire and it may be necessary to pre-form a curve on the stent and delivery system to achieve passage around a tight fixed curve, even with the degree of straightening achieved using a stiff guide-wire. This is especially a problem with the relatively stiff and bulky Memotherm; the key to success is to straighten the colon as much as possible; it may even be necessary to use two guide wires in tandem to achieve this. Most importantly, a short delivery system facilitates tracking the stent over the guide-wire because the guide-wire can exit the distal end of the delivery system and be 'fixed' by the radiologist or assistant. The major benefit of the Memotherm delivery system is its reasonable length. In contrast, although the Wallstent is more flexible and easier to track, its major disadvantage is its excessive length; 225 cm. This stent was originally designed for endoscopic delivery with the result that it is far to long for the guide-wires generally employed in radiology. With a system this long, it is impossible to pass the guide-wire out of the distal end of the delivery system and thus very difficult to track the stent far proximally. However, at the time of writing a shorter delivery system has been designed with radiologists in mind, which will overcome this major disadvantage. The author would generally choose the Memotherm excepting those circumstances where there is a comparatively distal tumour in combination with tracking difficulties, in which case the relative flexibility of the Wallstent is very advantageous and tracking is not likely to be much of a problem. The Wallstent must be used for any deployment through the endoscope.

Depending on the stricture morphology, the aim is to deploy the stent so that there is a good upstream 'flange', the aim of which is to prevent subsequent migration due to peristalsis. Indeed, for localised strictures approximately two-thirds of the stent should be upstream. If a mucosal clip has been placed, then this will facilitate accurate deployment of the distal stent margin relative to the stricture (Fig. 9.3). Balloon dilatation prior to deployment is not recommended because it potentially risks tumour perforation and dissemination. Deployment should be slow and careful. In the author's experience, it is helpful to deploy approximately one-third of the stent relatively upstream of the stricture and then to continue deployment with traction on the delivery system, with the effect that the stent is pulled into the stricture. This manoeuvre helps achieve both a stable position within the stricture and a good upstream flange. Because the aim is to deploy the distal aspect of the stent just beyond the tumour margin, deployment without some degree of traction can result in the stent springing above the stricture altogether. The Memotherm in particular has a tendency to leap upstream if deployment is too rapid and this should be borne in mind. However, the Memotherm does not shorten during deployment and its eventual position is thus probably easier to predict overall. Furthermore, the 'pistol-grip' deployment mechanism is easy and comfortable to use. The Memotherm stent cannot be

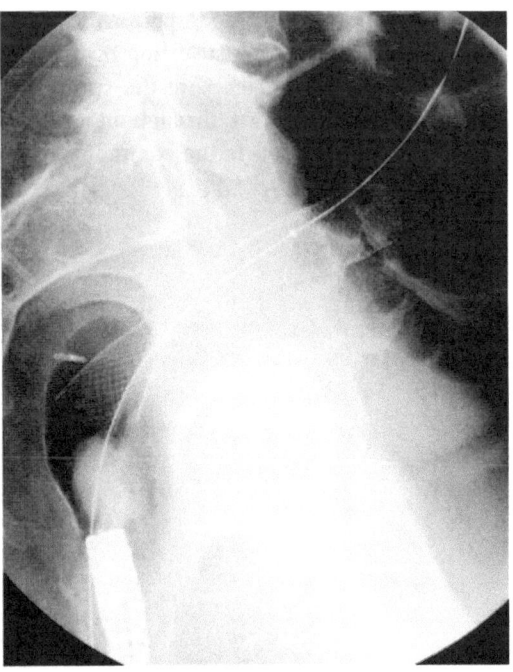

Fig. 9.3. In this case, stent deployment at the rectosigmoid junction is viewed using a colonoscope. Note the mucosal clip placed at the distal tumour margin, to aid positioning

retracted once delivery has commenced whereas it is possible to retract the Wallstent if no more than 50% of the stent has been released. However, the Wallstent delivery system is primitive and relatively difficult to use and the stent also shortens during delivery with the result that its final position can occasionally be difficult to predict. When the stricture length approaches the stent length it should be borne in mind that overlaying two stents may treat long strictures. For rectal tumours it should also be borne in mind that care should be taken so that the distal stent does not impinge on the anus, which can cause very distressing tenesmus. For this reason it is probably best to consider stenting only proximal ampullary tumours.

9.3
Aftercare and Complications

Adequate post procedural pain relief is vital especially since expansion occurs over the first 24 h after deployment. Just because a stent has been placed does not mean that clinical decompression definitely follows and the symptoms and signs of obstruction must still be monitored carefully. Patency can be checked using a water-soluble contrast enema. Stool softeners should be administered to prevent impaction within the stent. Perforation is serious and is related to excessive guide wire manipulation and balloon dilatation. It is sensible to perform a water-soluble enema if there is any suspicion of this and, for earlier detection, to make sure the stricture is well visualised with contrast throughout the procedure (Fig. 9.4). Migration is the commonest later

complication and often occurs within the first 24 h. An abdominal film the day following deployment is useful to check for this, to document stent expansion, and to monitor signs of obstruction (Fig. 9.5). Digital retrieval should be cautious since the stents have sharp ends that can easily puncture a gloved finger. Stent fracture is a reported late complication as is perforation into an adjacent viscus, the bladder for example (MARSHALL et al. 2001). Reobstruction due to tumour ingrowth can also occur and can be potentially treated by a second stent if necessary.

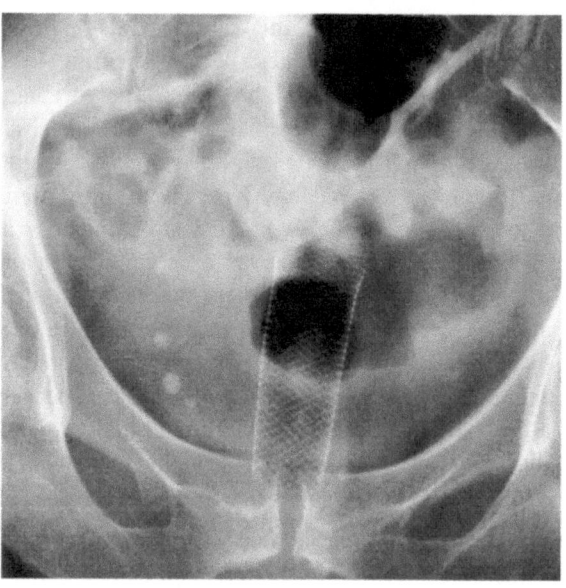

Fig. 9.5. An abdominal film the morning after stent deployment shows rectal migration in this patient

9.4
Literature Review

The first description of deployment of self-expanding metal stent to treat colonic carcinoma was a single case report in 1991 (DOHMOTO 1991). By 2001 there were 40 reports of the procedure in the literature, indicating rapid and widespread acceptance (HARRIS et al. 2001). In addition to the treatment of colonic obstruction due to primary colorectal cancer, there are now articles that focus specifically on palliative series (AVIV et al. 2002), patients with extrinsic malignant disease (MIYAYAMA et al. 2000) (Fig. 9.6), and benign indications (PAUL et al. 2002) (Fig. 9.7). The largest individual series to date comprises 80 patients (CAMUNEZ et al. 2000) but the problems of addressing the literature have largely been resolved

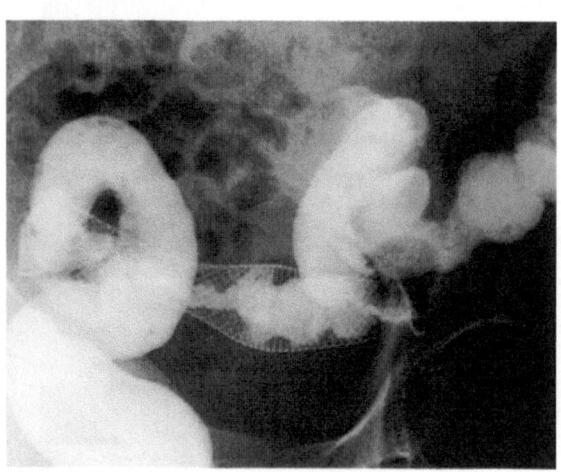

Fig. 9.4. Water soluble enema reveals a patent stent and good position

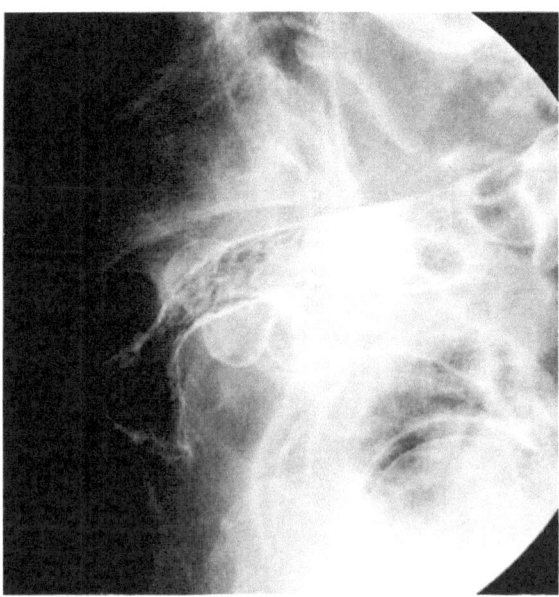

Fig. 9.6. A stent has been placed to palliate recurrent anastomotic rectal carcinoma

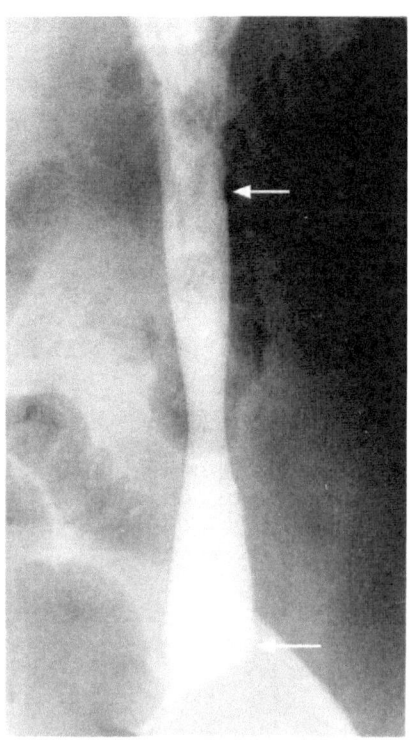

Fig. 9.7. A descending colon stent (*between arrows*) in a young woman with a benign stricture due to Crohn's disease

by a recent systematic review (KHOT et al. 2002). Technical success was achieved in 551 (92%) of 598 patients (90% were palliative procedures and in 85% deployment was as a 'bridge to surgery'). The commonest cause for technical failure was inability to cannulated the tumour ostium with a guide wire. Five percent of patients in whom technical success was achieved failed to clinically decompress. Three of 598 patients died, giving a mortality of 1%, which compares excellently with even the best operative mortality in this group. Fatalities were due to perforation and subsequent laparotomy. Indeed, perforation occurred in 4% of cases (10% of those where a balloon was used to predilate the stricture versus 2% where it was not). Migration occurred in 10% of deployments, half of these within 3 days. Interestingly, many of these required no further intervention.

9.5
Conclusion

Deployment of colorectal self-expanding metal stents is technically feasible and well within the capabilities of many interventional radiologists, especially those familiar with oesophageal procedures. It would seem that morbidity and mortality compare extremely well with surgery for potentially curative cases and there are clear benefits to avoiding surgery in those patients

who need palliation. Furthermore, there are likely to be considerable financial savings as well although no detailed economic analysis has been performed to date on both surgical and stented groups. The results of prospective randomised trials comparing stenting with surgery are awaited with great interest.

References

Aldridge MC, Phillips RK, Hittinger R et al (1986) Influence of tumour site on presentation, management and subsequent outcome in large bowel cancer. Br J Surg 73:663–670

Aviv RI, Shyamalan G, Watkinson A et al (2002) Radiological palliation of malignant colonic obstruction. Clin Radiol 57:347–351

Camunez F, Echen Agusia A, Simo G (2000) Malignant colorectal obstruction treated by means of self-expanding metallic stents: effectiveness before surgery and in palliation. Radiology 216:492–497

Dohmoto M (1991) Endoscopic implantation of rectal stent for palliation of malignant stenosis. Endosc Dig 3:1507–1512

Harris GJ, Senagore AJ, Lavery IC et al (2001) The management of neoplastic colorectal obstruction with colonic endoluminal stenting devices. Am J Surg 181:499–506

Khot UP, Wenk-Lang A, Murali K et al (2002) Systematic review of the efficacy and safety of colorectal stents. Br J Surg 89:1096–1102

Marshall MM, Suzuki N, Halligan S et al (2001) Self-expand-
   able metal stents for benign and malignant colonic
   obstruction. Eur Radiol 11:C14

McIntyre R, Reinbach D, Cuschieri RJ (1997) Emergency abdominal surgery in the elderly. J R Coll Edinb 42:173–178

Miyayama S, Matsui O, Kifune K et al (2000) Malignant colonic
   obstruction due to extrinsic tumour: palliative treatment
   with a self-expanding nitinol stent. AJR 175:1631–1637

Paul L, Pinto I, Gomez H et al (2002) Fernandez-Lobato R,

Moyano E. Metallic stents in the treatment of benign diseases
   of the colon: preliminary experience in 10 cases. Radiology
   223:715–722

Runkel NS, Schlag P, Schwarz V et al (1991) Outcome after
   emergency surgery for cancer of the large intestine. Br J
   Surg 78:183–188

Scott NA, Jeacock J, Kingston RD (1995) Risk factors in
   patients presenting as an emergency with colorectal cancer.
   Br J Surg 82:321

10 Endorectal Ultrasound in Rectal Carcinoma

Michael C. Hill

CONTENTS

10.1   Introduction   97
10.2   Ultrasound Equipment   97
10.3   Technique of Examination   98
10.4   Normal Anatomy of the Rectum   99
10.5   Endorectal Ultrasound Evaluation
        of Rectal Carcinoma   100
10.6   Endorectal Ultrasound Evaluation
        of Recurrent Rectal Carcinoma   105
10.7   Endorectal Ultrasound-Guided Biopsy of Locally
        Metastatic and Recurrent Rectal Carcinoma   106
        References   106

10.1
Introduction

The appropriate treatment of rectal carcinoma requires accurate staging of the initial tumor (KIM and WONG 2000). Small tumors confined to the rectal wall may be amenable to treatment by local transanal excision (TAE) (ORKIN et al. 1995; SENEGORE et al. 1988), which has a lesser morbidity and mortality than a low anterior resection or abdominoperineal resection. In a study of TAE in 334 patients, 236 adenomas, 98 carcinomas, MENTGES et al. (1996) had a complication rate of 5.5% and 8.0%, respectively, and an overall mortality rate of 0.3%. Large tumors and those that have invaded through the wall or into the anal sphincter, with or without local metastatic lymphadenopathy, will require a low anterior resection or abdominoperineal resection. Some cases may require preoperative treatment with chemotherapy and or radiation therapy (BERNINI et al. 1996; KIM and WONG 2000). The patients' overall prognosis is provided by the pathological staging of the postoperative tumor specimen using the Astler–Coller modification of the Dukes' staging system or the TNM system (Table 10.1) (ASTLER and COLLER 1954; SPIESSEL et al. 1982). This pathological staging also deter-

M. C. HILL, MB
Department of Radiology, The George Washington University Hospital, Medical Center, 900 23rd Street, NW, 1st Floor Suite Room 11104, Washington, DC 20037, USA

mines which patients need postoperative treatment with chemotherapy/radiation therapy.

Endorectal ultrasound (ERUS) has proven to be a useful tool in staging certain patients with rectal carcinoma (HAREWOOD and WIERSEMA 2002b; HILL 1999; HERIOT et al. 1999; KIM and WONG 2000). It can detect the presence or absence of local invasion through the rectal wall into the perirectal soft tissues and adjacent lymphadenopathy. In one study it was shown to change the surgical treatment approach in 31% of 80 patients (HAREWOOD et al. 2002).

ERUS cannot evaluate all cancers including those that are: (1) too high in the rectum, (2) large tumors, especially if they are polypoid, and (3) tumors that have ulcerations that trap air. Such tumors should be locally staged using CT or more preferably MRI (BLOMQVIST et al. 1997, 2000; BEETS-TAN et al. 2001, 2002; CHIESURA-CORONA et al. 2001; GUALDI et al. 2000; GAGLIARDI et al. 2002; HADFIELD et al. 1997; KIM et al. 1999, 2000; URBAN et al. 2000; WALLENGREN et al. 2000).

ERUS can also be used in the follow-up of patients treated by transanal excision or low anterior resection, looking for local recurrence in or adjacent to the rectal wall (ORKIN 1995; KIM and WONG 2000).

10.2
Ultrasound Equipment

Endorectal ultrasound probes can be of many types including radial array, mechanical sector, phased and linear probes, some of which are biplanar. The field of view for the rectal wall is maximal with radial array probes (360°) while mechanical sector, phased and linear probes have a field of view limited to 120–210° (Figs. 10.1 and 10.2). The frequency of the probes used varies from 7 to 10 MHz and the focal zone is from 2 to 5 cm. All of these probes are rigid and can only evaluate the rectum. Flexible echoendoscopes, which can evaluate the wall of the entire colon, will not be discussed in this chapter (TIO et al. 1995).

Table 10.1. Pathologic staging of rectal carcinoma

Astler-Coller[a]	TNM*	Description
Stage A1	T1 N0 M0	Tumors limited to the mucosa and submucosa; negative lymph nodes
Stage B1	T2 N0 M0	Tumors involving and limited to the muscularis propria; negative lymph nodes
Stage B2	T3 N0 M0	Tumor infiltration through the muscularis propria into the perirectal fat; negative lymph nodes
Stage C1	T2 N1 M0	Tumor limited to the bowel wall; positive lymph nodes
Stage C2	T3 N1 M0	Tumor infiltration through the muscularis propria into the perirectal fat; positive lymph nodes
	T4	Tumor invades other structures
Stage D	M1	Distant metastasis

[a] ASTLER and COLLER (1954) and SPIESSL et al. (1982)

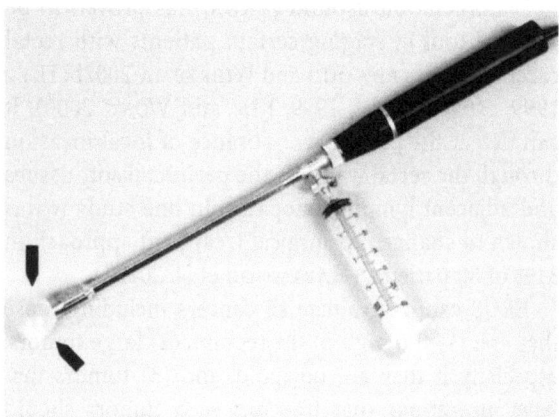

Fig. 10.1. Radial array probe with a 24-cm shaft and a rotating transducer (7–10 MHz) at its tip surrounded by a water-filled balloon (*arrows*). The amount of water in the balloon is controlled by the water-filled syringe at the base of the metal shaft

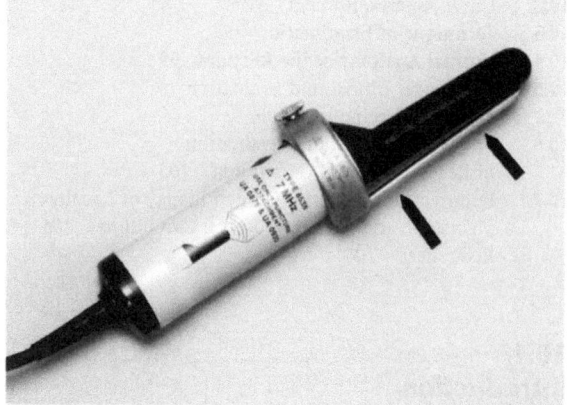

Fig. 10.2. End-fine probe (7 MHz) with the guided needle (*arrows*) attached

The best overall probe for evaluating rectal wall tumors is the radial array probe and the one most commonly used has a 24-cm metal shaft (Bruel and Kjaer Medical Systems Inc., Wilmington, MA, USA). This has a rotating 7–10-MHz transducer at its tip with a focal zone of 2–5 cm that provides an axial image of the entire circumference of the rectal wall (Figs. 10.1 and 10.3). Acoustic contact between the rotating transducer and the rectal wall is achieved by surrounding the transducer with a balloon that contains 30–50 cc of degassed water (tap water that is left to stand for a couple of minutes).

10.3
Technique of Examination

Before coming to the department for the study the patient should be requested to take an enema to clear excess stool from the rectum. The examination is performed with the patient in the left lateral decubitus

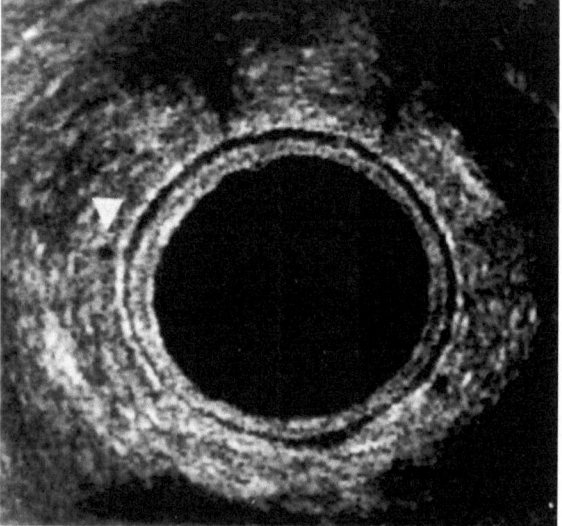

Fig. 10.3. Normal ultrasound anatomy of the rectal wall. *Inner white line*, interface between water-filled balloon and rectal mucosa; *inner black line*, mucosa and muscularis mucosa; *middle white line*, interface between the submucosa and the muscularis propria; *outer black line*, muscularis propria; *outer white line*, interface between muscularis propria and perirectal fat. A normal sized lymph node (*arrowhead*) is present along the right lateral wall of the rectum at 9 o'clock

position. Prior to inserting the probe into the rectum, a digital rectal examination (DRE) should be performed to determine the location of the tumor and make sure that it is not too stenotic to allow passage of the probe. The probe is coated with a liberal amount of warm gel prior to its insertion into the rectum. Most resistance is met at the level of the anal sphincter and gentle pressure should be used to overcome this. Once the probe tip is in the lower rectum it should be pushed superiorly, using the curve of the sacrum as a guide. In most patients the probe can be inserted to 10–14 cm from the anal verge. Once the probe has reached this level the balloon at the tip of the transducer should be inflated with degassed water and the transducer activated (Fig. 10.1). At this point, there should be good contact with the entire circumference of the rectal wall (Fig. 10.3). If there is not good contact with a portion or all of the rectal wall the balloon should be deflated and re-inflated again. The balloon can be distended with a maximum of 80 cc of water to achieve this. If this does not work the probe should be drawn down to the level of the anal sphincter and the balloon re-inflated with a maximum volume of 80 cc of water. Then, gently push the inflated balloon up the rectum and this will hopefully displace the air in the rectum superiorly. If this fails, the patient's position should be changed with the probe in the rectum so the lesion to be evaluated is in the dependent position. The offending air should move superiorly out of the way allowing visualization of the tumor.

Once the probe is at the highest level possible in the rectum its position needs to be checked. The transducer should be rotated until the patient's anterior is at 12 o'clock and the right side at 9 o'clock, just as if one was looking at an axial CT/MRI image. The probe should now be slowly withdrawn down the rectum and images should be obtained at 1-cm intervals. The tip of the probe should be maintained within the center portion of the lumen at all times. If contact with the rectal wall is lost at any level, the water-filled balloon should be deflated and re-inflated until acoustic contact is achieved. At the level of the tumor more closely spaced images should be taken and each image should be marked off in centimeters equating with the distance from the anal verge as marked on the metal shaft of the probe (Fig. 10.1). If the tumor is in the lower rectum, its distance from the superior portion of the anal sphincter should be documented. If sphincteric involvement is seen, the probe should be withdrawn down through the sphincter to document the extent of this finding. Upon completion of the examination the balloon is deflated and the probe withdrawn from the anorectum.

End-fire probes and biplane probes can be helpful in staging some rectal carcinomas as they allow a longitudinal view of the tumor (NIELSEN et al. 1993). This can be especially helpful in determining invasion of the anal sphincter and adjacent structures such as the prostate and seminal vesicles in the male and the vagina in the female. A transvaginal probe can also be used by scanning through the posterior wall of the vagina to determine invasion of its posterior wall. The radial array probe and its balloon can also be used in the vagina for this purpose (FEDYAEV et al. 1995; SANDRIDGE and THORP 1995). SCIALPI et al. (1996, 1999) have described using the transvaginal probe along with instilling 1–1.5 liters of warm water into the rectum in the pre-operative staging of stenotic rectal carcinomas. The use of end-fire and high frequency microprobes have also been described for this purpose (HUNERBEIN et al. 1996; HUNERBEIN and SCHLAG 1997; AKAHOSHI et al. 2000).

At the end of every procedure, the probe is cleaned with soap and warm water and then steeped in a cleansing solution [Cidex (R), Johnson and Johnson Company, 33 Technology Drive, Irvine, CA, USA 92618] for the appropriate amount of time before being used on the next patient.

10.4
Normal Anatomy of the Rectum

The long length of the normal rectum is 11–15 cm and its diameter is 4 cm. Throughout its length it is surrounded by fibrofatty tissue that contains blood vessels, nerves, small lymph nodes and lymphatics. Superiorly it joins with the sigmoid colon at the level of the third segment of the sacrum and courses inferiorly along the anterior aspect of the sacral curve to pass through the muscular pelvic floor to become the anal canal (Fig. 10.4) (GORDON and NIVATVONGS 1992). It is covered by pelvic peritoneum both anteriorly and laterally in its upper one third, while its middle third is only covered anteriorly. The pelvic peritoneum at this point curves anteriorly to cover the bladder in the male and the uterus in the female. The lower one third of the rectum is below the peritoneal reflection. In the male it is related anteriorly to the prostate, seminal vesicles and bladder base and in the female to the vagina, cervix and lower uterus.

The lymphatic drainage of the rectum occurs in a superior direction along the lymphatic chain that accompanies the superior rectal (hemorrhoidal) and inferior mesenteric arteries (Fig. 10.4). Lymphatic

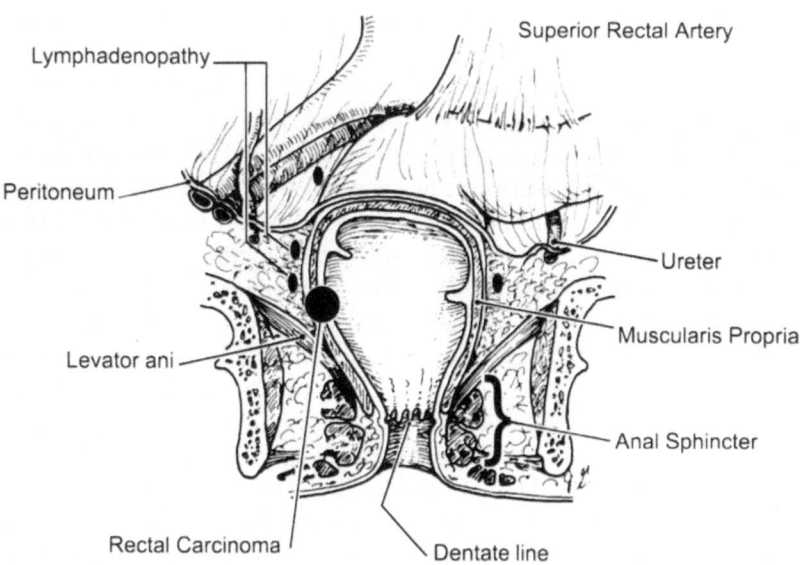

Fig. 10.4. Coronal diagram of the ano-rectum containing a T3 N1 rectal carcinoma – right lateral wall rectal carcinoma with invasion into the perirectal fat. Metastatic perirectal lymphadenopathy is seen extending superiorly above the level of the tumor

extension from rectal carcinoma only involves the internal iliac chain if the superior route is already obstructed by tumor.

Adequate visualization of the rectal wall on endorectal scanning requires good contact between the water balloon and rectal wall with the probe tip in its center lumen. The normal rectal wall is 2–3 mm thick and has a multilayered appearance composed of between five and seven hyperechoic/hypoechoic interfaces from inner to outer as described in detail in Fig. 10.3.

On occasion a thin echogenic line consisting of connective tissue can be seen within the hypoechoic muscularis propria; however, visualization of this line depends upon the degree of distension of the rectal lumen and will disappear with further distension. The surrounding perirectal tissues have an inhomogeneous echogenic appearance. Small lymph nodes measuring 2–3 mm can be seen and should be distinguished from tubular blood vessels cut in cross section by scanning back and forth (Fig. 10.3). Anteriorly the bladder, seminal vesicles and prostate can be seen in the male and the lower uterus, cervix and vagina in the female.

10.5
Endorectal Ultrasound Evaluation of Rectal Carcinoma

ERUS is used to determine the degree of wall penetration by rectal carcinoma and the presence or absence of perirectal lymphadenopathy. Rectal carcinomas have a hypoechoic appearance and the mass deforms the normal layered appearance of the rectal wall (Fig. 10.5). Very careful evaluation of the entire tumor is necessary for staging, as invasion may be limited to only a small portion of the tumor (Fig. 10.6). When tumor invasion is subtle it is indicated by a slight contour irregularity along the muscularis propria/perirectal fat interface. One should also look for submucosal spread of tumor in a superior and inferior direction. This is very important in low rectal carcinomas where a 2- to 3-cm margin of normal rectal wall above the anal sphincter is needed for surgical resection. The degree of intramural spread relates to the overall size of the tumor and degree of wall penetration and its prevalence ranges from 12% to 26%. In a study of 37 patients by YANAGI et al. (1996) intramural spread within 20 mm of the tumor margin was correctly diagnosed in 86%.

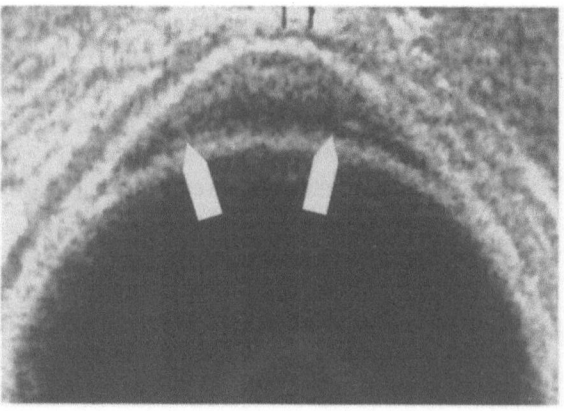

Fig. 10.5. T1 N0 anterior rectal wall hypoechoic carcinoma (*arrows*)

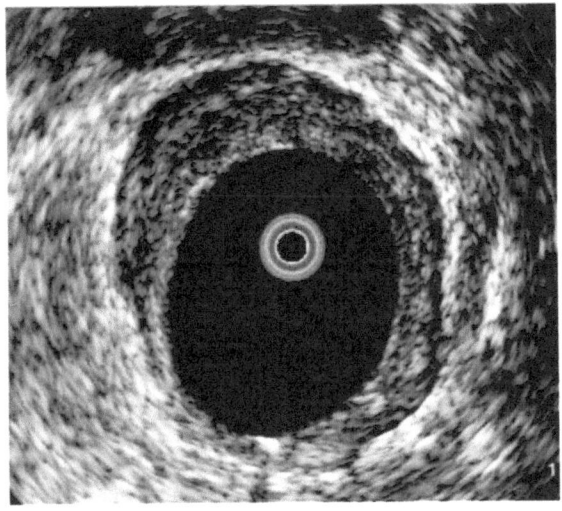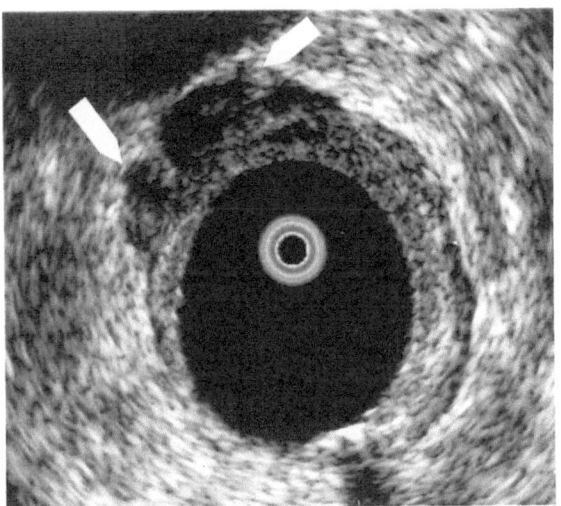

a   b

Fig. 10.6a,b. T3 N0 rectal carcinoma. **a** At this level the carcinoma appears to be within the muscularis propria. **b** At a slightly higher level the tumor can be seen invading into the perirectal fat (*arrows*)

However, they failed to diagnose intramural spread in 29%, and made an incorrect diagnosis in 37%.

Invasion of adjacent structures can be detected with the radial array probe; however, when this is in doubt an end-fire probe or linear array probe can be used to clarify the situation (Fig. 10.7). In the female patient, invasion of the posterior wall of the vagina can be assessed not only endorectally, but also by using the radial array probe in the vagina or a transvaginal probe (Fig. 10.8). If the tumor extends beyond the ultrasonic field of view, this extension should be evaluated with contrast-enhanced CT, or preferably an MRI scan (CHIESURA-CORONA et al. 2001; BEETS-TAN et al. 2000; BLOMQVIST et al. 2000; GUALDI et al. 2000; GAGLIARDI et al. 2002).

Some rectal wall tumors are difficult to evaluate with ERUS. This is especially true of small flat tumors and although they may be palpable on DRE, they can be difficult to see once the rectal wall is distended and stretched by the water-filled balloon. The same problem exists with partially resected polypoid tumors where only the base of the stalk may remain. If these areas can be identified on DRE and thoroughly evaluated with US for residual tumor in the wall and/or extension through the muscularis propria into the perirectal fat, then the tumor can be considered adequately evaluated. In contrast, full sonographic assessment is very difficult or even impossible in tumors that are large or ulcerated, especially if they are polypoid, and such patients should be referred for contrast-enhanced

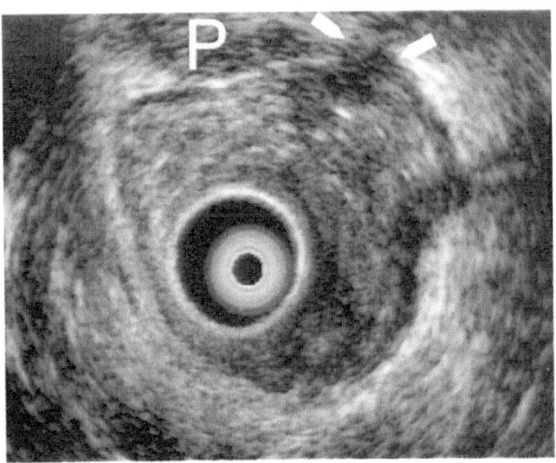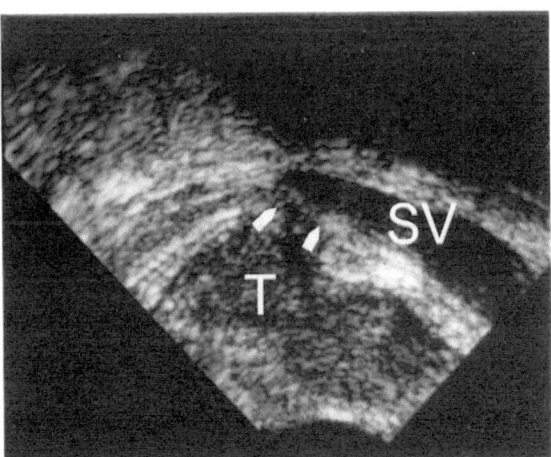

a   b

Fig. 10.7. T4 rectal carcinoma invading the left seminal vesicles. **a** Tumor is invading through the muscularis propria into the perirectal fat (*arrows*). P, prostate. **b** End-fire probe shows invasion of the tumor (*T*) into the seminal vesicles (*SV*) (*arrows*)

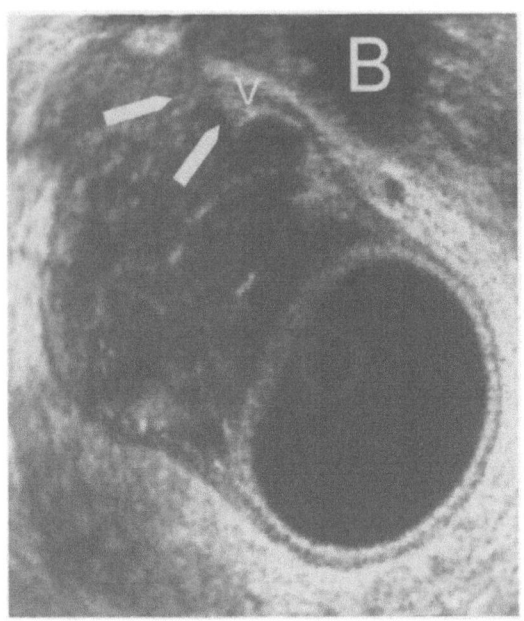

Fig. 10.8. T4 rectal carcinoma (*arrows*) invading the vagina (*V*). *B*, bladder

CT/MRI. The same can be true of stenotic cancers and the US probe should never be forced through a stenotic tumor to enable evaluation. HUNERBEIN et al. (1996) used a 3D end-fire probe (7–10 MHz) to locally stage such tumors and they accurately determined the depth of penetration in 78% of 26 patients with obstructing rectal carcinomas. NIELSEN et al. (1993) in a study of 28 patients achieved similar accuracy (82%). AKAHOSHI et al. (2000) used a 7.5-MHz probe with a 7.3 mm diameter shaft that they inserted through a colonoscope to evaluate 32 patients. The small diameter of this probe allowed it to be used in some stenotic cancers. They reported an accuracy in overall staging of 72%. In a similar study by HUNERBEIN et al. (2000b), they used a 12.5-MHz mini probe on 21 stenotic lesions, and had a staging accuracy of 86%.

Villous tumors of the rectum may have a typical sonographic appearance as the tumor may be divided up by linear echogenic lines due to its frond-like nature (Fig. 10.9). These tumors should be carefully evaluated as 30%–42% undergo malignant transformation and may invade through the muscularis propria into the perirectal fat (HENDRICKS et al. 1989; MOSNIER et al. 1990; PIKARSKY et al. 2000).

Rectal wall masses other than carcinoma can have a hypoechoic appearance. These masses include abscess, endometriosis, colitis cystica profunda and tumors such as leiomyomas, lymphoma and metastasis (HULSMAN et al. 1991). Solitary rectal ulcers can be polypoid, ulcerative or flat in appearance and although

they thicken the rectal wall, especially the third layer, they do not destroy its normal five-layered appearance (HIZAWA et al. 1994). Tumors arising outside the rectal wall can mimic rectal carcinoma and the one most likely to do this is prostate carcinoma (LORENTZEN et al. 1990). If there is any doubt about the diagnosis, a biopsy can be performed along with prostate specific antigen (PSA) staining of the tissue specimen to determine whether it is of prostate origin. Tail gut cysts, dermoids, teratomas and chordomas can also mimic rectal cancer (JOHNSON et al. 1986). Such mimics are usually not a diagnostic problem as most patients referred for ERUS staging of their tumors have a biopsy proven rectal carcinoma.

Normal perirectal lymph nodes are difficult to see with US as they only measure 2–3 mm in diameter (Fig. 10.4). When lymph nodes are larger than this and especially when multiple, metastatic disease has to be considered (Fig. 10.10). Lymph nodes of a normal size that contain metastatic disease cannot be detected by ERUS. Sonography also cannot distinguish enlarged inflamed nodes from those that are metastatic (AKASU et al. 1997). Inflamed lymph nodes tend to have a heterogeneous echo pattern while nodes with metastatic disease tend to be hypoechoic and more round than oval in shape. However, ERUS cannot reliably distinguish between the two. Since lymphatic drainage is in a superior

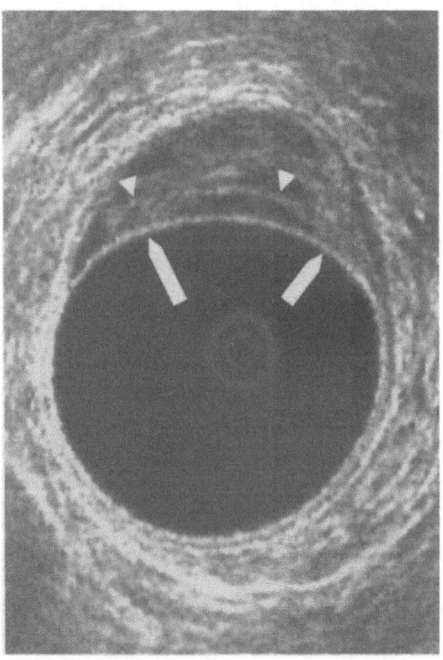

Fig. 10.9. T2 anterior rectal wall villous adenoma (*arrows*). Note the linear lace-like echogenic lines (*arrows heads*) within the tumor

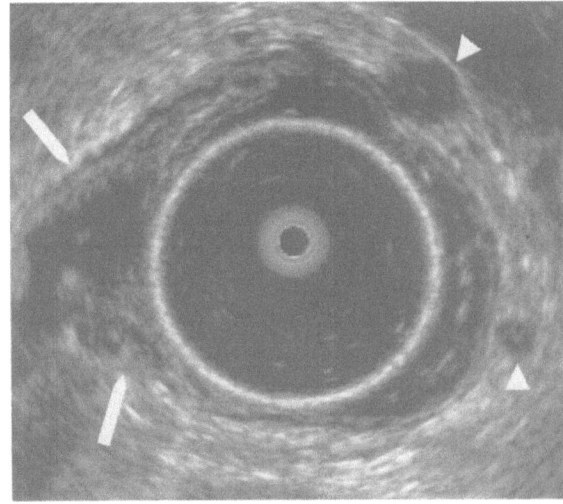

Fig. 10.10. T3 N1 rectal carcinoma. The hypoechoic tumor can be seen invading into the perirectal fat (*arrows*) with associated lymphadenopathy (*arrowheads*)

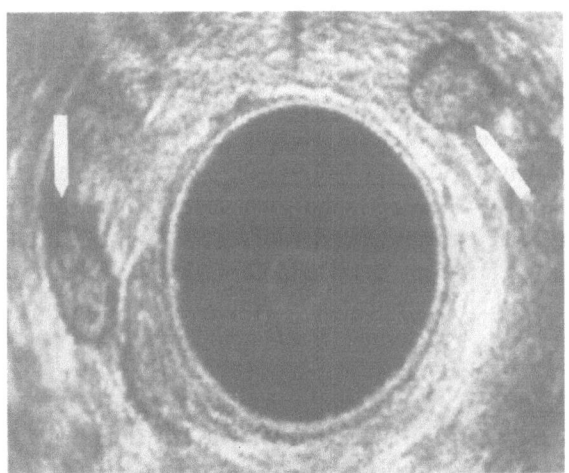

Fig. 10.11. Loops of bowel adjacent to the rectosigmoid junction with the appearance of lymphadenopathy (*arrows*)

direction it is very important to evaluate the perirectal tissues above the level of the tumor when looking for metastatic lymphadenopathy (Fig. 10.3). This should be done even if the tumor is confined to the rectal wall as metastatic adenopathy may be present in 10% of such cases (MORSON 1966). Be careful not to mistake loops of bowel anterior to the upper third of the rectum as enlarged lymph nodes (Fig. 10.11). This error can be avoided by scanning back and forth, thus demonstrating the tubular nature of the bowel, while the presence of peristalsis also helps.

The accuracy of ERUS in determining invasion of rectal carcinoma through the muscularis propria depends upon the skill of the examiner and varies

from 50% to 96% (BEYNON et al. 1986a; DERSHAW et al. 1990; GLASER et al. 1990; GOLDMAN et al. 1991; HENEGHAN et al. 1997; KIM et al. 1999; MARONE et al. 2000; MASSARI et al. 1998; NIELSEN et al. 1996; ORROM et al. 1990; OSTI et al. 1997; RIFKIN et al. 1989; SENEGORE et al. 1988; THALER et al. 1994; TIO et al. 1995; TSENG et al. 1999). Its specificity (accurate diagnosis of no invasion) varies from 76% to 97%, and its negative predictive value (accuracy of a negative study) is 25%–72% (BEYNON et al. 1986a; JOCHEM et al. 1990; KIM et al. 1999; MILSOM and GRAFFNER 1990; RIFKIN et al. 1989; YANASHITA et al. 1988). Ultrasound tends to overestimate (8%–17%) rather than underestimate (2%–6%) tumor invasion through the muscularis propria into the perirectal fat (AKASU et al. 1997; HUNERBEIN et al. 1996; JOCHEM et al. 1990; KIM et al. 1999; MAIER et al. 1997; YANASHITA et al. 1988). In one study, ANDERSON et al. (1994) found that the staging of A1/T1 tumors was more accurate than the staging of B1/T2 tumors where they under-staged up to 30%. As an overall policy it is better for ultrasound to overestimate rather than underestimate tumor invasion as it is never a good policy to undertreat carcinoma. An error can happen at the rectosigmoid junction where anteriorly the lower sigmoid wall is going away from the rectum, and the ultrasound beam cuts along the long axis of this muscular wall which can mimic a tumor (Fig. 10.12) (JOCHEM et al. 1990).

MAIER et al. (1997) did a prospective study on two groups of 40 patients. They compared the ERUS stage with the histological staging after surgical removal. In the first group of 40 patients the accuracy for tumor staging was 70%. In the second group of

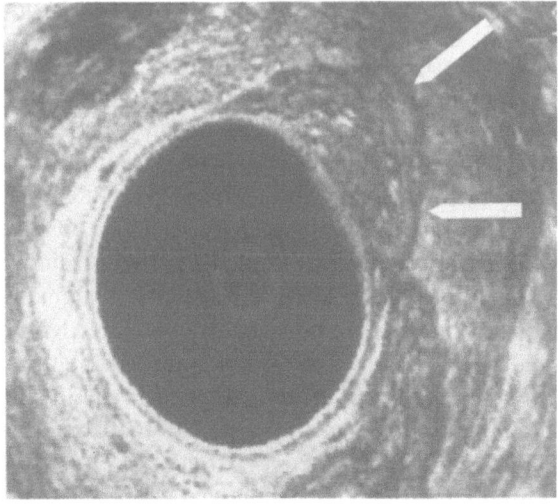

Fig. 10.12. Muscular wall of the sigmoid colon going away from the rectum mimics an anterior rectal wall tumor (*arrows*)

40 patients, they excluded the anechoic/hypoechoic peri-tumoral tissue reaction from their ERUS staging, and increased their accuracy to 95%.

The position and level of a tumor in the rectum does not appear to have an effect on tumor staging. SAILER et al. (1997b) studied 162 tumors in 154 patients to determine if the level (low, mid, high) or location (anterior, posterior, right or left lateral wall) of a tumor had any effect on the accuracy of ERUS staging. The study suggested that the accuracy was reduced in lower rectal wall lesions; however, the difference did not reach statistical significance.

The use of 3D ultrasound probably does not greatly increase the accuracy of ERUS staging. In a study by HUNERBEIN and SCHLAG (1997), they compared conventional ERUS to 3D ultrasound in 49 patients and found 3D to be only slightly more accurate in T staging (88% v 82%) and N staging (79% v 74%).

Ultrasound is not very accurate in demonstrating direct invasion of adjacent structures and here its accuracy ranges from 57% to 86% (Figs. 10 7 and 10.8) (DERSHAW et al. 1990; YANASHITA et al. 1988).

All of the imaging modalities (ERUS, CT, MRI) use size as a criterion to diagnose metastatic lymphadenopathy and their overall accuracy is not very good ranging from 50% to 88% (DE LANGE 1994; DERSHAW et al. 1990; GOLDMAN et al. 1991; JOCHEM et al. 1990; KIM et al. 1999; MARONE et al. 2000; MASSARI et al. 1998; MILSOM and GRAFFNER 1990; NIELSEN et al. 1996; ORROM et al. 1990; OSTI et al. 1997; RIFKIN et al. 1989; SAILER et al. 1997a; THALER et al. 1994; TIO et al. 1995; TSENG et al. 1999). The size of normal lymph nodes can be above the normal range (3 mm or less), while metastatic lymph nodes can vary from 2 to 13 mm and above (mean 7 mm) (GOLDMAN et al. 1991; BEYNON et al. 1989a). This overlap in size between benign and malignant lymph nodes reduces the accuracy of ultrasound in diagnosing metastatic lymphadenopathy. However, that said, the larger the lymph node the more likely it is to be malignant (Fig. 10.10). In a study by MILSOM and GRAFFNER (1990), ERUS had a sensitivity of 81%, a specificity of 80%, a positive predictive value of 74%, and a negative predictive value of 86% in predicting metastatic lymphadenopathy in 52 patients. In a study of resected lymph nodes by HULSMAN et al. (1992), they could only differentiate benign from malignant in 40% using the long axis diameter, a roundness index and the nodal echo pattern. HENEGHAN et al. (1997), using a node size of 7 mm had an accuracy of 83%. Using color flow and special Doppler analysis, they showed that a peak systolic velocity within a node greater than 20 cm/s classified it as malignant with 100% sensitivity, 62% specificity and 76% accuracy. When clinically indicated, an ERUS-guided biopsy can be performed upon a perirectal lymph node if it is 1 cm or greater.

In experienced hands the overall accuracy of ERUS in T and N staging of rectal carcinoma should be around 85% which is certainly better than DRE (BEYNON et al. 1986b; NICHOLLS et al. 1982). There is a learning curve in performing this examination and accuracy increases with experience (CARMODY and OTCHY 2000; MARUSCH et al. 2002). ERUS is slightly better than contrast enhanced CT and this is especially true for small tumors that are minimally invasive (BALTHAZAR et al. 1988; BEYNON et al. 1986b; FREENY et al. 1986; GOLDMAN et al. 1991; KIM et al. 1999; RIFKIN et al. 1989; THOMPSON et al. 1986). MRI is also more accurate than CT and is probably comparable in its accuracy to ERUS (CHAN et al. 1991; GUINET et al. 1988, 1990; HUNERBEIN et al. 2000a; IMAI et al. 1990; JOOSTEN et al. 1995; KIM et al. 1999, 2000; MEYENBERGER et al. 1995; SCHNALL et al. 1994; THALER et al. 1994; URBAN et al. 2000; WALLENGREN et al. 2000). In comparing US with MRI, the former is technically more difficult to perform and interpret while the latter is a more expensive and time-consuming study and cannot be used in patients who are claustrophobic or have cardiac pacemakers. We use MRI when the cancer is too large or ulcerated to be staged by ultrasound and when we need to determine invasion of adjacent structures including the pelvic side wall.

Rectal villous tumors deserve special mention as ERUS can play a major role in staging and so influence treatment. If ERUS shows no invasion through the muscularis propria then a TAE can be performed and more extensive surgery avoided. PIKARSKY et al. (2000) performed ERUS on 35 patients and correctly identified no invasions through the muscularis propria in 26 of 27 patients (96%). The one patient incorrectly staged as a T2 tumor was pathologically staged as T3 following TAE and was treated with radiation therapy. The eight patients that preoperatively had ERUS evidence of a T3 tumor had US-guided biopsies performed and the diagnosis was confirmed in seven of these eight patients. Post-operative pathological staging demonstrated a T3 tumor in seven, and a T2 tumor in the single patient with negative preoperative US-guided biopsies. SAILER et al. (1997a), in a study of 152 patients with 162 tumors of which 38 (24%) were adenomas had an overall T staging accuracy of 78% while that for N staging was 83%. They were able to accurately stage T1 tumors and adenomas but over-staged 17 of 299 T2 tumors where the sensitivity was 41% and the specificity was 92%.

If rectal carcinoma has invaded through the muscularis propria into the perirectal fat and/or if there is metastatic lymphadenopathy, the tumor can be down-staged before surgery by radiation therapy and/or chemotherapy. HAREWOOD and WIERSEMA (2002) demonstrated that a combination of ERUS and abdominal CT scanning were more cost effective than CT and MRI or CT alone in selecting patients for preoperative radiation therapy. In a study of 43 patients by BERNINI et al. (1996), down-staging occurred in 53% with perirectal fat involvement and 72% with lymph node metastasis resulting in an overall down-staging of 70%. However, this treatment results in a reduction of the overall staging accuracy of endorectal ultrasound as overstaging of the original tumor occurs due to the inflammatory changes produce by the treatment (BERNINI et al. 1996; WILLIAMSON et al. 1996).

10.6
Endorectal Ultrasound Evaluation of Recurrent Rectal Carcinoma

Following transanal excision or low anterior resection of a rectal carcinoma, ERUS can be used to detect local recurrences. Those treated by abdominoperineal resection need to be followed with CT and/or MRI (FREENY et al. 1986; THOMPSON et al. 1986; KIM and WONG 2000; MEYENBERGER et al. 1995; BAZZARINI et al. 1990). Follow-up with ERUS should be at 6-month intervals for a period of at least 2 years, as most local tumor recurrences (80%) occur during this time period. The incidence of local recurrence varies from 3% to 30% and is most likely in patients having locally invasive tumors and/or metastatic lymphadenopathy at the time of the initial diagnosis (HOJO 1986; PHILLIPS et al. 1984).

These local recurrences have a hypoechoic appearance (BEYNON et al. 1989b) and are usually found at the site of surgery but can occur at a more superior level. Small tumor recurrences may be missed on DRE and on endoscopy. In a study by MASCAGNI et al. (1989) of 120 patients followed-up using DRE, carcinoembryonic antigen (CEA), endoscopy, ERUS and CT there were 17 local recurrences. Six asymptomatic recurrences and four of 11 symptomatic recurrences were only detected by ERUS. MULLER et al. (2000) reported an accuracy

of 90% in detecting locally recurrent tumors with ERUS. Recurrence can be confined to the rectal wall or can invade the perirectal fat. When confined to the wall, they may be extramucosal and may not be visible during endoscopy. The mass in the wall may be focal in nature or may partially or completely involve the circumference producing an irregular area of hypoechoic thickening (Fig. 10.13). This should be distinguished from the smooth symmetrical thickening of the entire circumference of the wall produced by postoperative fibrosis or radiation therapy (Fig. 10.14) (DERSHAW et al. 1990). Metastatic lymph nodes may also be found with wall recurrences but may also occur in the absence of wall involvement.

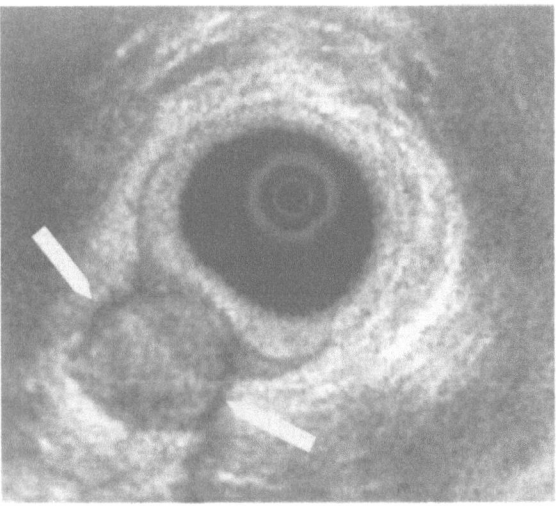

Fig. 10.13. Recurrent rectal carcinoma (*arrows*) in the rectal wall near the site of surgery. This did not involve the mucosa and was not visible endoscopically

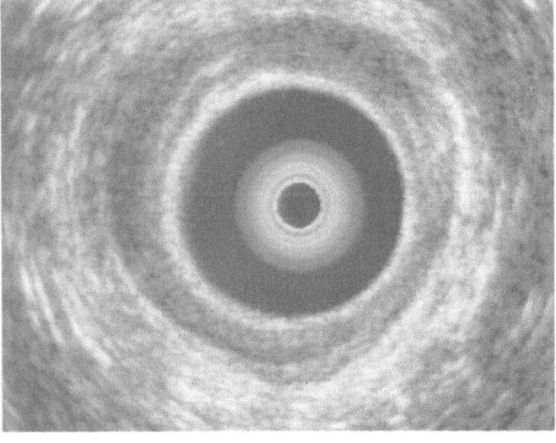

Fig. 10.14. Smooth symmetrical, circumferential rectal wall thickening due to radiation therapy for a resected rectal carcinoma

10.7
Endorectal Ultrasound-Guided Biopsy of Locally Metastatic and Recurrent Rectal Carcinoma

To prove that an extramucosal wall mass or an enlarged perirectal lymph node represent metastatic disease, an ERUS-guided biopsy can be performed using a biopsy guide and an 18-gauge automated cutting needle (Figs. 10.2 and 10.15) (QUAM et al. 1989). A broad spectrum antibiotic should be administered for 3 days starting the day before the biopsy and it is probably a good idea to have the patient take a cleansing enema several hours prior to the procedure.

HUNERBEIN et al. (2001) in the follow-up of 312 patients with sphincter-saving surgery, performed biopsies on 68 perirectal masses. Tumor recurrence was present in 22, absent in 41, while the biopsy failed in five patients. Recurrent tumor masses tend to be hypervascular whereas fibrotic change is hypovascular and color Doppler imaging may help distinguish between the two (ALEXANDER et al. 1994; SUDAKOFF et al. 1996).

Most local tumor recurrences are not surgically resectable and the overall 5-year survival is less than 5% (CHARNLEY et al. 1988). If surgery is being considered in such a patient, a CT or MRI of the abdomen and pelvis should be performed to confirm the extent of disease in the pelvis and look for metastatic disease in the retroperitoneum and liver (MARKUS et al. 1997). If distant metastases are present then surgical resection of the local recurrence might not be indicated.

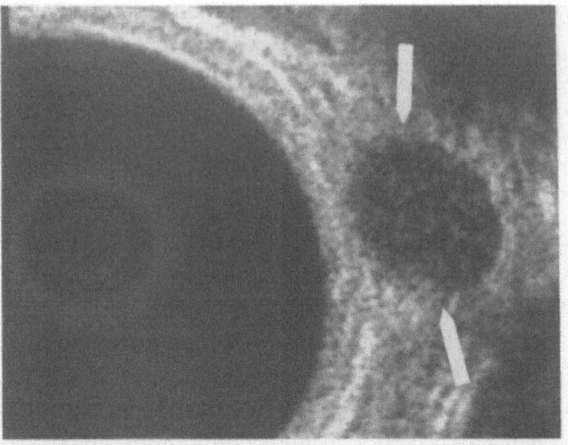

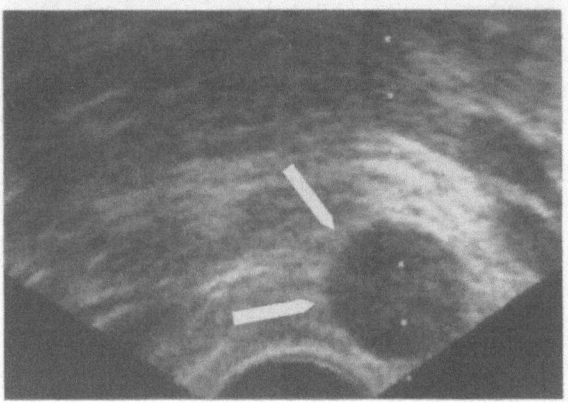

Fig. 10.15. Recurrent rectal wall carcinoma. **a** A 1-cm, extramucosal hypoechoic wall mass (*arrows*) superior to the site of a transanal excision of a small T2 N0 rectal carcinoma. **b** An ERUS end-fire probe biopsy of the mass (*arrows*) demonstrated recurrent rectal carcinoma

References

Akahoshi K, Kondoh A, Nagaie T, Koyanagi N, Nakanishi K, Harada N, Nawata H (2000) Preoperative staging of rectal cancer using a 7.5 MHz front-loading US Probe. Gastrointest Endosc 52:529–534

Akasu T, Sugihara K, Moriya Y, Fujita S (1997) Limitations and pitfalls of transrectal ultrasonography for staging of rectal cancer. Dis Colon Rectum 40 [Suppl 10]:S10–S15

Alexander AA, Liu JB, Palazzo JP, Jakob Z, Forsberg F, Ehrlich SM, Goldberg BB (1994) Endorectal color and duplex imaging of the normal rectal wall and rectal masses. J Ultrasound Med 13:509–515

Anderson BO, Hann LE, Enker WE (1994) Transrectal ultrasonography and operative selection for early carcinoma of the rectum. J Am Coll Surg 179:513–517

Astler VB, Coller FA (1954) The prognostic significance of direct extension of carcinoma of the colon and rectum. Ann Surg 139:846–851

Balthazar EJ, Megibow AJ, Hulnick DH, Naidich DP (1988) Carcinoma of the colon: detection and pre-operative staging by CT. AJR 150:301–306

Bazzarini L, Ceglia E, D'Ippolito G, Petrillo R et al (1990) Local recurrence of rectosigmoid cancer; what about the choice of MRI for diagnosis? Gastrointest Radiol 15:338–342

Beets-Tan RG, Beets GL, Borstlap AC, Oei TK, Teune TM, von Meyenfeldt MF, van Engelshoven JM (2000) Pre-operative assessment of local tumor extent in advanced rectal cancer: CT or high-resolution MRI? Abdom Imaging 5:533–541

Beets-Tan RG, Beets GL, Vliegen RF, Kessels AG, van Boven H, DeBruine A, von Meyenfeldt MF, Baeten CG, van Engelshoven JM (2001) Accuracy of magnetic resonance imaging in prediction of tumor-free resection margin in rectal cancer surgery. Lancet 357:497–504

Bernini A, Deen KI, Madoff RD, Wong WD (1996) Preoperative adjuvant radiation with chemotherapy for rectal cancer: its impact on stage of disease and the role of endorectal ultrasound. Ann Surg Oncol 3:131–135

Beynon J, Foy DMA, Roe AM, Temple LN, Mortensen NJ (1986a) Endoluminal ultrasound in the assessment of local invasion in rectal cancer. Br J Surg 73:474–477

Beynon J, Mortensen NJ, Foy DMA, Channer JL, Rigby H,

Virjee J (1986b) Preoperative assessment of local invasion of rectal cancer: digital examination, endoluminal sonography or computed tomography? Br J Surg 73:1015–1017

Beynon J, Mortensen NJ, Foy DM, Channer JL (1989a) Preoperative assessment of mesorectal lymph node involvement in rectal cancer. Br J Surg 76:276–279

Beynon J, Mortensen NJ, Foy DMA, Channer JL et al (1989b) The detection and evaluation of locally recurrent rectal cancer with rectal endosonography. Dis Colon Rectum 32:500–517

Blomqvist L, Holm T, Rubio C, Hindmarsh T (1997) Rectal tumors Ñ MR imaging with endorectal and/or phased-array coils, and histopathological staging on giant sections. A comparative study. Acta Radiol 38:437–444

Blomqvist L, Machado M, Rubio C, Gabrielsson N, Granqvist S, Goldman S, Holm T (2000) Rectal tumor staging: MR imaging using pelvic phased-array and endorectal coils vs endoscopic ultrasonography. Eur Radiol 10:653–660

Carmody BJ, Otchy DP (2002) Learning curve of transrectal ultrasound. Dis Colon Rectum 43:193–197

Chan TW, Kressel HY, Milestone B, Tomachefski J et al (1991) Rectal carcinoma: staging at MRI imaging with endorectal coil. Radiology 181:461–467

Charnley RM, Pyf G, Amar SS, Hardcastle JD (1988) The early detection of recurrent rectal carcinoma by rectal endosonography. Br J Surg 75:1232

Chiesura-Corona M, Muzzio PC, Giust G, Zuliani M, Pucciarelli S, Toppan P (2001) Rectal cancer: CT local staging with histopathologic correlation. Abdom Imaging 2:134–138

De Lange EE (1994) Staging rectal carcinoma with endorectal imaging: how much detail do we really need? Radiology 190:633–635

Dershaw DD, Enker WE, Cohen AM, Sigurdson ER (1990) Transrectal ultrasonography of rectal carcinoma. Cancer 66:2336–2340

Fedyaev EB, Volkova EA, Kuznetsova EE (1995) Transrectal and transvaginal ultrasonography in the preoperative staging of rectal carcinoma. Eur J Radiol 20:35–38

Freeny PC, Marks WM, Ryan JA, Bolen JW (1986) Colorectal carcinoma evaluation with CT: preoperative staging and detection of post operative recurrence. Radiology 158:347–353

Gagliardi G, Bayar S, Smith R, Salem RR (2002) Preoperative staging of rectal cancer using magnetic resonance imaging with external phase-arrayed coils. Arch Surg 137:447–451

Glaser F, Schlag P, Herfarth C (1990) Endorectal ultrasonography for the assessment of invasion of rectal tumors and lymph node involvement. Br J Surg 77:883–887

Goldman S, Arvidsson H, Norming U, Lagerstedt U (1991) Transrectal ultrasound and computed tomography in preoperative staging of lower rectal adenocarcinoma. Gastrointest Radiol 16:259–263

Gordon PH, Nivatvongs S (1992) Surgical anatomy of the colon, rectum and anal canal. Principles and practice of surgery for the colon, rectum and anus. Quality Medical Publishing, St Louis, pp 3–37

Gualdi GF, Casciani E, Guadalaxara A, d'Orta C, Polettini E, Pappalardo G (2000) Local staging of rectal cancer with transrectal ultrasound and endorectal magnetic resonance imaging: comparison with histologic findings. Dis Colon Rectum 3:338–345

Guinet C, Buy JN, Sezeur A, Mosnier H et al (1988) Preoperative assessment of the extension of rectal carcinoma: correlation of MR, surgical, and histopathologic findings. J Comput Assist Tomogr 12:209–214

Guinet C, Buy JN, Ghossain MA, Sezeur A et al (1990) Comparison of magnetic resonance imaging and computed tomography in the preoperative staging of rectal cancer. Arch Surg 125:385–388

Hadfield MB, Nicholson AA, MacDonald AW, Farouk R, Lee PW, Duthie GS, Monson JR (1997) Preoperative staging of rectal carcinoma by magnetic resonance imaging with pelvic phased-array coil. Br J Surg 4:529–531

Harewood GC, Wiersema MJ (2002a) Cost-effectiveness of endoscopic ultrasonography in the evaluation of proximal rectal cancer. Am J Gastroenterol 4:874–882

Harewood GC, Wiersema MJ, Nelson H, Maccarty RL, Olson JE, Clain JE, Ahlquist DA, Jondal ML (2002b) A prospective, blinded assessment of the impact of preopreative staging on the management of rectal cancer. Gastroenterology 123:24–32

Hendricks PJ, Keefe B, Wechsler RJ (1989) The value of CT in rectal villous tumors. J Comput Assist Tomogr 13:269–272

Heneghan JP, Salem RR, Lange RC, Taylor KJ, Hammers LW (1997) Transrcctal sonography in staging rectal carcinoma: the role of gray-scale, color-flow, and Doppler imaging analysis. AJR Am J Roentgenol 169:1247–1252

Heriot AG, Grundy A, Kumar D (1999) Preoperative staging of rectal carcinoma. Br J Surg 86:17–28

Hill MC (1999) Endoluminal ultrasound of the rectum and anus. In: Kane RA (ed) Intraoperative laparoscopic and endoluminal ultrasound. Churchill Livingston, Philadelphia, pp 184–199

Hizawa K, Iida M, Suekane H, Mibu R, Mochizuki Y, Yao T, Fujishima M (1994) Mucosal prolapse syndrome: diagnosis with endoscopic US. Radiology 191:527–530

Hojo K (1986) Anastomotic recurrence after sphincter saving resection for rectal cancer: length of distal clearance of the bowel. Dis Colon Rectum 29:11–14

Hulsmans FJH, Tio LT, Reeders JWA, Tytgat GNJ (1991) Transrectal US in the diagnosis of localized colitis cystica profunda. Radiology 181:201–203

Hulsman FH, Bosma A, Mulder PJ, Reeders JW, Tytgt GN (1992) Perirectal lymph nodes in rectal cancer: in vitro correlation of sonographic parameters and histopathologic findings. Radiology 184:553–560

Hunerbein M, Schlag PM (1997) Three-dimensional endosonography for staging of rectal cancer. Ann Surg 225:432–438

Hunerbein M, Below C, Schlag PM (1996) Three-dimensional endorectal ultrasonography for staging of obstructing rectal cancer. Dis Colon Rectum 39:636–642

Hunerbein M, Pegios W, Rau B, Vogl TJ, Felix R, Schlag PM (2000a) Prospective comparison of endorectal ultrasound, three-dimensional endorectal ultrasound, and endorectal MRI in the preoperative evaluation of rectal tumors. Preliminary results. Surg Endosc 14:1005–1009

Hunerbein M, Totkas S, Ghadimi BM, Schlag PM (2000b) Preoperative evaluation of colorectal neoplasms by colonoscopic miniprobe ultrasonography. Ann Surg 232:46–50

Hunerbein M, Totkas S, Moesta KT, Ulmer C, Handke T, Schlag PM (2001) The role of transrectal ultrasound-guided biopsy in the postoperative follow-up of patients with rectal cancer. Surgery 129:164–169

Imai Y, Kressel HY, Saul SH, Chao PW et al (1990) Colo-rectal tumors: an in vitro study of high-resolution MR imaging. Radiology 177:695–701

Jochem RJ, Reading CC, Dozois RR, Carpenter HA et al (1990)

Endorectal ultrasonographic staging of rectal carcinoma. Mayo Clin Proc 65:1571–1577

Johnson AR, Ros PR, Hjermstad BM (1986) Tailgut cyst: diagnosis with CT and sonography. AJR 147:1309–1311

Joosten FB, Jansen JB, Joosten HJ, Rosenbusch G (1995) Staging of rectal carcinoma using MR double surface coil, MR endorectal coil, and intrarectal ultrasound: correlation with histopathologic findings. J Comput Assist Tomogr 19:752–758

Kim NK, Wong WD (2000) Role of endorectal ultrasound in the conservative management of rectal cancers. Semin Surg Oncol 19:358–366

Kim NK, Kim MJ, Yun SH, Sohn SK, Min JS (1999) Comparative study of transrectal ultrasonography, pelvic computerized tomography, and magnetic resonance imaging in preoperative staging of rectal cancer. Dis Colon Rectum 42:770–775

Kim NK, Kim MJ, Park JK, Park SI, Min JS (2000) Preoperative staging of rectal cancer with MRI: accuracy and clinical usefulness. Ann Surg Oncol 7:732–737

Lorentzen T, Torp-Pedersen S, Nolsoe C (1990) Transrectal ultrasound findings of prostate cancer mimicking primary rectal tumor. Acta Radiol 31:625–626

Maier AG, Barton PP, Neuhold NR, Herbst F, Teleky BK, Lechner GL (1997) Peritumoral tissue reaction at transrectal US as a possible cause of overstaging in rectal cancer: histopathologic correlation. Radiology 203:785–789

Markus J, Morrissey B, de Gara C, Tarulli G (1997) MRI of recurrent rectosigmoid carcinoma. Abdom Imaging 22:338–342

Marone P, Petrulio F, de Bellis M, Battista Rossi G, Tempesta A (2000) Role of endoscopic ultrasonography in the staging of rectal cancer: a retrospective study of 63 patients. J Clin Gastroenterol 30:420–424

Marusch F, Koch A, Schmidt U, Zippel R, Kuhn R, Wolff S, Pross M, Wierth A, Gastinger I, Lippert H (2002) Routine use of transrectal ultrasound in rectal carcinoma: results of a prospective multicenter study. Endoscopy 34:385–390

Mascagni D, Corbellini L, Urciuoli P, di Matteo G (1989) Endoluminal ultrasound for early detection of local recurrence of rectal cancer. Br J Surg 76:1176–1180

Massari M, De Simone M, Cioffi U, Rosso L, Chiarelli M, Gabrielli F (1998) Value and limits of endorectal ultrasonography for preoperative staging of rectal carcinoma. Surg Laparosc Endosc 8:438–444

Mentges B, Buess G, Schafer D, Manncke K, Becker HD (1996) Local therapy of rectal tumors. Dis Colon Rectum 39:886–892

Meyenberger C, Huch Boni RA, Bertschinger P, Zala GF, Klotz HP, Krestin GP (1995) Endoscopic ultrasound and endorectal magnetic resonance imaging: a prospective, comparative study for preoperative staging and follow-up of rectal cancer. Endoscopy 27:469–479

Milsom JW, Graffner H (1990) Intrarectal ultrasonography in rectal cancer staging and in the evaluation of pelvic disease. Ann Surg 212:42–46

Morson BC (1966) Factors influencing the prognosis of early cancer of the rectum. Proc R Soc Med 59:607–608

Mosnier H, Guivarc'h M, Meduri B, Fritsch J, Outters F (1990) Endorectal sonography in the management of rectal villous tumors. Int J Colorectal Dis 5:90–93

Muller C, Kahler G, Scheele J (2000) Endosonographic examination of gastrointestinal anastomoses with suspected locoregional tumor recurrence. Surg Endosc 14:45–50

Nicholls RJ, Mason AY, Morson BC (1982) The clinical staging of rectal cancer. Br J Surg 69:404–409

Nielsen MB, Pedersen JF, Christiansen J (1993) Rectal endosonography in the evaluation of stenotic rectal tumors. Dis Colon Rectum 36:275–279

Nielsen MB, Qvitzau S, Pedersen JF, Christiansen J (1996) Endosonography for preoperative staging of rectal tumors. Acta Radiol 37:799–803

Orkin BA (1995) Local treatment of rectal neoplasms. In: Mazier WP, Levien DH, Luchtefeld MA, Senagore AJ (eds) Surgery of the colon, rectum and anus. Saunders, Philadelphia, pp 470–489

Orrom WJ, Wong WD, Rothenberger DA (1990) Endorectal ultrasound in the preoperative staging of rectal tumors. Dis Colon Rectum 33:654–659

Osti MF, Padovan FS, Pirolli C, Sbarbati S, Tombolini V, Meli C, Enrici RM (1997) Comparison between transrectal ultrasonography and computed tomgraphy with rectal inflation of gas in preoperaitis staging of lower rectal cancer. Eur Radiol 7:26–30

Phillips RK. Hittinger R, Blesovsky L, Fry JS, Fielding LP (1984) Local recurrence following "curative" surgery for large bowel cancer II. The rectum and rectosigmoid. Br J Surg 71:17–20

Pikarsky A, Wexner S, Lebensart P, Efron J, Weiss E, Nogueras J, Reissman P (2000) The use of rectal ultrasound for the correct diagnosis and treatment of rectal villous tumors. Am J Surg 179:261–265

Quam JP, Reading CC, Charboneau JW (1989) Transrectal sonographically guided biopsy of a perirectal lymph node in recurrent rectal carcinoma. AJR 153:1101

Rifkin MD, Ehrlich SM, Marks G (1989) Staging of rectal carcinoma: prospective comparison of endorectal US and CT. Radiology 170:319–322

Sailer M, Leppert R, Kraemer M, Fuchs KH, Thiede A (1997a) The value of endorectal ultrasound in the assessment of adenomas, T1 and T2-carcinomas. Int J Color Dis 12:214–219

Sailer M, Leppert R, Bussen D, Fuchs KH, Thiede A (1997b) Influence of tumor position on accuracy of endorectal ultrasound staging. Dis Colon Rectum 40:1180–1186

Sandridge DA, Thorp JM Jr (1995) Vaginal endosonography in the assessment of the anorectum. Obstet Gynecol 86:1007–1009

Schnall MD, Furth EE, Rosato EF, Kressel HY (1994) Rectal tumor staging: correlation of endorectal MR imaging and pathologic findings. Radiology 190:709–714

Scialpi M, Niccolini M, Zottele F, Dalla Palma F, Scialpi P (1996) A new method for study of the rectum using transvaginal ultrasound with water enema. Abdom Imaging 21:342–344

Scialpi M, Rotondo A, Angelelli G (1999) Water enema transvaginal ultrasound for local staging of stenotic rectal carcinoma. Abdom Imaging 24:132–136

Senegore A, Milsom JW, Talbott TM et al (1988) Intrarectal ultrasonography in the staging and management of rectal tumors. Am Surg 6:352–355

Spiessl B, Schiebe O, Wagner G (eds) (1982) UICC TNM atlas. Springer, Berlin Heidelberg New York

Sudakoff GS, Gasparaitis A, Michelassi F, Hurst R, Hoffmann K, Hackworth C (1996) Endorectal color Doppler imaging of primary and recurrent rectal wall tumors: preliminary experience. AJR 166:55–61

Thaler W, Watzka S, Martin F, La Guardia G, Psenner K, Bonatti G, Fichtel G, Egarter-Vigl E, Marzoli GP (1994) Preoperative staging of rectal cancer by endoluminal ultrasound vs. magnetic resonance imaging. Preliminary results of a prospective, comparative study. Dis Colon Rectum 37:1189–1193

Thompson WM, Halvorsen RA, Foster WL, Roberts L, Gibbons K (1986) Preoperative and postoperative CT staging of rectosigmoid carcinoma. AJR 146:703–710

Tio TL, Coene PPLO, van Delden OM, Tytgat NJ (1991) Colorectal carcinoma: preoperative TNM classification with endosonography. Radiology 179:165–70Tseng LJ, MO LR, Thian LT, Jao YT (1999) Pre-operative staging of recto-sigmoid colon carcinoma by upper gastrointestinal endoscopic ultrasonography. Hepatogastroenterology 46:891–893

Urban M, Rosen HR, Holbling N, Feil W, Hochwarther G, Hruby W, Schiessel R (2000) MR imaging for the preoperative planning of sphincter-saving surgery for tumors of the lower third of the rectum: use of intravenous and endorectal contrast materials. Radiology 214:503–508

Wallengren NO, Holtas S, Andren-Sanberg A, Jonsson E, Kristoffersson DT, McGill S (2000) Rectal carcinoma: double-contrast MR imaging for preoperative staging. Radiology 215:108–114

Wang KY, Kimmey MB, Nyberg DA et al (1987) Colorectal neoplasms: accuracy of US in demonstrating the depth of invasion. Radiology 165:827–829

Williamson PR, Hellinger MD, Larach SW, Ferrara A (1996) Endorectal ultrasound of T3 and T4 rectal cancers after preoperative chemoradiation. Dis Colon Rectum 39: 45–49

Yanagi H, Kusunoki M, Shoji Y, Yamamura T, Utsunomiya J (1996) Preoperative detection of distal intramural spread of lower rectal carcinoma using transrectal ultrasonography. Dis Colon Rectum 39:1210–1214

Yanashita Y, Machi J, Shirouzu K, Morotomi T, Isomoto H, Kakagawa T (1988) Evaluation of endorectal ultrasound for the assessment of wall invasion of rectal cancer. Dis Colon Rectum 31:617–653

11 Rectal Tumours – MRI

Regina G. H. Beets-Tan and Geerard L. Beets

CONTENTS

11.1 Introduction *111*
11.2 The Dutch TME Trial *112*
11.3 Rectal Cancer Imaging *112*
11.4 T Stage Determination with MRI *113*
11.4.1 The Relevance of Preoperative T Staging *115*
11.4.2 Determination of the Circumferential Resection Margin with MRI *115*
11.4.3 Assessment of Local Tumour Extent in Locally Advanced and Recurrent Rectal Cancer *116*
11.5 Difficulties in Reading Rectal Cancer MRI *116*
11.5.1 Prediction of Nodal Involvement *117*
11.5.2 Prediction of the Circumferential Resection Margin in Distal Rectal Cancer *118*
11.5.3 Prediction of the Circumferential Resection Margin in Irradiated Rectal Cancer *119*
11.6 Conclusions *121*
References *121*

11.1 Introduction

Colorectal cancer is a major health problem with over 7500 new cases diagnosed each year in the Netherlands (VISSER et al. 1996). One third of all colorectal cancers occur in the rectosigmoid. Rectal cancer carries a poor prognosis because of the risk of metastases and local recurrences. After curative resection of the rectum for rectal cancer, local recurrence rates can vary from 3%–32% (SAGAR and PEMBERTON 1996). Although local recurrence has a small impact on survival, it has a profound impact on quality of life as it is often debilitating from severe pain and immobility, and involves prolonged and multiple hospital admissions for surgery, radiation and chemotherapy.

Incomplete removal of lateral tumour spread is now accepted as the cause of the majority of such recurrences (ADAM et al. 1994; QUIRKE et al. 1986). QUIRKE et al. (1986) demonstrated that microscopi-

cally positive resection margins resulted in a local recurrence rate of 83%. Attention has therefore been mainly directed at defining the best treatment strategy for the primary tumour, in order to obtain optimal local control.

A large randomised Scandinavian trial has shown that a short course of preoperative radiotherapy (5×5 Gy) can reduce the local recurrence rate from 27% to 11% (INVESTIGATORS SWEDISH RECTAL CANCER TRIAL 1997). Progress has also been made in refining the surgical procedure as the generally accepted standard procedure has become the total mesorectal excision (TME), in which the rectum is removed by sharp dissection along the mesorectal fascia. This mesorectal fascia, or visceral rectal fascia, completely encloses the mesorectum, a distinct anatomical unit that comprises the rectum, the perirectal fat and the superior hemorrhoidal vessels, nerves and lymphatics. The rectal cancer, lymph nodes and perirectal tumour deposits are most often confined to the mesorectum, with the mesorectal fascia acting as a barrier to tumour growth (Fig. 11.1). A complete removal of the mesorectum along the mesorectal fascia results in overall local recurrence rates of well below 10% even without the help of radiotherapy (HEALD and RYALL 1986).

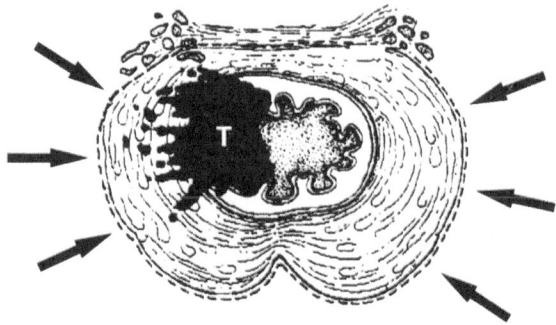

Fig. 11.1. Total mesorectal excision (TME) and its resection plane. Axial section through the mesorectum shows a rectal tumor (T) and its relation to the mesorectal fascia (*arrows*). Traditionally rectal cancer was resected through the mesorectal fat with the risk of leaving behind some tumour deposits. At TME the entire mesorectum is excised along the mesorectal fascia.

R. G. H. BEETS-TAN, MD, PhD; G. L. BEETS, MD, PhD
University Hospital Maastricht, P Debyelaan 25, PO Box 5800, 6202 AZ Maastricht, The Netherlands

The relative merits of both preoperative radiotherapy and total mesorectal excision in obtaining optimal local control have been tested in a large Dutch randomised trial (The Dutch TME Trial).

11.2
The Dutch TME Trial

This trial compared TME surgery with and without a preoperative short course of radiotherapy (KAPITEIJN et al. 2001). The trial showed that a short course of preoperative radiation therapy for all rectal cancer patients, with the exception of clinically obvious T4 tumours, reduces the local recurrence rate from 8.2% to 2.4% at 2 years. This implies that even with a properly performed TME resection patients with rectal cancer benefit from preoperative radiotherapy. However, if this treatment strategy was used for all rectal cancer patients, patients with stage I disease (T1/T2 N0M0) would be over treated because the local recurrence rate for this group is negligible (0.7% for the surgery arm versus 0.5% for the surgery and radiation arm). These are patients with tumour confined to the bowel wall and a wide circumferential resection margin (Fig. 11.2). Furthermore, the trial has shown that patients with stage II (T3N0) and III (TxN1) dis-

ease are at higher risk for local recurrence despite a short course of preoperative radiation therapy. These are patients with a close or involved resection margin and/or nodal disease who would benefit from a more extensive neoadjuvant treatment schedule (Fig. 11.3). At present it is unclear as to whether the ideal schedule should involve a short or long course of radiotherapy, with or without preoperative chemotherapy.

These findings suggest that different stages of rectal cancer have differing degrees of risk for local recurrence. On one side of the spectrum there is the low risk group, patients with superficial rectal cancer, that are adequately treated with surgery alone (a transanal resection or TME). At the other end of the spectrum there is a high risk group: patients with anticipated close or involved resection margin at TME, the very advanced tumours that probably require a longer course of chemo – radiotherapy and extensive surgery. Treatment selection depends on a reliable preoperative test that can distinguish between these groups.

11.3
Rectal Cancer Imaging

So far there has been no consensus as to the role of diagnostic imaging in the management of patients

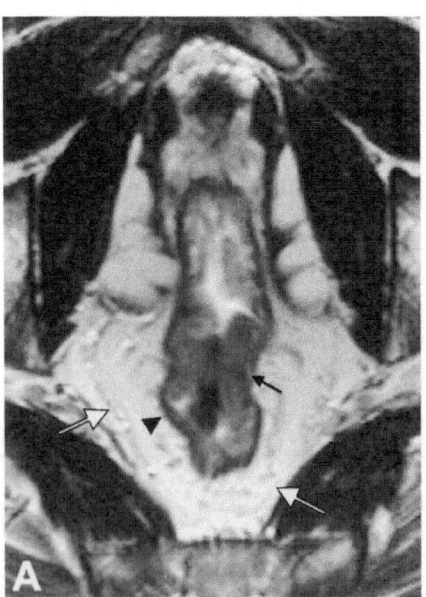
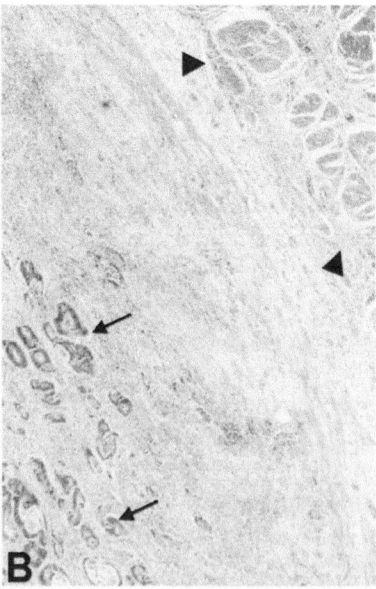

Fig.11.2a,b. T2 rectal cancer with a wide circumferential resection margin. **a** Axial T2W fast spin echo (TSE) MR image shows a thickening of the rectal wall, isointense (*small black arrow*) as compared to the intact hypointense rectal wall (*black arrowhead*). The distance from the tumour to the mesorectal fascia (*white arrows*) is more than 10 mm. This MR finding suggests a T2 rectal cancer with a wide circumferential resection margin. **b** Corresponding histology shows the tumour (*black arrows*) limited to the muscular rectal wall layers (*arrowheads*). The circumferential resection margin measured 9 mm at histology.

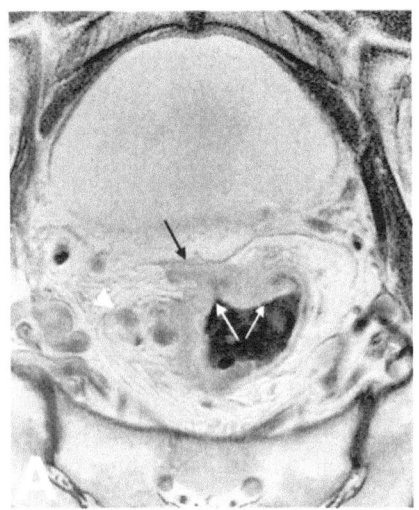

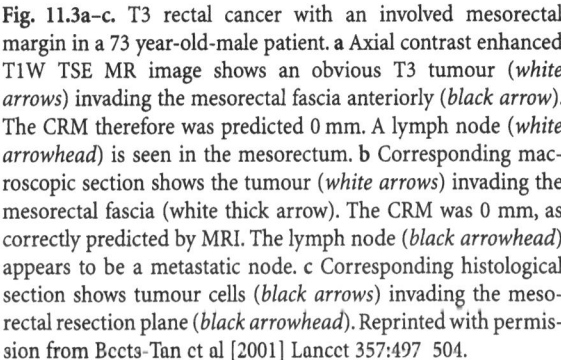

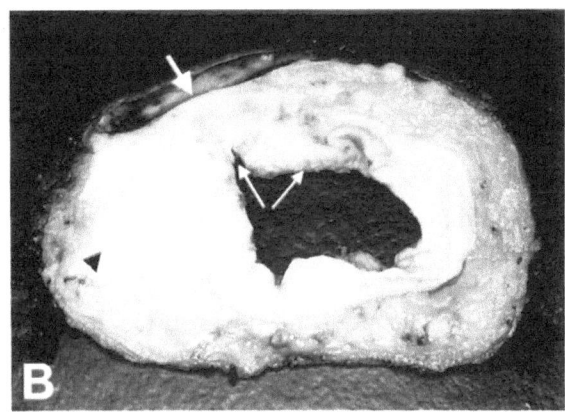

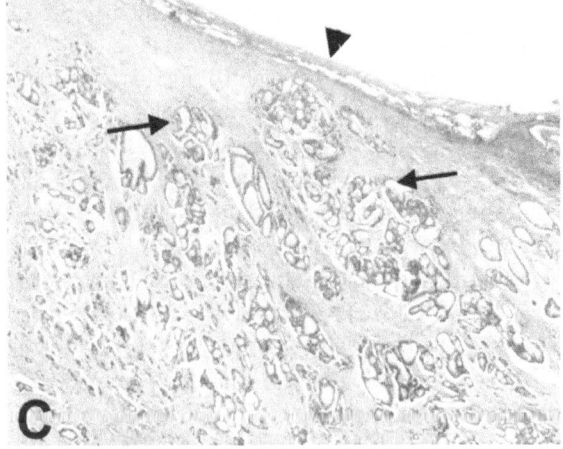

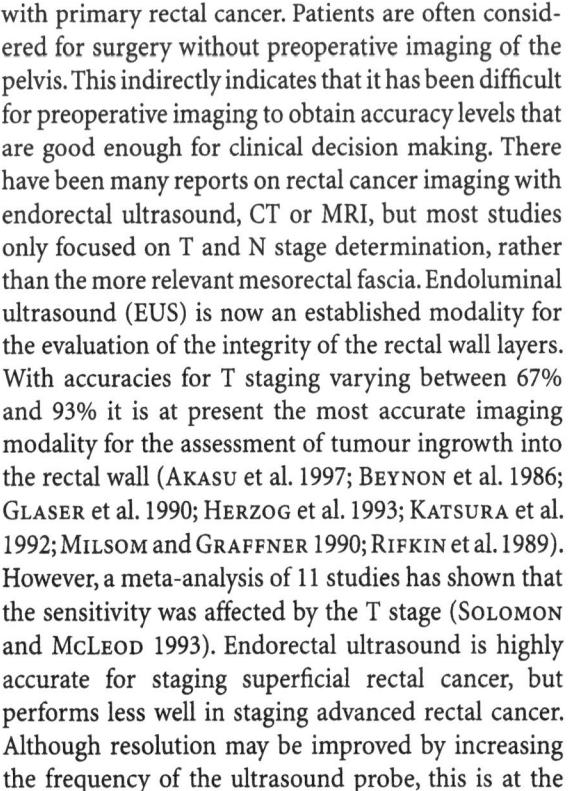

Fig. 11.3a–c. T3 rectal cancer with an involved mesorectal margin in a 73 year-old-male patient. **a** Axial contrast enhanced T1W TSE MR image shows an obvious T3 tumour (*white arrows*) invading the mesorectal fascia anteriorly (*black arrow*). The CRM therefore was predicted 0 mm. A lymph node (*white arrowhead*) is seen in the mesorectum. **b** Corresponding macroscopic section shows the tumour (*white arrows*) invading the mesorectal fascia (white thick arrow). The CRM was 0 mm, as correctly predicted by MRI. The lymph node (*black arrowhead*) appears to be a metastatic node. **c** Corresponding histological section shows tumour cells (*black arrows*) invading the mesorectal resection plane (*black arrowhead*). Reprinted with permission from Beets-Tan et al [2001] Lancet 357:497 504.

with primary rectal cancer. Patients are often considered for surgery without preoperative imaging of the pelvis. This indirectly indicates that it has been difficult for preoperative imaging to obtain accuracy levels that are good enough for clinical decision making. There have been many reports on rectal cancer imaging with endorectal ultrasound, CT or MRI, but most studies only focused on T and N stage determination, rather than the more relevant mesorectal fascia. Endoluminal ultrasound (EUS) is now an established modality for the evaluation of the integrity of the rectal wall layers. With accuracies for T staging varying between 67% and 93% it is at present the most accurate imaging modality for the assessment of tumour ingrowth into the rectal wall (AKASU et al. 1997; BEYNON et al. 1986; GLASER et al. 1990; HERZOG et al. 1993; KATSURA et al. 1992; MILSOM and GRAFFNER 1990; RIFKIN et al. 1989). However, a meta-analysis of 11 studies has shown that the sensitivity was affected by the T stage (SOLOMON and McLEOD 1993). Endorectal ultrasound is highly accurate for staging superficial rectal cancer, but performs less well in staging advanced rectal cancer. Although resolution may be improved by increasing the frequency of the ultrasound probe, this is at the

expense of tissue penetration and because of this the mesorectal fascia and surrounding structures are difficult to identify with endorectal sonography.

11.4
T Stage Determination with MRI

MRI provides images in multiple planes and with a high soft tissue contrast resolution, without the need for ionising radiation. Initial reports on magnetic resonance imaging of the pelvis were promising, and MRI was soon evaluated for rectal diseases. Conventional MR techniques using a body coil had a resolution that was still insufficient to differentiate the layers of the rectum. The overall accuracy reported for body coil MRI ranged from 59% to 95% (BUTCH et al. 1986; COVA et al. 1994; GUINET et al. 1990; HODGMAN et al. 1986; McNICHOLAS et al. 1994; OKIZUKA et al. 1993; STARCK et al. 1995; ZERHOUNI et al. 1996) and is no better than CT.

Efforts were therefore aimed at increasing the signal-to-noise ratio in order to obtain small voxel sizes. With the introduction of endoluminal coils, spatial resolution improved and detailed evaluation of the layers of the rectal wall was feasible (VOGL et al. 1998). This was also reflected in improved and more consistent accuracy for T staging ranging from 66% to 91% (CHAN et al. 1991; IMAI et al. 1990; INDIN-NIMEO et al. 1996; JOOSTEN et al. 1995; MALDJIAN et al. 2000; PEGIOS et al. 1996; SCHNALL et al. 1994; VOGL et al. 1997; ZAGORIA et al. 1997).

Although endorectal MRI is very accurate for the assessment of tumour ingrowth into the layers of the rectal wall and shows accuracies comparable to EUS, some problems remain. The major shortcoming of the endoluminal technique is the sudden signal drop off at short distance from the coil which limits its field of view. Therefore the mesorectal fascia and surrounding pelvic structures are difficult to visualise (DESOUZA et al. 1996). Furthermore, the positioning of an endoluminal device can be difficult or impossible in patients with high or stenosing tumours, and failure rates for insertion as high as 40% have been reported in patients with rectal cancer.

With the introduction of dedicated surface phased array coils, improved MRI performance was expected (BEETS-TAN et al. 1999, 2001a,c; BLOMQVIST et al. 2000; BROWN et al. 1999). A phased array coil consists of an arrangement of multiple surface coils that result in a considerable improvement in the signal to noise ratio and so images can be obtained with a high

spatial resolution and a large field of view. However, the first MRI studies involving the use of these coils reported an overall accuracy for T staging of only 55%–65% and showed no benefit as compared to the body coil MR technique or even to CT (HADFIELD et al. 1997; DE LANGE et al. 1989). The low performance of MRI in these studies could have been attributed to the low spatial resolution used but even when a higher spatial resolution was applied with the newer generation phased array coil MR techniques, the accuracy for T staging was not as high as anticipated with figures varying between 67% and 83% (BEETS-TAN et al. 2001b; BLOMVIST et al. 1997) and considerable interobserver variability (BEETS-TAN et al. 2001b). An exception to the above findings were those of BROWN et al. (1999) who reported a 100% accuracy and complete agreement between two independent readers for predicting tumour stage with phased array MRI.

Most staging failures with MRI occur in the differentiation of T2 from borderline T3 lesions with overstaging as the main cause of error. These staging difficulties apply to both the endoluminal and the phased array MR technique. Overstaging is often caused by desmoplastic reaction (BEETS-TAN et al. 2001b; MEYENBERGER et al. 1995; VOGL et al. 1997) as it is difficult to distinguish on MRI between spiculation in the perirectal fat caused by fibrosis alone (stage pT2) and spiculation caused by fibrosis that contains tumour cells (stage pT3) (BEETS-TAN et al. 2001b) (Figs. 11.4 and 11.5).

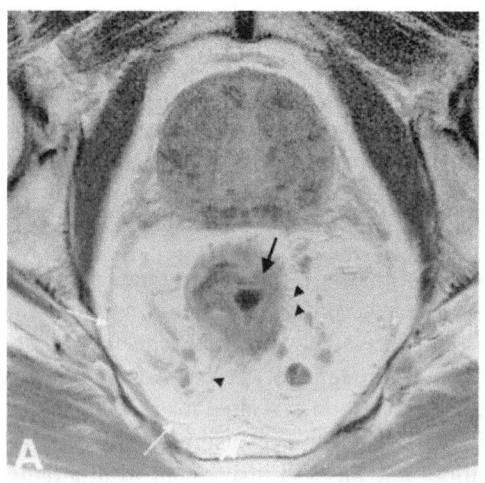
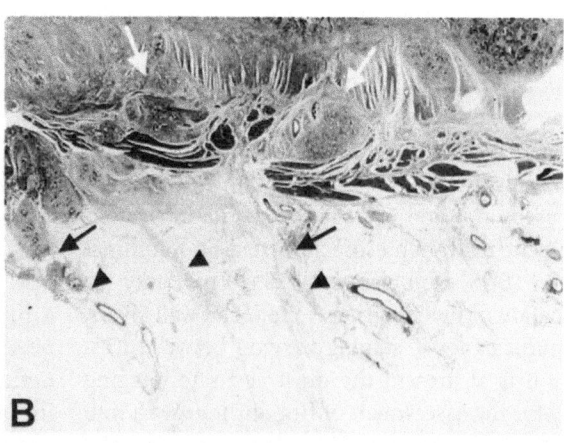

Fig. 11.4a,b. T3 rectal cancer in a 70-year-old male patient. **a** Axial contrast enhanced T1W TSE MR image shows a tumour (*black arrow*) with extramural stranding (*black arrowheads*), suggesting a T3 rectal cancer. The mesorectal fascia (*small white arrows*) and the presacral fascia (*white thick arrow*) are well visualized. An enlarged lymph node is seen in the mesorectum postero-lateral from the tumour. On these images a wide tumour free CRM was predicted both when measured from the tumour and from the lymph node. **b** Corresponding histology demonstrates that the spiculations consist of a desmoplastic reaction (*black arrowheads*). In contrast to the tumour shown in fig. 11.5 these fibrotic strands contain tumour cells (*black arrows*). The tumour penetrates the muscular rectal wall (*white arrows*) and is therefore staged T3. The lymph node contained malignant cells and the CRM was more than 10 mm. Fig. 11.4 and 11.5 illustrate that it can be difficult with MRI to distinguish between desmoplastic reaction with and without tumor cells. Reprinted with permission from Beets-Tan et al [2001] Lancet 357:497–504.

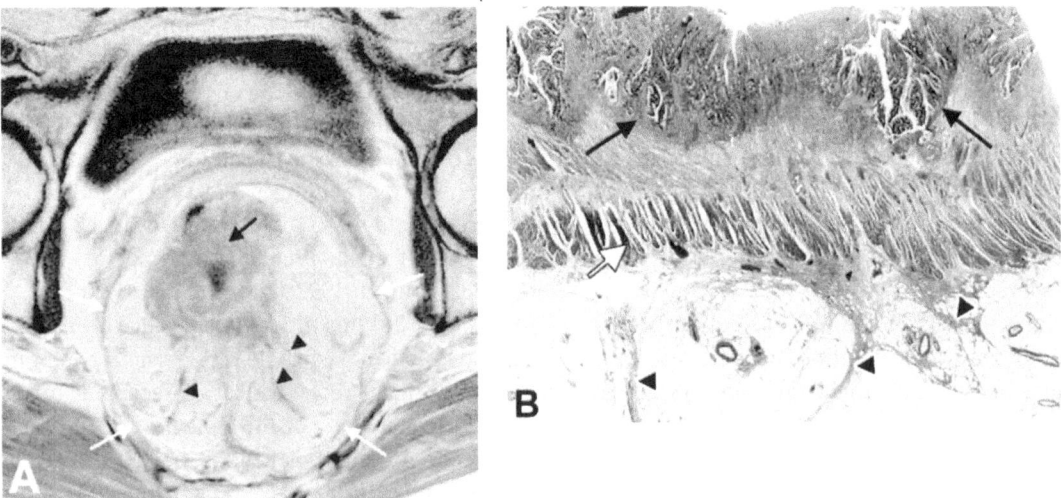

Fig. 11.5a,b. Histological T2 rectal cancer in a 67-year-old female patient, overstaged by MRI as a T3 tumour. a Axial contrast enhanced T1W TSE MR image shows an enhancing mass in the laterodorsal rectal wall (*black arrow*). Because of the extramural stranding from the tumour into the perirectal fat (*black arrowheads*) the tumor was staged as T3. The mesorectal fascia is clearly visualized (*white arrows*). A circumferential resection margin (CRM) of more than 10 mm was predicted. b Corresponding histology demonstrates that the spiculations are formed by desmoplastic reaction from the tumour. The fibrotic strands (*black arrowheads*) contain no tumour cells. The tumour (*black arrows*) does not penetrate the muscular rectal wall (*white arrow*) and is therefore staged T2. Although MRI overstaged the tumour, it correctly predicted a histological CRM of more than 10 mm. Reprinted with permission from Beets-Tan et al [2001] Lancet 357:497–504.

Endoluminal MR techniques using dynamic contrast enhanced sequences have been proposed to solve this problem as they can more reliably show complete rupture of the muscular rectal wall (Vogl et al. 1997). However, there is significant interobserver variability and so the reliability of this technique is in question (Drew et al. 1999).

11.4.1
The Relevance of Preoperative T Staging

Although the TNM staging system is a very reliable prognostic indicator, it does have its limitations. It may be valuable to preoperatively identify those patients with small superficial (T1) tumours that can be treated with transanal resection, but the majority of rectal cancer patients have T2 or T3 tumours, both of which require complete excision. A T3 tumour that has just breached the muscularis propria of the rectal wall and minimally penetrates the mesorectal fat (Fig. 11.4) will have a lower risk for recurrence than a T3 tumour that invades the mesorectal fascia (Fig. 11.3). Therefore there is little benefit in differentiating between tumours limited to the rectal wall (T2) and tumours that have just breached the wall (minimal T3) when this does not influence preoperative or operative management.

11.4.2
Determination of the Circumferential Resection Margin with MRI

It has been repeatedly shown that it is the distance from the tumour to the circumferential resection margin that is the most powerful predictor of local recurrence rate (Nagtegaal et al. 2002; Quirke and Dixon 1988; Wibe et al. 2002) and not the T stage. It would therefore be of far more importance to be able to identify preoperatively by imaging those tumours that will have a close resection margin so that they can be selected for more extensive neoadjuvant treatment and for more extensive surgery. Recent editorials in the *Lancet* and the *New England Journal of Medicine* have stressed the importance of tailoring treatment in rectal cancer and the need for an accurate method of selecting patients on the basis of risk factors (Nelson and Sargent 2001; Radcliffe and Brown 2001).

Prediction of the circumferential resection margins has not been the subject of many imaging studies. The reason is that radiologists were not acquainted with the concept of total mesorectal excision, and were not used to evaluating the mesorectal fascia as an anatomic border. The very first report on the identification of the mesorectal fascia by imaging was published in 1983 (Grabbe et al. 1983), but since then nothing has been published until very recently (BLOMQVIST et al. 1999; BROWN et al. 1999). In one report the mesorectal fascia was visualised with a high resolution phased array MR technique, and although the authors concluded that the depth of tumour extension could be predicted, the more relevant distance between tumour and fascia was not studied (BROWN et al. 1999). With postoperative MRI of resected specimens BLOMQVIST et al. (1999) were able to predict the tumour-free lateral resection margin with high accuracy.

A landmark study on the MR evaluation of circumferential resection margins in patients with rectal cancer was published in the *Lancet* early in 2001 (BEETS-TAN et al. 2001b). Using a high resolution phased array MR technique the authors reported a higher accuracy for the prediction of the circumferential resection margin in 76 rectal cancer patients than for the prediction of the T stage. An important finding is the high agreement of the measurements both between and within the observers in contrast to the only moderate intra- and interobserver agreement for the T stage determination. This indicates that phased array MRI is more reliable for the assessment of the circumferential resection margin than for the assessment of the T stage. These results were confirmed in a third study on the MR determination of the circumferential resection margins in 43 patients (BISSETT et al. 2001). The authors not only reported a 95% accuracy on the MR prediction of the tumour-free lateral resection margin with a phased array technique, they also proved in a cadaver study that the fascia that was visualised on high resolution phased array MRI was indeed the mesorectal fascia.

Although the value of a preoperative MRI in patient management is presently being evaluated in larger clinical trials, these findings already suggest that that the anatomical information provided by a high resolution MRI is detailed, reliable and easy to communicate.

11.4.3
Assessment of Local Tumour Extent in Locally Advanced and Recurrent Rectal Cancer

Approximately 10%–20% of rectal tumours are locally advanced and fixed to surrounding pelvic organs. In these cases the patient's best chance for cure is a radical en bloc resection of the tumour and the surrounding invaded structures (POEZE et al. 1995). Accurate and detailed anatomic information on tumour extent is essential not only for the selection of patients for an extensive course of chemoradiation to shrink the tumour but also for planning the optimal surgical

procedure. The same holds true for locally recurrent rectal cancer (SAGAR and PEMBERTON 1996).

In the imaging literature only a few studies have addressed the problem of predicting primary rectal cancer infiltration into neighbouring organs (BLOMQVIST et al. 1997; COVA et al. 1994; DE LANGE et al. 1989; POPVICH et al. 1993). Based on the initial optimistic results for CT in staging advanced rectal cancer (BUTCH et al. 1986; HODGMAN et al. 1986; MOSS 1989; THOENI 1997; THOENI et al. 1981; ZAUNBAUER et al. 1981) this modality has since been used in clinical practice to evaluate local tumour extent in patients with fixed rectal cancer or recurrent rectal cancer. The exact value of MRI has never fully been investigated. Although MRI has been extensively compared with CT for its accuracy in detecting local recurrences, only few publications exist comparing CT and MRI for the prediction of local tumour extent (BEETS-TAN et al. 2000; BLOMQVIST et al. 1996, 2002). In an early study BLOMQVIST et al. found a better prediction for organ invasion with pelvic phased array MRI (6/9) than with CT (3/9), but this was based on only a limited number of patients. The same author recently published the results of a study in 16 patients with advanced rectal cancer. This showed superior performance for MRI in the prediction of urinary bladder and uterine invasion (BLOMQVIST et al. 2002). BEETS-TAN et al. (2000) found phased array MRI far more accurate than CT in predicting pelvic floor invasion, piriform muscle invasion (Fig. 11.6) and subtle bone invasion (Fig. 11.7) but the large difference in outcome between the two modalities could partially be attributed to the fact that a state of the art high resolution MR technique was compared with conventional CT techniques.

Theoretically newer generation multislice spiral CT techniques with optimal bolus timing and reconstructions in multiple planes may perform better than conventional CT (CHIESURA-CORONA et al. 2001; HORTON et al. 2000). In a study of 105 rectal cancer patients undergoing a spiral CT an improved overall accuracy for T staging (82%) was reported (CHIESURA-CORONA et al. 2001). However this study only included four T4 lesions. Thus, to date, the role of multislice spiral CT in rectal cancer imaging has not been fully explored.

11.5
Difficulties in Reading Rectal Cancer MRI

Despite the accuracy of phased array MRI in the preoperative selection of different risk groups of rectal

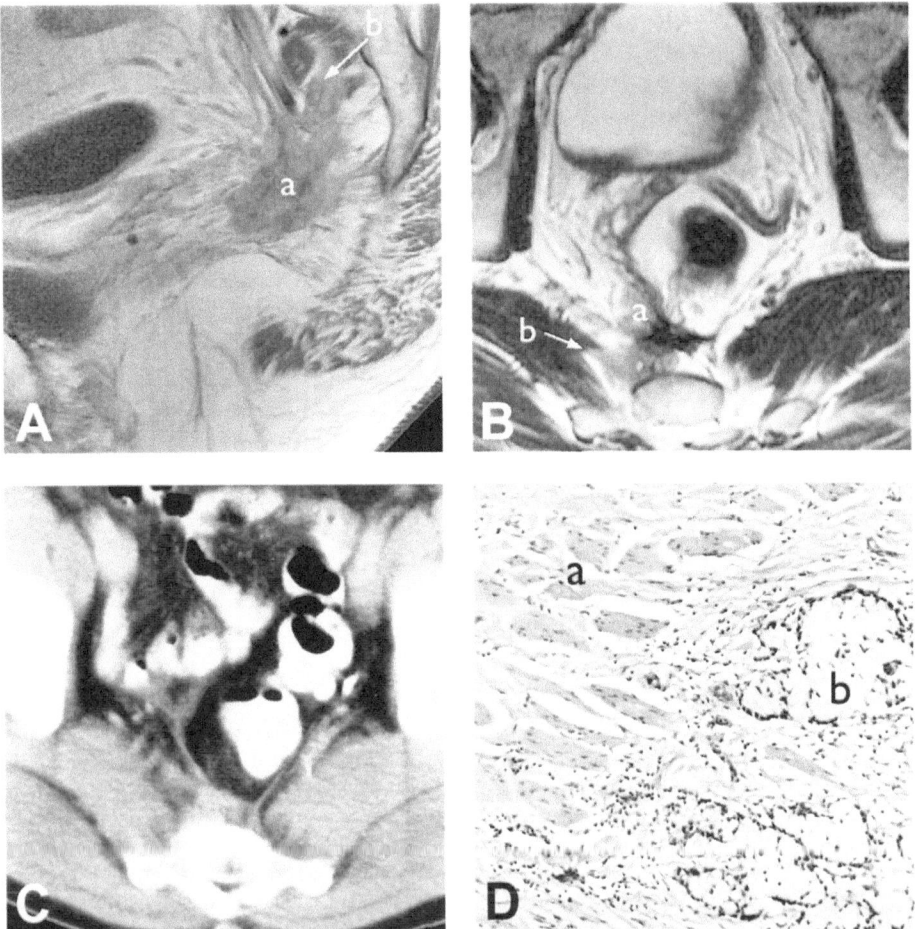

Fig. 11.6a–d. A 55-year-old male with recurrent rectal cancer in the presacral region. **a** Sagittal contrast-enhanced T1W TSE MRI accurately shows the tumor (**a**) invading the right piriform muscle (**b**). **b** Axial T2W TSE MRI also clearly visualizes the tumor (**a**) invading the presacral space and the right piriforin muscle (**b**). (The axial plane was angled perpendicular to the sacral bone.) **c** CT shows the tumor mass but fails to show the exact extent into the piriform muscle. **d** Corresponding histologic section through the right piriform muscle shows tumor (**b**) infiltrating the muscle fibers (**a**). Reprinted with permission from Beets-Tan et al [2000] Abdominal Imaging 25:533–541.

cancer patients there are some pitfalls. Difficulties may arise in the prediction of nodal involvement and in the prediction of the circumferential margins in distal and irradiated rectal cancer.

11.5.1
Prediction of Nodal Involvement

At present the exact relation between metastatic lymph nodes and local recurrence is not known. Nodal disease is an important prognostic indicator for overall survival. In some reports nodal disease was associated with a higher rate of local recurrence (KAPITEIJN et al. 2001; PHILLIPS et al. 1984), whereas in others there was no such association (CAWTHORN et al. 1990; DE HAAS-KOCK et al. 1996; HEALD and RYALL 1986; WIBE et al. 2002). Further trials will need to show whether lymph node involvement is an important prognostic indicator for local recurrence irrespective of the resection margins. If it is, then radiologists will face a problem as at the moment there is no imaging method that can reliably detect nodal metastases. The radiological assessment of nodal involvement generally relies on morphological criteria such as the size and shape of the node (CARRINGTON 1998; JAGER et al. 1996; WILLIAMS et al. 2001). As a consequence differentiation between enlarged reactive and metastatic nodes is difficult and micrometastases are easily missed in normal sized nodes. Most imaging studies have so far been performed in patients with nodal disease in urologi-

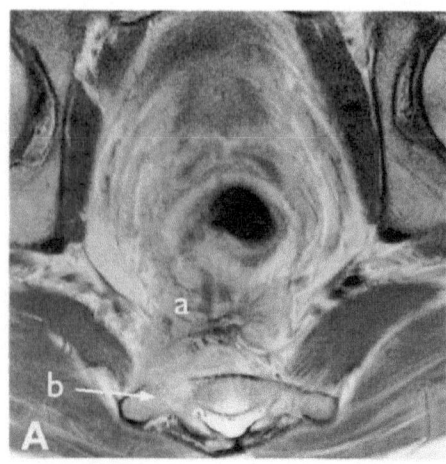
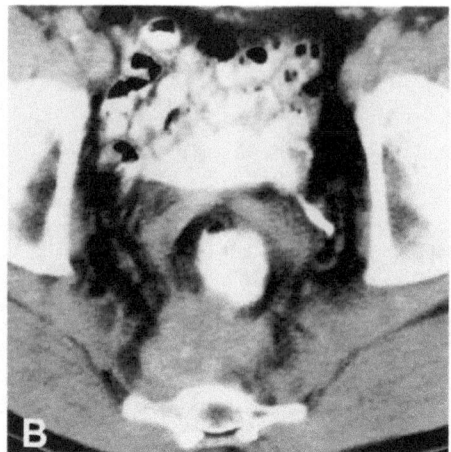
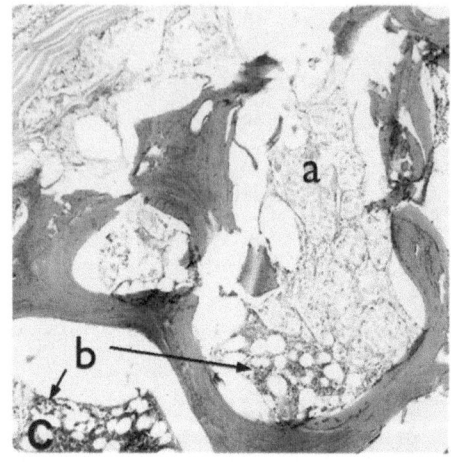

Fig. 11.7a–c. A 48-year-old male with recurrent rectal cancer in the presacral region. **a** Axial T2W TSE MRI shows the tumour (a) invading the bone marrow (b). **b** Axial CT at the level of the tumour fails to show bone invasion. The axial CT section may appear to be at a different level because of the slightly different angulation of the MR axial section (perpendicular to the sacral bone). **c** Histology confirms the tumour (a) invading the bone marrow (b). The trabecular bone is intact. Reprinted with permission from Beets-Tan et al [2000] Abdominal Imaging 25:533–541.

cal and gynaecological cancer and large studies in rectal cancer patients are lacking. An additional problem in rectal cancer as compared with other pelvic tumours is the high frequency of micrometastases in normal sized nodes (DWORAK 1989). It is therefore not surprising that a large variation in accuracy for nodal detection can be found in the imaging literature for EUS (62%–83%) (AKASU et al. 1997; BEYNON et al. 1989; GLASER et al. 1990; HERZOG et al. 1993; KWOK et al. 2000; RIFKIN et al. 1989; TIO et al. 1991), as well as for CT (22%–73%) (BALTHAZAR et al. 1988; GUINET et al. 1990; HOLDSWORTH et al. 1988; KWOK et al. 2000; SHANK et al. 1990; THOMPSON et al. 1986) and MRI (39%–95%) (BUTCH et al. 1986; DE LANGE et al. 1990; GUINET et al. 1990; HODGMAN et al. 1986; INDINNIMEO et al. 1996; KWOK et al. 2000; MCNICHOLAS et al. 1994; OKIZUKA et al. 1993; SCHNALL et al. 1994; THALER et al. 1994; ZAGORIA et al. 1997).

There have been some preliminary reports on studies with dynamic contrast enhanced MRI using ultra-small super paramagnetic iron oxide

contrast agents (USPIO) (BELLIN and BARENTSZ 2001). The addition of functional criteria to morphological criteria has been shown to improve detection accuracy of nodal metastases in patients with urological tumours (92% accuracy), but the role of USPIO enhanced MRI in rectal cancer patients has never been studied and certainly deserves investigation.

11.5.2
Prediction of the Circumferential Resection Margin in Distal Rectal Cancer

Tumours located in the distal rectum, specifically low and anteriorly located rectal cancer, can pose a problem for surgeons as well as for radiologists. These tumours generally show a higher rate of local recurrence (KAPITEIJN et al. 2001). The mesorectum contains less mesorectal fat ventrally and there is less fat distally by virtue of its tapered anatomy (Fig. 11.8). Technically it is more difficult for sur-

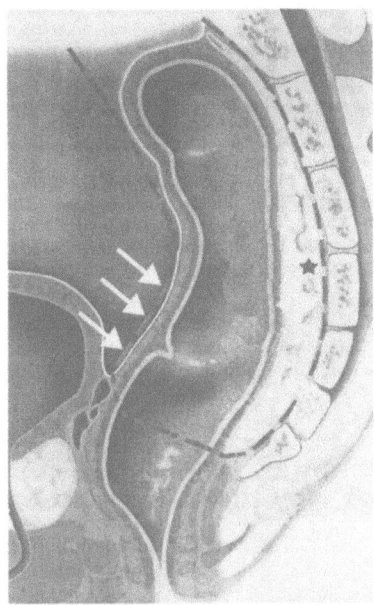

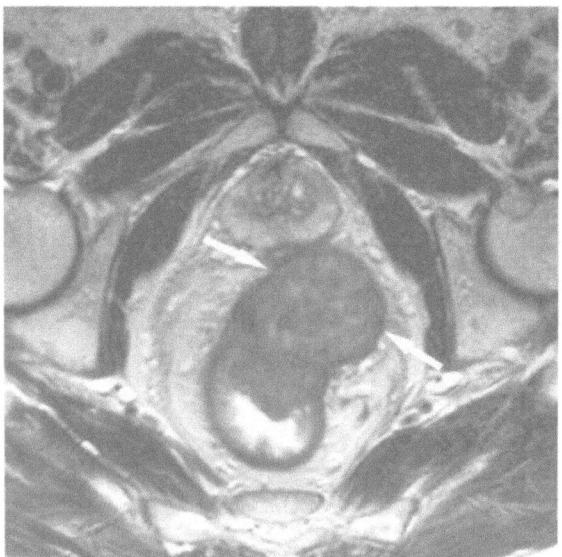

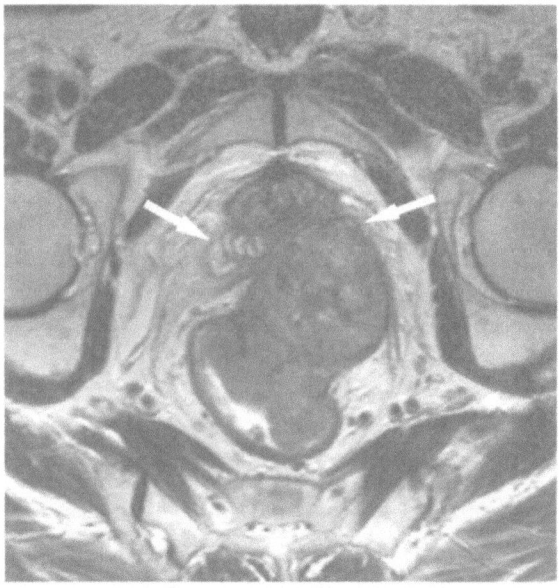

Fig. 11.8. Anatomy of the distal mesorectum. Sagittal section of the mesorectum shows the complex anatomy of the distal mesorectum. On the ventral and distal side the mesorectum contains less mesorectal fat (*arrows*) than on the posterior side (*asterisk*). It can therefore be more difficult for the surgeons to obtain a complete resection in these low rectal tumours. Caution is necessary when interpreting MR images of low and anterior tumours, as illustrated in figs 11. 9, 11.10 and 11.11.

Fig. 11.9a,b. Low and anterior T4 rectal cancer. **a** Axial T2W TSE MR image illustrates a rectal tumour that has penetrated the mesorectal fascia on the ventral side (*white arrows*) and **b** that has clearly invaded the seminal vesicles (*white arrows*). It is obvious that the mesorectal resection plane in this patient is involved. Based on these MR images the patient was selected for a long course of chemo-radiation before extensive surgery.

geons to completely resect these tumours. Also from an imaging point of view, there are problems in staging low rectal cancer as a consequence of the rectal anatomy. Even the best staging method, EUS, fails to accurately stage these tumours (HERZOG et al. 1993; SAILER et al. 1997) (Figs. 11.9–11.11). The main message is that one needs to be aware of a very close or involved anterior resection margin when dealing with low rectal tumours.

11.5.3
Prediction of the Circumferential Resection Margin in Irradiated Rectal Cancer

MR images of rectal cancer patients who have had a long course of radiotherapy may be difficult to interpret. Radiation therapy can induce fibrosis, both in normal tissue and in areas of tumour necrosis. MRI cannot reliably distinguish between fibrosis and fibrosis that contains tumour cells (BEETS-TAN et al. 2000; DE LANGE et al. 1989; KAHN et al. 1997).

This can pose diagnostic problems in predicting whether the cancer is close to or actually invading the mesorectal resection plane and surrounding organs. In order to minimise such problems the assessment of organ invasion should be made on a baseline MRI before radiotherapy (BEETS-TAN et al. 2000) (Figs. 11.12 and 11.13).

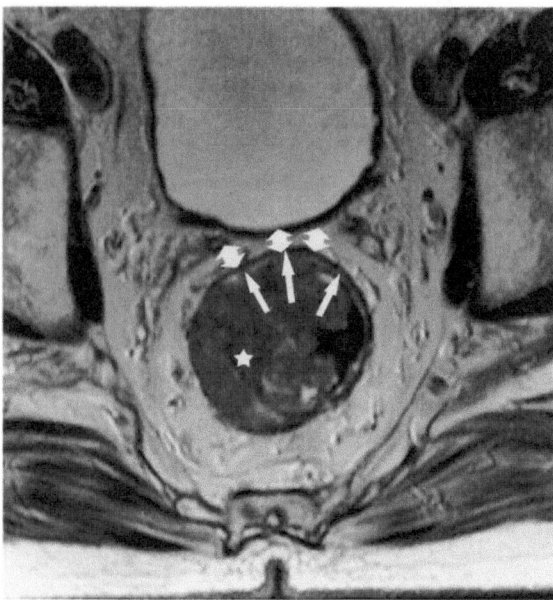

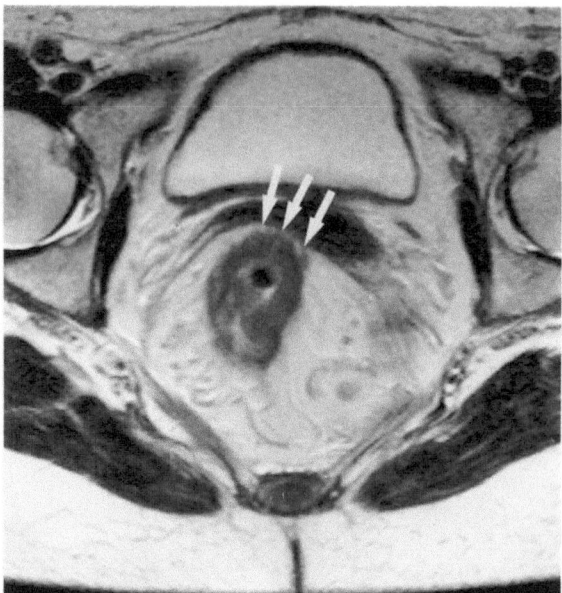

Fig. 11.10. Anterior rectal cancer with a close but tumor free resection margin. Axial T2W fast spin echo MR image shows the tumour (*asterisk*) and an intact hypointense rectal wall on the ventral side (*arrows*). The MR diagnosis of a T2 rectal cancer was confidently made and the surgeon told that although the margin on the anterior side would be close, it would be free (*double arrowheads*). This was confirmed at histology.

Fig. 11.11. Low anterior rectal cancer: Always be aware of a close resection margin! Axial T2W TSE MR image shows a rectal tumour anteriorly, which has just breached the rectal wall (*white arrows*). Interpretation difficulties can arise with these anterior tumours. Is it tumour or only desmoplastic reaction that you're looking at? However, no matter what the exact T stage (T2 or T3) of the tumour is, one always needs to be aware of a very close or involved anterior resection margin when dealing with these low cancers, so that the surgeon can anticipate the need for a wider excision.

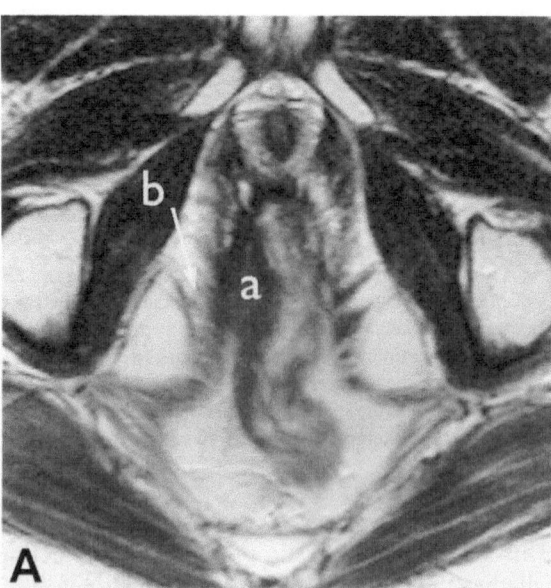

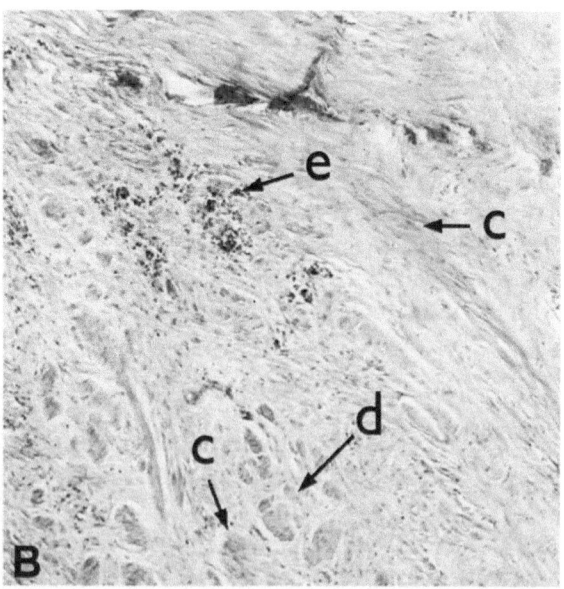

Fig. 11.12a,b. A 67-year-old male with rectal cancer involving the pelvic floor, after a full dose of preoperative radiotherapy. **a** Axial post irradiation T2W TSE MRI shows a hypointense thickening of the right latero-ventral rectal wall (**a**) extending into the right pelvic floor (**b**), suggesting fibrosis. **b** Corresponding histology shows fibrosis (**c**) between the muscle fibers (**d**). No tumor cells were seen. The tumour has responded well to radiotherapy and has been completely replaced by fibrosis. (**e**) inflammatory response. Reprinted with permission from Beets-Tan et al [2000] Abdominal Imaging 25:533–541.

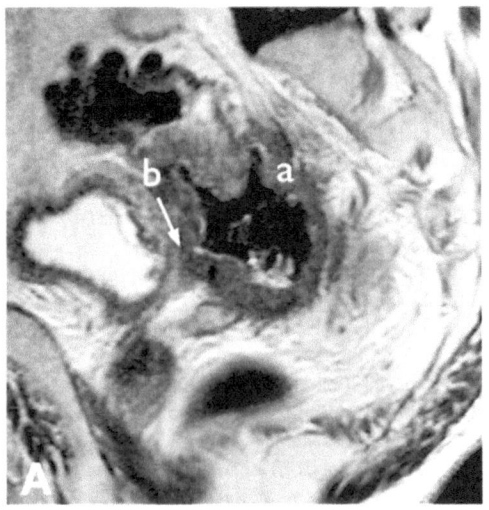
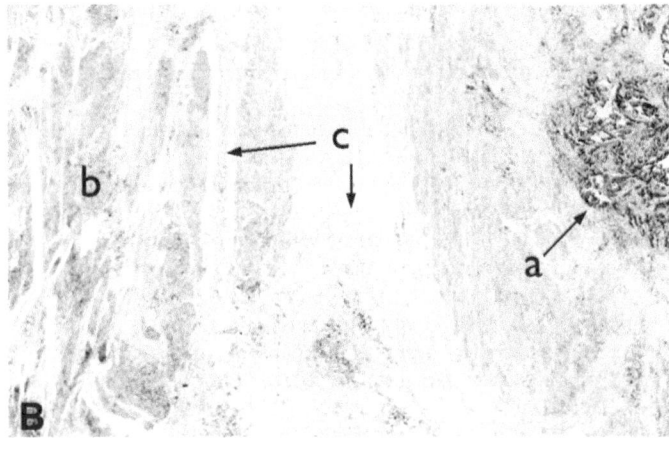

Fig. 11.13a,b. A 62-year-old male with primary rectal cancer involving the bladder, after a full dose of radiotherapy. **a** Sagittal T2W TSE MRI shows a hypointense thickening of the rectal wall (**a**) invading the dorsal bladder wall (**b**), suggesting fibrosis. **b** At histology there is still viable tumor in the rectal wall (**a**), surrounded by extensive fibrosis (**c**), that is invading the muscular bladder wall (**b**). This fibrosis may be tumor that has responded to radiotherapy. MRI was not able to distinguish between fibrosis and the tumor. Reprinted with permission from Beets-Tan et al [2000] Abdominal Imaging 25:533–541.

11.6
Conclusions

Since the recent introduction of new treatment strategies for rectal cancer (preoperative radiotherapy and total mesorectal excision) there is a growing need for an accurate method of imaging to select patients at different risk for local recurrence so that appropriate preoperative management decisions can be made.

For superficial rectal cancer that can be treated with surgery alone, EUS remains the most accurate staging modality for the assessment of tumour ingrowth into the muscular rectal wall. Endorectal MRI is as accurate as EUS but at present EUS remains the imaging modality of choice for staging superficial tumours because it is more readily available and less expensive. Although both endoluminal techniques provide clear detail of the rectal wall, EUS is less accurate for evaluating the outer border of the mesorectum: the mesorectal fascia and its relation to the tumour (the circumferential resection margin).

For all remaining mobile and fixed rectal cancers MRI, using a high resolution phased array coil, is at present the most reliable method of imaging the mesorectal plane and the circumferential resection margins. Preoperative identification of these margins allows selection of patients at different risk for recurrence so that each patient can be given the most appropriate treatment.

Despite the potential of multislice spiral CT, its role in rectal cancer imaging has yet to be fully explored.

References

Adam IJ et al (1994) Role of circumferential margin involvement in the local recurrence of rectal cancer (see comments). Lancet 344:707–711

Akasu T et al (1997) Limitations and pitfalls of transrectal ultrasonography for staging of rectal cancer. Dis Colon Rectum 40:S10–S15

Balthazar EJ et al (1988) Carcinoma of the colon: detection and preoperative staging by CT. AJR Am J Roentgenol 150: 301–306

Beets-Tan RG et al (1999) High-resolution magnetic resonance imaging of the anorectal region without an endocoil. Abdom Imaging 24:576–581; discussion 582–584

Beets-Tan RG et al (2000) Preoperative assessment of local tumor extent in advanced rectal cancer: CT or high-resolution MRI? Abdom Imaging 25:533–541

Beets-Tan RG et al (2001a) Preoperative MR imaging of anal fistulas: does it really help the surgeon? Radiology 218: 75–84

Beets-Tan RG et al (2001b) Accuracy of magnetic resonance imaging in prediction of tumour-free resection margin in rectal cancer surgery. Lancet 357:497–504

Beets-Tan RG et al (2001c) Measurement of anal sphincter muscles: endoanal US, endoanal MR imaging, or phased-array MR imaging? A study with healthy volunteers. Radiology 220:81–89

Bellin MF, Barentsz JO (2001) MR lymphography in pelvic cancer. Eur Radiol 11:A19

Beynon J et al (1986) Endoluminal ultrasound in the assessment of local invasion in rectal cancer. Br J Surg 73: 474–477

Beynon J et al (1989) Preoperative assessment of mesorectal lymph node involvement in rectal cancer. Br J Surg 76: 276–279

Bissett IP et al (2001) Identification of the fascia propria by magnetic resonance imaging and its relevance to preoperative assessment of rectal cancer. Dis Colon Rectum 44: 259–265

Blomqvist L et al (1996) MR imaging, CT and CEA scintigraphy in the diagnosis of local recurrence of rectal carcinoma. Acta Radiol 37:779–784

Blomqvist L et al (1997) Rectal tumours – MR imaging with endorectal and/or phased–array coils, and histopathological staging on giant sections. A comparative study. Acta Radiol 38:437–444

Blomqvist L et al (1999) Rectal adenocarcinoma: assessment of tumour involvement of the lateral resection margin by MRI of resected specimen. Br J Radiol 72:18–23

Blomqvist L et al (2000) Rectal tumour staging: MR imaging using pelvic phased-array and endorectal coils vs endoscopic ultrasonography (in process citation). Eur Radiol 10:653–660

Blomqvist L et al (2002) MR imaging and computed tomography in patients with rectal tumours clinically judged as locally advanced. Clin Radiol 57:211–218

Brown G et al (1999) Rectal carcinoma: thin-section MR imaging for staging in 28 patients. Radiology 211:215–222

Butch RJ et al (1986) Staging rectal cancer by MR and CT. AJR Am J Roentgenol 146:1155–1160

Carrington B (1998) Lymph nodes. In: Husband JES RR (ed) Imaging in oncology. Isis Medical Media, Oxford, England

Cawthorn SJ et al (1990) Extent of mesorectal spread and involvement of lateral resection margin as prognostic factors after surgery for rectal cancer (see comments). Lancet 335:1055–1059

Chan TW et al (1991) Rectal carcinoma: staging at MR imaging with endorectal surface coil. Work in progress. Radiology 181:461–467

Chiesura-Corona M et al (2001) Rectal cancer: CT local staging with histopathologic correlation. Abdom Imaging 26: 134–138

Cova M et al (1994) Computed tomography and magnetic resonance in the preoperative staging of the spread of rectal cancer. A correlation with the anatomicopathological aspects. Radiol Med (Torino) 87:82–89

De Haas-Kock DF et al (1996) Prognostic significance of radial margins of clearance in rectal cancer. Br J Surg 83: 781–785

De Lange EE et al (1989) Suspected recurrent rectosigmoid carcinoma after abdominoperineal resection: MR imaging and histopathologic findings. Radiology 170:323–328

De Lange EE et al (1990) Preoperative staging of rectal carcinoma with MR imaging: surgical and histopathologic correlation. Radiology 176:623–628

DeSouza NM et al (1996) High resolution magnetic resonance imaging of the anal sphincter using a dedicated endoanal coil. Comparison of magnetic resonance imaging with surgical findings. Dis Colon Rectum 39:926–934

Drew PJ et al (1999) Preoperative magnetic resonance staging of rectal cancer with an endorectal coil and dynamic gadolinium enhancement. Br J Surg 86:250–254

Dworak O (1989) Number and size of lymph nodes and node metastases in rectal carcinomas. Surg Endosc 3:96–99

Glaser F et al (1990) Endorectal ultrasonography for the assessment of invasion of rectal tumours and lymph node involvement. Br J Surg 77:883–887

Grabbe E et al (1983) The perirectal fascia: morphology and use in staging of rectal carcinoma. Radiology 149:241–246

Guinet C et al (1990) Comparison of magnetic resonance imaging and computed tomography in the preoperative staging of rectal cancer. Arch Surg 125:385–388

Hadfield MB et al (1997) Preoperative staging of rectal carcinoma by magnetic resonance imaging with a pelvic phased–array coil. Br J Surg 84:529–531

Heald RJ, Ryall RD (1986) Recurrence and survival after total mesorectal excision for rectal cancer. Lancet 1:1479–1482

Herzog U et al (1993) How accurate is endorectal ultrasound in the preoperative staging of rectal cancer? Dis Colon Rectum 36:127–134

Hodgman CG et al (1986) Preoperative staging of rectal carcinoma by computed tomography and 0.15T magnetic resonance imaging. Preliminary report. Dis Colon Rectum 29:446–450

Holdsworth PJ et al (1988) Endoluminal ultrasound and computed tomography in the staging of rectal cancer. Br J Surg 75:1019–1022

Horton KM et al (2000) Spiral CT of colon cancer: imaging features and role in management. Radiographics 20:419–430

Imai Y et al (1990) Colorectal tumors: an in vitro study of high-resolution MR imaging. Radiology 177:695–701

Indinnimeo M et al (1996) Endorectal magnetic resonance imaging in the preoperative staging of rectal tumors. Int Surg 81:419–422

Investigators Swedish Rectal Cancer Trial (1997) Improved survival with preoperative radiotherapy in resectable rectal cancer. Swedish Rectal Cancer Trial (see comments) (published erratum appears in N Engl J Med 1997, 336:1539). N Engl J Med 336:980–987

Jager GJ et al (1996) Pelvic adenopathy in prostatic and urinary bladder carcinoma: MR imaging with a three-dimensional TI-weighted magnetization-prepared-rapid gradient-echo sequence. AJR Am J Roentgenol 167:1503–1507

Joosten FB et al (1995) Staging of rectal carcinoma using MR double surface coil, MR endorectal coil, and intrarectal ultrasound: correlation with histopathologic findings. J Comput Assist Tomogr 19:752–758

Kahn H et al (1997) Preoperative staging of irradiated rectal cancers using digital rectal examination, computed tomography, endorectal ultrasound, and magnetic resonance imaging does not accurately predict T0,N0 pathology. Dis Colon Rectum 40:140–144

Kapiteijn E et al (2001) Preoperative radiotherapy combined with total mesorectal excision for resectable rectal cancer. N Engl J Med 345:638–646

Katsura Y et al (1992) Endorectal ultrasonography for the assessment of wall invasion and lymph node metastasis in rectal cancer. Dis Colon Rectum 35:362–368

Kwok H et al (2000) Preoperative staging of rectal cancer. Int J Colorectal Dis 15:9–20

Maldjian C et al (2000) Endorectal surface coil MR imaging as a staging technique for rectal carcinoma: a comparison study to rectal endosonography. Abdom Imaging 25:75–80

McNicholas MM et al (1994) Magnetic resonance imaging of rectal carcinoma: a prospective study. Br J Surg 81:911–914

Meyenberger C et al (1995) Endoscopic ultrasound and endorectal magnetic resonance imaging: a prospective, comparative study for preoperative staging and follow-up of rectal cancer. Endoscopy 27:469–479

Milsom JW, Graffner H (1990) Intrarectal ultrasonography in rectal cancer staging and in the evaluation of pelvic disease. Clinical uses of intrarectal ultrasound. Ann Surg 212:602–606

Moss AA (1989) Imaging of colorectal carcinoma (see comments). Radiology 170:308–310

Nagtegaal ID et al (2002) Circumferential margin involvement is still an important predictor of local recurrence in rectal carcinoma: not one millimeter but two millimeters is the limit. Am J Surg Pathol 26:350–357

Nelson H, Sargent DJ (2001) Refining multimodal therapy for rectal cancer. N Engl J Med 345:690–692

Okizuka H et al (1993) Preoperative local staging of rectal carcinoma with MR imaging and a rectal balloon. J Magn Reson Imaging 3:329–335

Pegios W et al (1996) MRI diagnosis and staging of rectal carcinoma. Abdom Imaging 21:211–218

Phillips RK et al (1984) Local recurrence following 'curative' surgery for large bowel cancer. II. The rectum and rectosigmoid. Br J Surg 71:17–20

Poeze M et al (1995) Radical resection of locally advanced colorectal cancer. Br J Surg 82:1386–1390

Popovich MJ et al (1993) The role of MR imaging in determining surgical eligibility for pelvic exenteration. AJR Am J Roentgenol 160:525–531

Quirke P, Dixon MF (1988) The prediction of local recurrence in rectal adenocarcinoma by histopathological examination. Int J Colorectal Dis 3:127–131

Quirke P et al (1986) Local recurrence of rectal adenocarcinoma due to inadequate surgical resection. Histopathological study of lateral tumour spread and surgical excision. Lancet 2:996–999

Radcliffe A, Brown G (2001) Will MRI provide maps of lines of excision for rectal cancer? Lancet 357:495–496

Rifkin MD et al (1989) Staging of rectal carcinoma: prospective comparison of endorectal US and CT. Radiology 170: 319–322

Sagar PM, Pemberton JH (1996) Surgical management of locally recurrent rectal cancer. Br J Surg 83:293–304

Sailer M et al (1997) Influence of tumor position on accuracy of endorectal ultrasound staging. Dis Colon Rectum 40: 1180–1186

Schnall MD et al (1994) Rectal tumor stage: correlation of endorectal MR imaging and pathologic findings (see comments). Radiology 190:709–714

Shank B et al (1990) A prospective study of the accuracy of preoperative computed tomographic staging of patients with biopsy-proven rectal carcinoma. Dis Colon Rectum 33:285–290

Solomon MJ, McLeod RS (1993) Endoluminal transrectal ultrasonography: accuracy, reliability, and validity. Dis Colon Rectum 36:200–205

Starck M et al (1995) Endoluminal ultrasound and low-field magnetic resonance imaging are superior to clinical examination in the preoperative staging of rectal cancer. Eur J Surg 161:841–845

Thaler W et al (1994) Preoperative staging of rectal cancer by endoluminal ultrasound vs. magnetic resonance imaging. Preliminary results of a prospective, comparative study. Dis Colon Rectum 37:1189–1193

Thoeni RF (1997) Colorectal cancer. Radiologic staging. Radiol Clin North Am 35:457–485

Thoeni RF et al (1981) Detection and staging of primary rectal and rectosigmoid cancer by computed tomography. Radiology 141:135–138

Thompson WM et al (1986) Preoperative and postoperative CT staging of rectosigmoid carcinoma. AJR Am J Roentgenol 146:703–710

Tio TL et al (1991) Colorectal carcinoma: preoperative TNM classification with endosonography. Radiology 179: 165–170

Visser O et al (1996) Incidence of cancer in the Netherlands 1996. Utrecht Association of Comprehensive Cancer Centres

Vogl TJ et al (1997) Accuracy of staging rectal tumors with contrast-enhanced transrectal MR imaging. AJR Am J Roentgenol 168:1427–1434

Vogl TJ et al (1998) Use and applications of MRI techniques in the diagnosis and staging of rectal lesions. Rec Res Cancer Res 146:35–47

Wibe A et al (2002) Prognostic significance of the circumferential resection margin following total mesorectal excision for rectal cancer. Br J Surg 89:327–334

Williams AD et al (2001) Detection of pelvic lymph node metastases in gynecologic malignancy: a comparison of CT, MR imaging, and positron emission tomography. AJR Am J Roentgenol 177:343–348

Zagoria RJ et al (1997) Assessment of rectal tumor infiltration utilizing endorectal MR imaging and comparison with endoscopic rectal sonography. J Surg Oncol 64:312–317

Zaunbauer W et al (1981) Computed tomography in carcinoma of the rectum. Gastrointest Radiol 6:79–84

Zerhouni EA et al (1996) CT and MR imaging in the staging of colorectal carcinoma: report of the Radiology Diagnostic Oncology Group II. Radiology 200:443–451

12 Staging and Follow-Up of Colorectal Cancer

J. ASHLEY GUTHRIE

CONTENTS

12.1   Introduction   *125*
12.2   Dissemination of Colorectal Cancer   *125*
12.3   Staging   *126*
12.4   Surveillance   *127*
12.4.1   Evidence for Post-operative Surveillance   *129*
12.4.2   Imaging Within a Surveillance Programme   *130*
12.4.3   Risk Adapted Surveillance   *131*
12.4.5   Overall Outcome   *132*
12.4.6   The Future   *133*
12.5   Conclusion   *133*
    References   *133*

12.1
Introduction

The prognosis of any neoplasm is dependant upon its extent of dissemination at the time of initial treatment and the efficacy of available therapies to eliminate all sites of disease. Staging and post-operative surveillance have the common goals of determining the extent of dissemination of the cancer so as to direct treatment. Staging is performed at presentation with the aim of giving a measure of the extent of local and metastatic disease and is now a fundamental part of oncological practice. Post-operative surveillance is performed for two purposes, firstly to identify metachronous tumours for which the patient is at increased risk and secondly to detect residual or recurrent cancer from the original tumour. The latter is much more contentious and is performed to compensate for failures of initial treatment and staging techniques with the intention of initiating further treatment. An understanding of the sites and mechanism of spread is useful in considering both staging and surveillance. The role of radiology for staging and post-operative surveillance of colorectal cancer will be examined. Follow-up to identify second primary tumours is usually performed by colonoscopy and will not be discussed in detail.

J. A. GUTHRIE, MRCP, FRCR
Consultant Radiologist, Clinical Radiology, St James's University Hospital, Beckett Street, LEEDS LS9 7TF, UK

12.2
Dissemination of Colorectal Cancer

Colorectal adenocarcinomas arise in the mucosa and grow to progressively invade the deeper layers of the bowel wall. As this growth continues uncontrolled, the muscularis and then serosa will ultimately be breached with extension into the pericolic fat and adjacent organs. If the involved colon is covered with peritoneum this can become invaded by tumour leading to trans-coelomic dissemination with the development of distant peritoneal and omental deposits. The commonest site of metastasis is the locoregional lymph nodes (AUGUST et al. 1984) occurring as a consequence of invasion of the local lymphatic plexus. Haematological dissemination may occur after vascular invasion. The final mechanism of spread is by implantation of tumour cells by the surgeon at the time of operation (GORE 1997).

Mechanisms of distant metastasis are complex and probably occur as a consequence of both non-random and random events. Malignant tumour cells leave the primary neoplasm as the result of several cellular processes and it is postulated that they are then disseminated via metastatic "cascades" (MORGAN-PARKES 1995; BAKER and PELLEY 1995). This involves malignant metastatic cells becoming established in one organ before spreading to the next and then becoming "generalised" into many organ systems. Necropsy based studies observing the distribution of distant metastases suggest hematogenous dissemination is probably the most important mechanism with colonic carcinomas. The proposed cascade of spread is via the portal venous system to the liver and then to the lungs before generalised dissemination. The distribution of observed organ involvement following lung metastases is approximately proportional to the organ blood flow with reduced representation in the thyroid and a higher than anticipated incidence in bones (WEISS et al. 1986). This suggests that not only blood flow but also local influences have an affect. Due to the venous drainage of the lower rectum, tumours at this site may bye-pass the liver and metastasise directly to the lungs.

The cascade pathways have clinical importance since there is a second opportunity for cure if the course is interrupted. Lymphatic invasion may also lead to widespread dissemination. Despite adequate surgical margins there is an increased incidence of local recurrence and distant metastases in patients with lymph node positive resections (AUGUST et al. 1984).

12.3
Staging

The premise upon which staging is undertaken is that it reflects prognosis. A staging system should aim to identify the major features that predict outcome so patients can be grouped into categories with a similar outcome. The most commonly used staging systems are the Dukes and TNM systems (Tables 12.1, 12.2, Fig. 12.1) Ideally this information can then be used to deliver stage specific treatment, with more advanced stages of disease warranting more aggressive treatment or palliation depending on the likely outcome of the treatments balanced against the morbidity of intensive therapy. The additional benefits of staging are that more valid comparisons can then be made between different forms of treatment, institutions or clinicians with the purpose of improving outcome.

The surgeon, pathologist and radiologist have complementary roles in the complete staging of a patient with colorectal cancer. The surgeon removes the primary tumour, the draining lymph nodes and a surrounding margin of tissue to reduce the risk of local recurrence. The peritoneal cavity and liver are examined and any possible peritoneal deposits sampled. The pathologist determines the extent of tumour growth through the bowel wall, the microscopic margin of clearance, involvement of lymph nodes and peritoneal surfaces. The timing and nature of radiological input is variable and in part dependent on the mode of presentation. If a pre-operative measure of the extent of disease will modify the surgery or result in therapy, such as radiotherapy being employed prior to surgery then clearly the imaging should take place first. This is most applicable to rectal cancer but there are advantages with colonic cancer. Preoperative imaging reduces the likelihood of unexpected findings at laparotomy. If the tumour is demonstrated to be more advanced than clinically suspected a more informed discussion can take place with regards to the extent of primary surgery, the need for additional surgery such as liver resection, the need for adjuvant chemotherapy and the post

Table 12.1. UICC TNM classification of malignant tumours (SOBIN and WITTEKIND 2002)

T	*Primary tumour*
T1	Tumour invades the submucosa
T2	Tumour invades the muscularis propria
T3	Tumour invades through the muscularis propria into the sub-serosa or into peri-colic/peri-rectal tissues
T4	Tumour directly invades other organs or perforates visceral peritoneum
N	*Regional lymph nodes*
N0	No regional lymph node metastases
N1	Metastases in 1–3 regional lymph nodes
N2	Metastases in 4 or more regional lymph nodes
M	*Distant metastases*
M1	No distant metastases
M2	Distant metastases

Table 12.2. Modified Dukes' classification system

Dukes' A	Penetration into but not through the bowel wall
Dukes' B	Penetration through the bowel wall
Dukes' C	Lymph node involvement regardless of extent of bowel wall penetration
Dukes' D	Distant metastases present

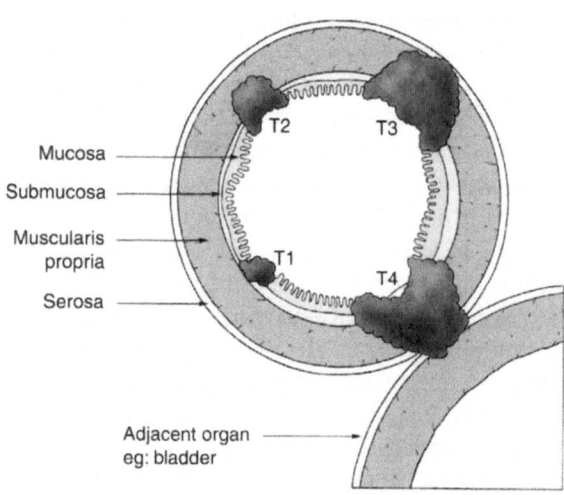

Fig. 12.1. Cross section of colon. Primary tumour (T) staging. See Table 12.1.

operative pathway can be streamlined. In patients with extensive disease and minimal local symptoms there is a case for systemic chemotherapy as the primary treatment, reserving surgery for symptoms that cannot be palliated by other means (SARELA et al. 2001).

Techniques for the local staging of rectal cancers are covered elsewhere (Chaps. 10 and 11). The principal distant organs for radiological assessment are the liver and lungs. The superiority of CT over the surgeon's hands in the assessment of the liver is well established (FINDLAY and MCARDLE 1986). The minimum examination should comprise an ultrasound of the liver and a chest radiograph. CT has the advantage of providing an overview of the primary tumour, the peritoneal cavity, distant nodal groups and gives a complete representation of the liver, which can also serve as a baseline for further follow-up. A role for FDG-PET scanning in staging has been proposed but is yet to be established. FDG-PET cannot provide local staging detail and staging of lymph nodes is poor (ARULAMPALAM et al. 2001). The site of maximal sensitivity is the liver (ARULAM-PALAM et al. 2001; KINKEL et al. 2002); however, CT has a reasonable sensitivity for liver metastases and can provide additional anatomical detail, making PET unlikely to replace CT and the cost benefit of an additional expensive test has to be questioned.

12.4
Surveillance

Typically the recurrence rates for carcinoma of the colon and rectum treated by surgery with curative intent are 33% and 42%, respectively (PIHL et al. 1981). There has been little change in these rates in the last few decades. The objective of surveillance is to identify asymptomatic recurrences after 'curative' surgery so that further treatment can be initiated and survival improved. Intuitively a recurrent tumour deposit will initially be undetectable and then become an asymptomatic detectable lesion before becoming a symptomatic lesion. The implicit assumption is that the pre-symptomatic detection of locally persistent tumour or metastases and the early initiation of further treatment lead to cure or a significant extension of life. If a surveillance program is to be of value there needs to be an effective means of identifying asymptomatic recurrent disease coupled with effective treatment.

The treatment options for patients with recurrent disease are largely dependent upon whether the disease is localised or generalised. An isolated site of recurrence may be amenable to further surgery whereas disseminated disease generally requires systemic chemotherapy or palliation. Isolated local recurrence occurs in 15% of colonic and 18% of rectal cancer patients (SAFI et al. 1993; CASS et al. 1976; FLOYD et al. 1965; MOSSA et al. 1975; POLK

and SPRATT 1971). In a large surgical series of colon cancer patients treated with curative intent distant metastases developed in the liver in 13%, lung 3%, lymph nodes 1%, peritoneum 4%, bone 0.9%, and brain 0.7% with higher incidences of pulmonary and bone metastases in patients treated with rectal cancer (PIHL et al. 1981).

The commonest site for isolated metastasis is the liver (PIHL et al. 1981; KIEVIT 2002). Symptoms occur late in the natural history of liver metastases and the median survival of untreated liver metastases is 6–12 months (BENGMARK and HAFSTRÖM 1969; JAFFE et al. 1968). Liver resection offers a second chance for curative surgery as there is an opportunity to remove all viable disease and interrupt the metastatic cascade. Refinements in surgical techniques allow liver resections to be performed with low morbidity and mortality rates. Five year survival rates following liver resection are typically 30%–40% (FONG et al. 1999; SUGIHARA and YAMAMOTO 2000). The best reported outcomes are for patients with solitary lesions, metastases smaller than 5 cm, and a disease free interval of at least 12 months (FONG et al. 1999). The traditional restrictive indications for resection have been challenged and some surgeons are now performing more extensive resections and second resections following the detection of further metastases in the remnant liver (PETROWSKY et al. 2002). Non-surgical techniques such as thermal ablation also show promise as an alternative or supplementary therapy to surgery (GILLAMS and LEES 2000).

Colorectal metastases are the commonest indication for liver resection and this demand has fuelled improvements in liver imaging. More is now known about the radiology of liver metastases from colorectal cancers than for any other malignancy. The prevalence of small lesions and the nature of the gold standard influence the accuracy of any investigation for the detection of liver metastases. Imaging resected liver specimens with helical CT the sensitivity for the detection of colorectal liver metastases above 1cm in diameter reaches 94% (SCOTT et al. 2001), although performance drops off for lesions below 1 cm. If the liver is the only site of metastases under consideration then ultrasound has the advantage of being cheap and does not involve a repeated radiation burden to those who are truly disease free. However, the sensitivity of ultrasound is less than CT in comparative studies (CARTER et al. 1996; CHARNLEY et al. 1991; KINKEL et al. 2002; LEEN et al. 1995; WERNECKE et al. 1991). It has been suggested that the performance of ultrasound can be improved with contrast agents to the extent that it may exceed that of CT (BLOMLEY et al. 1999; DALLA-PALMA et al. 1999), but the use of contrast detracts from the appeal of ultrasound for surveillance and adds to the cost. MR, particularly using superparamagnetic iron oxide (WARD et al. 1999) and PET (KINKEL et al. 2002; ARULAMPALAM et al. 2001; ZHAUANG et al. 2000) have greater accuracy but cost, availability and practical difficulties make them inappropriate investigations for surveillance of the entire post surgical colorectal population.

An alternative approach to identifying liver metastases whilst still small is to try and identify patients with occult disease by indirect means. Doppler ultrasound and nuclear medicine techniques have been used to exploit the changes in perfusion that occur as a result of the presence of metastases. The blood supply of colorectal liver metastases is predominantly arterial, even though they are generally considered hypovascular, and the presence of metastases causes a relative increase in liver arterial to portal flow. Some workers have found that changes in this ratio occur before deposits are visible radiologically (LEEN et al. 1995; LEVESON et al. 1985), but these techniques have not achieved their early promise (GLOVER et al. 2002).

The lungs are a common site of metastases but are uncommonly an isolated site for recurrence. Traditionally patients with pulmonary metastases are identified with CXR although CT is increasingly being used. The population suitable for pulmonary resection with curative intent is relatively small. Newer surgical techniques, such as video-assisted thoracoscopic surgery, have resulted in less invasive approaches than the traditional lobectomy. Typically, 5 year survival in relatively large series is 30%–40% (INOUE et al. 2000; TURK et al. 1993; MCAFEE et al. 1992). The prognosis is better in the absence of mediastinal lymphadenopathy and with a normal serum carcinoembryonic antigen (CEA) (INOUE et al. 2000). More aggressive surgeons will resect both liver and lung metastases if the lung metastases are limited in number and distribution (HAMY et al. 2001).

Local recurrence reflects, in part, inadequate primary surgery. With rectal cancer the appreciation of the value of a microscopic lateral resection margin of at least 1 mm (QUIRKE et al. 1986) has resulted in modifications in surgical (MACFARLANE et al. 1993) and adjuvant therapeutic approaches (SWEDISH RECTAL CANCER GROUP 1997; GOLDBERG et al. 1994) to reduce local treatment failure rates. Most surveillance studies antedate these treatment changes. Local and the less frequent anastomotic recurrences are usually extra-luminal with mucosal invasion occurring late (KRESTIN 1997) and both are more common

after resection of rectal tumours. The nature of these lesions is different from metachronous tumours, which these patients are also at risk of developing. The strategy used to identify anastomotic recurrences therefore needs to differ from that to identify second cancers. Colonoscopy performed every 3–5 years is recommended to identify metachronous tumours (BERMAN et al. 2000), but even when performed more frequently it is a poor means of identifying local or anastomotic recurrence (SCHOEMAKER et al. 1998; AUDISIO et al. 1996). The extra-mucosal nature of the lesion in the early stages of recurrence accounts for the poor sensitivity of faecal occult blood testing (AHLQUIST et al. 1993; SAFI et al. 1993). Alternative means of identifying local recurrence are digital rectal examination, CT, MRI, endorectal ultrasound and FDG-PET. In justifying surveillance for local recurrence the poor results from further surgery have to be considered. Despite optimistic reviews suggesting that intensive follow up and aggressive therapy for locally recurrent disease is beneficial (AUGUST et al. 1984), co-existent distant disease is frequently present in these patients and the prognosis is generally poor (KRESTIN 1997). Potentially curative resections are achievable in only a small proportion of patients although 5 year survival rates of 27% in selective series have been achieved (GOLDBERG et al. 1998; DELPERO et al. 1998). However, surgery is associated with substantial morbidity (DELPERO et al. 1998).

The radiology of local recurrence is difficult. The site at greatest risk is the pelvis and following surgery at this site there is frequently a residual inflammatory mass. Differentiating inflammatory from malignant tissue is problematic, particularly as the two may co-exist. A baseline post operative CT scan 3 months after surgery is of value in identifying recurrence on subsequent examinations (KELVIN et al. 1983; THOMPSON et al. 1986). MR is more reliable in differentiating fibrotic inflammatory masses from recurrent tumour (PEMA et al. 1994; MARKUS et al. 1997) but is generally used for problem solving rather than surveillance. If radiotherapy or a major resection is to be performed many clinicians will only act once histology has been obtained. CT has reported to have sensitivities between 69%–88% for identifying recurrent disease (BERMAN et al. 2000) but the clinical setting will influence this performance. Higher sensitivities are likely to be achieved in a population of patients with symptoms or raised CEA levels than in an asymptomatic post-operative population. In follow-up studies when CT was performed 6 monthly the detection rate of curable recurrences was disappointingly low (OHLSSON et al. 1995).

Whilst anastomotic recurrences may be palpable (NORTHOVER 2000), or visible with endoscopy (STAIB et al. 2000), endoscopic ultrasound has the advantage of being able to detect extra-mucosal recurrences within the bowel wall. However, fibrosis can result in false positives and pelvic side wall recurrence is difficult to identify. The potential of FDG-PET for identification of extra-hepatic disease not be identifiable with other imaging techniques may provide the stimulus for its use (ARULAMPALAM et al. 2001; ZHAUANG et al. 2000; JOHNSON et al. 2001; IMDAHL et al. 2000). The availability of PET scanning in the UK is limited but as the role of PET is proven its availability should increase and costs reduce. FDG-PET is likely to have a selective role in identification of recurrent disease and in differentiating benign from recurrent malignant pelvic masses (KEOGAN et al. 1997).

Although surgery may be required for palliation, surgery with curative intent for disease at other sites is uncommon as it usually reflects generalised disease. Disseminated disease is treated with chemotherapy. 5-Fluorouracil based agents have been the principle treatment for many years and extend life by 3-6 months (NHS EXECUTIVE 1997; INTERNATIONAL POOLED ANALYSIS OF B2 COLON CANCER TRIALS 1999). There are newer regimens that make use of oxaliplatin and irinotecan which show promise with higher response rates (ROUGIER et al. 1997; LEVI et al. 1992), although the median increase in life expectancy is still in the order of months. Patients have a better quality of life if chemotherapy is initiated as soon as metastatic disease is identified rather than waiting until symptoms develop (NORDIC GASTROINTESTINAL TUMOUR ADJUVANT THERAPY GROUP 1992; ALLEN-MERSH et al. 1994). There are therefore benefits other than 5-year survival for patients with recurrence identified early.

Having established that there are investigations that are sensitive in identifying recurrent disease and that there are effective treatments, the critical question is how would outcome be affected by screening a large post-operative population. The population in a surgically based series will inevitably differ from a screening population, as in a screening population additional selection criteria will be applied between the identification of recurrence and re-operation; some patients that initially appear to have resectable disease will not undergo resection due to other factors thus reducing the number in the surveillance population likely to be cured. Offset against this is that in moving from a symptomatic to an asymptomatic population a greater proportion of patients should theoretically have a smaller

volume of less disseminated and therefore resectable disease. In considering surveillance there are several key issues. Is there any evidence that post-operative surveillance is effective? Should imaging play any part in a surveillance program, and if imaging is to be employed which techniques and how often? There is also a cost to be borne both in economic terms to society and psychologically by the patient. Can a selective approach reduce these burdens and increase the effectiveness of a program?

12.4.1
Evidence for Post-operative Surveillance

Screening post-operative patients to identify asymptomatic recurrence, particularly liver metastases, may seem worthwhile but is there any evidence of a benefit in following up this population? Five studies have been published, and subjected to meta-analysis, in which a total of 1342 patients believed to be disease free following surgery were randomised to intensive and non-intensive surveillance regimens (KJELDSEN et al. 1997a,b; MÄKELÄ et al. 1995; OHLSSON et al. 1995; PIETRA et al. 1998; SCHOEMAKER et al. 1998). These studies were recruited in the late 1980s and published between 1995 and 1998. The differences between the control and intensive arms of the studies were very variable; the follow up regimens in the non-intensive arms would be regarded as intensive by some, whilst in two studies patients were referred back to the community primary health care services (KJELDSEN et al. 1997a,b; OHLSSON et al. 1995). The use of radiology in the surveillance protocols was also variable with one not using any radiological investigation other than CXR even in the intensive arm (KIELDSEN et al. 1997b). The studies with the most intensive follow up regimens also tended to have the most intensive control regimens. Only one of these 5 studies concluded that intensive follow up resulted in a significant improvement in outcome (PIETRA et al. 1998). However, there was a trend to an increased 5-year survival in all five studies. Two meta-analyses of these studies have been published and both concluded that there was a survival benefit at 5 years in the intensive follow-up arm (RENEHAN and O'DWYER 2000; JEFFERY et al. 2002). Recurrences were identified on average 8.5 months earlier in the intensive group and were more likely to be at a single site (RENEHAN and O'DWYER 2000). The principal failing of all of these five studies is that the numbers of patients recruited are too small to reach valid statistical conclusions. The study populations range from 106 to 697 patients which would not be able to detect a statistical difference in survival of less than 20%, it is estimated that 1000 patients would need to be randomised to demonstrate a 9% difference between groups (OHLSSON et al. 1995).

There have also been several non-randomised studies, which have used non-compliant patients or historic groups as controls. A complex meta-analysis of post-operative colorectal cancer surveillance series published between 1972 and 1996 attempted to incorporate both randomised and non-randomised studies (ROSEN et al. 1998). The studies were subdivided into two; firstly randomised and comparative cohort studies, which comprised 2005 patients and secondly single cohort studies compared with historic controls, reflecting the outcome of a further 6641 patients. There was a 2.5-fold increase in curative resections in the first group and 1.9-fold increase in the single cohort group. Compared with the controls in the first group the cumulative 5-year survival rate was 16% greater in the intensive follow up arms and 13% in the single cohort group. These results are comparable to the absolute reduction in mortality of 9%–13% calculated in one of the meta-analyses of the 5 controlled trials. Since this analysis there have been other controlled (SECCO et al. 2002) and non-controlled studies in which the authors advocate intensive follow up regimens to detect asymptomatic recurrence, leading to a greater proportion of patients suitable for further surgery with curative intent (GOLDBERG et al. 1998; STAIB et al. 2000) and improved median survival (GOLDBERG et al. 1998). The net benefit from intensive follow up should therefore lead to a reduction in mortality in the order of 10%–15% which compares favourably with a benefit of 6% from adjuvant chemotherapy for Dukes' C tumours (NHS EXECUTIVE 1997; DUBE et al. 1997).

12.4.2
Imaging Within a Surveillance Programme

If one accepts that there is an argument for surveillance the question arises as to whether radiology should form part of the program. National bodies have reached differing conclusions. The members of the American Society of Clinical Oncology (BENSON et al. 2000) argue against the use of any imaging whereas French bodies recommend liver ultrasound 3–6 monthly for 3 years and then annually with an annual CXR (CONSENSUS CONFERENCE 1998; O'DWYER et al. 2001). The Association of Coloproctol-

ogy of Great Britain and Ireland take a more ambivalent view suggesting it is reasonable to perform liver imaging in fit patients for 2 years without actually making a recommendation (GUIDELINES FOR THE MANAGEMENT OF COLORECTAL CANCER 2001). The mainstay of most follow up regimens is the serial measurement of CEA. Approximately 80% of patients have an elevated CEA and it usually returns to normal after resection. Failure to return to normal or a rising CEA suggests recurrent disease. In a study of asymptomatic post-operative patients in which a single CEA measurement was made and compared with several imaging tests performed at the same time, CEA was a less sensitive means of identifying patients with liver metastases than CT or ultrasound (GLOVER et al. 2002). Evidence relating to the efficacy of serial CEA measurement is contradictory. A meta-analysis of non-randomised studies demonstrated a 9% improved 5-year survival for those monitored with serial CEA measurement (BRUINNELS et al. 1994), but there are studies that have shown no improvement in outcome (BERMAN et al. 2000). Recommendations for CEA measurements are usually for every 2–3 months (BENSON et al. 2000; CONSENSUS CONFERENCE 1998; KIEVIT 2002). CEA as the most frequently performed examination was usually the initial indicator of 'asymptomatic' recurrence in the controlled trials. However, it should be appreciated that patients initially believed to be asymptomatic have often noticed new symptoms on closer questioning. In a study in which patients had CEA levels performed monthly, 18% of the 58% 'asymptomatic' recurrences subsequently admitted to having noticed rectal bleeding or a change in bowel habit (NHS EXECUTIVE 1997). Serial CEA measurement is a better indicator of liver and widespread disease than other sites of disease (BERGAMASCHI and ARNAUD 1996) but far from ideal in identifying patients for liver resection. In Goldberg's series 50% of patients undergoing liver resection as a consequence of elevated CEA levels had metastases ranging from 4–10 cm in diameter (GOLDBERG et al. 1998). The use of CEA is clearly limited as a post-operative screening investigation to identify patients with resectable liver disease. To maximise the likelihood of identifying curable recurrence CEA needs to be supplemented or replaced.

It is often difficult to determine the contribution of imaging to the initial diagnosis of recurrent disease. A substantial proportion of patients present with symptoms even within surveillance programmes (GOLDBERG et al. 1998) and since CEA measurement is the most frequent investigation used it is unsurprising that CEA most commonly identifies recurrence. The proportion of patients in whom a positive imaging test is the only evidence of recurrence when CEA is also measured is generally small although in De Salvo's series 41.5% of distant metastases were identified by liver ultrasound and CXR (DE SALVO et al. 1997). Jeffery's meta-analysis of five of the randomised studies would also support the use of radiology finding that mortality was significantly reduced when liver imaging was performed (JEFFREY et al. 2002).

There is most to gain in identifying patients with liver metastases because they occur commonly, develop symptoms late and have a greater cure rate than other sites of recurrence. If the identification of patients with liver metastases were to be the primary objective of surveillance then imaging of the liver alone would be sufficient. There is some evidence from non-randomised studies that frequent ultrasound (DE SALVO et al. 1997; HOWELL et al. 1999; SECCO et al. 2002) could be used to effect, the attraction being that it is relatively cheap and non-invasive enabling a high frequency of investigation in the initial high-risk period. Frequent liver ultrasound forms part of the French surveillance recommendations (O'DWYER et al. 2001). It is noteworthy that, in one study, even when ultrasound was performed 3 monthly for 2 years and 6 monthly thereafter to five years 43% of patients identified as having liver metastases were only diagnosed on the annual CT (HOWELL et al. 1999). CT is generally reported to have a higher sensitivity than US in identifying patients with liver metastases (GLOVER et al. 2002; KINKEL et al. 2002). In a comparative study of CT, MRI, US, CEA and perfusion based techniques (Doppler and isotope) in the identification of asymptomatic colorectal liver metastases, CT had the highest sensitivity, almost 50% greater than US and double that of CEA (GLOVER et al. 2002).

CT would seem more attractive than the other investigations for identifying liver metastases because it can be extended to cover the pelvis and coupled either with CXR or chest CT to cover the other major areas of treatable recurrence. CT techniques have progressed considerably since the published programmes, most of which were performed in the pre-helical CT era. Liver metastases have been observed to double in diameter on unenhanced CT between 90 and 1109 days (FINLAY et al. 1988). Theoretically the distribution of even the most aggressive liver metastases should be revealed with 6 monthly examinations with little effect on local operability. There is little data with regards the timing of spread to other sites and therefore the influence of such an

interval on the ability to achieve cure. The use of CT within randomised studies has been limited to date and appears to have had little impact on outcome. In a study by SCHOEMAKER et al. (1998) in which annual CT was performed, ten patients were discovered to have asymptomatic metastases confined to the liver but only three underwent liver resection which was similar to the control group. The reasons why the other seven patients did not undergo resection are not apparent. In a study by OHLSSON et al. (1995) the use of pelvic CT after abdominoperineal resection resulted in the identification of few curative resections that were unidentified by other means. These findings have led to commentators advising against its use on current evidence (BERMAN et al. 2000), whether current CT scanning techniques will prove to be more effective remains to be seen.

The use of CXR has also been argued against as the yield is low (BENSON et al. 2000). In SCHOEMAKER et al.'s study (1998) 633 CXRs were performed for one patient to achieve a 4-year plus disease-free survival following surgery. However, in a follow up study of 1247 patients all 20 patients who had pulmonary surgery with curative intent were identified with chest radiography (GOLDBERG et al. 1998), and whilst the diagnostic yield may be low so is the cost. The use of endoscopic ultrasound (EUS) as a primary surveillance investigation for the assessment of the pelvis following resection of rectal carcinomas has been the subject of little investigation. In Germany it has been suggested that EUS be used as an alternative to flexible proctosigmoidoscopy as part of the follow-up regimen for patients at high risk of local recurrence (HERMANEK et al. 1999; STAIB et al. 2000). The cost and availability of MR and FDG-PET make them unfeasible as a first line surveillance investigation and there is little data available with regard performance in this context. Both could have specific roles in the assessment of patients either suspected of having recurrence when other investigations are negative or in whom a second resection is being contemplated.

12.4.3
Risk Adapted Surveillance

In the US, as in the European Community, approximately 137,000 people are diagnosed as having colorectal cancer each year (AUDISIO and ROBERTSON 2000; PARKER et al. 1997). Public health resources are finite and the cost of follow up is potentially extremely large. There is considerable variation in follow-up practice (BRUINVELS et al. 1995; RICHERT-BOE 1995), which is not surprising given the conflicting published evidence and advice; one costing found a 28-fold difference in expense between regimens with little evidence of difference in outcome (VIRGO et al. 1995). The risk of developing recurrent or metastatic disease is not uniform. There is interest in stratifying patients into groups which reflect the risk of recurrence on the basis of features identified at initial staging and subjecting the highest risk patients to a more intensive follow up regimen. The objective would be to maximise the use of limited resources whilst preserving sensitivity for treatable recurrence. Clearly care must be taken not to adversely prejudice the outcome of patients with indolent disease who may have most to gain from the identification of recurrence and for a programme to be successfully applied it should not be too complex.

An assessment of a patients risk of recurrence is made on the basis of pathological features within the surgical specimen. At least 22 pathological parameters have been reported to confer prognostic significance (SHEPHERD and QUIRK 1997; HERMANEK et al. 1999). It would be unfeasible to make use of all of these in a risk assessment, and some reported parameters are of questionable value. The major indicators of outcome include depth of penetration of tumour through the bowel wall, lateral resection margin clearance, lymph node involvement, vascular invasion and mucinous differentiation. If follow-up is to be determined by histological features then accuracy of pathological examination and reporting will be critical. The detection of positive lymph nodes, for example, at least in part reflects the total number isolated from the resection specimen. When a low number of lymph nodes are harvested there is the potential to misclassify a high risk tumour as low. Universal high quality pathological examinations and reports cannot be assumed, a regional audit from the UK suggested that a quarter of cases were understaged (SHEPHERD and QUIRK 1997). Poor histological staging would undermine attempts to risk adapt follow-up as well as deny patients the benefits of adjuvant chemotherapy. The risk of recurrence is also greatest in the first 2 years following surgery and most surveillance programmes reflect this, the most intense monitoring occurring during this period with most regimens continuing for a further 3 years with reduced investigation.

Using a risk analysis approach, and dividing patients into those with rectal and colonic cancer, STAIB et al. (2000) estimate that costs can be reduced by 50%–60% when compared with a universally applied intensive programme. There is some prospective evidence that a risk-adapted approach can be used to reduce surveillance costs and improve outcome. SECCO et al. (2002) performed a study comprising four arms with patients stratified into high and low risk groups and then randomised into intensive and minimal follow-up arms. High risk was defined as low rectal tumours, T3 colonic tumours, positive lymph nodes, poor histological differentiation, CEA >7.5 ng/ml and mucinous tumours. The imaging component of both the high and low risk intensive follow-up was ultrasound and unlike other tests employed there was little difference in the frequency of use (there was one fewer ultrasound examination in the 5 year follow up period in the low risk group). The rate of recurrence was relatively high and the authors demonstrated an improvement in 5-year survival with intensive follow-up and cost savings in the low risk group.

12.4.5
Overall Outcome

When considering the outcome of colorectal cancer it should be appreciated that surveillance will have a limited impact on overall 5-year survival. Approximately 75 of 100 patients presenting with colorectal cancer will be treated with curative intent, and of these approximately a third will develop recurrent disease. Of these 25 patients many will be elderly with other co-morbidity, typically 16% (i.e. four) will undergo further surgery and only 20% of these will be alive at 5 years (5-year survival in the non-surgical group is <5%). From the initial cohort of 100 one will be cured as a result of a second operative intervention after the initial "curative" surgery. Conversely 99% of patients have either incurable disease or are disease free. If intensive surveillance protocols with aggressive treatment regimens were adopted and salvage surgery rates were to rise to 40% (GOLDBERG et al. 1998) with consequent improvements in 5-year survival to say 30%, this would lead to a three-fold increase in cure as a result of surgery for recurrent disease but the overall improvement in the 5-year survival of the initial 100 patients will be only 2%. If there are higher rates of recurrence, as has been observed in some surveillance studies, the effect of intensive follow-up will be amplified yielding greater benefits. Intensive follow-up should also be restricted to patients fit enough for aggressive treatment of recurrent disease which will improve the cost benefits of surveillance.

Whilst cure and 5-year survival may be ideal goals these targets should not be over-emphasised. Lesser prolongation of quality life is of value and can be achieved by identifying recurrence early (NORDIC GASTROINTESTINAL TUMOUR ADJUVANT THERAPY GROUP 1992). Contrary to the view taken by some that follow-up merely provides a reminder to patients that they have or have had cancer (NORTHOVER 2000), patients value follow-up, even if they are aware that it may not lead to early detection of recurrence (STIGGELBOUT et al. 1997).

12.4.6
The Future

There is still a need for well designed trials to assess follow-up programmes. The populations recruited must be large enough to draw statistically valid conclusions. Many would find it difficult to enter patients into randomised studies in which patients are returned to the community with no formal follow-up. The principle issues that need to be considered are overall outcome, indicators of increased risk of recurrence, the relative costs and benefit of each component and quality of life. I would favour testing an intensive follow up arm comprising 3 monthly CEA measurements, 6 monthly CT of the abdomen and pelvis and annual CXR for the first 2 years with a reduced frequency of all tests for the following 3 years. In addition colonoscopy would need to be performed every 3 years to identify any metachronous tumours. Whether current CT techniques will outperform those of the past in a surveillance setting remains to be seen. The greatest scope for alternative investigations is in the detection of extra-hepatic disease. FDG-PET shows potential but its application would need to be restricted to those at particularly high risk due to cost. EUS following resection of rectal cancer could also have a role. There are currently 2 studies (one in Italy and one in the UK) which are intending to recruit 2920 and 4890 patients respectively to address some of these issues.

12.5
Conclusion

There are advantages for patients with colorectal cancer from both accurate staging and post-operative surveillance. Staging offers a more informed tailored approach to the primary treatment. Surveillance will benefit some

patients with an extended life of high quality but the numbers cured by further surgery will be small and the cost high. There are many strategies that could be adopted and the options will increase as new investigations develop. The relative benefits of follow-up will constantly alter. More complete initial staging, changes to primary therapeutic interventions with improved surgical techniques, adjuvant or neoadjuvant chemotherapy with or without radiotherapy will decrease the potential value of surveillance whereas improvements in surveillance investigations and treatments of recurrence should have the converse effect. Controversy regarding what form surveillance will take and the role of the various radiological modalities within follow-up regimens will continue for a long time to come.

References

Ahlquist DA, Weiand HS, Moertel CG et al (1993) Accuracy of fecal occult blood screening for colorectal neoplasia. A prospective study using Hemoccult and HemoQuant tests. JAMA 269:1262–1267

Allen-Mersh TG, Earlam S, Fordy C et al (1994) Quality of life and survival with continuous hepatic artery floxuridine infusion for colorectal liver metastases. Lancet 344:1255–1260

Arulampalam TH, Costa DC, Loizidou M et al (2001) Positron emission tomography and colorectal cancer. Br J Surg 88: 176–189

Audisio RA, Robertson (2000) Colorectal cancer follow-up: perspectives for future studies. Eur J Surg Oncol 26:329–337

Audisio RA, Setti-Carraro P, Segala M et al (1996) Follow-up in colorectal cancer patients: a cost-benefit analysis. Ann Surg Oncol 3:349–57

August DA, Ottow RT, Sugarbaker PH (1984) Clinical perspective of human colorectal cancer metastasis. Cancer Metast Rev 3:303–324

Baker ME, Pelley R (1995) Hepatic metastases: basic principles and implications for Radiologists. Radiology 197:329–337

Bengmark S, Hafström L (1969) The natural history of primary and secondary malignant tumors of the liver. The prognosis for patients with hepatic metastases from colonic and rectal carcinoma by laparotomy. Cancer 23:198–202

Benson AB 3rd, Desch CE, Flynn PJ et al (2000) Update of American Society of clinical oncology colorectal surveillance guidelines. J Clin Oncol 8:3586–3588

Bergamaschi R, Arnaud JP (1996) Routine compared with nonscheduled follow-up of patients with "curative" surgery for colorectal cancer. Ann Surg Oncol 3:464–469

Berman JM, Cheung RJ, Weinberg DS (2000) Surveillance after colorectal cancer resection. Lancet 355:395–399

Blomley MJ, Albrecht T, Cosgrove DO et al (1999) Improved imaging of liver metastases with stimulated acoustic emission in the late phase of enhancement with the US contrast agent DHU 508A: early experience. Radiology 210:409–416

Bruinvels DJ, Stiggelbout AM, Kievit J et al (1994) Follow-up of patients with colorectal cancer: Ameta-analysis. Ann Surg 219:174–182

Bruinvels DJ, Stiggelbout AM, Klaassen MP et al (1995) Follow-up after colorectal cancer: current practice in The Netherlands. Eur J Surg 161:827–831

Carter R, Hemingway D, Cooke TG et al (1996) A prospective study of six methods for detection of hepatic colorectal metastases. Ann R Coll Surg Engl 78:27–30

Cass AW, Million RR, Pfaff WW (1976) Patterns of recurrence following surgery alone for adenocarcinoma of the colon and rectum. Cancer 37:2861–2865

Charnley RM, Morris DL, Dennison AR et al (1991) Detection of colorectal liver metastases using intraoperative ultrasonography. Br J Surg 78:45–48

Consensus Conference (1998) Prevention, diagnosis and treatment of colon cancer (French). Gastroentérol Clin Biol 22:205–218

Dalla-Palma L, Bertolottom, Quaia E et al (1999) Detection of liver metastases with pulse inversion harmonic imaging: preliminary results. Euro Radiol 9 [Suppl 3]:S382–S387

Delpero JR, Pol B, Le Treut P et al (1998) Surgical resection of locally recurrent colorectal adenocarcinoma. Br J Surg 85:372–376

De Salvo L, Razzetta F, Arezzo A et al (1997) Surveillance after colorectal cancer surgery. Eur J Surg Oncol 23:522–525

Dube S, Heyen F, Jenicek M (1997) Adjuvant chemotherapy in colorectal carcinoma: results of a meta-analysis. Dis Colon Rectum 40:35–41

Findlay IG, McArdle CS (1986) Occult hepatic metastases in colorectal carcinoma. Br J Surg 73:732–735

Finlay IG, Meek D, Brunton F et al (1988) Growth rate of hepatic metastases in colorectal carcinoma. Br J Surg 75:641–644

Floyd EC, Corley RG, Chon J (1965) Local recurrence of carcinoma of the colon and rectum. Am J Surg 109:150–159

Fong Y, Fortner J, Sun RL et al (1999) Clinical score for predicting recurrence after hepatic resection for metastatic colorectal cancer analysis of 1001 consecutive cases. Ann Surg 230:309–321

Gillams AR, Lees WR (2000) Survival after percutaneous, image-guided, thermal ablation of hepatic metastases from colorectal cancer. Dis Colon Rectum 43:656–661

Glover MA , Douse P, Kane P et al (2002) Accuracy of investigations for asymptomatic colorectal liver metastases. Dis Colon Rectum 45:476–484

Goldberg PA, Nicholls RJ, Porter NH et al (1994) Long-term results of a randomised trial of short-course low-dose adjuvant pre-operative radiotherapy for rectal cancer: reduction in local treatment failure. Eur J Cancer 30A:1602–1606

Goldberg RM, Fleming TR, Tangen CM et al (1998) Surgery for recurrent colon cancer: strategies for identifying resectable recurrence and success rates after resection. Eastern Cooperative Oncology Group, North Central Cancer Treatment Group, and the Southwest Oncology Group. Ann Intern Med 129:27–35

Gore RM (1997) Colorectal cancer clinical and pathologic features. Radiol Clin North Am 35:403–429

Guidelines for the Management of Colorectal Cancer (2001) The Association of Coloproctology of Great Britain and Ireland

Hamy A, Baron O, Bennouna J et al (2001) Resection of hepatic and pulmonary metastases in patients with colorectal cancer. Am J Clin Oncol 24:607–609

Hermanek P, Junginger T, Hossfeld DK et al (1999) Follow-up and rehabilitation for patients with gastrointestinal tumours. Dtsch Arztebl 96a:2084–2088

Howell JD, Wotherspoon H, Leen E et al (1999) Evaluation of a follow-up programme after curative resection for colorectal cancer. Br J Cancer 79:308–310

Imdahl A, Reinhardt MJ, Nitzsche EU et al (2000) Impact of 18-FDG-positron emission tomography for decision making in colorectal cancer recurrences. Langenbecks Arch Surg 385:129–134

Inoue M, Kotake Y, Nakagawa K et al (2000) Surgery for pulmonary metastases from colorectal carcinoma. Ann Thorac Surg 70:380–383

International Multicentre Pooled Analysis of B2 Colon Cancer Trials (IMPACT B2) (1999) Efficacy of adjuvant fluorouracil and folinic acid in B2 colon cancer. J Clin Oncol 17:1356–1363

Jaffe BM, Donegan WL, Watson F et al (1968) Factors influencing survival in patients with untreated hepatic metastases. Surg Gynecol Obstet 127:1–11

Jeffery GM, Hickey BE, Hider P (2002) Follow-up strategies for patients treated for non-metastatic colorectal cancer (Cochrane Review). Cochrane Library, issue 2, Oxford: Update Software

Johnson K, Bakhsh A, Young D et al (2001) Correlating computed tomography and positron emission tomography scan with operative findings in metastatic colorectal cancer. Dis Colon Rectum 44:354–357

Kelvin FM, Korobkin M, Heaston DK et al (1983) The pelvis after surgery for rectal carcinoma: serial CT observations with emphasis on nonneoplastic features. AJR Am J Roentgenol 141:959–964

Keogan MT, Lowe VJ, Baker ME et al (1997) Local recurrence of rectal cancer: evaluation with F18-fluoredeoxyglucose PET imaging. Abdom Imaging 22:332–337

Kievit J (2002) Follow-up of patients with colorectal cancer: numbers needed to test and treat. Eur J Cancer 38:986–999

Kinkel K, Lu Y, Both M et al (2002) Detection of hepatic metastases from cancers of the gastrointestinal tract using noninvasive imaging methods (US, CT, MR Imaging, PET): a meta-analysis. Radiology 224:748–756

Kjeldsen BJ, Kronborg O, Fenger C et al (1997)a A prospective randomized study of follow-up after radical surgery for colorectal cancer. Br J Surg 84:666–669

Kjeldsen BJ, Kronborg O, Fenger C et al (1997)b The pattern of recurrent colorectal cancer in a prospective randomised study and the characteristics of diagnostic tests. Int J Colorectal Dis 12:329–334

Krestin GP (1997) Is magnetic resonance imaging the method of choice in the diagnosis of recurrent rectal carcinoma? Abdom Imaging 22:343–345

Leen E, Angerson WJ, Wotherspoon H et al (1995) Detection of colorectal liver metastases: comparison of laparotomy, CT, US and Doppler perfusion index and evaluation of postoperative follow-up results. Radiology 195:113–116

Leveson SH, Wiggins PA, Giles GR et al (1985) Deranged blood flow patterns in the detection of liver metastases. Br J Surg 72:128–130

Levi F, Misset JL, Brienza S et al (1992) A chronopharmacologic phase II clinical trial with 5-flurouracil, folinic acid, and oxaliplatin using ambulatory multichannel programmable pump. High antitumor effectiveness against metastatic colorectal cancer. Cancer 69:893–900

McAfee MK, Allen MS, Trastek VF et al (1992) Colorectal lung metastases: results of surgical excision. Ann Thorac Surg 53:780–785

Mäkelä JT, Laitinen SO, Kairaluoma MI (1995) Five-year follow-up after radical surgery for colorectal cancer. Results of a prospective randomized trial. Arch Surg 130: 1062–1067

Markus J, Morrissey B, DeGara C et al (1997) MRI of recurrent rectosigmoid carcinoma. Abdom Imaging 22:338–342

Morgan-Parkes JH (1995) Metastases: mechanisms, pathways, and cascades. AJR 164:1075–1082

Mossa AR, Ree PC, Marks JE et al (1975) Factors influencing local recurrence after abdominoperineal resection for cancer of the rectum and rectosigmoid. Br J Surg 62:727–730

NHS Executive (1997) Guidance on commissioning cancer services. Improving outcomes in colorectal cancer. The research evidence

Nordic Gastrointestinal Tumour Adjuvant Therapy Group (1992) Expectancy or primary chemotherapy in patients with advanced asymptomatic colorectal cancer: a randomized trial. J Clin Oncol 10:904–911

Northover J (2000) Which type of follow-up? Hepatogastroenterology 47:335–336

O'Dwyer PJ, Stevenson JP, Haller DG et al (2001) Follow-up of stage B and C colorectal cancer in the United States and France. Semin Oncol 28 [Suppl 1]:45–49

Ohlsson B, Breland U, Ekberg H et al (1995) Follow-up after curative surgery for colorectal carcinoma. Randomized comparison with no follow-up. Dis Colon Rectum 38: 619–626

Parker Sl, Tong T, Bolden S et al (1997) Cancer statistics. CA Cancer J Clin 47:5–27

Pema PJ, Bennett WF, Bova JG et al (1994) CT vs MRI in diagnosis of recurrent rectosigmoid carcinoma. J Comput Assist Tomogr 18:256–261

Petrowsky H, Gonen M, Jarnagin W et al (2002) Second liver resections are safe and effective treatment for recurrent hepatic metastases from colorectal cancer: a bi-institutional analysis. Ann Surg 235:863–871

Pietra N, Sarli L, Costi R et al (1998) Role of follow-up in management of local recurrences of colorectal cancer: a prospective, randomised study. Dis Colon Rectum 41:1127–1133

Pihl E, Hughes ES, McDermott FT et al (1981) Disease-free survival and recurrence after resection of colorectal carcinoma. J Surg Oncol 16:333–341

Polk HC, Spratt JS (1971) Recurrent colorectal carcinoma. Detection, treatment and other considerations. Surgery 69:9–23

Quirke P, Durdey P, Dixon MF et al (1986) Local recurrence of rectal adenocarcinoma due to inadequate surgical resection: histological study of lateral tumour spread and surgical excision. Lancet ii:996–999

Renehan AG, O'Dwyer ST (2000) Surveillance after colorectal cancer resection. Lancet 355:1095–1096

Richert-Boe KE (1995) Heterogeneity of cancer surveillance practices among medical oncologists in Washington and Oregon. Cancer 75:2605–2612

Rosen M, Chan L, Beart RW et al (1998) Follow-up of colorectal cancer a meta-analysis. Dis Colon Rectum 41:1116–1126

Rougier P, Bugat R, Douillard JY et al (1997) Phase II study of irinotecan in the treatment of advanced colorectal cancer in chemotherapy-naïve patients and patients pretreated with fluorouracil-based chemotherapy. J Clin Oncol 15:251–260

Safi F, Link KH, Beger HG (1993) Is follow-up of colorectal cancer patients worthwhile? Dis Colon Rectum 36: 636–644

Sarela AI, Guthrie JA, Seymour MT et al (2001) Non-operative management of the primary tumour in patients with incurable stage IV colorectal cancer. Br J Surg 88:1352–1356

Schoemaker D, Black R, Giles L et al (1998) Yearly colonoscopy, liver CT, and chest radiography do not influence 5-year survival of colorectal cancer patients. Gastroenterology 114:7–14

Scott DJ, Guthrie JA, Arnold P et al (2001) Dual phase helical CT versus portal venous phase CT for the detection of colorectal liver metastases: correlation with intra-operative sonography, surgical and pathological findings. Clin Rad 56:235–242

Secco GB, Fardelli R, Gianquinto D et al (2002) Efficacy and cost of risk – adapted follow-up in patients after colorectal cancer surgery: a prospective, randomised and controlled trial. Eur J Surg Oncol 28:418–423

Shepherd NA, Quirke P (1997) Colorectal cancer reporting: are we failing the patient? J Clin Pathol 50:266–267

Sobin LH, Wittekind C (2002) TNM classification of malignant tumours, 6th edn. Wiley-Liss, New York, pp 72–76

Staib L, Link KH, Beger HG (2000) Follow-up in colorectal cancer: cost-effectiveness analysis of established and novel concepts. Langenbecks Arch Surg 385:412–420

Stiggelbout AM, de Haes JC, Vree R et al (1997) Follow-up of colorectal cancer patients: quality of life and attitudes towards follow-up. Br J Cancer 75:914–920

Sugihara K, Yamamoto J (2000) Surgical treatment of colorectal liver metastases. Ann Chir Gynaecol 89:221–224

Swedish Rectal Cancer Group (1997) Improved survival with pre-operative radiotherapy rectal cancer. N Eng J Med 336: 980–987

Thompson WM, Halvorsen RA, Foster WL Jr (1986) Preoperative and postoperative CT staging of rectosigmoid carcinoma. Am J Roentgenol 146:703–710

Turk PS, Wanebo HJ (1993) Results of surgical treatment of nonhepatic recurrence of carcinoma. Cancer 71 (12 Supply):4267–4277

Virgo KS, Vernava AM, Long WE et al (1995) Cost of patient follow-up after potentially curative colorectal cancer treatment. JAMA 273:1837–1841

Ward J, Naik KS, Guthrie JA et al (1999) Hepatic lesion detection: comparison of MR imaging after the administration of superparamagnetic iron oxide with dual-phase CT by using alternative-free response receiver operating characteristic analysis. Radiology 210:459–466

Weiss L, Grundmann E, Torhorst J et al (1986) Haematogenous metastatic patterns in colonic carcinoma: an analysis of 1541 necropsies. J Pathol 150:195–203

Wernecke K, Rummeny EJ, Bongartz G et al (1991) Detection of hepatic masses in patients with carcinoma: comparative sensitivities of sonography, CT and MR imaging. Am J Roentgenol 157:731–739

Zhauang H, Sinha P, Pourdehanad M et al (2000) The role of positron emission tomography with fluorine-18-deoxyglucose in identifying colorectal cancer metastases to liver. Nuci Med Commun 21:793–798

13 Positron Emission Tomography in the Management of Colon Cancer

Stephen J. Skehan

CONTENTS

13.1   Introduction   137
13.2   Biological Considerations   137
13.3   PET Physics   137
13.4   Imaging Technique   138
13.5   Staging Prior to Hepatic Resection   138
13.6   Diagnosis of Pelvic Recurrence   141
13.7   Diagnosis of Recurrence with Rising CEA   142
13.8   Diagnosis of Primary Disease and Screening   143
13.9   Monitoring the Effect of Therapy   144
13.10 Conclusions   144
       References   145

13.1
Introduction

Positron emission tomography (PET) has been extensively studied in patients with colorectal carcinoma and it is clear that it offers the highest diagnostic accuracy of all imaging modalities in certain clinical settings (Gambhir et al. 2001). Despite the high costs associated with PET, its availability is increasing as its benefits become more widely appreciated by radiologists and oncologists. PET is no longer only a research tool limited to large academic centres and all physicians involved in the care of patients with colorectal cancer are likely to require some knowledge of the applications and limitations of the technique. This chapter begins with a brief discussion of the physical and biological basis for PET. The accepted clinical applications of PET in colorectal cancer will then be discussed. These include pre-operative assessment of patients with potentially resectable colorectal metastases to the liver, evaluation of residual pelvic masses following surgery for colorectal cancer and investigation of the patient with an elevated carcinoembryonic antigen (CEA) level. The impact of PET on the management of patients, both in terms of treatment decisions and cost implications, will also be discussed. The chapter will finish with a discussion of

the less well established role of PET in diagnosis and staging of primary disease.

13.2
Biological Considerations

The metabolism of malignant cells differs in several important ways from that of normal cells and these metabolic differences underlie the use of PET in oncology. Malignant cells use more glucose than normal cells. This is brought about by an increase in the number of glucose transporters on the surface of malignant cells and by increased expression of the hexokinase enzyme within malignant cells (Brown et al. 2002; Higashi et al. 1998). The radiopharmaceutical ^{18}F-fluorodeoxyglucose (hereafter referred to as FDG) is an analogue of glucose that can be readily manufactured from ^{18}F, a radioisotope produced in a type of accelerator known as a cyclotron. When FDG is taken up by a malignant cell it is converted to FDG-6-phosphate. Unlike its natural analogue, glucose-6-phosphate, FDG-6-phosphate cannot be further metabolised along the glycolytic pathway and is therefore trapped within the malignant cell. Excess accumulation of the radioactive tracer in malignant tissues compared with normal tissues forms the biological basis for FDG imaging in oncology. Other tracers, such as ^{11}C-labelled amino acids, also accumulate preferentially in malignant cells. They have also been used in oncology imaging, but the shorter half-life of ^{11}C (20 min) compared with ^{18}F (126 min) makes them less useful in routine clinical practice. One of the main advantages of PET is this use of "biological" molecules, unlike the artificial tracers used in routine radionuclide imaging.

13.3
PET Physics

The radioisotopes used in PET, such as ^{18}F, decay by emitting a positron. A positron is a tiny particle

S. J. Skehan, MD
Consultant Radiologist, St Vincent's University Hospital, Elm Park, Dublin 4, Ireland

with the same mass as an electron but the opposite charge. Almost as soon as a positron is emitted from the decaying nucleus it collides with an electron in the adjacent tissues. The two particles annihilate each other and their mass is converted to energy in the form of two gamma rays that travel in diametrically opposite directions from the point of annihilation. These gamma rays are detected by crystals of bismuth germanate or lutetium orthosilicate placed in a ring around the patient. Detection of the site of annihilation (which essentially equates to the site of positron emission) depends on two detectors detecting gamma rays within a very short time window, typically less than 10 ns. These two events are assumed to have arisen from the same annihilation and the imaging computer draws an imaginary "line of response" joining the site of detection of the two coincident gamma rays in the opposing detectors. A composite map of these "lines of response" is then used to build a three-dimensional image of the distribution of the tracer within the patient. PET is an exquisitely sensitive technique. The use of coincidence detection rather than lead collimation to determine the site of origin of the annihilation event improves sensitivity. The short half-life of ^{18}F-FDG also allows a relatively high dose to be administered, which allows for a high count rate in a short period of time. The typical dose to the patient is in the order of 5–10 mSv, depending on the administered dose of FDG .

13.4
Imaging Technique

Patients are injected with 185–370 MBq FDG after a 4-h fast. This is followed by a 45-min uptake period during which the patient should lie quietly in a relaxing environment to avoid excessive muscle uptake. Bowel cleansing is not necessary. Administration of frusemide at the time of injection helps to clear urinary activity from the field of view. Bladder catheterisation has also been advocated, but in the author's experience it is rarely required, except occasionally for clarification of a small soft tissue abnormality immediately adjacent to the bladder (MIRALDI et al. 1998). Scan times vary according to equipment, ranging from 25 to 45 min for a typical whole-body study. Images are ideally acquired with correction for the attenuation of activity arising from deeper structures within the patient. PET images must be reviewed in conjunction with CT or other relevant images. The most recent and expensive tomographs combine a CT and PET scan, so

that image registration is automatically achieved. It is important to recognise normal FDG uptake in stomach, colon, stomas (Fig. 13.1), kidneys, ureters, bladder and recent laparotomy wounds (ZEALLEY et al. 2001). More unusual mimics of abnormal pelvic activity such as the menstruating retroverted uterus and pelvic kidneys have also been reported (BHARGAVA et al. 2002; CHANDER et al. 2002).

13.5
Staging Prior to Hepatic Resection

Hepatic resection for metastases from colorectal carcinoma is technically feasible in approximately 10%–20% of patients with hepatic metastases (REES and JOHN 2001). The 5-year survival rate is reported at 35%–55% following this procedure, representing a marked improvement in prognosis compared with non-surgical approaches (BELLI et al. 2002; CHOTI et al. 2002; FONG et al. 1999a; HARDY et al. 1998; NAKA-MURA et al. 1999; OHLSSON et al. 1998; YAMAMOTO et al. 1999). There is also a trend towards better results in more recent years, compared with the earlier experience (CHOTI et al. 2002). The number and distribution of metastases within the liver is clearly critical in determining the feasibility of resection. The other major determinant is the presence or absence of extrahepatic disease. In follow-up of surgical series approximately half of recurrences are in the unresected liver and the other half involve extrahepatic sites (YAMADA et al. 2001). Therefore, inability to detect disease at these sites before surgery is the main cause of treatment failure. The major challenge for diagnostic imaging is to identify these patients when they are being assessed for surgery. The morbidity and mortality associated with major surgery can then be avoided in those patients where such an operation is unlikely to result in long-term benefits because of untreated disease elsewhere.

Pre-operative imaging varies depending on local equipment and expertise. Portal phase, helical or multidetector CT scans are standard in most institutions, but MRI and ultrasound can also be used to evaluate the liver. CT of the thorax and of the remainder of the abdomen and pelvis are also routinely performed to exclude extrahepatic disease. Numerous studies have now been published showing that PET detects additional sites of disease in a significant number of patients who appear to have resectable disease after imaging with CT, MRI and ultrasound (Fig. 13.2). In one prospective study of 40 patients

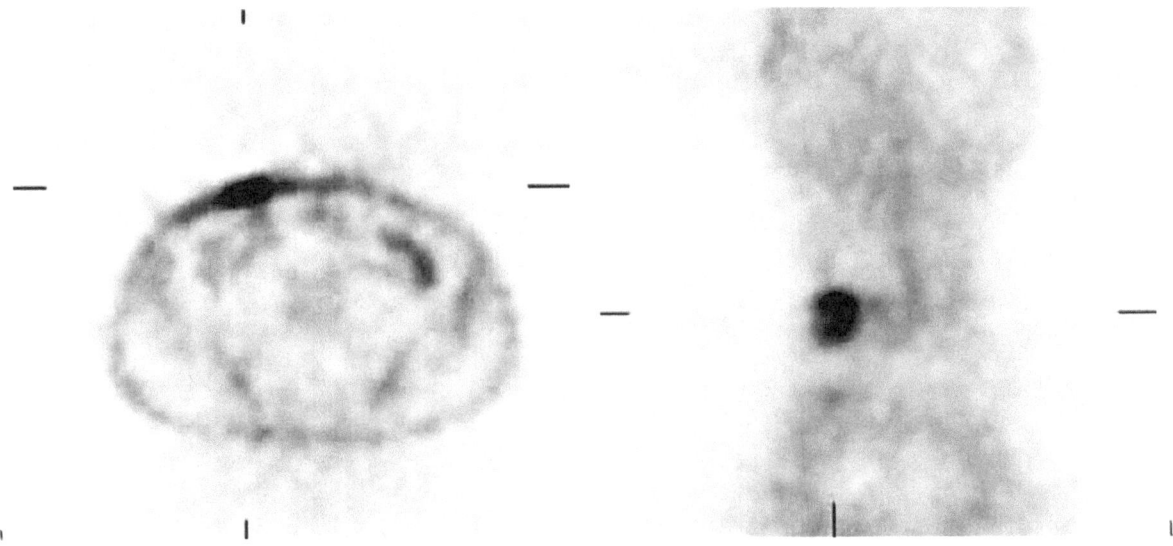

Fig. 13.1a,b. Normal uptake of FDG in a colostomy seen in the axial (**a**) and coronal (**b**) planes

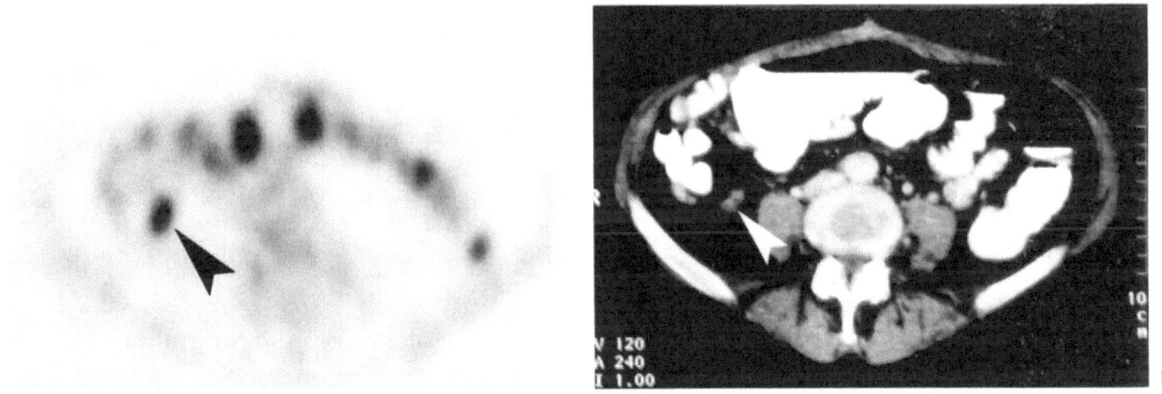

Fig. 13.2a,b. a Axial FDG PET image through the lower abdomen showing an abnormal focus of increased uptake (*arrowhead*) that was separate from normal bowel activity visible anteriorly. The typical serpiginous pattern of bowel activity is easier to appreciate by viewing the multiple axial images at a workstation. **b** Corresponding axial CT image confirming a peritoneal nodule (*arrowhead*) in the right iliac fossa

considered resectable with anatomical imaging, PET demonstrated additional disease precluding curative resection in nine patients (FONG et al. 1999b). Sub-centimetre peritoneal metastases were missed with PET in three patients (7.5%) in the same study. Sensitivity for extrahepatic disease in another study was 94% for PET and 64% for anatomical imaging (WHITEFORD et al. 2000). Of 91 patients with hepatic disease in a study by TOPAL et al. (2001), ten were found to have additional disease with PET that precluded resection. A false negative rate of 7.7% was noted in the same study for small intra-abdominal lesions. VALK et al. (1999) found tumour at additional sites in 23 (29%) of 78 preoperative studies in which CT showed a single site of recurrence. Therefore, PET appears to offer the most accurate means of diagnosing unresectable disease although a small but definite false negative rate of less than 10% must be acknowledged. False positive uptake also occurs, making correlation with anatomical imaging extremely important (Fig. 13.3).

In addition to its role in detecting extrahepatic disease, PET is also useful for diagnosing hepatic abnormalities (Fig. 13.4). A recent meta-analysis has evaluated ultrasound, CT, MRI and PET for accuracy in diagnosing liver metastases from gastrointestinal primary tumours (KINKEL et al. 2002). In this study the authors set a lower threshold of 85% to represent the lowest clinically useful specificity of a diagnostic test for evaluating liver lesions. In studies with a spe-

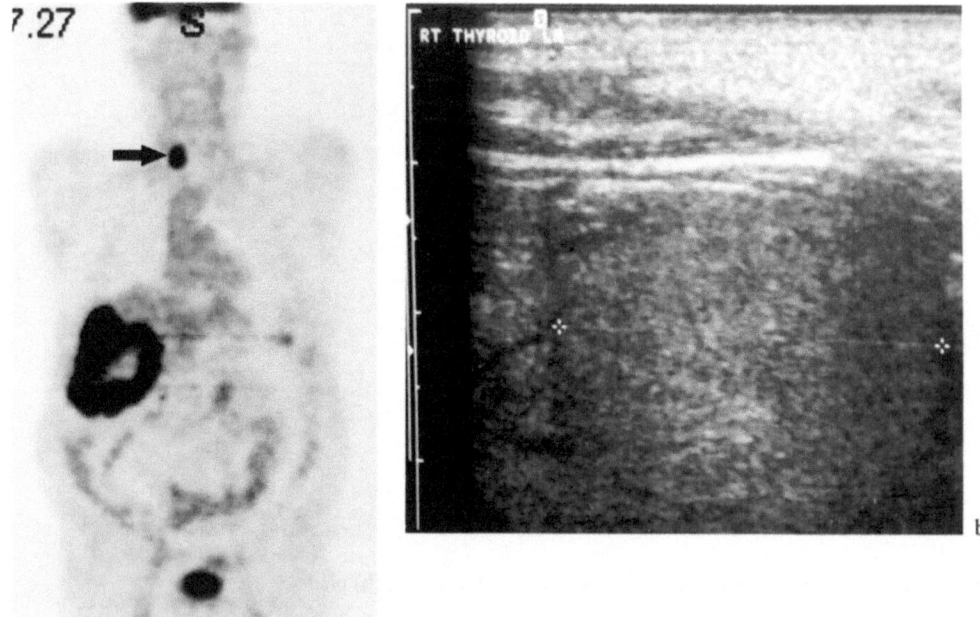

Fig. 13.3a,b. a Coronal FDG PET image showing a large solitary hepatic metastasis and further focus of abnormal uptake in the right supraclavicular region. **b** Sagittal ultrasound image of the thyroid in the same patient confirmed a solid, hypoechoic nodule that proved benign on fine needle cytology

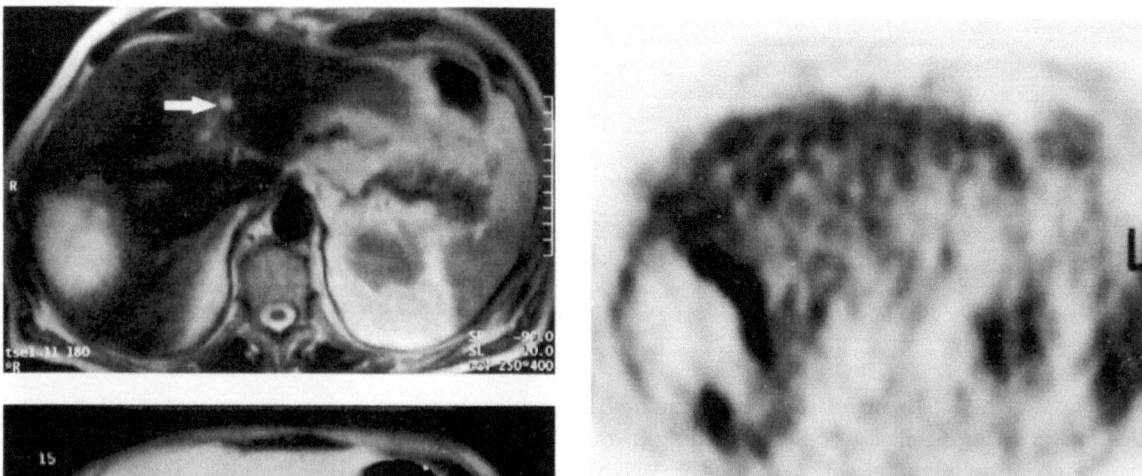

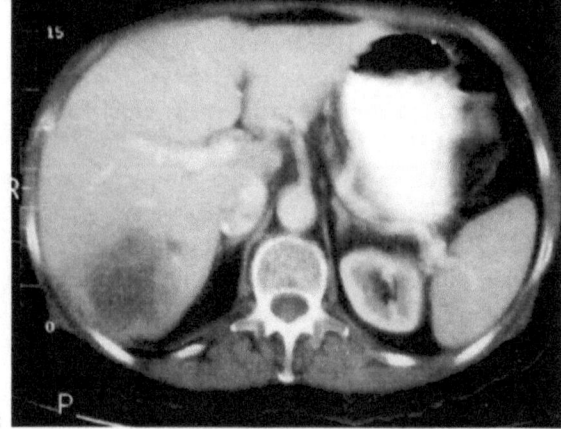

Fig. 13.4a–c. a Axial T2-weighted MR image showing a large partly necrotic metastasis in the right lobe of the liver, with a smaller high signal lesion in segment 4 (*arrow*). **b** Corresponding axial FDG PET image with a ring of increased uptake in the viable part of the metastasis, but no abnormal uptake in the other lesion which was a simple cyst and remained stable on follow-up. The activity between liver and spleen is normal upper pole of left kidney. **c** Corresponding CT image

cificity higher than 85%, the mean weighted sensitivity was 55% for ultrasound [95% confidence intervals (CI): 41, 68], 72% for CT (95% CI: 63, 80), 76% for MRI (95% CI: 57, 91), and 90% for FDG PET (95% CI: 80, 97). As with all diagnostic tests for evaluating liver metastases, small lesions are more difficult to identify with PET. RUERS et al. (2002) demonstrated a sensitivity of only 65% for PET compared with 80% for CT for liver lesions, with size being the most important factor in non-detection of lesions. In another study only 25% of hepatic lesions smaller than 1 cm were detected by PET, while 85% of lesions larger than 1 cm were detected (FONG et al. 1999b). In practice it is best to perform PET with MRI or portal-phase CT of the liver, the former for greatest accuracy in lesion detection and characterisation and the latter for optimal segmental lesion localisation.

This additional diagnostic accuracy of PET has a major effect on management planning for patients with hepatic metastases. Planned management changed in 11%–29% of patients in a variety of prospective and retrospective studies when compared with the management plan based on anatomical imaging (FONG et al. 1999b; LAI et al. 1996; RUERS et al. 2002; TOPAL et al. 2001; VALK et al. 1999; VITOLA et al. 1996). The change in management was most often a change from surgical to non-surgical treatment due to the detection of disease that would not have been treated by local hepatic resection.

It is interesting in the light of the above data to consider the role of PET in preoperative assessment in terms of its contribution to the patient management process. A hierarchical structure has been described for assessing the efficacy of an imaging technique in overall patient care (FRYBACK and THORNBURY 1991). Demonstration of efficacy at each lower level in this hierarchy is logically necessary, but not sufficient, to assure efficacy at higher levels. The diagnostic accuracy of PET is undoubtedly superior to other imaging modalities in the pre-resection setting. This represents level 2 of the hierarchy of efficacy (how well can we see it?). The efficacy of PET at level 3 (effect on diagnostic thinking) and level 4 (effect on the patient's management plan) is also proven. Level 5 studies measure the effect of the imaging procedure on patient outcome. There are very few studies demonstrating the efficacy of PET at level 5. There are no randomised outcome studies as yet of patients managed with and without pre-operative PET. In one published study 43 patients referred for resection on the basis of conventional staging with CT subsequently underwent preoperative PET (STRASBERG et al. 2001). Additional disease was found in ten patients

and six of those were considered inoperable on the basis of the PET result. Median follow-up was only 24 months in this study. The Kaplan-Meier estimate of 3-year survival for operable patients was 77% and the lower 95% confidence limit of this estimate of survival was 60%. Actual 3-year survival rates of 61%–65% have been reported without using PET for preselection (FINCH et al. 1998; YAMAMOTO et al. 1999). Therefore, improvement in survival as an outcome measure when PET is used pre-operatively has not yet been proven in spite of the obvious efficacy at lower levels in the hierarchy. It is worth noting that this criticism of PET is also true for most other imaging tests in most clinical settings, as the vast majority of radiology research only investigates the lower levels of this hierarchy. In addition, survival is not the only important outcome measure in this setting and a well-designed level-5 study would also take into account quality-of-life measures for all patients.

13.6
Diagnosis of Pelvic Recurrence

The residual presacral mass in patients who have had surgery and often radiotherapy for rectal cancer gives rise to much diagnostic difficulty. Post-therapy scarring and fibrosis result in a great variety of chronic presacral CT abnormalities, ranging from stranding of the presacral fat to frank mass formation. The clinical presentation is often with pelvic discomfort, which can be due to benign or malignant causes. With anatomical imaging there are two main options for determining the nature of a residual mass. The first option is to repeat the examination after an interval of several weeks to months in order to assess any change in the mass – obviously a malignant lesion will tend to enlarge. This approach results in a delay in diagnosis and may render any salvage therapy impossible (Fig. 13.5). Alternatively, CT can be used to direct a biopsy of the presacral abnormality, although this is not always technically feasible.

PET offers a particularly useful solution to this problem in that residual active tumour shows uptake of the tracer, while post-therapy scar tissue does not (Fig. 13.6). An early paper reported 100% sensitivity and specificity for PET in differentiating scar and recurrent tumour in 15 patients (ITO et al. 1992). A total of 18 patients with presacral masses or streaking were investigated with PET in a later study (KEOGAN et al. 1997) in which PET had a sensitivity of 92.3% (95% confidence limits 63.9% to 99.8%) for detection

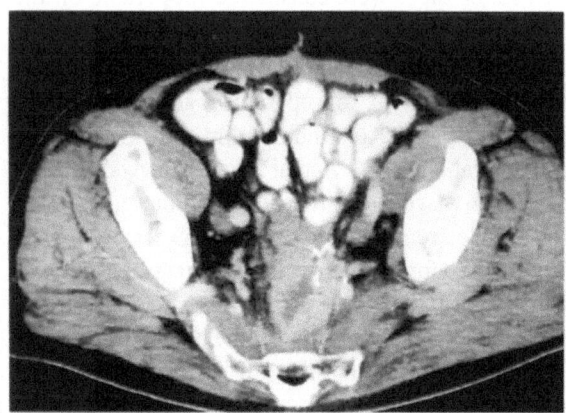
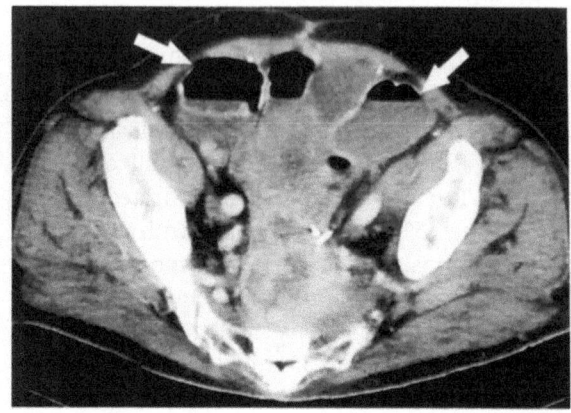

Fig. 13.5a,b. a Axial CT image showing a presacral soft tissue mass containing some surgical clips in a patient with pelvic pain and previous resection of a rectal tumour. **b** Axial CT at the same level obtained 3 months later. The presacral mass has enlarged and is now causing small bowel obstruction (*arrows*)

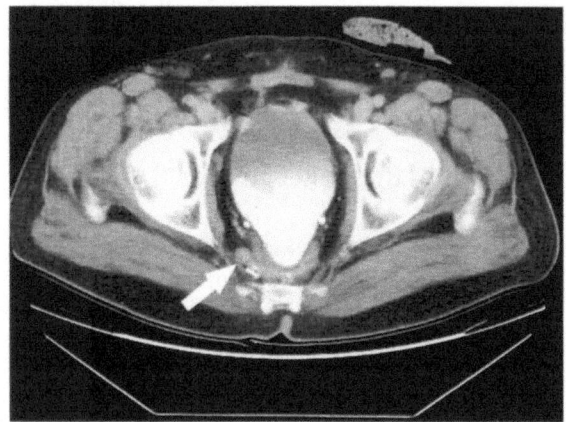
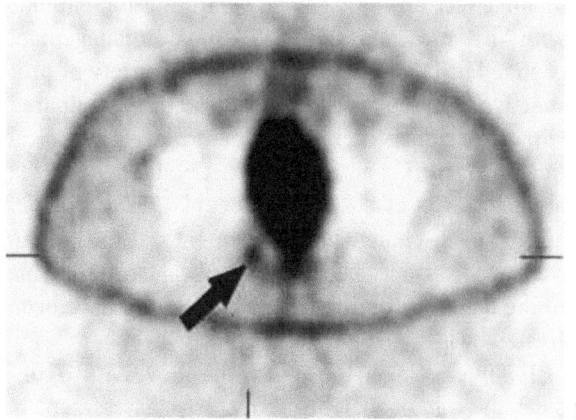

Fig. 13.6a,b. a Axial CT in a patient with a tiny soft tissue nodule (*arrow*) adjacent to a surgical clip post rectal resection. **b** Corresponding axial FDG PET image showed increased uptake in the nodule (*arrow*) indicating active disease. Urinary activity is seen anteriorly in the bladder

of recurrent disease and a specificity of 80% (95% confidence limits; 28.3%, 99.4%). In a different study PET was found to be 91% sensitive and 100% specific for detection of local pelvic recurrence (OGUNBIYI et al. 1997). Correlation with CT or MRI is essential in this area to ensure that urinary activity is not mistaken for local pelvic recurrence. Bladder catheterisation is usually not necessary, even for detection of small lesions close to the bladder (Fig. 13.6). It is important to know the timing of previous radiation when interpreting a PET examination as increased uptake may be seen in a tumour for several months after radiotherapy. There is a lack of scientific data on the exact time course of this finding, but most experts agree that increased uptake more than 6 months after radiotherapy indicates active malignant disease (DELBEKE 1999).

13.7
Diagnosis of Recurrence with Rising CEA

CEA is a serum marker of disease activity in colorectal cancer that can detect recurrence with a sensitivity of 59% and a specificity of 84% (MOERTEL et al. 1993). Some surgeons routinely measure CEA levels during follow-up of patients with previously treated colorectal cancer. The rationale is that a rise in the serum marker may herald an early recurrence that can be successfully treated. A recent meta-analysis of randomised trials (intensive versus minimal follow-up) has concluded that 5-year survival is improved by intensive follow-up (RENEHAN et al. 2002). The use of CT and frequent measurement of CEA resulted in a reduction of cancer-related mortality by 9%–13%. The authors noted that "this survival benefit was partly attributable to the earlier detection of all recurrences, particularly the increased detection of isolated recurrent disease".

One of the difficulties that arises when using CEA to detect recurrent disease is localisation of the site of recurrence in the presence of rising CEA. PET has proven extremely useful in locating disease in this setting (Fig. 13.7). FLANAGAN et al. (1998) performed PET on 22 patients with rising CEA and normal anatomical imaging; 17 had positive PET studies (of whom 15 proved true positive) and disease was resected with curative intent in four of these patients. All five patients with negative PET examinations remained free of disease on follow-up. In another study of 15 patients with rising CEA and normal anatomical imaging, 14 had abnormal PET examinations (ZERVOS et al. 2001). Nine of these were considered potentially curable by surgery and six underwent successful operative procedures. Two of the nine had more extensive disease at exploratory surgery than was predicted by PET and in one case PET was falsely positive. FLAMEN et al. (2001) studied 50 consecutive patients with rising CEA and normal or equivocal anatomical imaging examina-

tions. PET identified recurrent disease in 43 patients and 14 subsequently underwent surgery with curative intent. To summarise: the role of PET is to direct laparotomy when recurrent disease appears isolated and to avoid unnecessary second-look laparotomy when disease clearly involves several sites. A conservative, watchful waiting approach is suggested when PET is negative (LIBUTTI et al. 2001).

13.8
Diagnosis of Primary Disease and Screening

PET is not currently recommended for the diagnosis of primary colorectal neoplasms, although there is no doubt that the technique can detect primary tumours with very high sensitivity (96%–100%) (ABDEL-NABI et al. 1998; MUKAI et al. 2000). Endoscopy and biopsy, supported by CT and barium studies, are likely to remain the diagnostic techniques of choice for this purpose. The appearances of primary tumours with

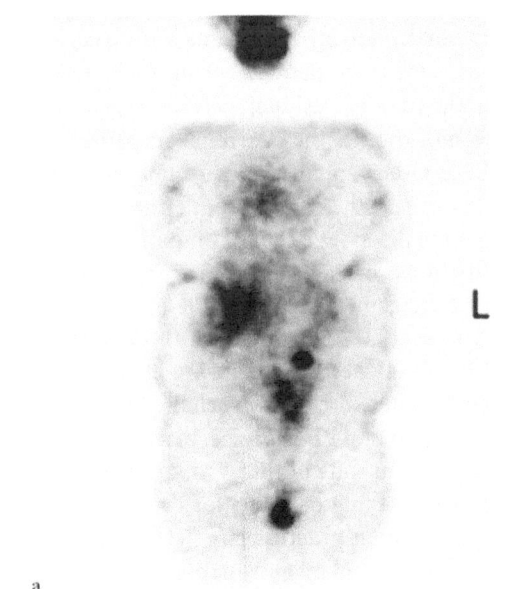

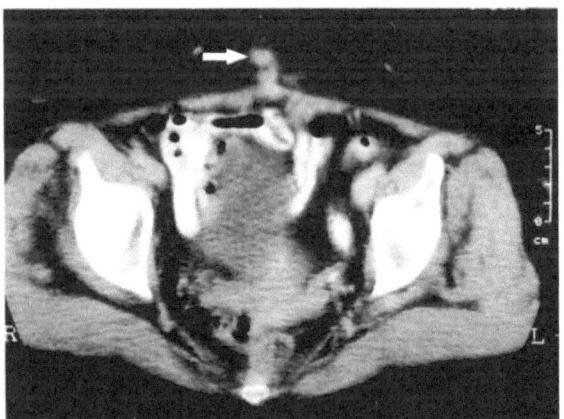

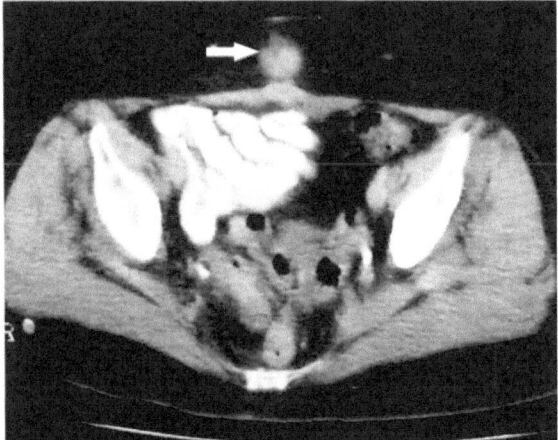

Fig. 13.7a–c. a Coronal FDG PET image in a patient with rising CEA. Two foci of increased uptake are seen in the anterior abdominal wall. **b** Axial CT image through the pelvis confirmed a soft tissue nodule (*arrow*) related to the previous laparotomy scar, which enlarged on subsequent repeat CT (**c**)

PET are nevertheless important as they may be noted on a PET study performed for other purposes. Normal colon demonstrates a variable signal up to the intensity of bone marrow (Skehan et al. 1999). Increased colonic uptake can be seen with inflammation or with neoplasm (Drenth et al. 2001; Skehan et al. 1999). In a cohort of 39 patients who underwent both PET and colonoscopy (mostly for follow-up of colorectal cancer), PET had sensitivity of 74% and specificity of 84% for the detection of polyps greater than 3 mm and carcinomas (Drenth et al. 2001). The authors of another study investigated the pattern of colonic uptake (nodular, segmental or diffuse) in 27 patients with a history of colorectal cancer undergoing PET (Tatlidil et al. 2002). They found that nodular high FDG uptake implied at least a 79% chance (lower 95% CI) that an adenoma or carcinoma would be found at endoscopy. Segmental increased uptake predicted colitis in five out of six patients in whom it was found.

In Japan whole body PET is now being used as part of health screening for asymptomatic individuals. In a study of 110 patients from such a population who underwent both PET and colonoscopy, the sensitivity of PET for detecting adenomas was only 24% (14/59) (Yasuda et al. 2001). However, the sensitivity was 90% for polyps greater than 12 mm in diameter. A false positive rate of 5.5% (6/110) was noted in this study. Certainly in countries with limited PET resources there is insufficient evidence to suggest that PET should be used in any way for this type of screening.

13.9
Monitoring the Effect of Therapy

For several years much has been spoken about the potential of PET to act as a very early marker of response or lack of response to oncological therapies. It has been suggested that decisions about therapeutic efficacy or the need to change to alternative therapy can be made after a single course of chemotherapy or at a very early stage in radiotherapy, rather than waiting for several weeks to months as is the current practice (Shields et al. 1998). However, relatively few studies have yet been published that confirm this role in a routine clinical setting for any malignancy.

In a limited study of ten patients with non-resectable hepatic metastases from colorectal cancer, FDG uptake was quantified prior to and 72 h after a single infusion of 5-fluorouracil and folinic acid (Bender et al. 1999). Patients were followed for 6 months to determine outcome. The six patients with a sustained response to therapy showed a statistically significant reduction in FDG uptake (-22±10%) at 72 h while those with disease progression had enhanced FDG uptake (13±17%). In another study of neoadjuvant chemoradiation for rectal carcinoma, PET was performed before and 4–5 weeks after treatment (Guillem et al. 2000). All 15 patients had a pathological response to treatment and this was predicted by PET in all cases, but in only 7 of 9 patients who also underwent CT. The degree of pathological response was predicted in nine of the 15 patients by a PET parameter known as the visual response score.

While PET shows a certain degree of promise for assessing treatment response in colorectal cancer, there is clearly a lack of evidence to suggest any clinically useful role at this time.

13.10
Conclusions

FDG PET has three well-defined applications in the management of patients with colorectal cancer: assessment of patients prior to hepatic resection, evaluation of residual pelvic masses and localisation of the site of recurrence in patients with rising CEA. Other applications are not well established at this time. When PET is added to anatomical imaging for the assessment of all patients with known or suspected disease recurrence, it results in a change in management in 28%–61% of patients (Arulampalam et al. 2001; Beets et al. 1994; Delbeke et al. 1997; Kalff et al. 2002; Staib et al. 2000; Valk et al. 1999). There are obvious challenges associated with provision of a PET service, particularly related to its expense. In spite of this, Valk et al. (1999) have estimated a saving of $3003 for every preoperative PET study in their practice, largely due to the saving arising from avoidance of inappropriate major surgery. As noted in the section on hepatic metastases above, these results need to be interpreted with caution until more outcome data are available for patients imaged with PET. However, even without such data, it is reasonable to suggest that for the three indications outlined above PET represents the present standard of care.

References

Abdel-Nabi H, Doerr RJ, Lamonica DM et al (1998) Staging of primary colorectal carcinomas with fluorine-18 fluorodeoxyglucose whole-body PET: correlation with histopathologic and CT findings. Radiology 206:755–760

Arulampalam T, Costa D, Visvikis D et al (2001) The impact of FDG-PET on the management algorithm for recurrent colorectal cancer. Eur J Nucl Med 28:1758–1765

Beets G, Penninckx F, Schiepers C et al (1994) Clinical value of whole-body positron emission tomography with [18F]fluorodeoxyglucose in recurrent colorectal cancer. Br J Surg 81:1666–1670

Belli G, D'Agostino A, Ciciliano F et al (2002) Liver resection for hepatic metastases: 15 years of experience. J Hepatobil Pancreat Surg 9:607–613

Bender H, Bangard N, Metten N et al (1999) Possible role of FDG-PET in the early prediction of therapy outcome in liver metastases of colorectal cancer. Hybridoma 18:87–91

Bhargava P, Zhuang H, Hickeson M et al (2002) Pelvic kidney mimicking recurrent colon cancer on FDG positron emission tomographic imaging. Clin Nucl Med 27:602–603

Brown RS, Goodman TM, Zasadny KR et al (2002) Expression of hexokinase II and Glut-1 in untreated human breast cancer. Nucl Med Biol 29:443–453

Chander S, Meltzer CC, McCook BM (2002) Physiologic uterine uptake of FDG during menstruation demonstrated with serial combined positron emission tomography and computed tomography. Clin Nucl Med 27:22–24

Choti MA, Sitzmann JV, Tiburi MF et al (2002) Trends in long-term survival following liver resection for hepatic colorectal metastases. Ann Surg 235:759–766

Delbeke D (1999) Oncological applications of FDG PET imaging: brain tumors, colorectal cancer, lymphoma and melanoma. J Nucl Med 40:591–603

Delbeke D, Vitola JV, Sandler MP et al (1997) Staging recurrent metastatic colorectal carcinoma with PET. J Nucl Med 38:1196–1201

Drenth JP, Nagengast FM, Oyen WJ (2001) Evaluation of (pre-)malignant colonic abnormalities: endoscopic validation of FDG-PET findings. Eur J Nucl Med 28:1766–1769

Finch MD, Crosbie JL, Currie E et al (1998) An 8-year experience of hepatic resection: indications and outcome. Br J Surg 85:315–319

Flamen P, Hoekstra OS, Homans F et al (2001) Unexplained rising carcinoembryonic antigen (CEA) in the postoperative surveillance of colorectal cancer: the utility of positron emission tomography (PET). Eur J Cancer 37:862–869

Flanagan FL, Dehdashti F, Ogunbiyi OA et al (1998) Utility of FDG-PET for investigating unexplained plasma CEA elevation in patients with colorectal cancer. Ann Surg 227:319–323

Fong Y, Fortner J, Sun RL et al (1999a) Clinical score for predicting recurrence after hepatic resection for metastatic colorectal cancer: analysis of 1001 consecutive cases. Ann Surg 230:309–318; discussion 318–321

Fong Y, Saldinger PF, Akhurst T et al (1999b) Utility of 18F-FDG positron emission tomography scanning on selection of patients for resection of hepatic colorectal metastases. Am J Surg 178:282–287

Fryback DG, Thornbury JR (1991) The efficacy of diagnostic imaging. Med Decis Making 11:88–94

Gambhir SS, Czernin J, Schwimmer J et al (2001) A tabu-lated summary of the FDG PET literature. J Nucl Med 42:1S–93S

Guillem JG, Puig-La Calle J Jr, Akhurst T et al (2000) Prospective assessment of primary rectal cancer response to preoperative radiation and chemotherapy using 18-fluorodeoxyglucose positron emission tomography. Dis Colon Rectum 43:18–24

Hardy KJ, Fletcher DR, Jones RM (1998) One hundred liver resections including comparison to non-resected liver-mobilized patients. Aust NZ J Surg 68:716–721

Higashi T, Tamaki N, Torizuka T et al (1998) FDG uptake, GLUT-1 glucose transporter and cellularity in human pancreatic tumors. J Nucl Med 39:1727–1735

Ito K, Kato T, Tadokoro M et al (1992) Recurrent rectal cancer and scar: differentiation with PET and MR imaging. Radiology 182:549–552

Kalff V, Hicks RJ, Ware RE et al (2002) The clinical impact of (18)F-FDG PET in patients with suspected or confirmed recurrence of colorectal cancer: a prospective study. J Nucl Med 43:492–499

Keogan MT, Lowe VJ, Baker ME et al (1997) Local recurrence of rectal cancer: evaluation with F-18 fluorodeoxyglucose PET imaging. Abdom Imaging 22:332–337

Kinkel K, Lu Y, Both M et al (2002) Detection of hepatic metastases from cancers of the gastrointestinal tract by using noninvasive imaging methods (US, CT, MR imaging, PET): a meta-analysis. Radiology 224:748–756

Lai DT, Fulham M, Stephen MS et al (1996) The role of whole-body positron emission tomography with [18F]fluorodeoxyglucose in identifying operable colorectal cancer metastases to the liver. Arch Surg 131:703–707

Libutti SK, Alexander HR Jr, Choyke P et al (2001) A prospective study of 2-[18F] fluoro-2-deoxy-D-glucose/positron emission tomography scan, 99mTc-labeled arcitumomab (CEA-scan), and blind second-look laparotomy for detecting colon cancer recurrence in patients with increasing carcinoembryonic antigen levels. Ann Surg Oncol 8:779–786

Miraldi F, Vesselle H, Faulhaber PF et al (1998) Elimination of artifactual accumulation of FDG in PET imaging of colorectal cancer. Clin Nucl Med 23:3–7

Moertel CG, Fleming TR, Macdonald JS et al (1993) An evaluation of the carcinoembryonic antigen (CEA) test for monitoring patients with resected colon cancer. JAMA 270:943–947

Mukai M, Sadahiro S, Yasuda S et al (2000) Preoperative evaluation by whole-body 18F-fluorodeoxyglucose positron emission tomography in patients with primary colorectal cancer. Oncol Rep 7:85–87

Nakamura S, Suzuki S, Konno H (1999) Resection of hepatic metastases of colorectal carcinoma: 20 years' experience. J Hepatobil Pancreat Surg 6:16–22

Ogunbiyi OA, Flanagan FL, Dehdashti F et al (1997) Detection of recurrent and metastatic colorectal cancer: comparison of positron emission tomography and computed tomography. Ann Surg Oncol 4:613–620

Ohlsson B, Stenram U, Tranberg KG (1998) Resection of colorectal liver metastases: 25-year experience. World J Surg 22:268–276; discussion 276–267

Rees M, John TG (2001) Current status of surgery in colorectal metastases to the liver. Hepatogastroenterology 48:341–344

Renehan AG, Egger M, Saunders MP et al (2002) Impact on survival of intensive follow up after curative resection for colorectal cancer: systematic review and meta-analysis of randomised trials. BMJ 324:813

Ruers TJ, Langenhoff BS, Neeleman N et al (2002) Value of positron emission tomography with [F-18]fluorodeoxyglucose in patients with colorectal liver metastases: a prospective study. J Clin Oncol 20:388–395

Shields AF, Mankoff DA, Link JM et al (1998) Carbon-11-thymidine and FDG to measure therapy response. J Nucl Med 39:1757–1762

Skehan SJ, Issenman R, Mernagh J et al (1999) 18F-fluorodeoxyglucose positron tomography in diagnosis of paediatric inflammatory bowel disease (letter). Lancet 354:836–837

Staib L, Schirrmeister H, Reske SN et al (2000) Is (18)F-fluorodeoxyglucose positron emission tomography in recurrent colorectal cancer a contribution to surgical decision making? Am J Surg 180:1–5

Strasberg SM, Dehdashti F, Siegel BA et al (2001) Survival of patients evaluated by FDG-PET before hepatic resection for metastatic colorectal carcinoma: a prospective database study. Ann Surg 233:293–299

Tatlidil R, Jadvar H, Bading JR et al (2002) Incidental colonic fluorodeoxyglucose uptake: correlation with colonoscopic and histopathologic findings. Radiology 224:783–787

Topal B, Flamen P, Aerts R et al (2001) Clinical value of whole-body emission tomography in potentially curable colorectal liver metastases. Eur J Surg Oncol 27:175–179

Valk PE, Abella-Columna E, Haseman MK et al (1999) Whole-body PET imaging with [18F]fluorodeoxyglucose in management of recurrent colorectal cancer. Arch Surg 134:503–511; discussion 511–503

Vitola JV, Delbeke D, Sandler MP et al (1996) Positron emission tomography to stage suspected metastatic colorectal carcinoma to the liver. Am J Surg 171:21–26

Whiteford MH, Whiteford HM, Yee LF et al (2000) Usefulness of FDG-PET scan in the assessment of suspected metastatic or recurrent adenocarcinoma of the colon and rectum. Dis Colon Rectum 43:759–767; discussion 767–770

Yamada H, Kondo S, Okushiba S et al (2001) Analysis of predictive factors for recurrence after hepatectomy for colorectal liver metastases. World J Surg 25:1129–1133

Yamamoto J, Shimada K, Kosuge T et al (1999) Factors influencing survival of patients undergoing hepatectomy for colorectal metastases. Br J Surg 86:332–337

Yasuda S, Fujii H, Nakahara T et al (2001) 18F-FDG PET detection of colonic adenomas. J Nucl Med 42:989–992

Zealley IA, Skehan SJ, Rawlinson J et al (2001) Selection of patients for resection of hepatic metastases: improved detection of extrahepatic disease with FDG PET. Radiographics 21 (Spec No):S55–S69

Zervos EE, Badgwell BD, Burak WE Jr et al (2001) Fluorodeoxyglucose positron emission tomography as an adjunct to carcinoembryonic antigen in the management of patients with presumed recurrent colorectal cancer and nondiagnostic radiologic workup. Surgery 130:636–643; discussion 643–634

14 Sonography and Appendicitis in Adults: Current Status

Etienne M. Danse, Bernhard E. Van Beers, Patrice Taourel

CONTENTS

14.1 Introduction *147*
14.2 Clinical Findings *147*
14.3 Cross-Sectional Imaging of Acute Appendicitis *148*
14.4 Sonographic Technique and Normal Findings *148*
14.5 Sonographic Findings in Acute Appendicitis *149*
14.6 Differential Diagnosis *150*
14.7 Strategy *152*
14.7.1 Indications for Sonography *152*
14.7.2 How to Manage Sonographic Results *153*
14.8 Conclusion *153*
References *153*

14.1 Introduction

Sonography as a means of diagnosing acute appendicitis was first described in 1986 (Puylaert 1986; Puylaert et al. 1987). Since then it has gained acceptance and with the use of high frequency probes, graded compression and colour Doppler imaging there have been many reports emphasizing an increasing role for sonography in the initial diagnostic work-up of patients with acute abdominal symptoms. Meanwhile, numerous publications have shown an increasing role for body computed tomography in this field and some papers have compared sonography with computed tomography. Computed tomography wins the battle as it does not depend on operator experience, body habitus, or the presence of gaseous interfaces (Wilson et al. 2001; Pena et al. 2000; Horton et al. 2000; Sivit et al. 2000; Wise et al. 2001).

Despite the superior accuracy of computed tomography, sonography is still considered the first method to use when a patient is seen in the emergency room with acute pain in the right iliac fossa (Puylaert 1990, 1994, 2001; Puylaert et al. 1997;

E. M. Danse, MD; B. E. Van Beers, MD, PhD
Department of Medical Imaging, Cliniques Universitaires St-Luc, Avenue Hippocrate, 10, 1200 Brussels, Belgium
P. Taourel, MD, PhD
Service de Radiologie Hopital la Peyronie, CHU de Montpellier, 2 Avenue Berlin Sans, 34295 Montpellier Cedex 5, France

Rioux 1995). This chapter reviews the main clinical and sonographic findings of appendicitis in adults.

14.2 Clinical Findings

Acute appendicitis is one of the commonest causes of surgery for the acute abdomen (Puylaert et al. 1987; Doherty and Lewis 1989). Inflammation of the appendix results from obstruction of its lumen (Birnbaum and Wilson 2000) from stercoliths, foreign bodies, lymphoid hyperplasia, parasites or tumours (primary or metastatic) (Birnbaum and Wilson 2000; Hermans et al. 1993; Jeffrey et al. 1988). The initial description of the normal and pathologic vermiform appendix was made in the 16th century (Williams and Myers 1994), and during this century, the first clinical report of acute appendicitis was made by the French physician, Jean Fernel (Doherty and Lewis 1989). Before the advent of cross-sectional imaging of the abdomen, surgery was based only on suggestive clinical and laboratory findings (Taourel 2001). Classically, appendicitis occurs in young male patients, aged 7–45 years, who present with acute periumbilical pain, mild fever, nausea, vomiting and anorexia (Doherty and Lewis 1989; Williams and Myers 1994; Horton et al. 2000). After some hours, the pain migrates to McBurney's point in the right iliac fossa.

Up to 40% of patients with a final diagnosis of acute appendicitis have non-specific symptoms. When surgery is based solely on clinical data an inconclusive laparotomy can be expected in 20%–35% of cases (Puylaert et al.1987; Rioux 1992; Taourel 2001). The leucocyte count is often higher than 10,000/mm³ and it has been shown that the probability of acute appendicitis is related to a leucocyte count (higher than 11,500/mm³) and to the sex and age of the patient (male patients under 25) (Roth et al. 2001), whereas if both leucocyte count and C-reactive protein are normal at the time of admission and remain so during follow-up, appendicitis can reasonably be excluded (GRÖNROOS and GRÖNROOS 2001).

14.3
Cross-Sectional Imaging of Acute Appendicitis

The superiority of cross-sectional imaging over clinical judgement for the diagnosis of appendicitis has been demonstrated in several studies. Sonography is very helpful for providing a prompt diagnosis but there is still debate about the contribution of imaging to prognosis and duration of hospital stay (CHEN et al. 2000; DOUGLAS et al. 2000; GARCIA-AGUAYO and GIL 2000). By using sonography and computed tomography, the diagnosis of acute appendicitis is made earlier, often before perforation has occurred and the number of non-contributory laparotomies drops to below 11% (PUYLAERT 1994, 1990; PUYLAERT et al. 1987, 1997; GARCIA-AGUAYO and GIL 2000; HORTON et al. 2000; RAMAN et al. 2002; RETTENBACHER et al. 2002; RAO et al. 1998). Sonography has a sensitivity of 75%–90%, a specificity of 86%–100% and an accuracy of 87%–96% (BIRNBAUM and WILSON 2000).

Sonography is the imaging method of choice for young, thin patients. Computed tomography is required in obese patients or when there is uncertainty regarding the sonographic finding (PUYLAERT et al. 1987; MINDELZUN and JEFFREY 1999). Sonography can also diagnose diseases that mimic acute appendicitis by causing right iliac fossa pain such as ileocaecitis, acute renal colic, tubo-ovarian inflammation or torsion, right sided or sigmoid diverticulitis, epiploic appendagitis, caecal tumours, bowel obstruction, and ischaemic bowel diseases (PUYLAERT 1994, 2001; PUYLAERT et al. 1987, 1997; RIOUX 1995; GARCIA-AGUAYO and GIL 2000).

Sometimes, sonography and computed tomography are inconclusive and clinical examination and laboratory tests have to be relied upon for making an appropriate management decision (WEYANT et al. 2000).

14.4
Sonographic Technique and Normal Findings

When sonography of the appendix is performed, the bladder should not be distended, as this results in further discomfort when abdominal wall compression is applied with the linear probe. Appendiceal sonography does not require any oral or colonic preparation. The improvement in the visualisation of the appendix obtained by using a saline enema seems to be of little value in routine practice (HAN 2002). The examination of patients with acute pain in the right iliac fossa begins with a global survey of the abdomen, by using a convex or sector low frequency probe (RIOUX 1995). Solid organs should be scanned, as well as the biliary tract, aorta, and main portal and mesenteric vessels. The detection of free fluid in Morison's pouch, the pelvis and the paracolic gutters is part of this initial evaluation. After this, higher frequency probes are selected and a focused examination of the right iliac fossa is performed (PUYLAERT 1990; RIOUX 1995). PUYLAERT (1990) described the method of graded compression to improve visualization of the appendix; a gentle and progressive compression of the anterior abdominal wall is applied with a linear probe.

Compression is usually initiated in the mid part of the abdomen, in front of the aortoiliac bifurcation. The probe is then moved slowly to the site of maximum tenderness (PUYLAERT 1990; BIRNBAUM and WILSON 2000). As the probe is moved laterally the anterior wall of the caecum and the ileocaecal junction can be identified. It has been recently suggested that by combining graded compression with posterior manual compression visualisation of the appendix is improved by 10% (LEE et al. 2002).

The sonographic diagnosis of acute appendicitis can also be improved by asking the patient to identify the point of maximum tenderness (CHESBROUGH et al. 1993), whereas the use of drugs to relieve pain can decrease the performance of sonography (VERMEULEN et al. 1999).

The wall thickness of normal intestine is less than 4 mm (HATA et al. 1992, 1994; LEDERMAN et al. 2000; WILSON 1996). Using high frequency probes (5–13 MHz) the five layers of the intestinal wall can be seen (LEDERMAN et al. 2000; WILSON 1996). The first layer is hyperechoic and corresponds to the interface between the intestinal content and the mucosa. The second layer is hypoechoic and consists of deep mucosa and muscularis mucosa. The hyperechoic submucosa forms the third layer. The fourth layer consists of hypoechoic muscularis propria. The serosal surface and adventitia are hyperechoic and form the fifth layer. The colon can be differentiated from the small bowel because the colon has a peripheral location and peristalsis is not seen (LIM et al. 1994). The ileocaecal valve is recognised by its pseudo-tumoral shape, bulging into the caecal lumen (Fig. 14.1) (RIOUX 1994). The appendix is in direct continuity with the caecum and

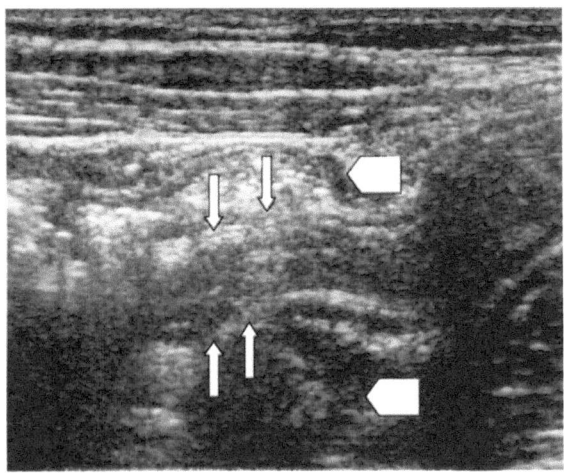

Fig. 14.1. Longitudinal view of the ileocaecal junction: the distal ileum (*white arrows*) is bulging into the caecal lumen (*white arrowheads*)

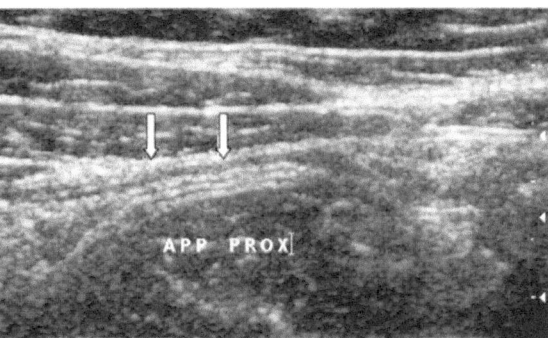

Fig. 14.2. Longitudinal view of the caeco-appendicular junction: the appendix (*white arrows*) is in the continuity of the caecum

has no valve (Fig. 14.2). Starting from the caecal tip, the normal appendix appears as a blind-ended tubular structure with a mean diameter of less than 6 mm. Its length is quite variable, ranging from 2 to 25 cm (WILLIAMS and MYERS 1994). The thickness of the appendiceal wall is less than 3 mm (SIMONOSVKY 2002). The appendix is mobile and can have different locations. The most frequent are retrocaecal, retroileal, preileal, and pelvic (WILLIAMS and MYERS 1994; BIRNBAUM and WILSON 2000). The normal appendix is compressible and is not peristaltic. The appendiceal lumen contains hyperechoic foci corresponding to gas and faeces (RETTENBACHER et al. 2000), but is hypoechoic when fluid-filled (WILSON 1996; PUYLAERT et al. 1987; PULYAERT 2001). The appendix cannot be considered normal unless its tip has been demonstrated (LIM et al. 1996b).

When Doppler sonographic parameters are optimised to detect low-velocity flow then flow is detected in the normal intestinal wall, but not in the normal appendix (JEFFREY et al. 1994; QUILLIN and SIEGEL 1994a,b).

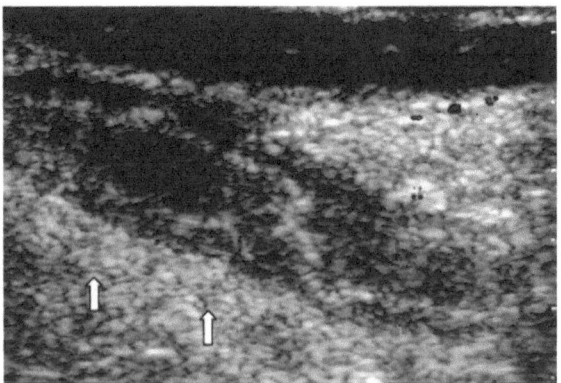

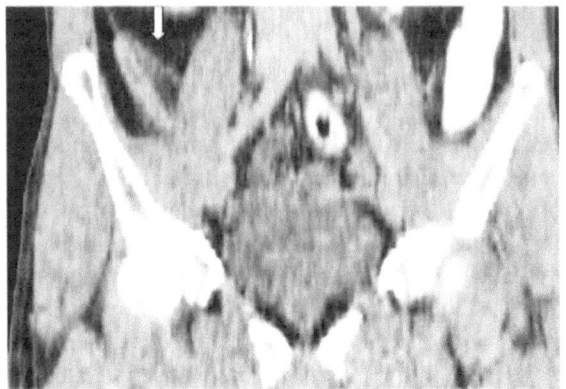

Fig. 14.3a,b. Typical acute appendicitis: (a) sonographic and (b) reformatted computed tomography of the inflamed appendix; there is inflammation of the surrounding fat tissue (*white arrows*)

14.5
Sonographic Findings in Acute Appendicitis

The sonographic diagnosis of acute appendicitis is based on the detection of a blind-ended, non-compressible, non-peristaltic, intestinal structure arising from the end of the caecum, with a maximum transverse diameter of 6 mm or more (Fig. 14.3) (BIRNBAUM and WILSON 2000; PUYLAERT 1986; PUYLAERT et al. 1987; RIOUX 1992; VIGNAULT et al. 1990). An obstructing appendicolith may be seen as a hyperechoic structure within the appendicular lumen (Fig. 14.4). Colour Doppler is useful in patients with borderline appendices

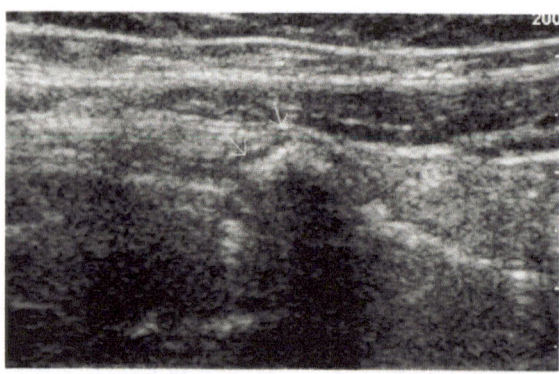

Fig. 14.4. Longitudinal view of the appendix containing an appendicolith (*white arrows*)

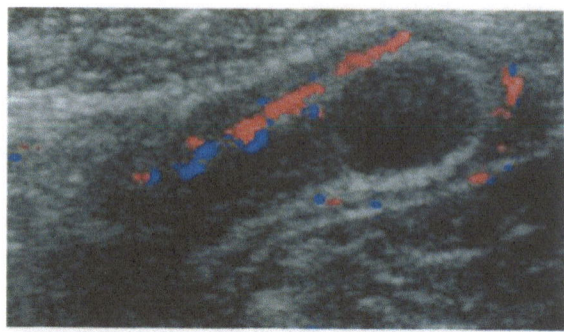

Fig. 14.5. Longitudinal view of an enlarged and inflamed appendix: increased mural flow is related to the acute inflammation

with an outer diameter of 5–6 mm as increased mural flow is suggestive of appendicitis (Fig. 14.5) (GUTIERREZ et al. 1999; QUILLIN and SIEGEL 1992, 1994; LIM et al. 1996a). Periappendiceal changes include hyperechoic fat, a small amount of fluid, and enlarged lymph nodes. Hypoechoic peri-appendiceal abscesses can also be detected. Perforation can be predicted when the submucosal hyperechoic layer has disappeared or when a loculated fluid collection is visible around the inflamed appendix (Fig. 14.6) (BIRNBAUM and WILSON 2000; GUTIERREZ et al. 1999; QUILLIN et al. 1992). Absence of mural flow in a thickened and inflamed appendix is suggestive of gangrenous appendicitis (LIM et al. 1996a).

In complicated appendicitis, the sensitivity of sonography is low at 28% (Fig. 14.7) (PUYLAERT et al. 1987). Poor performance is usually explained by overlying gas in bowel loops masking the inflamed appendix (Fig. 14.8).

Appendiceal mucocele is a condition mimicking acute appendicitis and defined as a mucin-filled dilatation of the appendix related to a benign or malignant hyperplasia of the appendicular epithelium (WILLIAMS and MYERS 1994; SOUEÏ-MHIRI et al. 2001). At sonography, this unusual diagnosis is suggested when a round or oval mass of 3–6 cm diameter is observed in the right iliac fossa, closely related to the caecum. This structure, which can be up to 40 cm in size, is fluid-filled, contains internal echoes which may layer or have „onion-peel" appearance or it may show septation or contain internal tumorous foci (PUYLAERT 1990; SOUEÏ-MHIRI et al. 2001). The diagnosis of appendiceal mucocele should be made before surgery to avoid peritoneal dissemination at operation leading to pseudomyxoma peritonei (WILLIAMS and Myers 1994; SOUEÏ-MHIRI et al. 2001).

Acute appendicitis may be secondary to luminal obstruction caused by primary or secondary ileocaecal tumours. Sonographic findings suggestive of a

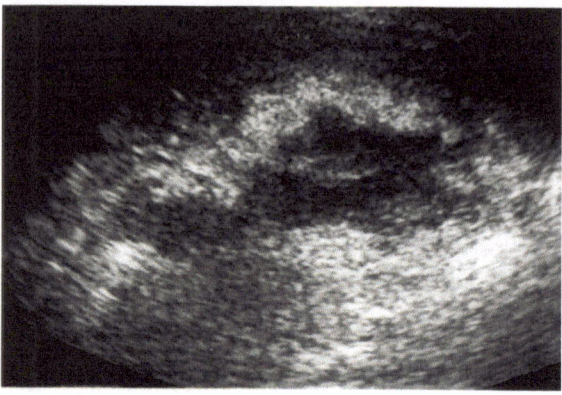

Fig. 14.6. Longitudinal view. Perforated acute appendicitis with periappendiceal collection. The hyperechoic submucosal layer has disappeared

colonic tumour include a short length (<10 cm) of wall thickening (>10 mm) with loss of stratification (LEDERMAN et al. 2000; LIM 1996; TRUONG et al. 1998; BOZKURT et al. 1994).

14.6
Differential Diagnosis

The most frequent alternative diagnosis to appendicitis is acute inflammation of the ileocaecal junction, caused by various infectious agents such as Salmonella enteritidis, Yersinia enterolitica and Campylobacter jejuni (Fig. 14.9) (QUILLIN et al. 1992; RIOUX 1994; TRUONG et al. 1998; LEDERMAN et al. 2000; PUYLAERT 1990, 2001; PUYLAERT et al. 1997). The appendix is normal but there are enlarged lymph nodes and there is thickening of the ileal and caecal wall with increased mural flow. The same sonographic findings are seen in neutropenic typhlitis, a non-specific inflammation

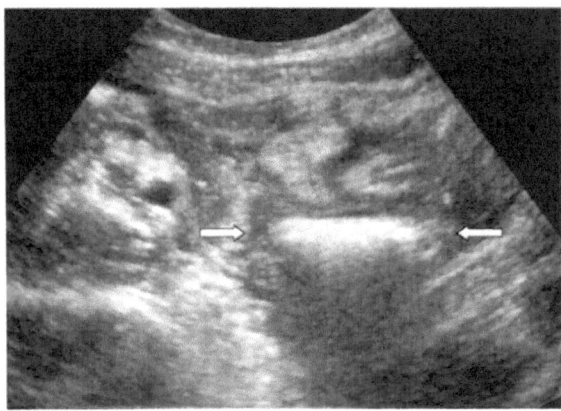
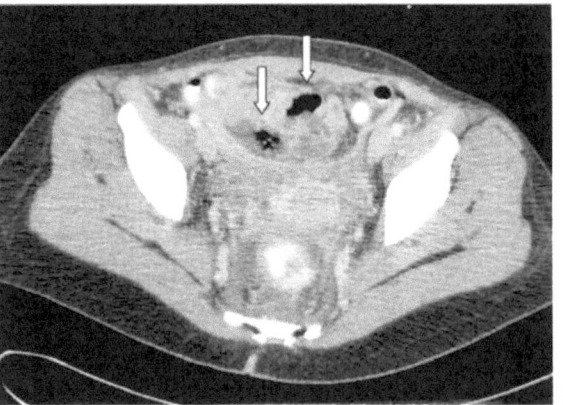

Fig. 14.7a,b. Perforated appendicitis: diffuse inflammation of the fatty tissue of the pelvis and gas-containing collection (*white arrows*) centrally located in the pelvis: (**a**) transverse sonogram, and (**b**) computed tomography of the pelvis. The appendix is not clearly visualised at this stage of the disease

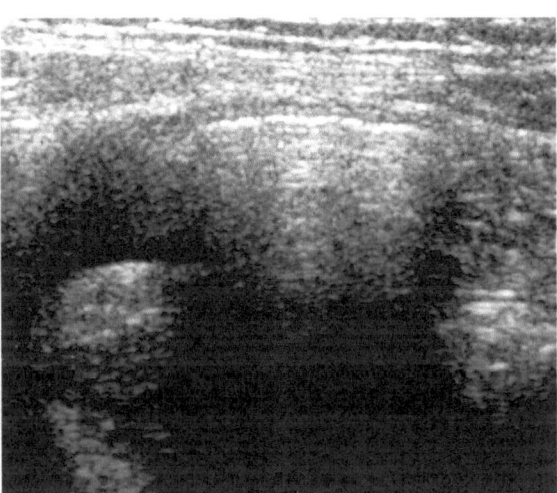
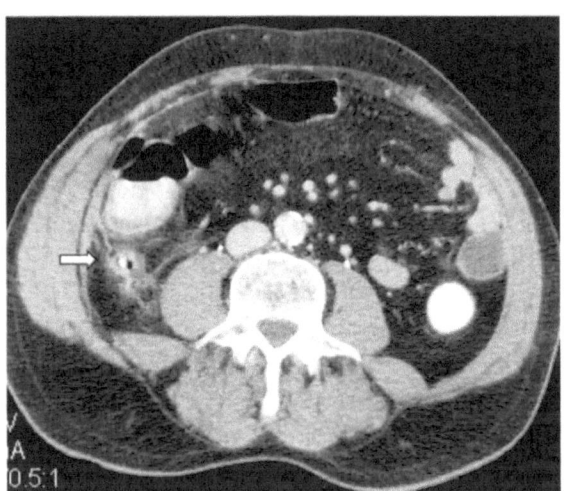

Fig. 14.8a,b. Acute right iliac fossa pain due to acute appendicitis with an obstructing appendicolith: (**a**) inconclusive sonography showing a small amount of fluid in the right paracolic gutter and a large acoustic shadow masking the appendix; (**b**) computed tomography showing severe inflammation of the appendix and the surrounding fatty tissue; the appendiceal lumen is obstructed by an appendicolith (*white arrow*)

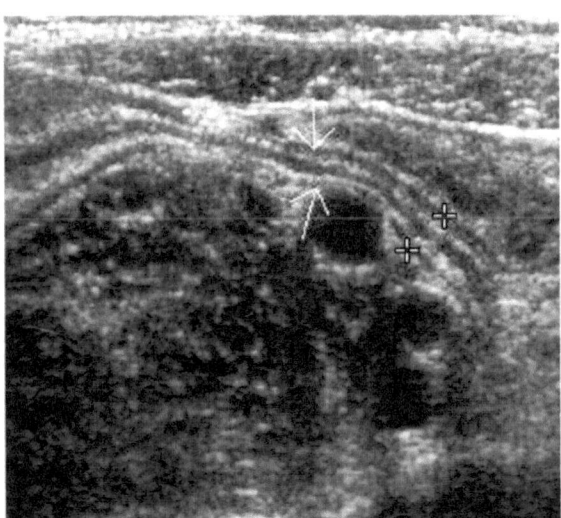
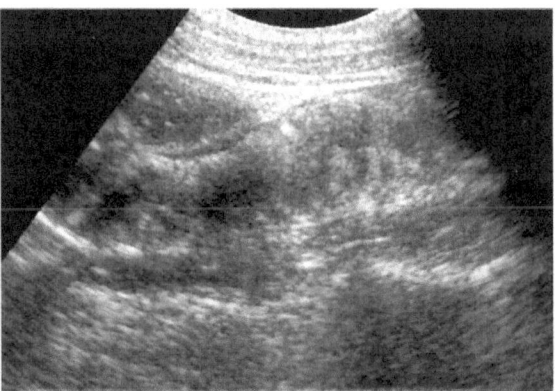

Fig. 14.9a,b. Sonogram performed in a case of acute right iliac fossa pain contributes by showing a normal appendix (**a**); the caecum and the ascendant colon (**b**) are thickened due to an acute infective colitis

of the ileum and the caecum that occurs in immuno-compromised patients (SUAREZ et al. 1995).

In patients with inflammatory bowel disease affecting the ileocaecal junction there is limited or extensive intestinal wall thickening (range 6–12 mm) (BOZKURT et al. 1994; SCHWERK et al. 1992a; HATA et al. 1992, 1994). Colour Doppler sonography will show increased wall flow that is related to the activity of the disease (JEFFREY et al. 1994; QUILLIN and SIEGEL 1994). Transmural caecal and small bowel involvement with surrounding changes, such as fistulae and abscesses, suggests Crohn's disease (LEDERMAN et al. 2000; WILSON 1996). Transmural spread of the inflammatory process is suspected when interruption of the hyperechoic submucosal ring is seen (RIOUX and LANGIS 1994) and helps differentiate Crohn's disease from infection of the ileocaecal junction. Intestinal strictures, fistulae, and intra-abdominal abscesses are all detectable with sonography (LEDERMAN et al. 2000; WILSON 1996; RIOUX and LANGIS 1994; SCHWERK et al. 1992a; HATA et al. 1992, 1994; GASHE et al. 1999).

Right sided colonic diverticulitis may cause symptoms mimicking appendicitis. The sonographic diagnosis of diverticulitis is based on the detection of a thickened colonic wall (>4 mm) and on the identification of at least one inflamed diverticulum (Fig. 14.10) (IDE et al. 1994; WILSON and TOI 1990; SCHWERK et al. 1992b; PUYLAERT et al. 1997). Inflamed diverticula are hypoechoic, oval or round shaped outpouchings closely related to a thickened colonic wall. Bright hyperechoic foci of gas may be seen in the centre of these outpouchings. The inflamed pericolic fat appears hyperechoic whereas a pericolic abscess appears as a hypoechoic mass.

Right sided epiploic appendagitis is an ischaemic disorder caused by spontaneous torsion of an epiploic appendix. Epiploic appendices are fatty pouches seen along the serosal surface of the colon and are adherent to the taenia coli (LYNN et al. 1956; GHAHERMANI et al. 1992; JENNINGS and COLLINS 1987; RIOUX 1994; MOLLA et al. 1998). The sonographic findings of epiploic appendagitis are a hyperechoic mass with internal anechoic zones and a hypoechoic border that lies adjacent to a colonic wall which is of normal thickness (Fig. 14.11) (GHAHERMANI et al. 1992; JENNINGS and COLLINS 1987; RIOUX 1994; MOLLA et al. 1998; HOLLERWERGER et al. 1996; DANSE et al. 2001). As this is an ischaemic disorder colour Doppler shows absent flow within the hyperechoic mass (MOLLA et al. 1998; DANSE et al. 2001). In contrast, arterial flow is usually observed in the fatty tissue infiltration seen around diverticulitis, appendicitis and acute Crohn's disease (DANSE et al. 2001).

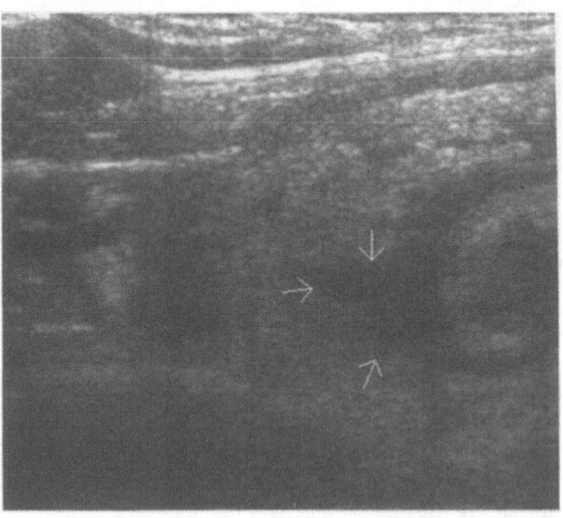

Fig. 14.10. Right sided colonic diverticulitis detected with sonography. An inflamed diverticulum is seen as a hypoechoic outpouching (*arrows*) arising from a thick walled colon; the fatty tissue adjacent to the colon has become hyperechoic as a result of the inflammation

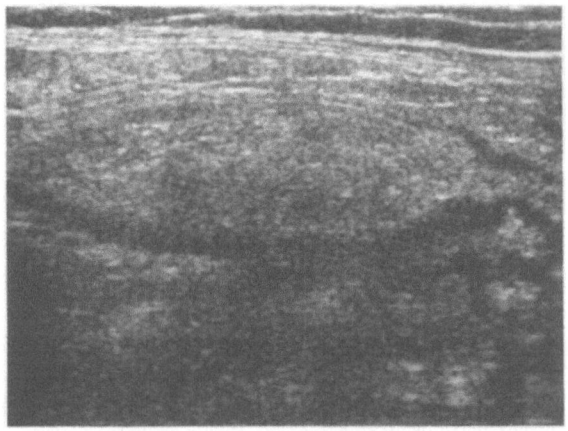

Fig. 14.11. Sonographic findings in a case of acute epiploic appendagitis. An ovoid hyperechoic mass with a thin hypoechoic border is seen at the outer margin of the descendant colon

14.7
Strategy

14.7.1
Indications for Sonography

Sonography is a powerful imaging tool that substantially improves diagnostic accuracy in patients with suspected appendicitis. However, its exact role as a diagnostic aid is still being defined; opinion varies as to whether it should be reserved for selected patients with atypical or confusing clinical presentations or whether it should be performed in all patients suspected of having acute appendicitis. Supporters of the restrictive use of sonography underline that knowing that this technique has both a high sensitivity and a high specificity is not as important as determining whether it provides new information to add to the clinical picture. A meta-analysis, that included more than 3300 patients, reported a sensitivity of 84.7% and a specificity of 92.1%, demonstrated the impact of sonography on determining the probability of disease. In a group of patients with high prevalence of appendicitis (80%, usually operated on clinical grounds), a negative sonography had a negative predictive value of only 59.5%. Conversely, in a group with low prevalence of appendicitis (2%, usually discharged home), a positive test had a positive predictive value of only 19.5%. So, it was concluded that sonography is useful in patients with an intermediate probability of disease and should be avoided in patients with high or low likelihood of disease due to the respective low negative and positive predictive values (ORR et al. 1995).

Supporters of the extensive use of imaging note that routine use of computed tomography in patients with suspected appendicitis is efficient and cost-effective as it averts unnecessary appendectomy, reduces delay before surgical treatment, and eliminates unnecessary hospital observation (RAO et al. 1998). However, other cost-effectiveness studies are needed to confirm these results in countries other than North America and with other imaging modalities such as sonography. In a recent study BENDECK et al. (2002) proposed that imaging should be part of the routine evaluation of women suspected of having acute appendicitis since the negative appendectomy rate was significantly lower in women who underwent preoperative imaging as compared to women who did not. Conversely, in men and in boys and girls it was recommended that preoperative imaging be reserved for patients with confusing clinical symptoms and signs.

14.7.2
How to Manage Sonographic Results

After sonography, three different management situations need to be considered:

- Appendicitis is confirmed with sonography: surgery is required. However, in selected cases the clinical condition favours conservative treatment, during which the symptoms subside. The diagnosis of spontaneously resolving appendicitis,

which is a component of over-diagnosed appendicitis (MIGRAINE et al. 1997), can be confirmed by follow-up sonographic examinations which will show the return of sonographic features to normal. However, it must be kept in mind that patients with spontaneous resolution of appendicitis are at risk of recurrences (COBBEN et al. 2000).

- The entire length of the normal appendix is seen at sonography or an alternative diagnosis has been demonstrated; appendicitis may be ruled out with a high level of confidence.
- Sonography cannot identify the appendix and does not suggest an alternative diagnosis: the strategy depends on the pre-sonographic probability of appendicitis being present and the likelihood of appendiceal perforation. In patients with low or intermediate probability, discharge or hospital observation should be recommended depending on the patient's clinical condition. Computed tomography must be performed where there is a high suspicion of appendicitis or perforation because of the severity of the clinical findings or in the elderly where misdiagnosis and delayed diagnosis is common.

14.8
Conclusion

The diagnosis of acute appendicitis has been improved by cross-sectional imaging and particularly by sonography. These techniques also allow other causes of acute pain in the right iliac fossa to be accurately diagnosed. The liberal use of sonography in suspected appendicitis reduces the number of unnecessary laparotomies and delayed surgical decisions.

References

Bendeck SE, Nino-Murcia M, Berry GJ et al (2002) Imaging for suspected appendicitis: negative appendectomy and perforation rates. Radiology 225:131–136

Birnbaum BA, Wilson SR (2000) Appendicitis at the Millenium. Radiology 215:337–348

Bozkurt T, Richter F, Lux G (1994) Ultrasonography as a primary diagnostic tool in patients with inflammatory disease and tumors of the small intestine and large bowel. J Clin Ultrasound 22:85–91

Chen SC, Wang HP, Hsu HY et al (2000) Accuracy of ED sonography in the diagnosis of acute appendicitis. Am J Emerg Med 18:449–452

Chesbrough RM, Burkhard TK, Balsara ZN et al (1993) Self-localization in US of appendicitis: an addition to graded compression. Radiology 187:349–351

Cobben LPJ, de van Otterloo AM, Puylaert JBCM (2000) Spontaneous resolving appendicitis: frequency and natural history in 60 patients. Radiology 215:349–352

Danse EM, van Beers BE, Baudrez V et al (2001) Epiploic Appendagitis: color Doppler sonographic findings. Eur Radiol 11:183–186

Doherty GM, Lewis FR (1989) Appendicitis: continuing diagnostic challenge. Emerg Med Clin North Am 7:537–553

Douglas CD, Maepherson NE, Davidson PM et al (2000) Randomised controlled trial of ultrasonography in diagnosis of acute appendicitis incorporating the Alvarado Score. BMJ 321:919–922

Garcia-Aguayo FJ, Gil P (2000) Sonography in acute appendicitis: diagnosis utility and influence upon management and outcome. Eur Radiol 10:1886–1893

Gasche C, Moser G, Turetschek K et al (1999) Transabdominal bowel sonography for the detection of intestinal complications in Crohn's disease. Gut 44:112–117

Ghahermani GG, White EM, Hoff FL et al (1992) Appendices epiploicae of the colon: radiologic and pathologic features Radiographics 12:59–77

Grönroos JM, Grönroos P (2001) Diagnosis of acute appendicitis Radiology 219:297–298

Gutierrez CJ, Mariano MC, Faddis DM et al (1999) Doppler ultrasound accurately screens patients with appendicitis. Am Surg 65:1015–1017

Han TI (2002) Improved sonographic visualisation of the appendix with a saline enema in children with suspected appendicitis. J Ultrasound Med 21:511–516

Hata J, Haruma K, Suenaga K et al (1992) Ultrasonographic assessment of inflammatory bowel disease. Am J Gastroenterol 87:443–447

Hata J, Haruma K, Yamanaka H et al (1994) Ultrasonographic evaluation of the bowel wall in inflammatory bowel disease: comparison of in vivo and in vitro studies. Abdom Imaging 19:395–399

Hermans JJ, Hermans AL, Risseeuw GA et al (1993) Appendicitis caused by carcinoid tumor. Radiology 188:71–72

Hollerweger A, Rettenbacher Th, Macheiner P et al (1996) Spontaneous fatty tissue necrosis of the omentum and epiploic appendices: clinical, ultrasonic and CT findings. Forschr Röntgenstr 165:529–534

Horton MD, Counter SF, Florence MG et al (2000) A prospective trial of computed tomography and ultrasonography for diagnosing appendicitis in the atypical patient. Am J Surg May 179:305–306

Ide C, Van Beers B, Pauls C et al (1994) Diagnosis of acute colonic diverticulitis : comparison of US and CT. JBR-BTR 77:262–267

Jeffrey RB Jr, Sommer G, Debatin JF (1994) Color Doppler sonography of focal gastrointestinal lesions: initial clinical experience. J Ultrasound Med 13:473–478

Jeffrey RB, Laing FC, Towsend RR (1998) Acute appendicitis: sonographic criteria based on 250 cases. Radiology 167:327–329

Jennings CM, Collins MC (1987) The radiological findings in torsion of an appendix epiploica. Br J Radiol 60:508–509

Lederman HP, Börner N, Strunk H et al (2000) Bowel wall thickening on transabdominal sonography. AJR 174:107–117

Lee JH, Jeong YK, Hwang JC et al (2002) Graded compression sonography with adjuvant use of a posterior manual compression technique in the sonographic diagnosis of acute appendicitis. AJR 178:863–868

Lim JH, Ko YT, Lee DH et al (1994) Determining the site and causes of colonic obstruction with sonography. AJR 163:1113–1117

Lim HK, Lee WJ, Kim TH et al (1996a) Appendicitis: usefulness of color Doppler US. Radiology 201:221–225

Lim HK, Lee WJ, Lee SJ et al. (1996b) Focal appendicitis confined to the tip: diagnosis at US. Radiology 200:799–801

Lim JH (1996) Colorectal cancer: sonographic findings. AJR 167:45–47

Lynn TE, Dockerty MB, Waugh JM (1956) A clinical and pathological study of the epiploic appendagitis. Surg Gynecol Obstet 103:423–433

Migraine S, Atri M, Bret PM et al (1997) Spontaneously resolving acute appendicitis: clinical and sonographic documentation. Radiology 205:55–58

Mindelzun RE, Jeffrey RB (1999) The acute abdomen: current CT imaging techniques. Semin Ultrasound CT MRI 20:63–67

Molla E, Ripolles T, Martinez MJ et al (1998) Primary epiploic appendagitis: US and CT findings. Eur Radiol 8:435–438

Orr RK, Porter D, Hartman D (1995) Ultrasonography to evaluate adults for appendicitis: decision making based on meta-analysis and probabilistic reasoning. Acad Emerg Med 2:644–650

Pena BM, Taylor GA, Fishman SJ et al (2000) Costs and effectiveness of ultrasonography and limited computed tomography for diagnosing appendicitis in children. Pediatrics 106:672–676

Puylaert JB (1986) Acute appendicitis: US evaluation using graded compression. Radiology 158:355–360

Puylaert JB (1990) Ultrasound of appendicitis and its differential diagnosis. Springer, Berlin Heidelberg New York

Puylaert JB (1994) When it doubt, sound it out Radiology 191:320–321

Puylaert JB (2001) Ultrasound of acute GI tract conditions. Eur Radiol 10:1867–1877

Puylaert JB, Rutgers PH, Lalisang RI et al (1987) A prospective study of ultrasonography in the diagnosis of appendicitis. N Engl J Med 317:666–669

Puylaert JB, van der Zant FM, Rijke AM (1997) Sonography and the acute abdomen: practical considerations. AJR 168:179–186

Quillin SP, Siegel MJ (1992) Appendicitis in children: color Doppler sonography. Radiology 184:745–747

Quillin SP, Siegel MJ (1994a) Gastrointestinal inflammation in children: color Doppler ultrasonography. J Ultrasound Med 13:751–756

Quillin SP, Siegel MJ (1994b) Appendicitis: efficacity of color Doppler sonography. Radiology 191:557–560

Quillin SP, Siegel MJ, Coffin CM (1992) Acute appendicitis in children: value of sonography in detecting perforation. AJR 159:1265–1268

Raman SS, Lu DSK, Kadell BM et al (2002) Accuracy of nonfocused helical CT for the diagnosis of acute appendicitis: a 5-year review. AJR 178:1319–1325

Rao PM, Rhea JT, Novelline RA, Mostafavi AA et al (1998) Effects of computed tomography of the appendix on treatment of patients and use of hospital resources. NEJM 338:141–146

Rettenbacher T, Hollerweger A, Macheiner P et al (2000) Presence of gas in the appendix: additional criteria to rule out or confirm acute appendicitis-evaluation with US. Radiology 214:183–187

Rettenbacher T, Hollerweger A, Gritzmann N et al (2002) Appendicitis: should diagnostic imaging be performed if the clinical presentation is highly suggestive of the disease. Gastroenterology 123:992–998

Rioux M (1992) Sonographic detection of the normal and abnormal appendix. AJR 158:773–778

Rioux M (1994) Echographie digestive: aspects échographiques des iléo-colites. Feuill Radiol 34:267–283

Rioux M (1995) Echographie digestive. L'échographie de l'appendice, normal ou anormal, et ses pièges. Feuill Radiol 35:87–107

Rioux M, Langis P (1994) Primary epiploic appendagitis. Clinical, US, and CT findings in 14 cases. Radiology 191: 523–526

Roth C, Tello R, Ptak T (2001) The predictive value of clinical data in the examination of patients with abdominal pain. AJR [Suppl] 176:96

Schwerk WB, Beckh K, Raith M (1992a) A prospective evaluation of high resolution sonography in the diagnosis of inflammatory bowel disease. Eur J Gastroenterol Hepatol 4:173–182

Schwerk WB, Schwarz S, Rothmund M (1992b) Sonography in acute colonic diverticulitis. A prospective study. Dis Colon Rectum 35:1077–1084

Simonosvsky V (2002) Normal appendix: is there any significant difference in the maximal mural thickness at US between pediatric and adult population. Radiology 224:333–337

Sivit CJ, Applegate KE, Stallion A et al (2000) Imaging evaluation of suspected appendicitis in a pediatric population: effectiveness of sonography versus CT. AJR 175:977–980

Soueï-Mhiri M, Tlili-Graies K, Cherifa LB et al (2001) Les mucocoèles appendiculaires. Etude rétrospective à propos de 10 cas. J Radiol 82:463–468

Suarez B, Kalifa G, Adamsbaum C et al (1995) Sonographic diagnosis and follow-up of diffuse neutropenic colitis: case report of a child treated for osteogenic sarcoma. Pediatr Radiol 25:373–374

Taourel P (2001) Work-up of appendicitis with imaging: the end of certainty. J Radiol 82:443–444

Truong M, Atri M, Bret PM et al (1998) Sonographic appearance of benign and malignant conditions of the colon. AJR 170:1451–1455

Vermeulen B, Morabia A, Unger PF et al (1999) Acute appendicitis: influence of early pain relief on the accuracy of clincial and US findings in the decision to operate – a randomized trial. Radiology 210:639–643

Vignault F, Filiatraut D, Brandt ML et al (1990) Acute appendicitis in children: evaluation with US. Radiology 176: 501–504

Weyant MJ, Eachempati SR, Maluccio MA et al (2000) Interpretation of computed tomography does not correlate with laboratory or pathologic findings in surgically confirmed acute appendicitis. Surgery 128:145–152

Williams RA, Myers P (1994) Pathology of the appendix and its surgical treatment. Chapman and Hall, London

Wilson EB, Cole C, Nipper ML et al (2001) Computed tomography and ultrasonography in the diagnosis of appendicitis. When they are indicated? Arch Surg 136:670–675

Wilson SR (1996) Gastrointestinal tract sonography. Abdom Imaging 21:1–8

Wilson SR, Toi A (1990) The value of sonography in the diagnosis of acute diverticulitis of the colon. AJR 154: 1199–1202

Wise SW, Labuski MR, Kasales CJ et al (2001) Comparative assessment of CT and sonographic techniques for appendiceal imaging. AJR 176:933–941

15 CT of Appendicitis

ABRAHAM A. GHIATAS and NICK KRITIKOS

CONTENTS

15.1   Introduction   157
15.2   Anatomy   157
15.3   Pathology   157
15.4   Epidemiology   158
15.5   Clinical Findings   158
15.6   Computed Tomography of Appendicitis   158
15.6.1 Introduction – Comparison with Other Imaging
        Modalities   158
15.6.2 Technique   158
15.6.3 Normal CT Findings   159
15.6.4 Findings in Appendicitis   159
15.6.5 CT classification of appendicitis   161
15.6.6 Differential Diagnosis   162
15.6.7 CT Limitations   162
        References   162

15.1
Introduction

Appendicitis may be acute or chronic. Acute appendicitis is the commonest surgical abdominal emergency in the western world. The low residue western diet is likely to be an etiological factor as the inflammatory process is secondary to obstruction to the narrow lumen of the appendix.

Chronic appendicitis is rare and may be seen in cystic fibrosis, where mucoid material occupies the lumen of the appendix. It is also seen with recurrent episodes of acute appendicitis or when the appendix has been incompletely removed (BAERT 1999).

Prompt and accurate diagnosis reduces the morbidity and mortality of acute appendicitis. Computed tomography (CT), because of its high sensitivity and specificity, is becoming the preferred imaging modality for suspected acute appendicitis, particularly in adults, and provides guidance for non-surgical management of this disease.

A. A. GHIATAS, MD
Director of Medical Imaging, Iaso Hospital, Voutsina 1A, Ekali, Athens 145–78, Greece
N. KRITIKOS, MD
Iaso Hospital, Voutsina 1A, Ekali, Athens 145–78, Greece

This chapter concentrates primarily on the CT features of acute appendicitis, the acute disease being by far the commonest form.

15.2
Anatomy

The appendix is a hollow, narrow, worm-like diverticular structure that arises from the postero-medial aspect of the caecum, 2.5–3.0 cm below the ileocecal valve. It is covered by peritoneum and has a short triangular mesentery that joins the mesentery of the ileum. Its average length is 9 cm (range 4–25 cm). The position of the tip of the appendix varies and may be retrocecal (66%), pelvic (31%), paracolic (in the sulcus on the outer side of the cecum), pre-ileal, post-ileal, promontoric (pointing towards the sacral promontory) and subcecal (Fig. 15.1). The appendix may even be located in the left lower quadrant if there is visceral transposition. Congenital absence and duplication of the appendix have been reported but are rare. The blood supply is provided by a branch of the ileocolic artery, the appendicular artery, which is its only feeding vessel and so occlusion of this vessel results in gangrene and perforation. The appendicular vein drains into the ileocolic vein which empties into the superior mesenteric vein (VOIGHT 1953; BALTHAZAR and GADE 1976; ELLIS and NATHANSAN 1997).

15.3
Pathology

Acute appendicitis is caused by obstruction to its lumen which leads to mucus stasis and secondary infection. Distension of the lumen with pus and inflammation of the wall may result in venous stasis and ischaemia with necrosis, abscess formation, rupture and peritonitis.

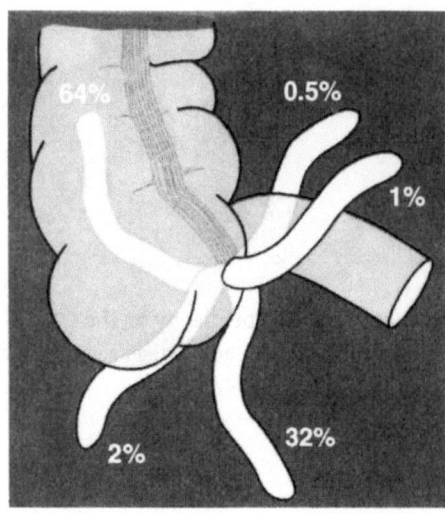

Fig. 15.1. Locations of the appendix. [Reproduced from DURAN et al. (1997) with permission]

15.4
Epidemiology

Acute appendicitis is more common in males than females (ratio 3:2) and the lifetime risk for developing the disease is 7%. Appendicitis under the age of 2 is rare and the disease increases in frequency during childhood to peak in young adult life. The mortality is less than 1:100,000 although it is 6:1000 from gangrenous appendicitis and 1:20 for perforated appendicitis (BERRY and MALT 1984; CONDON 1986, 1990).

15.5
Clinical Findings

A prompt and accurate diagnosis of acute appendicitis significantly decreases mortality and morbidity (BROWN 1991; ANDERSEN et al. 1980; GOLDMAN 1992).

The diagnosis of acute appendicitis may be strongly suspected from the clinical history and physical examination. Typically the patient develops centrally located colicky abdominal pain which is followed by nausea and several episodes of vomiting. A few hours later the pain shifts to the right lower quadrant and becomes continuous and severe. There may be constipation or diarrhoea. A fever generally develops within 24 h and in most patients there is mild leukocytosis. Tenderness and guarding develops at McBurney's point but extreme rigidity denotes the onset of peritonitis.

Although clinical symptoms and signs may strongly suggest a diagnosis of acute appendicitis,

in 20% of cases the clinical presentation is atypical, while in another 20% the condition is misdiagnosed. The clinical picture in children is often atypical with generalized rather than localized abdominal pain, and in the elderly there is a wider differential diagnosis than in the younger population because of the frequency of age-related diseases such as diverticulitis. The diagnosis may also be delayed in the elderly as they complain less of pain and clinical signs are less pronounced. There is also an increased risk of misdiagnosis in young females as gynaecological diseases may mimic acute appendicitis.

15.6
Computed Tomography of Appendicitis

15.6.1
Introduction –
Comparison with Other Imaging Modalities

CT has greatly facilitated the diagnosis of acute appendicitis with a reported decrease in the negative appendectomy rate from approximately 20% to 4% without any significant increase in perforation rate (BALTHAZAR et al. 1998).

CT is able to directly visualise the appendix, the periappendiceal area and the more remote parts of the abdomen which may be effected by appendicitis, such as the left lower quadrant and upper abdomen. The severity and extent of the inflammation are better appreciated by CT than by other imaging modalities, such as plain abdominal radiography and barium enema. Ultrasound (US) is useful for diagnosing acute appendicitis but is heavily dependent on the skill of the operator. Comparison of CT and US in the diagnosis of acute appendicitis shows CT to be superior to US in sensitivity (96% versus 76%) and accuracy (94% versus 83%) and almost equal in specificity (89% versus 91%). CT imaging tailored to evaluate acute appendicitis has proven particularly successful with a sensitivity of 100%, specificity of 95%, positive predictive value of 97%, negative predictive value of 100% and accuracy of 98% (BALTHAZAR et al. 1994; KAISER et al. 2002; RAO et al. 1997c).

15.6.2
Technique

A standard technique utilising helical scanning consists of thin, 5- to 7-mm, contiguous slices from the level of the T12 vertebra to the pubic symphysis during a single breath-hold. The patient is prepared with 800–1000 cc of oral contrast medium 60–90 min prior to scanning for bowel opacification. The scan is performed supine following an intravenous injection of 100–120 cc of iodinated contrast medium at a rate of 3 cc/s with a scan delay of approximately 60 s. Depending on the patient's condition some parameters may need to be modified such as the delay time, injection rate and volume of contrast medium. If the degree of urgency does not permit the administration of bowel contrast medium or if venous access cannot be obtained then the examination may be performed without oral or intravenous contrast medium without significantly compromising diagnostic accuracy. However, the combination of oral contrast medium and intravenous contrast medium provides the most information about the inflamed appendix and the surrounding tissues. Rectal contrast medium may also be administered immediately before scanning in a volume of 0.5–1.5 l in order to opacify the large bowel and appendix (FUNAKI et al. 1998; KAMEL et al. 2002; LANE et al. 1999; RAMAN et al. 2002; RAO et al. 1997c).

15.6.3
Normal CT Findings

The normal appendix may be demonstrated by CT in over 80% of cases depending upon the technique used and the presence of periappendiceal fat. The diameter of the appendix, outer to outer wall, does not exceed 6 mm and the lumen may contain fluid,

fecal material, air or contrast medium. An appendicolith may be present within the lumen of the appendix in asymptomatic patients. The wall of the appendix is well depicted by the surrounding fat and is thin, measuring less than 1 mm in thickness (BALTHAZAR 1994a; DURAN et al. 1997).

15.6.4
Findings in Appendicitis

The inflamed appendix shows a variable degree of distension, has a diameter measuring anything from 6 to 40 mm and wall thickness of 1–3 mm. The wall is usually asymmetrically thickened and enhances after the intravenous contrast medium (Fig. 15.2). If the periappendiceal fat is involved in the inflammatory process then it shows an increased haziness (dirty fat), streaky densities and/or fluid collections (Fig. 15.3). As the disease progresses a periappendiceal inflammatory mass called a phlegmon may develop. This is ill-defined, inhomogeneous, of soft tissue density with variable contrast enhancement (Fig. 15.4). The presence of fluid density areas or pockets of gas within the phlegmon indicates abscess formation (Fig. 15.5).

Thickening and enhancement after intravenous contrast medium may also be observed in the adjacent wall of the caecum or ileum if they are involved in the inflammatory process (Fig. 15.6). The demonstration of a calcified appendicolith with inflammatory changes is associated with a higher risk of complications, such as abscess formation and perforation (Fig. 15.7). Perforation of the appendix

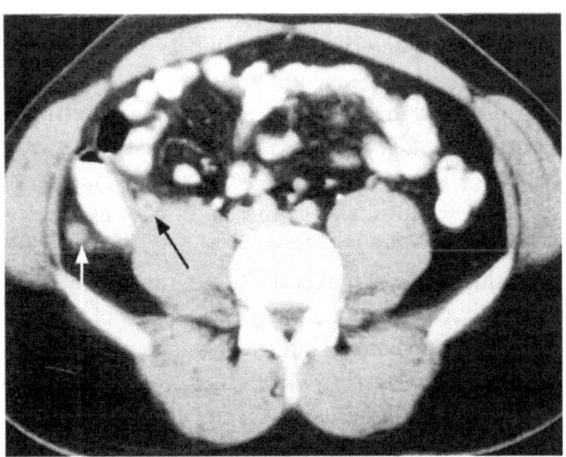

Fig. 15.2. Thickened appendix wall (*arrows*) with homogenous enhancement after intravenous contrast medium. [Reproduced from GHIATAS et al. (1977) with permission]

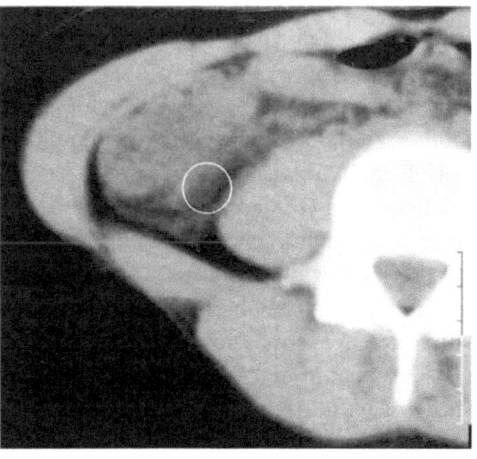

Fig. 15.3. CT in acute appendicitis without oral or intravenous contrast media. Note the "dirty fat" (*ringed*). Small portion of appendix is circled

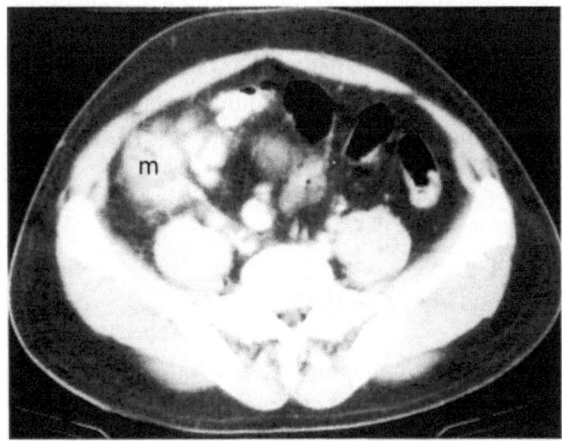

Fig. 15.4. Soft tissue periappendiceal mass (*m*) with variable enhancement in acute appendicitis, representing a phlegmon

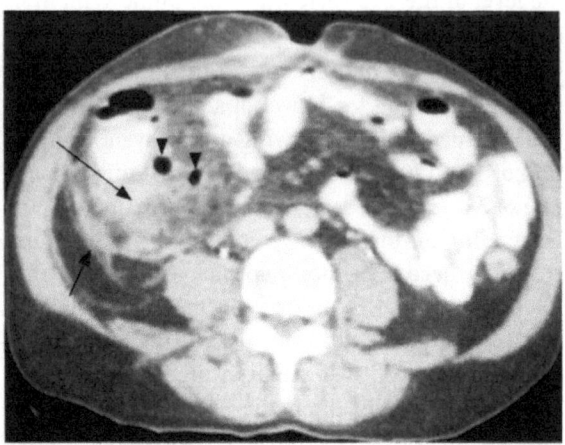

Fig. 15.5. Developing appendiceal abscess: an area of ill-defined and variable enhancement (*long arrow*) with pockets of extraluminal gas (*arrowheads*). There is thickening of the pericecal fascia (*short arrow*)

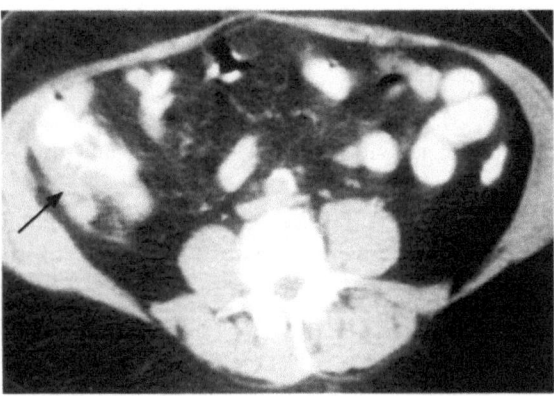

Fig. 15.6. Appendicitis: inflammatory changes thicken the cecal wall (*arrow*) and involve the pericecal fat

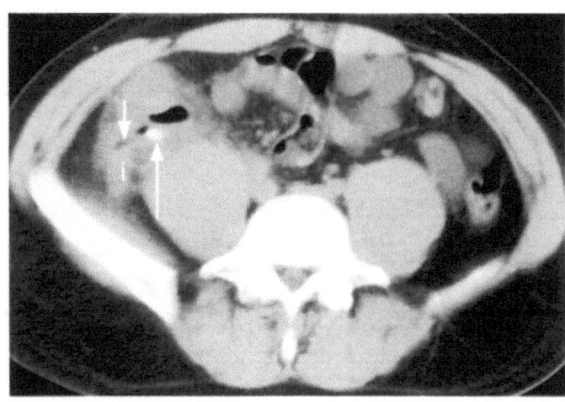

Fig. 15.7. Non-enhanced CT demonstrating an appendicolith (*long arrow*) and an inflammatory process (*i*) surrounding the appendiceal lumen (*short arrow*)

occurs in approximately 20% of the cases. Progression of the inflammatory process may lead to findings that range from a sealed off abscess to widespread intra-abdominal inflammatory seeding with multiple abscesses (Fig. 15.8). Abscesses may vary in size and be of low attenuation with an ill-defined outline. An abscess with a well-defined border usually indicates chronicity (from a few days to a few weeks) and the presence within it of air bubbles or air – fluid levels indicate the presence of gas forming micro-organisms (Fig. 15.9) or communication of the abscess with bowel. The presence of free peritoneal air, as seen with other bowel perforations, is uncommon as the neck of the appendix is usually obstructed and the perforation is usually sealed and localised. If there is free air it is usually minimal and not easily detected. Although

usually under the right hemidiaphragm, the air may collect elsewhere depending on the location of the appendix and may be retroperitoneal with a retroperitoneal appendix (BALTHAZAR 1994b; BALTHAZAR et al. 1988; DURAN et al. 1997; RAO et al. 1997c).

The arrowhead sign is present in 30% of cases of appendicitis and has 100% specificity. It describes focal thickening of the cecal wall around the root of the appendix, which funnels towards the point of obstruction of the appendiceal lumen. This appearance resembles an arrowhead (Fig. 15.10) (RAO et al. 1997a).

In cases of perforation, the appendix may not be seen if its lumen is empty or a phlegmon or abscess has developed. Inflammatory changes in the periappendiceal fat and the presence of an appendicolith strongly suggest a diagnosis of appendicitis. The hallmark

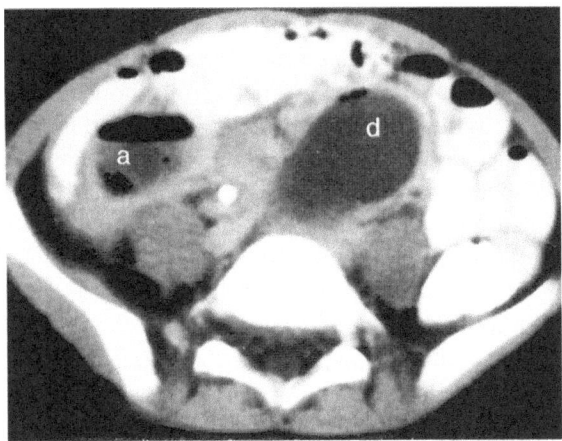

Fig. 15.8. An appendiceal abscess (*a*) and an abscess distant to the appendix (*d*). Small amount of contrast

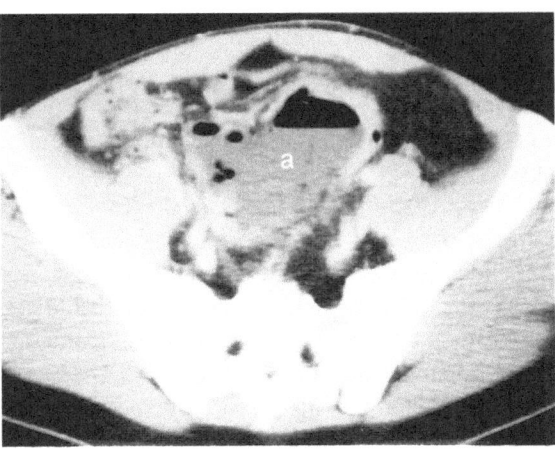

Fig. 15.9. Acute appendicitis with pelvic abscess (*a*). The air-fluid levels within the abscess indicate the presence of gas forming microorganisms

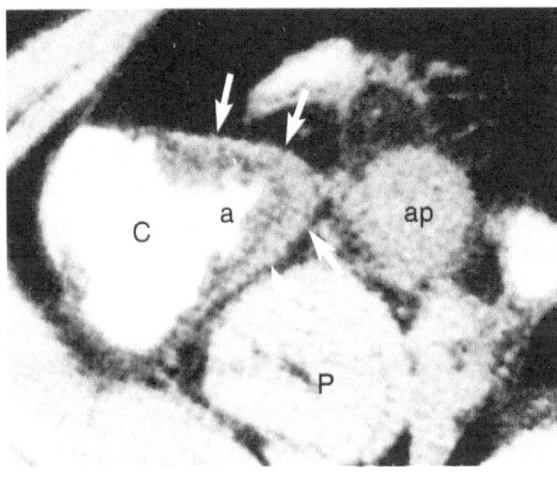

Fig. 15.10. Arrowhead sign in appendicitis. Axial CT image shows symmetric thickening of the medial side of the cecum (*arrows*), with contrast medium funnelling to the point of occlusion (*a*). Note the enlarged appendix (*ap*) with adjacent fat stranding. *C*, cecum; *P*, psoas muscle. [Reproduced from RAO et al. (1977) with permission]

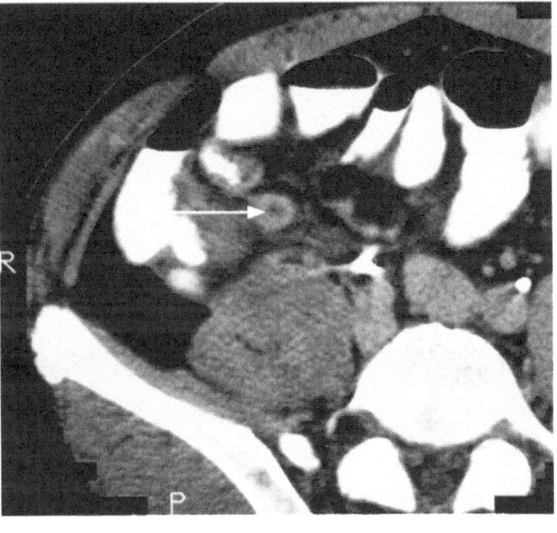

Fig. 15.11. The cardinal CT findings in acute appendicitis are an abnormal appendix with a distended lumen and an inflamed thickened wall (*arrow*) and changes in the periappendiceal fat

of the CT diagnosis is the presence of an abnormal appendix (distended lumen and inflamed thickened wall) and particularly the inflammatory changes in the periappendiceal fat which are seen in 93% of cases of acute appendicitis (Fig. 15.11) (RAO et al. 1997b).

15.6.5
CT classification of appendicitis

Based on CT findings, acute appendicitis may be classified into four categories of increasing severity (GHIATAS et al. 1997):

Category 1:
Simple appendicitis: This is the most subtle appearance of the disease and most challenging to diagnose. The findings are limited to the appendix. The lumen of the appendix may be distended with a thick and enhancing wall. Inflammatory changes in the periappendiceal fat are minimal.

Category 2:
Appendix with periappendiceal inflammatory changes: Inflammatory changes in the periappendiceal fat strongly suggest the presence of appendicitis. This is a specific sign for appendicitis and

suspicion of appendicitis should be raised even if the appendix is not visualised.

Category 3:
Appendicitis with periappendiceal phlegmon and/or abscess.

Category 4:
Appendicitis with distant inflammatory changes. This is the most severe type of appendicitis indicating perforation of the appendix with dissemination of the inflammatory process.

In addition to the high sensitivity, specificity and accuracy in establishing the diagnosis, CT helps plan both percutaneous aspiration (Fig. 15.12) and surgery by defining the exact site of the inflammation; it may also be used for follow-up.

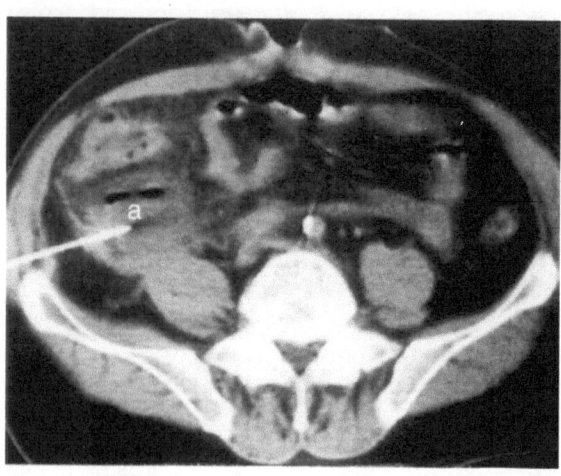

Fig. 15.12. Appendiceal abscess (*a*) in the process of being drained under CT guidance

15.6.6
Differential Diagnosis

A number of pathological conditions may mimic appendicitis on CT imaging. In right sided diverticulitis there is focal cecal wall thickening with adjacent pericecal inflammatory changes. Cecal carcinoma is usually asymptomatic unless complicated by perforation, obstruction or intussusception. Differentiating a perforated cecal carcinoma from a perforated appendix can be difficult, although the presence of a soft tissue mass involving the wall of the caecum with surrounding inflammatory changes should raise the suspicion of carcinoma.

In Crohn's colitis there is circumferential thickening of the colon wall and if, as is usually the case, there is an associated terminal ileitis, then the mural thick-

ening is most evident in the terminal ileum. Other features include mesenteric inflammation, fibrofatty proliferation separating small bowel loops and local lymphadenopathy. The hallmark of diagnosis of this disease is the presence of sinus tracks and fistula. The presence of a complicating abscess or phlegmon in relation to the cecal pole may mimic appendicitis.

Ileocolic lymphadenopathy may suggest a diagnosis of mesenteric adenitis, but it should be remembered that enlarged reactive nodes may be seen with both Crohn's disease and appendicitis.

Pelvic inflammatory disease, complicated ovarian cysts, endometriosis and ectopic pregnancy may all be difficult to differentiate from acute appendicitis (DURAN et al. 1997).

15.6.7
CT Limitations

The presence of periappendiceal fluid may obscure the appendix but fluid can be displaced and the inflamed appendix identified by scanning in a decubitus position. Radiation dose limits the use of CT imaging in pregnancy and for young women and children (RAO 1998).

References

Anderson M, Lilia T, Lundell L et al (1980) Clinical and laboratory findings in patients subjected to laparotomy for suspected acute appendicitis. Acta Chir Scand 146:55–63

Baert LA (1999) Appendicitis, chronic. In: Pettersson H (ed) The encyclopedia of medical imaging. Nicer Institute, Oslo, p 41

Balthazar EJ (1994a) Disorders of the appendix. In: Gore RM, Levine MS, Laufer I (eds) Textbook of gastrointestinal radiology. Saunders, Philadelphia, pp 1318–1319

Balthazar EJ (1994b) Disorders of the appendix. In: Gore RM, Levine MS, Laufer I (eds) Textbook of gastrointestinal radiology. Saunders, Philadelphia, pp 1319–1325

Balthazar EJ, Gade M (1976) The normal and abnormal development of the appendix. Radiology 121:599–604

Balthazar EJ, Megibow AJ, Gordon RB (1988) Computed tomography of the abnormal appendix. J Comput Assist Tomogr 12:1335–1340

Balthazar EJ, Birnbaum BA, Yee J et al (1994) CT and US correlation in 100 patients. Radiology 190:31–35

Balthazar EJ, Rofsky NM, Zucker R (1998) Appendicitis. The impact of computed tomography imaging on negative appendectomy and perforation rates. Am J Gastroenterol 93:768–771

Berry J Jr, Malt RA (1984) Appendicitis near its centenary. Ann Surg 200:567–575

Brown JJ (1991) Acute appendicitis. The radiologist's role. Radiology 180:13–14

Condon RE (1986) Appendicitis. In: Sabiston DC (ed) Text-book of surgery. Saunders, Philadelphia, pp 967–982

Condon RE (1990) Appendicitis. In: Moody FG (ed) Surgical treatment of digestive disease. Year Book Medical Publishers, Chicago, pp 719–739

Duran JC, Beidle TR, Perret R et al (1997) CT imaging of acute right lower quadrant disease. AJR Am J Roentgenol 168: 411–416

Ellis H, Nathanson LK (1997) Appendix and appendectomy. In: Zinner MJ, Schwartz SI, Ellis H (eds) Maigot's abdominal operations. Appleton and Lange, Stanford, Connecticut, pp 1191–1201

Funaki B, Grosskreutz SR, Funaki CN (1998) Using unehanced helical CT with enteric contrast material for suspected appendicitis in patients treated at a community hospital. AJR Am J Roentgenol 171:997–1001

Ghiatas AA, Chopra S, Chintipalli KN et al (1997) Computed tomography of normal appendix and acute appendicitis. Eur Radiol 7:1043–1047

Goldman LD (1992) Appendicitis. In: Taylor MD (ed) Gastrointestinal emergencies. Williams and Wilkins, Baltimore, pp 426–432

Kaiser S, Freckner B, Jorulf HK (2002) Suspected appendicitis in children: US and CT – a prospective randomized study. Radiology 223:633–638

Kamel RI, Goldberg SN, Keogan MT et al (2002) Right lower quadrant pain and suspected appendicitis: nonfocused appendiceal CT-review of 100 cases. Radiology 217:159–163

Lane MJ, Lim DM, Huynh MD et al (1999) Suspected acute appendicitis: nonenhanced helical CT in 300 consecutive patients. Radiology 213:341–346

Raman SS, Lu KD, Kadell BM et al (2002) Accuracy of nonfocused helical CT for the diagnosis of acute appendicitis: a 5-year review. AJR Am J Roentgenol 178:1319–1325

Rao PM (1998) Technical and interpretative pitfalls of appendiceal CT imaging. AJR Am J Roentgenol 171:419–425

Rao PM, Mueller PR (1998) Clinical and pathological variants of appendiceal disease: CT features. AJR Am J Roentgenol 170:1335–1340

Rao PM, Wittenberg J, McDowell KR et al (1997a) Appendicitis: use of arrowhead sign for diagnosis at CT. Radiology 202:363–366

Rao PM, Rhea JT, Novelline RA et al (1997b) Helical CT combined with contrast material administered only through the colon for imaging of suspected appendicitis. AJR Am J Roentgenol 169:1275–1280

Rao PM, Rhea JT, Novelline RA et al (1997c) Helical CT technique for the diagnosis of appendicitis: prospective evaluation of a focused appendix CT examination. Radiology 202:139–144

Voight AE (1953) Embryology and anatomy of the appendix. Southwest Med 34:285–287

16 CT of Diverticulitis

Abraham A. Ghiatas and Georgia P. Economou

CONTENTS

16.1   Introduction   165
16.2   Etiology, Pathology and Epidemiology   165
16.3   Clinical Findings   166
16.4   Computed Tomography of Diverticulitis   166
16.4.1 Introduction   166
16.4.2 Comparison with Other Imaging Modalities   166
16.4.3 Techniques   166
16.4.4 Findings   167
16.4.5 CT Staging and Differentiation from Colon
       Cancer   169
16.4.6 Limitations   169
       References   170

16.1
Introduction

There are three phases to diverticular disease:

The *prediverticular phase* describes thickening of the colon wall (myochosis) as a result of thickening of both the circular muscular coat and the taenia coli.

Diverticulosis describes outpouchings or herniations of the colon wall at sites where nutrient vessels penetrate the muscle coat. The term was first proposed by Case and de Quervain in 1914. The outpouchings usually comprise mucosa and muscularis mucosa and are covered by the serosa.

Diverticulitis describes inflammation of the peridiverticular tissues resulting from perforation of one or more diverticula (Baert 1999; Steinhagen and Aufses 1990).

A. A. Ghiatas, MD
Director of Medical Imaging, Iaso Hospital, Voutsina 1A, Ekali, Athens, 145–78, Greece
G. P. Economou, MD
Iaso Hospital, Voutsina 1A, Ekali, Athens, 145–78, Greece

16.2
Etiology, Pathology and Epidemiology

Colonic diverticulosis is common in the western world. Autopsy reports show that diverticulosis has increased from 5% in 1910 to 50% in 1980 and this is believed to be related to increased longevity and to a change in diet. By the age of 50, 5% of the population will suffer from diverticulosis, increasing to 50% by the age of 80. Although primarily affecting older people, the disease is increasingly seen in younger patients. Prevalence varies from country to country being greatest in the West and lowest in Africa, Latin America and Asia. This is believed to be due to differences in diet. In the West the diet is low in fiber resulting in low volume tenacious fecal material requiring a high propulsive force to move it through the colon and it is the resultant increase in colonic endoluminal pressure that predisposes to the formation of diverticula. In countries with a high fiber diet the prevalence of this condition is low but in time a similar prevalence of diverticulosis is developed in those who migrate from such countries to countries with a low fiber diet. Although dietary habit may be the most important predisposing factor, others have been proposed, such as reduced compliance of the colonic musculature (Balthazar 1994; Minardi et al. 2001; Parks 1997).

In the West almost 95% of diverticulosis occurs in the left colon. The commonest location is the sigmoid colon, followed by the junction of descending and sigmoid colon and then the descending colon. The least common site is the cecum which is affected in approximately 3% of patients.

Between 10% and 35% of patients with diverticulosis develop diverticulitis and of these 25% will require some kind of surgical intervention. The incidence of diverticulitis increases if diverticulosis is widely distributed throughout the colon, if the diverticula are numerous and if they have been present for more than 10 years (Balthazar 1994; Kircher et al. 2002).

In diverticular disease, the diverticula are not true diverticula but pseudodiverticula as their wall consists of just mucosal and submucosal layers. In diverticulitis, inspissated fecal material located within a diverticulum erodes the mucosa and initiates an inflammatory reaction, which may progress to ulceration, suppuration and finally perforation of the diverticulum. If the process remains confined to the colon wall an intramural abscess may form. If the inflammation spreads beyond the bowel wall, the pericolic fat becomes inflamed and an extramural abscess may form. In either case, fever, abdominal pain and tenderness may be accompanied by a palpable abdominal or rectal mass.

Peritoneal involvement may produce adhesions, which help to localize and seal off an abscess. Abscesses may fistulate to the skin or adjacent structures such as the bladder or vagina and if the inflammatory process is not localized or sealed off a generalized peritonitis results (BAERT 1999; PARKS 1997; SLACK 1962).

16.3
Clinical Findings

Sigmoid diverticulitis typically presents with fever, left lower quadrant pain and tenderness and a leukocytosis. These manifestations are similar to those of acute appendicitis except that the pain and tenderness are located to the left lower quadrant and for this reason the condition is sometimes referred to as 'left sided appendicitis'. Physical examination reveals tenderness in the left lower quadrant and it is not uncommon to palpate a mass. There may be abdominal distention and in 25% there is rectal bleeding. The course of the disease may be more aggressive in younger patients. As symptoms and clinical findings can be similar to those of colonic carcinoma, an initial diagnosis of colonic carcinoma may be entertained in 32% of patients with diverticulitis (CIMA and YOUNG-FADOK 2001; PARKS 1997; SLACK 1962).

16.4
Computed Tomography of Diverticulitis

16.4.1
Introduction

CT allows the extent, severity and complications of diverticulitis to be accurately assessed and also allows the disease to be followed during treatment and provides guidance for interventional therapeutic maneuvers (NEFF and VAN SONNENBERG 1989).

16.4.2
Comparison with Other Imaging Modalities

Plain films of the abdomen may demonstrate free or loculated air, ileus or an ill-defined pelvic inflammatory mass. However, these findings are non-specific, and often absent, so plain films of the abdomen are not part of the routine diagnostic work-up of diverticulitis.

The contrast enema has for a long time been the method of choice for diagnosing diverticulitis. It will show diverticula, narrowing of the lumen of the colon (stricture or spasm) and fistula. The extracolonic manifestations of diverticulitis such as phlegmon, abscess or peritonitis may be demonstrated indirectly. The study is uncomfortable, there is the slight risk of perforation and of barium spilling into the peritoneal cavity at the time of surgery. In addition the presence of barium in the colon precludes CT by creating artifacts that impair the quality of the examination (AMBROSETTI et al. 2002; BALTHAZAR et al. 1990; HAN and TISLER 1982; STEFANSON et al. 1997).

Ultrasound may image the inflammatory mass or abscess and demonstrate the bowel wall thickening, but access is limited and the study may be non-diagnostic in patients with free air, widespread ileus or gas containing abscesses. It is usually employed for the evaluation of non-specific abdominal pain or for patients where radiation is best avoided.

Magnetic resonance imaging is at present an expensive and time-consuming imaging modality that is unsuitable for certain patients, such as those with pacemakers or cerebral aneurysm clips, and lacks the sensitivity and specificity of CT.

CT is superior to other imaging modalities for establishing a diagnosis of diverticulitis and for demonstrating other pathology which may present with similar clinical symptoms. It has a sensitivity, specificity, positive and negative predictive value and overall accuracy of 99% (KIRCHER et al. 2002).

16.4.3
Techniques

Bowel preparation is recommended but as the disease often presents as an emergency it is not routine. If circumstances permit, the patient receives oral contrast (1000 cc of diluted barium or water soluble contrast medium) 60–90 min prior to the examination. The patient is placed supine on the CT table and intravenous contrast medium administered (150 cc at 2–3 cc/s with a time delay of 65–70 s).

Alternatively the study may be performed after the administration of rectal contrast medium (500–800 cc of water-soluble contrast medium administered rectally with a gravity drip). Intravenous contrast medium is administered but oral contrast is not. A third technique uses a combination of oral, rectal and intravenous contrast medium.

The study should cover the entire abdomen from the diaphragm to the pubic symphysis with 5–7 mm collimation. A non-contrast study may be performed if intravenous contrast medium is contraindicated (AMBROSETTI et al. 1997; HORTON et al. 2000; HULNICK et al. 1984; RAO et al. 1998).

16.4.4
Findings

The CT findings of diverticulitis may be summarized as follows:
- *Diverticula* are easily identified on CT presenting as outpouchings of the bowel wall, which are filled with air, contrast medium, fecal material or any combination of the three (Fig. 16.1).
- *Bowel wall thickening:* The wall of the large bowel is considered thickened when its width exceeds 4 mm. In diverticulitis the wall thickens from a combination of muscular hypertrophy and inflammation and may reach or exceed 20 mm. The length of colon affected varies depending on the severity of the disease. Intravenous contrast medium produces homogeneous enhancement of the inflamed bowel wall (Fig. 16.2).
- *Pericolonic fat changes:* Inflammatory changes involving the pericolonic fat are considered one of the most important and characteristic CT findings in diverticulitis. They usually consist of linear or non-linear densities within the fat adjacent to the inflamed or perforated diverticulum (Fig. 16.3).
- *Pericolonic edema:* Fat adjacent to the involved colon is of increased attenuation due to the inflammatory edema (Fig. 16.4).
- *Fluid:* Free fluid may be present in small quantities and this usually gravitates to the root of the mesentery (Fig. 16.5).
- *Extracolonic and free peritoneal air:* Air from a perforated diverticulum is usually confined to the area of inflammation or in the adjacent pericolic fat, although rarely air can be seen spreading from the pericolic fat to the retroperitoneum. If a diverticulum perforates into the peritoneal cavity adhesions and the omentum will usually localize

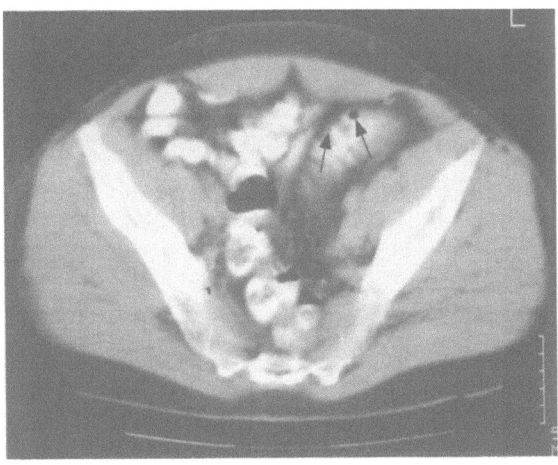

Fig. 16.1. CT showing diverticula (*arrows*)

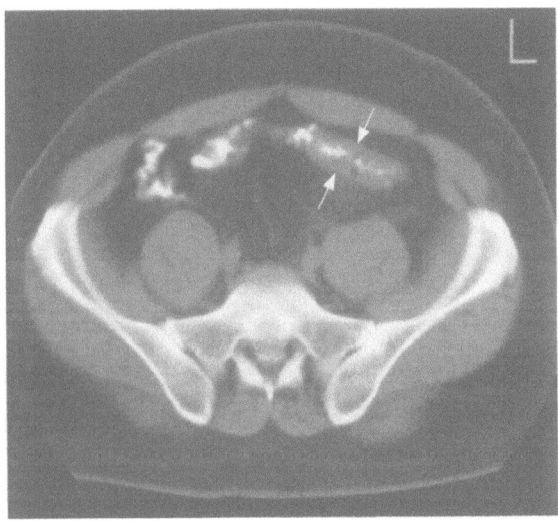

Fig. 16.2. Diverticulitis: bowel wall thickening (*arrows*)

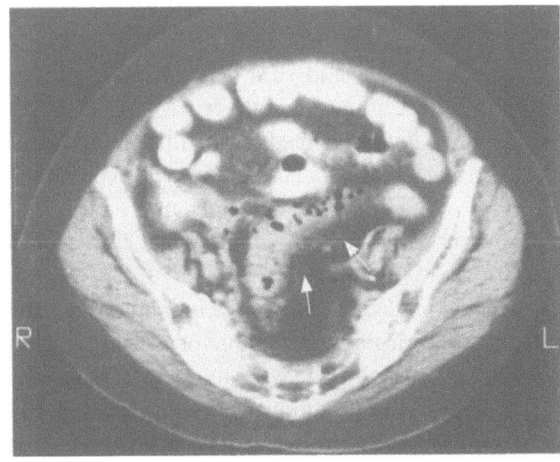

Fig. 16.3. Multiple diverticula and linear and non-linear densities indicating inflammatory changes involving the pericolonic fat (*arrows*)

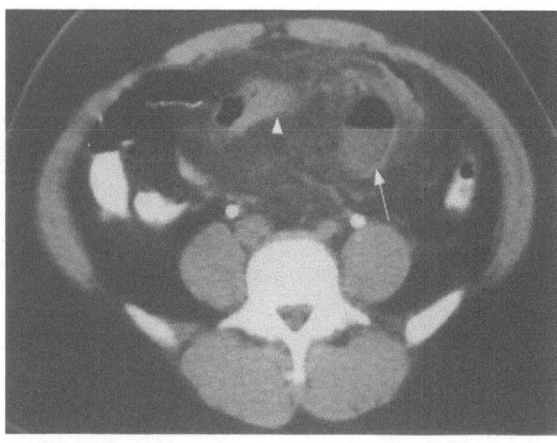

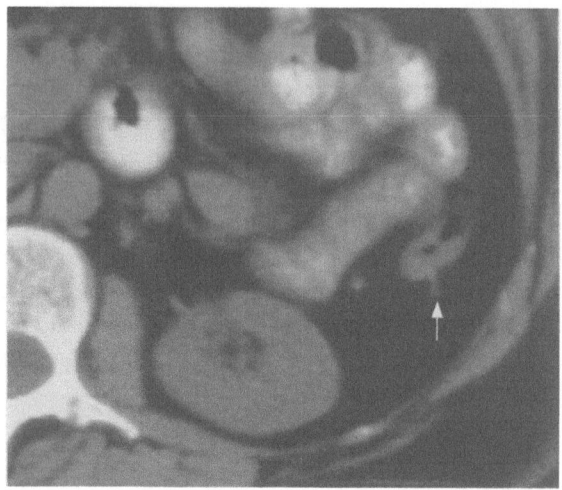

Fig. 16.4. Diverticulitis. There is bowel wall thickening (*arrowhead*), increased attenuation of pericolonic fat of the sigmoid mesocolon and a pericolic abscess (*arrow*)

Fig. 16.6. Deformed diverticulum due to inflammation (*arrow*)

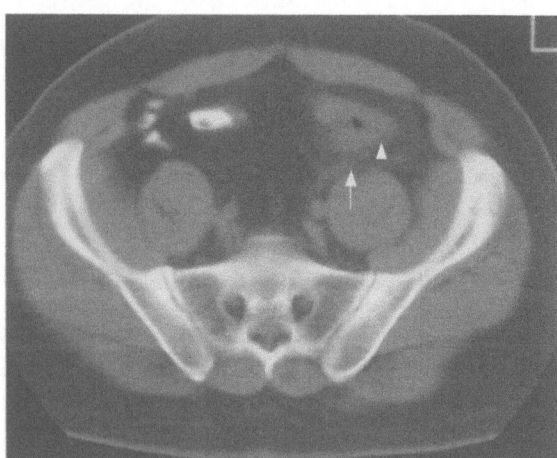

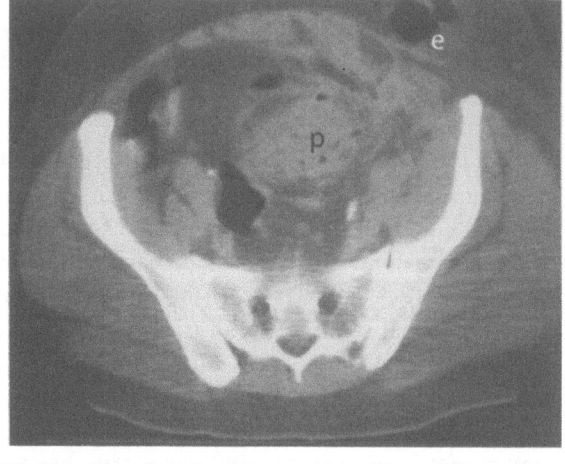

Fig. 16.5. Diverticulitis. A small amount of fluid has gravitated to the root of the mesentery (*arrow*) of a thick-walled sigmoid colon (*arrowhead*)

Fig. 16.7. Diverticulitis: phlegmon (*p*) with extension of the inflammatory process to the abdominal wall where there is a gas-filled abscess (*e*)

the perforation and so a generalized peritonitis with free peritoneal air is rare.

- *Inflamed diverticulum:* Infrequently CT may demonstrate the inflamed or ruptured diverticulum as a deformed out pouching which may have a small amount of air (small bubble) at its apex (site of rupture) (Fig. 16.6).
- *Phlegmon/abscess:* Should the inflammation progress, a pericolonic inflammatory mass develops (phlegmon) which may form an abscess, characterized by air and fluid within the mass (Fig. 16.7, 16.8). These findings may also develop at a distance from the original site of inflammation.
- *Fistula:* It is very uncommon to demonstrate a fistula on CT unless it is to the skin (Fig. 16.9).

However, the presence of a fistula may be inferred if contrast medium is seen in a viscus into which the fistula opens, such as the urinary bladder (Fig. 16.10).

- *Other signs:* Intramural air and intramural sinus tracts may occasionally be appreciated on CT scans. Thrombosis of the mesenteric and portal veins from pyelophlebitis may be recognized on contrast-enhanced scans. In pyelophlebitis air may rarely be seen within the veins and hepatic abscesses may develop.

Bowel wall thickening and inflammatory changes in the peridiverticular fat are the most frequent CT features of diverticulitis and have a sensitivity of

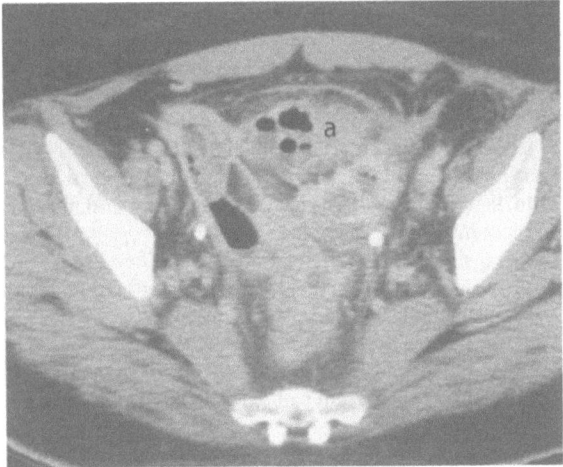

Fig. 16.8. Pelvic abscesses (*a*) in a patient with diverticulitis

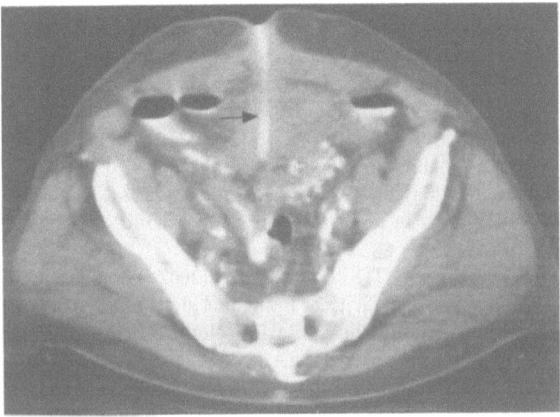

Fig. 16.9. CT fistulogram. A fistula tract (*arrow*) is demonstrated in a patient with a pericolic diverticular abscess that has ruptured to the skin

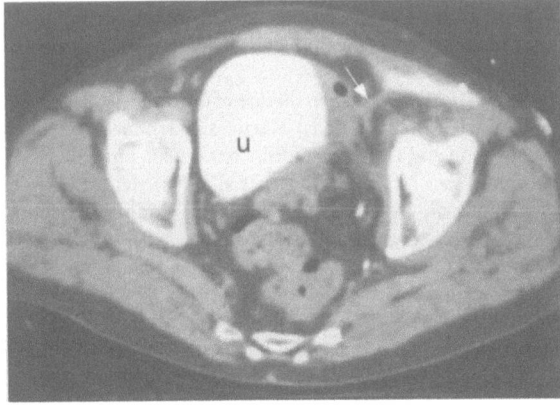

Fig. 16.10. Fistulation between diverticular abscess, urinary bladder (*u*) and abdominal wall (*arrow*). The inflammatory process has thickened the bladder wall

96% and 95% respectively and a specificity of 91% and 90%. Other CT features are the presence of diverticula, fluid in the root of the mesentery, an inflamed diverticulum, a phlegmon or abscess and free peritoneal air (HULNICK et al. 1984; KIRCHER et al. 2002).

16.4.5
CT Staging and Differentiation from Colon Cancer

Staging of diverticulitis by CT assists in management and helps determine prognosis.
- Stage 0: Mural thickening and minimal inflammation of the peridiverticular fat. Treatment for this stage is usually with antibiotics.
- Stage 1: Inflammation of the pericolonic fat with a small, up to 3-cm diameter, abscess. Treatment is with antibiotics and intervention is seldom required.
- Stage 2: Abscess or abscesses measuring 5–10 cm in diameter but confined within the pelvis. At this stage percutaneous drainage may be useful as a prelude to surgery.
- Stage 3: The abscess has grown beyond the confines of the pelvis and treatment is surgical.
- Stage 4: The CT appearances are similar to stage 3 but the patient's clinical condition has deteriorated with peritonitis and immediate surgical intervention is required (AMBROSETTI et al. 2002; BALTHAZAR 1994; KLOMRJEN and KAPUSTA 1990; NEFF et al. 1987).

It is important to attempt to differentiate between diverticulitis and colon cancer as their treatment differs. The CT features overlap but there are statistically significant differences in the frequency in which certain CT findings appear in these two conditions. By utilizing strict diagnostic criteria 50% of the cases will be diagnosed by CT as diverticulitis or colon cancer with high confidence and will not require further diagnostic evaluation. The absence of pericolonic lymph nodes and the presence of inflammatory changes, edema and fluid adjacent to the involved thickened colonic segment strongly favor a diagnosis of diverticulitis, while enlargement of local lymph nodes and no or minimal inflammatory changes, strongly suggests colon cancer (Fig. 16.11, 16.12). The longer the involved segment the less likely colon cancer, whereas the presence of shouldering or an intraluminal mass favors colon cancer. Of course the possibility of the two pathologies coexisting should be always kept in mind (CHINTAPALLI et al. 1997, 1999; PADIDAR et al. 1994).

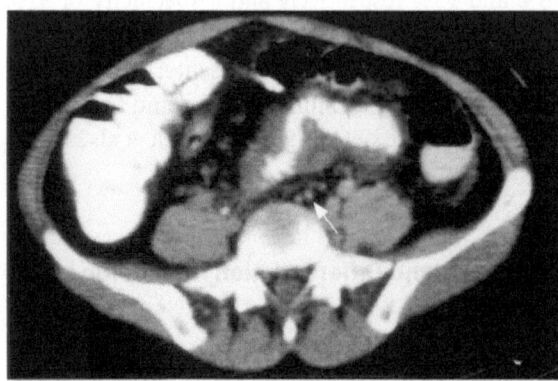

Fig. 16.11. Colon cancer. There is bowel wall thickening with small lymph nodes (*arrow*) in the pericolic fat

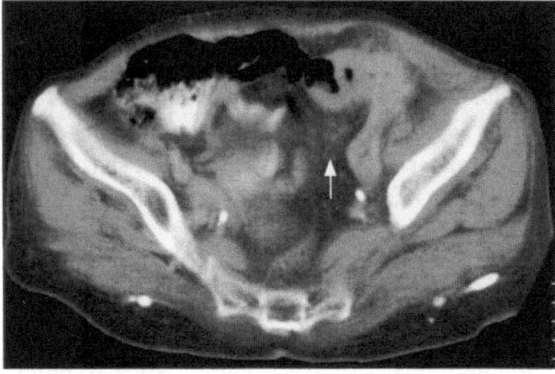

Fig. 16.12. Colon cancer. There is not only bowel wall thickening with adjacent small lymph nodes (*arrow*) but also some mild inflammatory change in the pericolonic fat

16.4.6
Limitations

CT is the best imaging modality for the diagnosis and management of diverticulitis although radiation restricts its use in pregnancy.

The accuracy of CT in depicting sinus and fistula tracts is low and when diverticulitis develops close to the appendix, it may not be possible to differentiate it from appendicitis. The presence of small amounts of fluid or small abscesses may escape CT detection and the differentiation from colon cancer may prove difficult or impossible. Nevertheless, despite these limitations, CT is superior to all other imaging modalities for the diagnosis of colonic diverticulitis (BALTHAZAR et al. 1990; BALTHAZAR 1994).

References

Ambrosetti P, Grossholz M, Becker C et al (1997) Computed tomography in acute left colonic diverticulitis. Br J Surg 84:532–534

Ambrosetti P, Jenny A, Becker C et al (2000) Acute left colonic diverticulitis – compared performance of computed tomography and water soluble contrast enema: prospective evaluation of 420 patients. Dis Colon Rectum 43:1363–1367

Ambrosetti P, Becker C, Terrier F (2002) Colonic diverticulitis: impact of imaging on surgical management – a prospective study of 542 patients. Eur Radiol 12:1145–1149

Baert LA (1999) Diverticulitis, colon and diverticulosis, colon. In: Petterson H (ed) The encyclopedia of medical imaging. Nicer Institute, Oslo, pp 117–121

Balthazar EJ (1994) Diverticular disease. In: Gore RM, Levine MS, Laufer I_(eds) Textbook of gastrointestinal radiology. Saunders, Philadelphia, pp 1072–1097

Balthazar EJ, Megibow AJ, Schinell RA et al (1990) Limitations in the CT diagnosis of acute diverticulitis: comparison of CT, contrast enema and pathologic findings in 16 patients. AJR 154:281–285

Chintapali KN, Chopra S, Ghiatas AA et al (1999) Diverticulitis versus colon cancer: differentiation with helical CT findings. Radiology 210:429–435

Chintapalli KN, Esola CC, Chopra S et al (1997) Pericolic mesenteric lymphnodes: an aid in distinguishing diverticulitis from colon cancer. AJR 169:1253–1255

Cima RR, Young-Fadok TM (2001) New developments in diverticular disease. Curr Gastroenterol Rep 3:420–424

Han SY, Tisler JM (1982) Perforation of the colon above peritoneal reflection during barium enema evaluation. Radiology 25:253–255

Horton KM, Corl MF, Fishman EK (2000) CT evaluation of the colon: inflammatory disease. Radiographics 20:399–418

Hulnick DH, Megibow AJ, Balthazar EJ et al (1984) Computed tomography in the evaluation of diverticulitis. Radiology 152:491–495

Kircher MF, Rhea JT, Kihiszak D et al (2002) Frequency, sensitivity and specificity of individual signs of diverticulitis on thin-section helical CT with colonic contrast material: experience with 312 cases. AJR 178:1313–1318

Klompjen G, Kapusta GR (1990) Options in the treatment of diverticular disease in the colon. Curr Prob Surg 7:479–485

Minardi AJ Jr, Johnson LW, Sedon JK et al (2001) Diverticulitis in the young patient. Am Surg 67:458–461

Neff CC, van Sonnenberg E (1989) CT of diverticulitis: diagnosis and treatment. Radiol Clin North Am 27:743–752

Neff CC, van Sonnenberg E, Casola G et al (1987) Diverticular abscess: percutaneous drainage. Radiology 163:15–18

Padidar AM, Jeffrey RB Jr, Mindelzun ER et al (1994) Differentiating sigmoid diverticulitis from carcinoma on CT scans: mesenteric inflammation suggests diverticulitis. AJR 163:81–83

Parks TG (1997) Diverticular disease of the colon. In: Zinner MJ, Schwartz SI, Ellis H (eds) Maigot´s abdominal operations. Appleton and Lange, Stanford, Connecticut, pp 1229–1234

Rao PM, Rhea JT, Novelling RA et al (1998) Helical CT with only colonic contrast material for diagnosing diverticulitis: prospective evaluation of 150 patients. AJR 170:1445–1449

Slack WW (1962) The anatomy, pathology and some clinical features of diverticulitis of the colon. Br J Surg 50: 185–194

Stefanson T, Nyman R, Nilsson S et al (1997) Diverticulitis of the sigmoid colon. A comparison of CT, colonic enema and laparoscopy. Acta Radiol 38:313–319

Steihagen RM, Aufses AH (1990) Diverticular disease of the colon. In: Moody FG (ed) Surgical treatment of digestive disease. Year Book Medical Publishers, Chicago, pp 740–753

17 Diagnosing Inflammatory Bowel Disease – Is There Still a Case for Barium Enema?

MARIA SHERIDAN

CONTENTS

17.1   Introduction   *171*
17.2   Barium Enema Appearances of Ulcerative
       Colitis   *171*
17.3   Barium Enema Appearances of Crohn's Disease   *172*
17.4   Barium Enema versus Colonoscopy   *174*
17.5   Barium Enema versus Cross-Sectional Imaging   *175*
17.6   Conclusion   *175*
       References   *175*

17.1
Introduction

Inflammatory bowel disease refers to the two chronic idiopathic inflammatory diseases, ulcerative colitis and Crohn's disease. The diagnosis is usually suggested on the basis of clinical symptoms and signs and confirmed by the typical appearances at double contrast barium enema (DCBE) or the endoscopic appearance plus typical histological features from colonoscopic biopsies. With the increase in requirement for histological evidence, the barium enema may be seen as obsolete as patients are going to require colonoscopy. However, in recent years, with the increasingly widespread availability of colonoscopy, some of the strengths and advantages of the DCBE in this setting have been overlooked. The barium appearances of both diseases have been well described on DCBE (GORE and LAUFER 1994). This chapter will briefly review the appearances of these conditions and then look at specific instances where the barium enema is of particular importance for diagnosis and assessment.

M. SHERIDAN, MRCP, FRCR
Consultant Radiologist, Department of Clinical Radiology, St James's University Hospital, Beckett Street, Leeds LS9 7TF, UK

17.2
Barium Enema Appearances of Ulcerative Colitis

Ulcerative colitis is an inflammatory condition limited to the mucosa and submucosa of the colon. The rectum is always involved in patients who have not received treatment. About 30% of patients have disease that is limited to the rectum at presentation, 40% have disease that extends proximally but not beyond the hepatic flexure and the remaining 30% have pancolitis. Those patients who have disease limited to the rectum may go on to develop more proximal disease in about 10% of cases.

The earliest barium enema change in the mucosa is development of a rather diffuse granularity and loss of the normal sharp colonic margin with the development of a blurred or indistinct margin. Slight thickening of the haustral folds may also be identified at this stage. As the inflammatory process proceeds, crypt abscesses develop which erode into the colonic lumen and these are seen as mucosal stippling, where tiny flecks of barium are adherent to the base of the abscesses (Fig. 17.1). With progression of the crypt abscesses, ulceration extends into the submucosa and spreads laterally to produce collar button ulcers (Fig. 17.2). Should ulceration progress, much of the mucosa may be lost and any remaining oedematous mucosa protrudes into the colonic lumen as pseudo-polyps.

In a small number of patients who have had chronic ulcerative colitis affecting the whole colon the distal 5–20 cm of the ileum may also be abnormal. In these patients, the ileocecal valve is patulous and barium refluxes easily into the terminal ileum revealing a rather granular mucosa and loss of the normal fold pattern. This is referred to as backwash ileitis and it has been suggested that reflux of colonic content is the cause rather than the underlying bowel inflammatory disease as the terminal ileum returns to normal after colectomy in these patients.

Those patients with long-standing ulcerative colitis also have a number of characteristic appearances on barium enema. The colon becomes shortened and

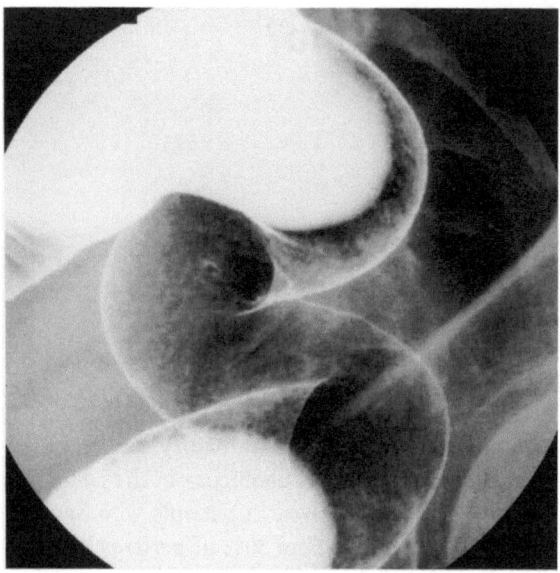

Fig. 17.1. Rectosigmoid junction showing mucosal stippling

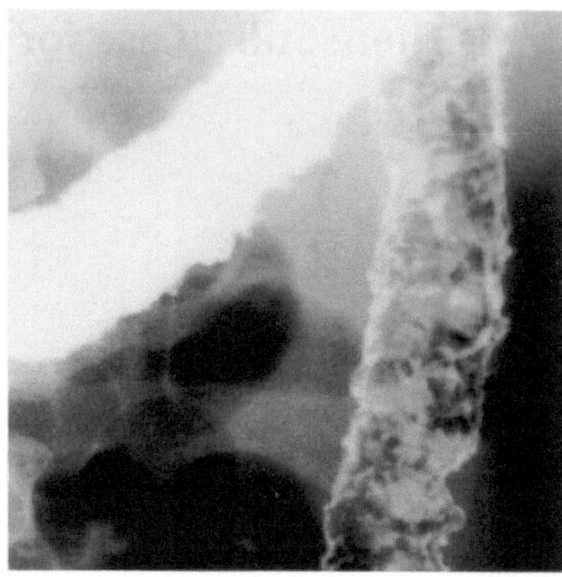

Fig. 17.2. Collar button ulcers in a patient with extensive shedding of the mucosa producing a pseudo-polypoid appearance

rather rigid due to the marked hypertrophy of the muscularis mucosa. In addition, for reasons that are unclear, the taenia coli relax and so the normal haustral pattern is lost, resulting in a featureless appearance to the colon.

Following an acute episode of severe ulcerative colitis, with loss of much of the mucosa, the bare areas are covered by granulation tissue. In some patients, overgrowth of the regenerating mucosa leads to the formation of post inflammatory pseudopolyps (Fig. 17.3). These have a variety of appearances, from small and round to long and filiform. These may be the only evidence of a previous episode of acute ulcerative colitis.

One of the most serious consequences of longstanding colitis is the development of colorectal cancer. The risk increases both with chronicity of disease and with extent of colonic involvement. The majority of patients who develop colorectal cancer have pancolitis although those who have colitis limited to the left side of the colon are at a slightly increased risk compared to the general population. It is recognised that carcinoma develops from areas of dysplasia in the colonic mucosa. Whilst the appearances of dysplasia have been described at DCBE, it is generally acknowledged that DCBE alone is not sufficiently sensitive for early identification (HOOYMAN et al. 1987; MATSUMO et al. 1996). Dysplasia may not be recognised even at endoscopy and accurate diagnosis usually requires multiple biopsies and these need to be examined by an experienced pathologist. (EADEN et al. 2001).

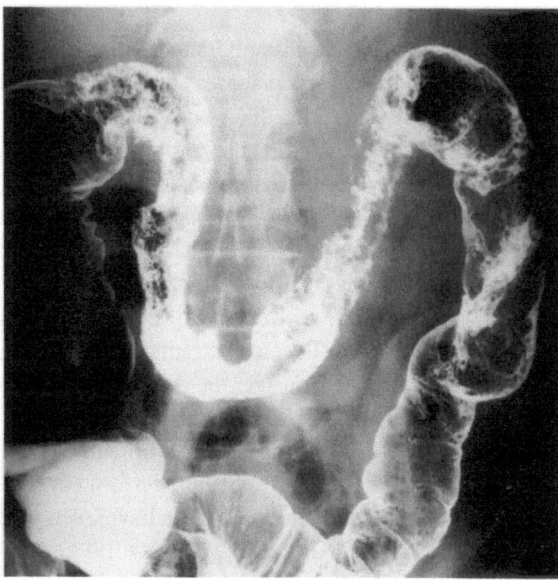

Fig. 17.3. Extensive post-inflammatory pseudopolyps

17.3
Barium Enema Appearances of Crohn's Disease

Crohn's disease is a transmural granulomatous inflammatory process, which can involve any part of the gastrointestinal tract. Both the terminal ileum and colon are involved in just over 50% of cases. The colon alone is involved in about 15% and the terminal ileum alone in 14%. Involvement of the gastrointestinal tract is not continuous and there are macroscopically normal areas of bowel between "skip" lesions. In the early stages of the disease, areas of ulceration are surrounded by normal looking mucosa. This is in contrast to ulcerative colitis where the whole of the involved mucosa looks abnormal. In Crohn's disease there is a particular predilection for the mesenteric border of the gastrointestinal tract.

There are a number of characteristic features that might be seen on a barium enema. Aphthous ulcers are small, superficial areas of ulceration that overlie enlarged lymphoid follicles. On a barium enema these are seen as small barium collections surrounded by a radiolucent halo (Fig. 17.4). The collection represents a superficial ulcer and the halo, the oedematous mucosa surrounding the ulcer. Aphthous ulcers are usually multiple and asymmetric in distribution, involving one side of the bowel wall more than the other. The mucosa between the ulcers is normal.

Deep ulceration penetrating the submucosa and the muscularis propria is a characteristic feature of Crohn's disease. These ulcers are referred to as rose-thorn ulcers (Fig. 17.5). The area of ulceration may enlarge and the longitudinal and transverse orientation of these deep clefts result in the typical cobblestone appearance (Fig. 17.5). The mucosa between these deep ulcerations may be oedematous but otherwise normal contributing to the cobblestone-like effect. Longitudinal ulceration along the mesenteric border of the colon is particularly suggestive of Crohn's disease.

As the ulceration deepens to penetrate the full thickness of the colonic wall, sinus tracts may develop and extend out into the peri-colic soft tissues (Fig. 17.6).

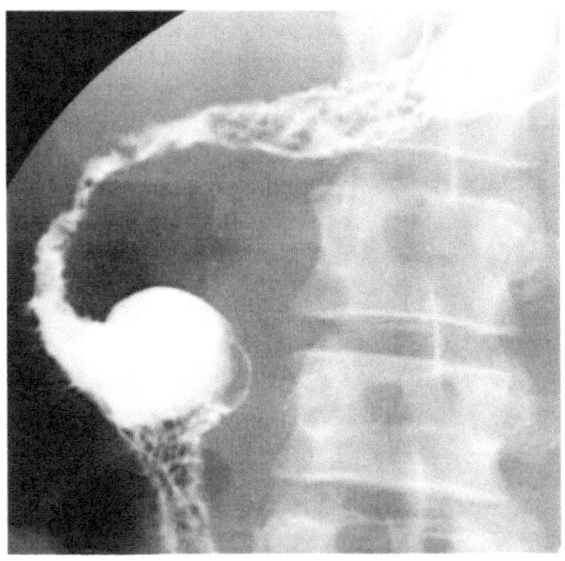

Fig. 17.5. Hepatic flexure showing deep ulceration which is both longitudinal and transverse producing a "cobblestone" appearance and pseudosacculation

Fistulae also develop if sinus tracts communicate with other structures such as bladder, vagina or other adjacent bowel loops.

Since Crohn's disease is a transmural process the wall thickening and subsequent fibrosis can lead to significant luminal narrowing and produce strictures (Fig. 17.7). Because of the asymmetric involvement of the bowel wall, the strictures are often asymmetric rather than circumferential. In some cases, healing of the bowel wall by fibrosis causes shortening and rigidity of that section of the wall. The non-involved section (usually the anti-mesenteric border) may

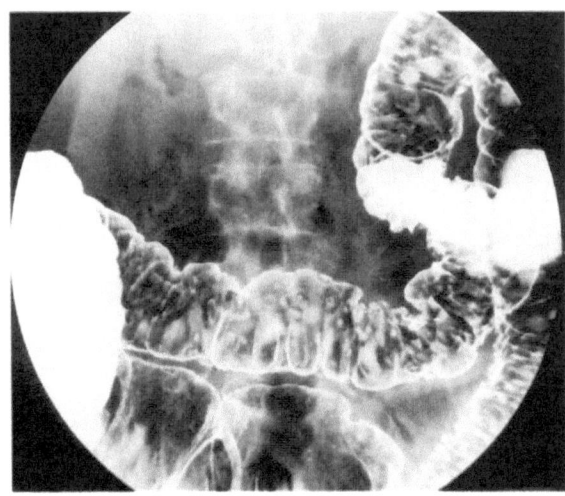

Fig. 17.4. Aphthous ulcers in the transverse colon

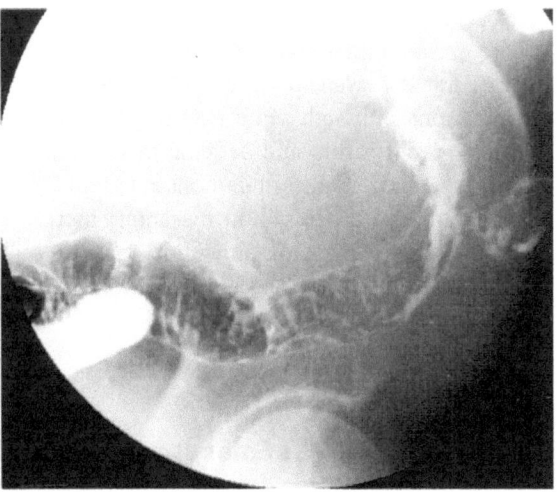

Fig. 17.6. Colonic Crohn's disease with a sinus track extending into the peri-colic soft tissues

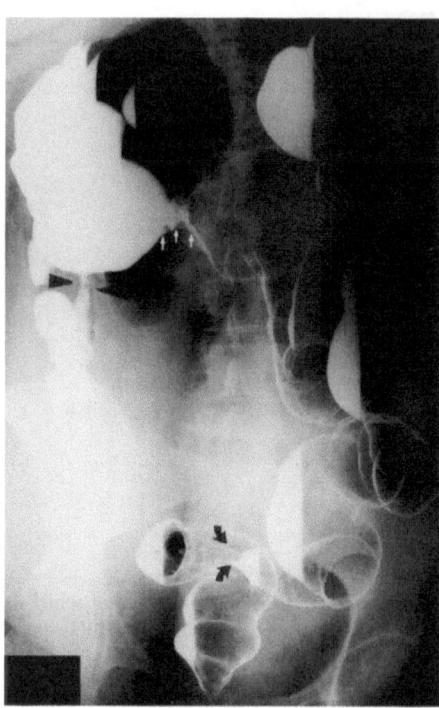

Fig. 17.7. Multiple short strictures in the sigmoid colon (*black curved arrows*), transverse colon (*white arrows*) and ascending colon (*black arrowheads*). At colonoscopy, it was not possible to intubate beyond the most distal stricture

then balloon outwards producing the appearance of pseudosacculation.

The anal canal is involved in about two thirds of patients with Crohn's colitis and this may antedate colonic involvement by several years. These perianal and perirectal fissures may be seen on barium enema in patients with an otherwise normal colon and non-specific symptoms (Fig. 17.8). They appear as short barium filled channels extending out from the anal canal. It is unusual to see the true extent on barium enema.

The extra-luminal abnormalities of Crohn's disease are not at all well appreciated on barium enema examinations, although some may be inferred. The fibrofatty proliferation and oedema in the adjacent mesentery is extremely well demonstrated on CT. As the inflammatory process in the mesentery increases, an inflammatory mass or phlegmon may be seen which may then go on to abscess formation.

17.4
Barium Enema versus Colonoscopy

Despite major advances in cross-sectional imaging techniques, DCBE and colonoscopy remain the prin-

cipal means of examining the colon. The diagnostic accuracy of DCBE and colonoscopy alone are similar when experienced operators perform the examinations. The major advantage of colonoscopy, however, is the ability to take biopsies at the time of the diagnostic examination. There is now general recognition that this is the most accurate method of establishing the presence and the nature of the inflammatory bowel disease (HOLDSTOCK et al. 1984). Therefore where there is a high index of suspicion, the patient is likely to be referred for colonoscopy as the first investigation. Biopsies obtained at colonoscopy are small and superficial. Granuloma formation is the pathological hallmark of Crohn's disease, however it is absent in up to 30% of cases (THOMPSON 1990). Deeper biopsies may increase the sensitivity for granuloma detection and can be obtained at rigid sigmoidoscopy in those with distal disease. In isolated right colonic disease, however, deep biopsies may not be possible. In these cases correlation with barium enema appearances is helpful to define the type of colitis since the radiological features of ulcerative colitis and Crohn's disease allow the correct diagnosis to be reached in the majority of cases (GORE and LAUFER 1994; DIJKSTRA et al. 1995). In some cases there is considerable diagnostic overlap between types of colitis, even when adequate tissue is available for histological examination, and a definite diagnosis cannot be established (TSANG 1999). In these cases, correlation with the barium enema

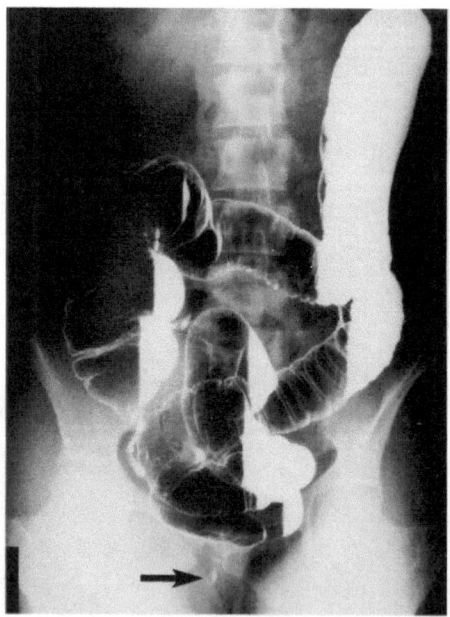

Fig. 17.8. Perianal fissure (*arrow*) in a patient with Crohn's disease. Note the aphthous ulceration of the sigmoid colon

appearances or endoscopic features is valuable in establishing the correct diagnosis. Moreover DCBE is superior to colonoscopy in its ability to demonstrate the whole of the colon and barium reflux into the terminal ileum occurs in up to 85% allowing assessment of the distal small bowel at the same examination (RUBESIN et al. 2001) In ulcerative colitis this is seldom of clinical relevance, since, in the untreated patient, the rectum is involved and biopsies can be performed easily using a rigid sigmoidoscope. It is, however of much greater importance in Crohn's disease, where its discontinuous nature and right-sided predominance make incomplete colonoscopy problematic (DIJKSTRA et al. 1995).

In Crohn's disease there are specific situations where DCBE is superior to colonoscopy. The first of these are those patients who have a colonic stricture due to Crohn's disease and active disease more proximally. In such patients, passage of the colonoscope to examine the proximal colon may not be possible.

DCBE is also more accurate than colonoscopy for determining the path of fistulae and sinuses. The luminal opening may be seen at colonoscopy, but DCBE will allow the extent and complexity of fistulous tracts to be assessed, which is of importance in planning surgical intervention.

Whilst it is outside the scope of this chapter, it is worth remembering the very important contribution barium examinations of the small bowel make when a patient has a colitis of uncertain aetiology.

17.5
Barium Enema versus Cross-Sectional Imaging

Cross-sectional imaging, in particular computed tomography (GORE et al. 1996) and sonography (SHERIDAN et al. 1993; PRADEL et al. 1997) have become increasingly important in the assessment of patients with inflammatory bowel disease, especially patients with Crohn's disease. The major advantage of cross-sectional imaging is its ability to demonstrate the extra-luminal components of the disease, such as inflammatory masses and abscesses (GORE et al. 1996). The mucosal detail, however, is considerably inferior to barium radiology and the major finding of wall thickening is non-specific for all types of colitis. Early disease, with only mild mucosal abnormalities, may be underestimated. For the most part, barium radiology is probably the most effective means to demonstrate fistulae or sinus tracts. A large track

may be identifiable on CT by the use of orally or rectally administered contrast, but more subtle tracks and complex fistulae are more easily appreciated at barium enema (PICKHARDT et al. 2002).

17.6
Conclusion

DCBE and colonoscopy are similar in diagnostic accuracy for Crohn's disease and ulcerative colitis. The major advantage of colonoscopy is the ability to biopsy the colonic mucosa. However, DCBE may still be valuable in histologically "indeterminate" cases, examining the colon proximal to strictures in patients with Crohn's disease and to establish the presence and complexity of fistulae and sinuses.

Although cross-sectional imaging techniques mainly provide information about the extraluminal components of the disease, recent advances have continued to challenge barium radiology as the initial radiological procedure. The information derived from DCBE, colonoscopy and cross-sectional imaging is largely complimentary and the decision as to which is the most appropriate investigation should be made on a patient by patient basis.

References

Dijkstra J, Reeders JWAJ, Tytgat GNJ (1995) Idiopathic Inflammatory bowel disease: endoscopic-radiologic correlation Radiology 197:369–375

Eaden J, Abrams K, McKay H et al (2001) Inter-observer variation between general and specialist gastrointestinal pathologists when grading dysplasia in ulcerative colitis. J Pathol 194:152–157

Gore RM, Laufer I (1994) Ulcerative colitis and granulomatous colitis: idiopathic inflammatory bowel disease. In: Gore RM, Levine MS, Laufer I (eds) Textbook of gastrointestinal radiology. Saunders, Philadelphia, pp 1098–1141

Gore RM, Balthazar EJ, Ghahremani GG et al (1996) CT features of ulcerative colitis and Crohn's disease. AJR 167:3–15

Holdstock G, DuBoulay CE, Smith CL (1984) Survey of the use of colonoscopy in inflammatory bowel disease. Dig Dis Sci 29:751–754

Hooyman JR, MacCarty RL, Carpenter HA et al (1987) Radiographic appearance of mucosal dysplasia associated with ulcerative colitis. AJR 149:47–51

Matsumoto T Iida M, Kuroki F et al (1996) Dysplasia in ulcerative colitis: is radiography adequate for diagnosis? Radiology 1999:85–90

Pickhardt PJ, Bhalla SV, Balfe DM (2002) Acquired gastrointestinal fistulas: classification, etiologies and imaging evaluation. Radiology 224:9–23

Pradel JA, David XR, Taourel P et al (1997) Sonographic assessment of the normal and abnormal bowel wall in nondiverticular ileitis and colitis. Abdom Imaging 22:167–172

Rubesin SE, Scotiniotis I, Birnbaum BA et al (2001) Radiologic and endoscopic diagnosis of Crohn's disease. Surg Clin North Am 81:39–70

Sheridan MB, Nicholson DA, Martin DF (1993) Transabdominal ultrasonography as the primary investigation in patients with suspected Crohn's disease or recurrence. Clin Radiol 48:402–404

Thompson H (1990) Histopathology of Crohn's disease. In: Allan RN, Keighley MRB, Alexander-Williams J, Hawkins C (eds) Inflammatory bowel diseases. Churchill Livingstone, London, pp 263–285

Tsang P (1999) Biopsy diagnosis of colitis: possibilities and pitfalls. Am J Surg Pathol 23:423–430

18 Ultrasound of Colitis

Robert James Peck

CONTENTS

18.1 Introduction 177
18.2 The Normal Colon 177
18.3 Crohn's Disease 178
18.3.1 Description 178
18.3.2 Complications 179
18.4 Ulcerative Colitis 179
18.4.1 Description 179
18.4.2 Complications 180
18.5 Accuracy 181
18.5.1 Sensitivity 181
18.5.2 Specificity 181
18.5.3 Activity of Disease 181
18.6 Infectious Colitis 182
18.7 Pseudomembranous Colitis 182
18.8 Typhlitis (Neutropenic Enterocolitis) 182
18.9 Ischaemic colitis 182
18.10 Other Techniques 183
18.10.1 Hydrocolonic Sonography 183
18.10.2 Endoluminal Rectal Ultrasound 183
References 183

18.1
Introduction

Ultrasound is increasingly recognised for its value in the assessment of bowel pathology. With the increasing speed and sensitivity of modern multi-slice CT, there is no doubt that the diagnostic potential of CT has increased significantly, but with an increase in radiation dose. For young patients who require repeated assessments of their inflammatory bowel disease non-radiation techniques such as ultrasound are of particular value. In addition, as colitis frequently presents in young people as a non-specific abdominal and pelvic complaint, the first imaging test obtained is frequently an ultrasound scan. Therefore, it is important for the sonographer to take a general overview of the abdomen and pelvis and be able to recognise bowel pathology when it is present.

Ultrasound may demonstrate the anatomical transition from normal to abnormal bowel in an affected individual, the changes that occur over time with treatment, the development of chronic changes, and the presence of complications such as abscesses and fistulae. Doppler techniques also provide an estimate of disease activity.

18.2
The Normal Colon

The normal colon typically contains faeces and air and its wall is most commonly seen as a thin layer between the luminal echo-bright air and the peritoneum adjacent to the anterior abdominal wall. The normal colon wall is just 2–3 mm thick (Fig. 18.1) and generally it is a layer which receives little attention.

High-frequency ultrasound can demonstrate the typical five-layer structure seen throughout the bowel, representing the different layers and interfaces (Fig. 18.2).

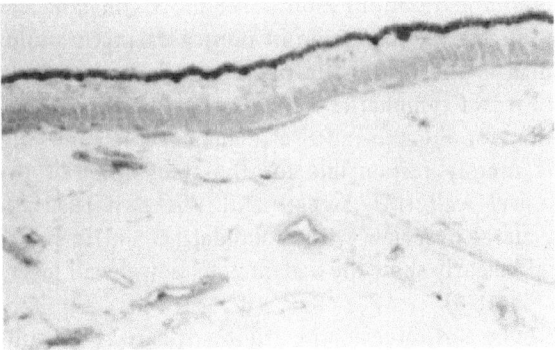

Fig. 18.1. Normal colon, histological specimen

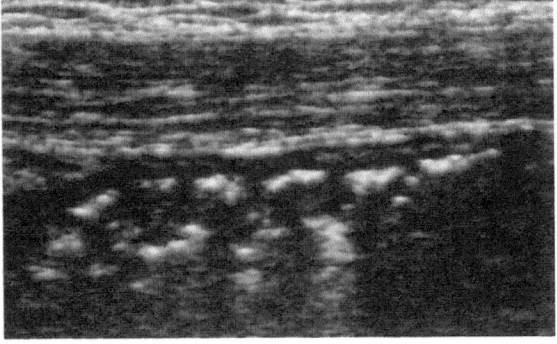

Fig. 18.2. Five-layered structure, normal wall

R. J. Peck
Royal Hallamshire Hospital, Glossop Road, Sheffield S10 2JF, United Kingdom

When there is inflammation these layers become thickened and then are visible when using standard abdominal probes at 3.5–5 MHz. Therefore, a routine abdominal scan will frequently detect abnormal bowel which can then be scanned at higher resolution if further detail is required.

18.3
Crohn's Disease

18.3.1
Description

Crohn's disease is a chronic inflammatory disease which has a peak age of onset between 15 and 25 years of age. Some series show a second, lesser peak between 55 and 65 years of age (YAMADA et al. 1995). The site most commonly involved is the terminal ileum, but the colon may be primarily affected in approximately 25% of cases (KIRSNER 2000). Unlike ulcerative colitis, Crohn's disease may just involve the right colon.

Histologically, this is an inflammatory process that involves all layers of the gut wall (i.e. transmural) and may extend into the mesentery. Focal lymphocytic infiltration is the most constant feature and the formation of non-caseating granulomas is the diagnostic pathological marker. Both obstruct lymphatics which is the likely explanation for the sub-mucosal oedema which initially, is mainly responsible for the thickening of the bowel wall (MacSWEEN and WHALEY 1992). A general overview with a standard 3.5 MHz probe will clearly show the oedematous bowel wall layers (Fig. 18.3).

The earliest lesion of Crohn's disease is the aphthoid ulcer, which is a mucosal lesion representing ulceration overlying lymphoid follicles (Figs. 18.4 and 18.5). These ulcers are non-specific and may occur in other conditions such as amoebiasis, salmonellosis and shigellosis (MacSWEEN and WHALEY 1992). Another important feature, which is highly characteristic, is the formation of deep fissure ulcers that traverse the bowel wall. (Figs. 18.6 and 18.7). Crohn's disease is also recognised by skip lesions, and so the visualisation of normal bowel between affected areas contributes towards establishing the diagnosis.

Disease progression and chronicity results in a number of manifestations. Inflammation that

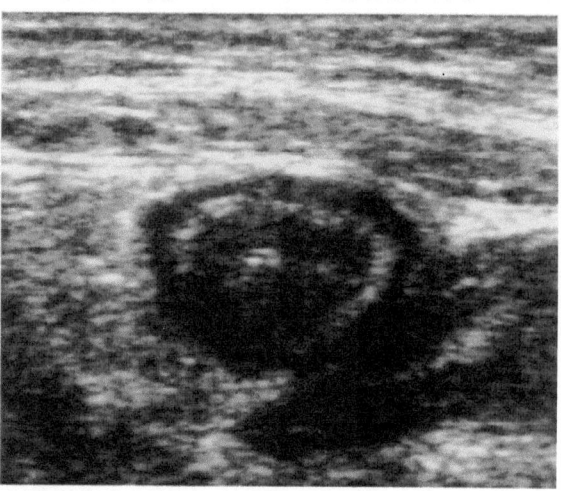

Fig. 18.3. Transverse section. Oedematous bowel involving all layers

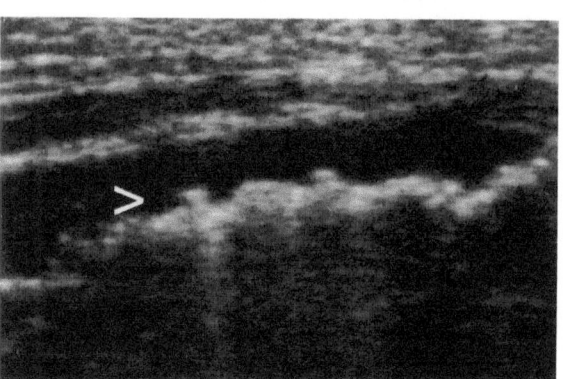

Fig. 18.4. Aphthoid ulcer (*arrowhead*)

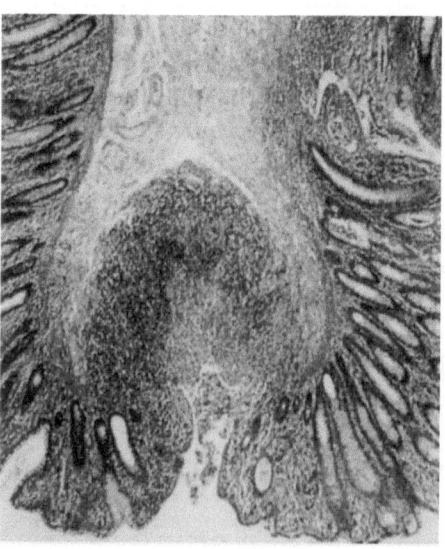

Fig. 18.5. Aphthoid ulcer, pathology

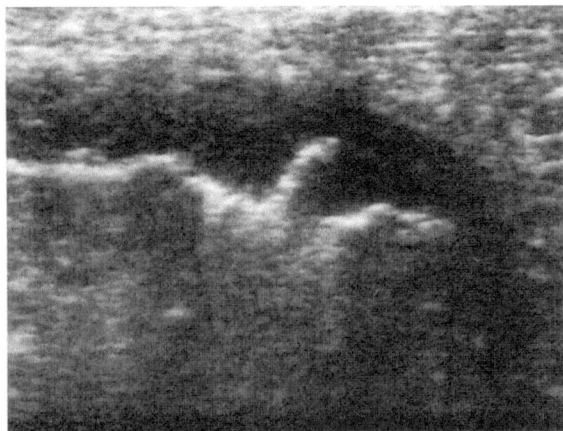

Fig. 18.6. Deep fissure ulcer, ultrasound

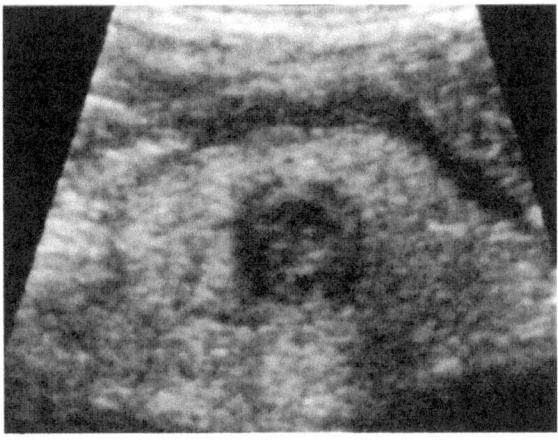

Fig. 18.8. Creeping fat; an echogenic halo surrounds bowel

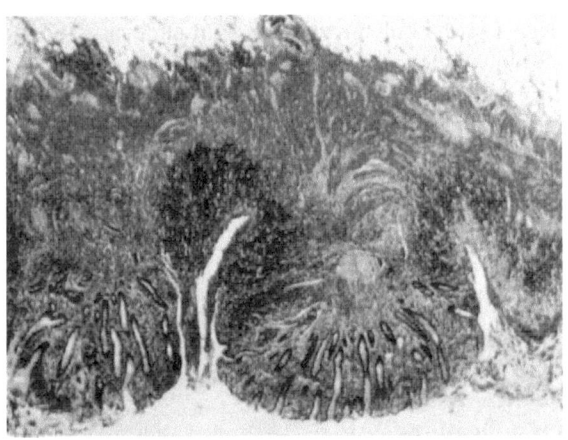

Fig. 18.7. Deep fissure ulcer, pathology

18.3.2
Complications

Perforation of deep fissure ulcers through the serosal surface can lead to abscess formation. Abscess recurrence or continuing drainage of abscess content after percutaneous drainage indicates continuing underlying inflammation and fistula formation, the latter being a characteristic feature of Crohn's disease. These abscesses and fistulae may be the presenting clinical feature of the disease. Various other types of fistulae may also be seen in Crohn's disease. These include entero-enteric (Fig. 18.9), or intra-mural which is characteristic in Crohn's, where there is longitudinal extension along the intra-mural portion of the bowel wall (Figs. 18.10 and 18.11). Stricture formation with resultant obstruction is more a feature of small bowel than large bowel Crohn's disease.

extends into the mesentery will cause thickening of the peri-enteric fat which spreads over the serosal surface of the colon - "creeping-fat". This is a non-specific feature of Crohn's disease which may also be seen in other inflammatory conditions of the large bowel. It frequently develops in diverticulitis and occasionally in pseudomembranous and ischemic colitis. It is seen as a halo of echo bright material surrounding the bowel (Fig. 18.8).

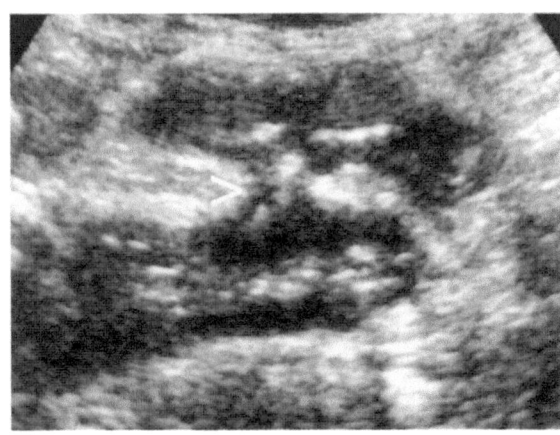

Fig. 18.9. Entero-enteric fistula (*arrowhead*) between two diseased small bowel loops

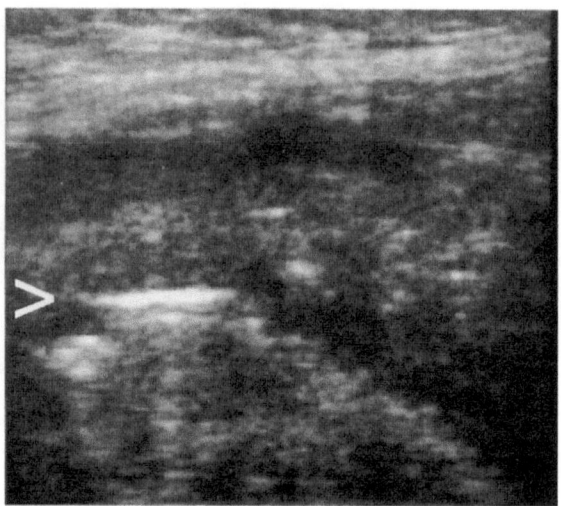

Fig. 18.10. Intra-mural fistula, gas line within bowel wall (*arrowhead*)

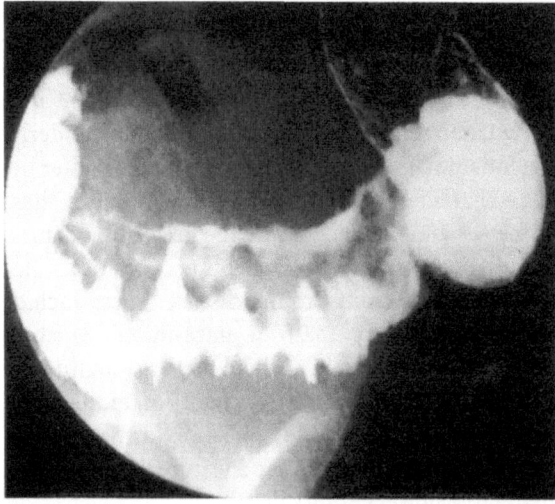

Fig. 18.11. Intra-mural fistula, same patient as in Fig. 18.10 showing barium tracking within the wall

18.4
Ulcerative Colitis

18.4.1
Description

Ulcerative colitis is a chronic granulomatous condition with a similar peak age of onset between 15 and 25 years. The similarities between Crohn's disease and ulcerative colitis in geographic distribution, racial and ethnic distribution, sex ratio, and age of onset support the idea that the two diseases are related (YAMADA et al. 1995). Histologically, the disease primarily affects

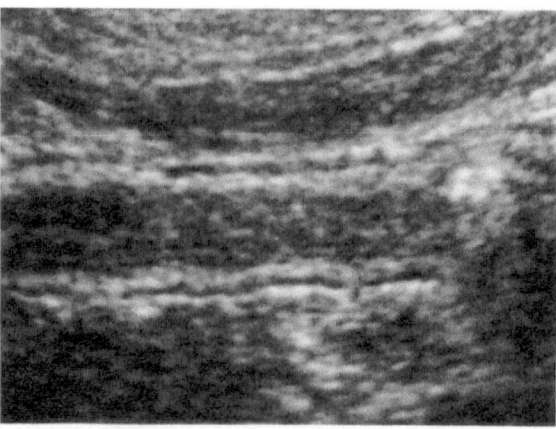

Fig. 18.12. Ulcerative colitis, inflammation in superficial layers

the rectum and sigmoid. The entire colon is affected in 40% of cases. Microscopically the inflammation is largely confined to the mucosa and sub-mucosa, with deeper layers only involved in fulminant cases. Sonographically the superficial layers of the bowel can be seen to be thickened with relatively normal deeper layers (Fig. 18.12). However, oedema may be present in deeper layers in severe acute inflammation. There is usually no increase in the pericolic fat. When only a portion of colon is involved a precise cut-off between normal and abnormal bowel can be seen (Figs. 18.13 and 18.14).

18.4.2
Complications

The most frequent acute complication of ulcerative colitis is toxic megacolon. This is a diagnosis most

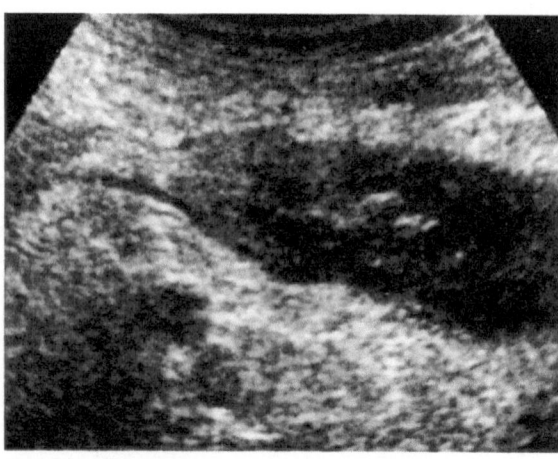

Fig. 18.13. Transition from abnormal to normal bowel in transverse colon

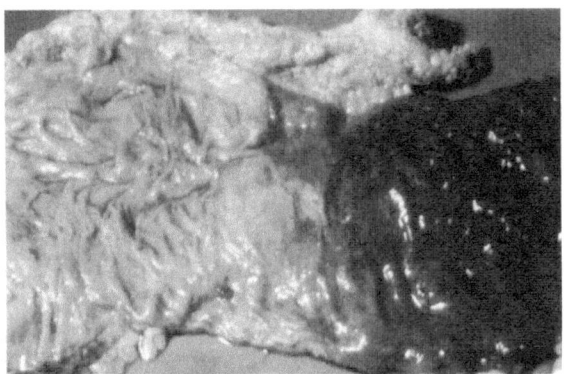

Fig. 18.14. Transition from abnormal to normal bowel, pathological specimen (different patient see fig 18.13)

frequently made on clinical evaluation and plain x-ray (LAMONT and KANDEL 1986). There is only one report of ultrasound detection of toxic megacolon, which found wall thinning, loss of haustration and colonic dilatation (ARIENTI et al. 1996). Carcinoma is a serious long-term complication of ulcerative colitis, the risk becoming appreciable 8–10 years after the onset of the disease. This may be discovered at ultrasound examination, particularly in those patients who have not been appropriately followed up by surveillance colonoscopy.

18.5
Accuracy

18.5.1
Sensitivity

Numerous studies have looked at the sensitivity of ultrasound in the initial diagnosis of inflammatory bowel disease, and for the detection of complications. A bowel wall thickness of 3 mm or more is considered to be pathological (GASCHE et al. 1999; SOLVIG et al. 1995). Sensitivities of 91%–96% have been shown for the diagnosis of bowel inflammation in Crohn's disease (SCHWERK et al. 1992; SONNENBERG et al. 1982). The same authors showed a slightly lower sensitivity for ulcerative colitis at 84%–86%.

Diagnosis of fistulas and abscesses can be made with an accuracy of 66%–90% (MACONI et al. 1996; REIMUND et al. 1999; PARENTE et al. 2002). Some of the variability arises from the different definitions of abscesses and fistulae. The higher levels of sensitivity are well replicated in other studies such as those by GASCHE et al. (1999), who also demonstrated a 100%

sensitivity for strictures in a series of patients in which there was surgical correlation.

18.5.2
Specificity

Most studies looking at inflammatory bowel disease have either looked to see if inflammation, extent and complications are detectable in a broad group of patients, or looked at disease processes in a series of patients with established diagnoses. Few studies have looked at the specificity of ultrasound in differentiating the major types of inflammatory bowel disease, including infectious colitis, but LIM et al. (1994) and VALETTE et al. (2001) found that the overlap of signs was significant. The latter made a diagnosis of Crohn's disease and ulcerative colitis with a specificity of 87% and 35%, respectively, on a retrospective analysis of taped examinations. They concluded that there can be confusion between infectious and ulcerative colitis which can appear similar in the early stage of the disease. In particular, tuberculous colitis may be confused with Crohn's disease clinically, endoscopically, radiologically and even histologically (ARNOLD et al. 1998; BOUDIAF et al.1998).

18.5.3
Activity of Disease

Numerous studies have looked at the correlation between various imaging parameters and clinical or laboratory activity of inflammatory bowel disease, although there are contradictory results between the various studies. Assessment of wall thickness or measurement of the Doppler flow indices of the mesenteric arteries and portal vein have given inconsistent results in relation to clinical progress, endoscopic activity, or serological measurements such as C-reactive protein (RUESS et al. 2000; MAYER et al. 2000; LUDWIG et al. 1999; MACONI et al. 1998). One value that has been found to be useful in Crohn's ileitis is measurement of the superior mesenteric artery blood flow volume (VAN OOSTAYEN et al. 1998; BYRNE et al. 2001). To date there have been only three publications looking at the inferior mesenteric artery in colitis, but the results have all been positive (MIRK et al. 1999; LUDWIG et al. 1999; SIGIRCI et al. 2001). These authors looked at patients with ulcerative, Crohn's, and infectious colitis. All the studies showed that flow velocity, flow volume and/or the pulsatility index were positively correlated with other imaging or clinical measurements.

Vessel density on colour Doppler has also been looked at as a parameter for assessing disease activity (Spalinger et al. 2000). Qualitative differences have been shown, along with bowel wall thickness, to reflect disease activity, but it is unclear whether this could provide useful quantitative and clinical information.

18.6
Infectious Colitis

The appearances of inflammatory bowel disease often overlap with those of infectious colitis. Diagnosis is most frequently confirmed by stool culture. Tuberculosis, however, can frequently be suggested when there are associated findings such as ascites, lymphadenopathy, or peritoneal thickening (Kedar et al. 1994; Jain et al. 1995; Sheikh et al. 1999). Percutaneous fine needle aspiration of gastrointestinal tract lesions has been shown to be an effective method of diagnosing bowel pathology including tuberculosis, even when patients have had negative colonoscopic biopsies (Das and Pant 1994; Suri et al. 1998; Javid et al. 1999).

18.7
Pseudomembranous Colitis

Pseudomembranous colitis (PMC) is an antibiotic-associated colitis caused by clostridium difficile. This organism is so-named because it was considered "difficult" to grow and isolate by its discoverers. Diarrhoea and cramp-like abdominal pain often start within the first week of antibiotic therapy. Raised yellow-white plaques may be seen at endoscopy, these pseudomembranes can become confluent and cover the entire mucosa. In fulminant PMC there is transmural extension of the disease which can result in bowel perforation. Ultrasound can show a markedly oedematous mucosa and sub-mucosa, with complete effacement of the lumen in some cases (Fig. 18.15).

The diagnosis can be strongly suggested in the presence of these features in a patient with the appropriate history. However, as with the well-described CT "accordion" sign, imaging features alone are non-specific (Macari et al. 1999).

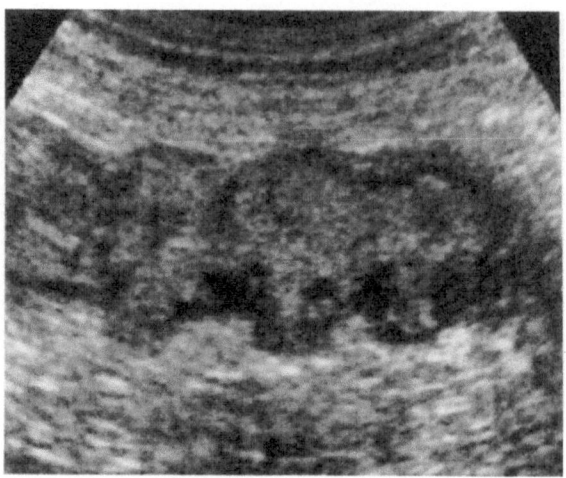

Fig. 18.15. Pseudomembranous colitis. Oedematous mucosa and submucosa effaces the lumen

18.8
Typhlitis (Neutropenic Enterocolitis)

Typhlitis (from the Greek "typhlos" meaning blind sac) is an acute necrotizing colitis involving the caecum (Yamada et al. 1995) and is a condition primarily seen in immunosuppressed patients with leukaemia. The pathogenesis is unknown. Ultrasound typically shows marked wall thickening, averaging 10 mm and centred on the caecum (Fig. 18.16).

It has been shown that in this disease the morbidity and mortality can be related to the bowel wall thickness (Cartoni et al. 2001).

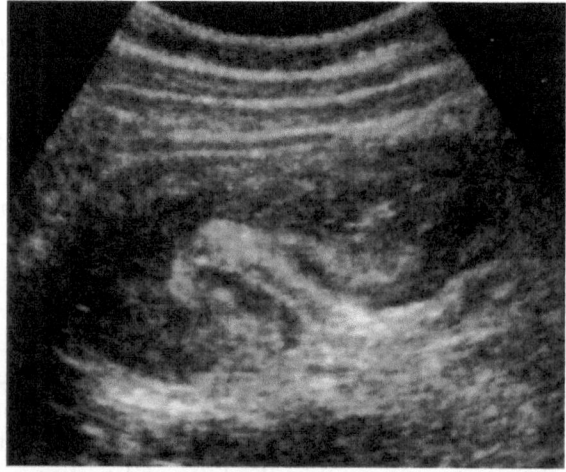

Fig. 18.16. Typhlitis in leukemic patient. Transverse scan shows the ileocecal valve protruding into a thick walled caecum

18.9
Ischaemic colitis

A number of studies have shown that ischemic colitis may be diagnosed and differentiated from inflammatory colitis using sonography (TEEFAY et al. 1996; SIEGEL et al. 1997). Absence of arterial flow in the wall of the ischemic colon suggests an unfavourable outcome and it has been proposed that this is more closely associated with outcome than the early clinical and laboratory findings (DANSE et al. 2000).

18.10
Other Techniques

18.10.1
Hydrocolonic Sonography

Instillation of water to carry out hydrocolonic sonography was a technique first described in 1992 for the diagnosis of colonic tumours (LIMBERG 1992). It is a technique that has not been widely adopted, despite having good sensitivity for the detection and diagnosis of inflammatory bowel disease. Sensitivities of between 91% and 100% have been obtained for the detection of active disease with an accuracy of 87% for estimating disease extent (LIMBERG and OSWALD 1994; BRU et al. 2001).

18.10.2
Endoluminal Rectal Ultrasound

Endorectal ultrasound will provide high resolution imaging of bowel wall layers. In a small pilot study, increased thickness of the first to third layers of the rectal wall was demonstrated to be associated with an increased relapse rate in patients with known ulcerative colitis (HIGAKI et al. 2002). However, the clinical application of this technique has not been fully established.

References

Arienti V, Campieri M, Boriani L et al (1996) Management of severe ulcerative colitis with the help of high resolution ultrasonography. Am J Gastroenterol 87:2163–2169

Arnold C, Moradpour D, Blum HE (1998) Tuberculous colitis mimicking Crohn's disease. Am J Gastroenterol 93:2294–2296

Boudiaf M, Zidi SH, Soyer P (1998) Tuberculous colitis mim-

icking Crohn's disease: utility of computed tomography in the differentiation. Eur Radiol 8:1221–1223

Bru C, Sans M, Defelitto MM (2001) Hydrocolonic sonography for evaluating inflammatory bowel disease. Am J Roentgenol 177:99–105

Byrne MF, Farrell MA, Abass et al (2001) Assessment of Crohn's disease activity by Doppler sonography of the superior mesenteric artery, clinical evaluation and the Crohn's disease activity index: a prospective study. Clin Radiol 56:973–978

Cartoni C, Dragoni F, Micozzi A et al (2001) Neutropenic enterocolitis in patients with acute leukaemia: prognostic significance of bowel wall thickening detected by ultrasonography. J Clon Oncol 19:756–761

Danse EM, van Beers BE, Jamart J et al (2000) Prognosis of ischaemic colitis: comparison of colour doppler sonography with early clinical and laboratory findings. Am J Roentgenol 175:1151–1154

Das DK, Pant CS (1994) Fine needle aspiration cytologic diagnosis of gastrointestinal tract lesions. A study of 78 cases. Acta Cytol 38:723–729

Gasche C, Moser G, Turetschek K et al (1999) Transabdominal sonography for the detection of intestinal complications of Crohn's disease. Gut 44:112–117

Higaki S, Nohara H, Saitoh Y et al (2002) Increased rectal wall thickness may predict relapse in ulcerative colitis: a pilot follow-up study by ultrasonographic colonoscopy. Endoscopy 34:212–219

Jain R, Sawhney S, Bhargava DK et al (1995) Diagnosis of abdominal tuberculosis: sonographic findings in patients with early disease. Am J Roentgenol 165:1391–1395

Javid G, Gulzar GM, Khan B et al (1999) Percutaneous sonography-guided fine needle aspiration biopsy of colonoscopic biopsy-negative colonic lesions. Indian J Gastroenterol 18: 146–148

Kedar RP, Shah PP, Shivde RS et al (1994) sonographic findings in gastrointestinal and peritoneal tuberculosis. Clin Radiol 49:24–29

Kirsner JB (2000) Inflammatory bowel disease, 5th edn. Saunders, Philadelphia

Lamont JT, Kandel GP (1986) Toxic megacolon in ulcerative colitis. Early diagnosis and management. Hosp Pracr (off Ed) 21:102A–102M passim

Lim JH, Ko YT, Lee DH et al (1994) Sonography of inflammatory bowel disease: findings and value in differential diagnosis. AJR 163:343–347

Limberg B (1992) Diagnosis and staging of colonic tumours by conventional abdominal sonography as compared with hydrocolonic sonography. N Engl J Med 327:65–69

Limberg B, Osswald B (1994) Diagnosis and differential diagnosis of ulcerative colitis and Crohn's disease by hydrocolonic sonography. Am J Gastroenterol 89:1051–1057

Ludwig D, Wiener S, Bruning A et al (1999) Mesenteric blood flow is related to disease activity and risk of relapse in ulcerative colitis: a prospective follow-up study. Gut 45:546–552

Macari M, Balthazar EJ, Megibow AJ (1999) The accordion sign at CT: a non-specific finding in patients with colonic edema. Radiology 211:743–746

Maconi G, Bollani S, Bianchi Porro G (1996) Ultrasonographic detection of intestinal complications in Crohn's disease. Dig Dis Sci 41:1643–1648

Maconi G, Parente F, Bollani S et al (1998) Factors affecting splanchnic haemodynamics in Crohn's disease: a prospective controlled study using Doppler ultrasound. Gut 43: 645–650

Mayer D, Reinshagen M, Mason RA et al (2000) Sonographic assessment of thickened bowel wall segments as a quantitative parameter for activity in inflammatory bowel disease. Z Gastroenterol 38:295–300

MacSween RNM, Whaley K (1992) Muir's textbook of pathology, 13th edn. Arnold, London

Mirk P, Palazzoni G, Gimondo P (1999) Doppler sonography of hemodynamic changes of the inferior mesenteric artery in inflammatory bowel disease: preliminary data. Am J Roentgenol 173:381–387

Parente F, Maconi G, Bollani S et al (2002) Bowel ultrasound in assessment of Crohn's disease and detection of related small bowel strictures: a prospective comparative study versus x-ray and intraoperative. Gut 50:490–495

Reimund JM, Jung Chaigneau E, Chamouard P et al (1999) Diagnostic value of high resolution sonography in Crohn's disease and ulcerative colitis. Gastroenterol Clin Biol 23:740–746

Ruess L, Blask AR, Bulas DI et al (2000) Inflammatory bowel disease in children and young adults: correlation of sonographic and clinical parameters during treatment. AJR 175:79–84

Schwerk WB, Beckh K, Raith M (1992) A prospective evaluation of high sonography in the diagnosis of inflammatory bowel diseases. Eur J Gastrenterol 4:173–1182

Sheikh M, Moosa I, Hussein FM et al (1999) Ultrasonographic diagnosis in abdominal tuberculosis. Austr Radiol 43: 175–179

Siegel MJ, Friedland JA, Hildebolt CF (1997) Bowel wall thickening in children: differentiation with ultrasound. Radiology 203:631–635

Sigirci A, Baysal T, Kutlu R et al (2001) Doppler sonography of the inferior and superior mesenteric arteries in ulcerative colitis. J Clin Ultrasound 29:130–139

Solvig J, Ekberg O, Lindgren S et al (1995) Ultrasound evaluation of the small bowel: comparison with enteroclysis in patients with Crohn's disease. Abdom Imaging 20:323–326

Sonnenberg A, Erckenbrecht J, Peter P et al (1982) Detection of Crohn's disease by ultrasound. Gastroenterology 83: 430–434

Spalinger J, Patriquin H, Miron MC et al (2000) Doppler ultrasound in patients with Crohn disease: vessel density in the diseased bowel reflects disease activity. Radiology 217:787–791

Suri R, Gupta S, Gupta SK et al (1998) Ultrasound guided fine needle aspiration cytology in abdominal tuberculosis. Br J Radiol 71:723–727

Teefay SA, Roarke MC, Brink JA (1996) Bowel wall thickeneing: differentiation of inflammation from ischaemia with colour Doppler and duplex ultrasound. Radiology 198:547–551

Valette P-J, Rioux M, Pilleul F et al (2001) Ultrasonography of chronic inflammatory bowel disease. Eur Radiol 11: 1859–1866

Van Oostayen JA, Wasser MN, Griffoen G et al (1998) Activity of Crohn's disease assessed by measurement of superior mesenteric artery flow with Doppler ultrasound. Neth J Med 53:S3–S8

Yamada T, Alpers DH, Owyang C (1995) Textbook of gastroenterology, 2nd edn. Lippincott, Philadelphia

19 CT of Colitis

Ruedi F. Thoeni

CONTENTS

19.1   Introduction   185
19.2   Idiopathic Inflammatory Bowel Disease   185
19.2.1   Ulcerative Colitis   185
19.2.2   Crohn's Colitis   187
19.3   Infectious Colitis   188
19.3.1   Bacterial Colitis   188
19.3.1.1 Campylobacteriosis   188
19.3.1.2 Escherichia coli colitis   188
19.3.1.3 Salmonellosis   189
19.3.1.4 Shigellosis   189
19.3.1.5 Yersinia colitis   189
19.3.1.6 Tuberculosis   189
19.3.2   Viral Colitis   190
19.3.2.1 Cytomegalovirus (CMV) Colitis   190
19.3.3   Parasitic Colitis   190
19.3.3.1 Cryptosporidiosis   190
19.3.3.2 Amebiasis   191
19.3.4   Fungal Colitis   191
19.4   Noninfectious Colitis   191
19.4.1   Typhlitis   192
19.4.2   Eosinophilic Colitis   192
19.4.3   Graft-Versus-Host Disease   193
19.4.4   Ischemic Colitis   193
19.5   Exogenous Causes of Colitis   194
19.5.1   Pseudomembranous Colitis   194
19.5.2   Drug-Induced Colitis   194
19.5.3   Caustic Colitis   195
19.6   Epiploic Appendagitis   195
19.7   Differential Diagnosis and Summary   196
         References   197

19.1
Introduction

Patients with appendicitis, diverticulitis, inflammatory and infectious colitis frequently present with abdominal pain. Computed tomography (CT) of appendicitis and diverticulitis are discussed in Chaps. 15 and 16, respectively. In many of these patients, the nature of the abdominal pain is nonspecific and CT is usually the initial radiologic test ordered for their evaluation. For the radiologist, one of the most commonly encountered causes for colonic inflammation is idiopathic inflammatory bowel disease. However, many other inflammatory conditions exist and occur with variable frequency. Some, such as pseudomembranous colitis, ischemic colitis or AIDS-related colitis are seen commonly in a busy clinical practice, but others are infrequently encountered or only rarely need imaging for their diagnosis. CT can assess the colonic wall and its changes as well as those of the surrounding fat, mesentery and peritoneum thus providing important clues to help make a specific diagnosis. It also can detect complications and assist in patient management. With multidetector CT, scan times are very short, slices as thin as 1–1.25 mm can be obtained and contrast boluses optimized. This leads to improved visualization of the inflammatory changes. Therefore today, CT has a pivotal role in the diagnostic work up and follow-up of patients with colitis.

The colon responds to injury in a limited number of ways. Nevertheless, the morphologic appearance, the severity, the distribution and progression of the inflammatory changes often can be used to make a specific diagnosis. Pericolonic changes and involvement of bowel other than the colon are also important features that need to be considered. The presence or absence of rectal involvement, asymmetrical involvement and diffuse versus focal disease are important characteristics when differentiating between ulcerative colitis and Crohn's disease and the various diseases that can mimic them. This chapter describes the CT signs of various colitides and provides up-to-date guidelines to help distinguish between them.

19.2
Idiopathic Inflammatory Bowel Disease

19.2.1
Ulcerative Colitis

Ulcerative colitis is characterized by changes in the mucosa and submucosa that include ulceration and

R. F. Thoeni, MD
Professor of Radiology, University of California, San Francisco, Box 0628, San Francisco, CA 94143, USA

extensive inflammation of the mucosa associated with edema or fatty infiltration of the submucosa. The disease begins in the rectum and extends proximally in a continuous fashion. In contrast to Crohn's disease, the involvement of the mucosa is symmetrical, circumferential, diffuse and contiguous. Early inflammatory changes may not be visible on CT but once the disease progresses, submucosal edema or in later phases fat appears which leads to stratification of the wall (the target sign). With progression of the disease, the inner colonic wall becomes denuded of mucosa and inflammatory pseudopolyps may be visualized as polypoid protrusions into the lumen. Subacute and chronic disease are characterized by marked thickening of the colonic wall and narrowing of the colonic lumen (MACARI and BALTHAZAR 2001).

In chronic ulcerative colitis, the muscularis propria becomes hypertrophied (MARCARI and BALTHAZAR 2001). Strong contraction of this layer results in diffuse or segmental narrowing of the lumen and also causes foreshortening of the colon. The submucosa becomes thickened from edema in the acute and subacute phases and from deposition of fat in the chronic phase; all contributing to the luminal narrowing. On CT, these changes give the wall a target or halo appearance as several concentric rings can be seen: the inner soft tissue ring represents the mucosa and thickened muscularis mucosa; the middle low-density ring represents the edematous submucosa with or without fatty infiltration and the outer soft tissue ring is formed by the muscularis propria (Fig. 19.1).The target sign is not specific for ulcerative colitis as it can also be seen in Crohn's disease, ischemia, some of the infectious colitides and graft-versus-host disease. However, when seen it is highly suggestive of ulcerative colitis and in one study, was seen in 61% of patients with chronic ulcerative colitis but in only 8% of chronic granulomatous disease (PHILPOTTS et al. 1994).

Other CT features of ulcerative colitis are symmetry and contiguous disease, moderate wall thickening and sparing of the small bowel except for backwash terminal ileitis. This form of ileitis leaves the terminal ileum dilated with a gaping ileocecal valve and at times a shaggy thin wall; narrowing of the ileal lumen is not a feature of ulcerative colitis. The outer margin of the colon is smooth in 95% of patients with ulcerative colitis, as it is not a transmural disease. In contrast, patients with Crohn's disease have an irregular outer colonic margin in 80% as the disease is usually transmural in extent (DURAN et al. 1997). Rectal narrowing, thickening of the wall and increased presacral space are typical for chronic ulcerative colitis and are well depicted by CT. These features result

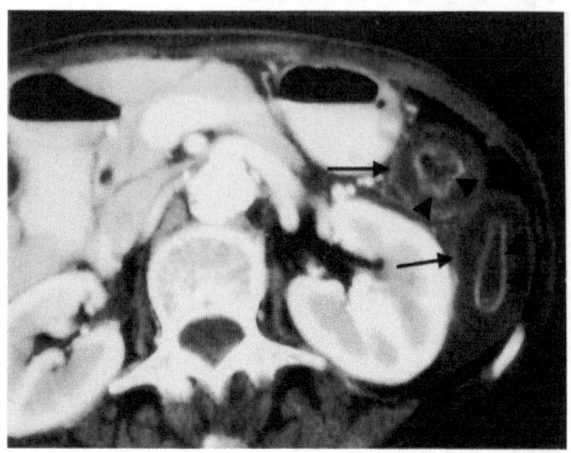

Fig. 19.1. Patient with acute ulcerative colitis. The left colon is markedly thickened creating the target sign. The inner most enhanced ring (*arrowheads*) consists of inflamed mucosa and the outer enhanced ring (*arrows*) represents the muscularis propria and serosa. The low-attenuation area between the two enhanced rings represents the edematous submucosa

from the mural thickening and proliferation of the perirectal fat. This fat has a slightly increased attenuation (10–20 HU) compared to normal mesenteric fat (–55 to –75) and is traversed by nodular and streaky soft tissue densities. This results from lipodystrophy with an influx of inflammatory cells and edema and often enlarged lymph nodes.

One of the most feared complications is toxic megacolon (TMC). CT typically demonstrates marked colonic dilatation with intraluminal air and/or fluid and a distorted luminal colonic contour or an ahaustral pattern. Often the colonic wall appears thinned with an ill-defined and nodular inner margin and some ascites may be present. Toxic megacolon also may occur in Crohn's disease and in some of the infectious and non-infectious types of colitis (Table 19.1). In severe ulcerative colitis, persistent colonic distension predicts a subgroup of patients who will demonstrate a poor response to medical therapy and who are at higher risk for TMC and are in need for surgery (LATELLA et al. 2002). Even though CT can readily detect all these abnormalities, it cannot be used to predict the clinical outcome unless complications are

Table 19.1. Disease in which toxic megacolon may occur

Ulcerative colitis
Crohn's disease
Amebiasis
Pseudomembranous colitis
Campylobacteriosis
Ischemic colitis
Salmonellosis

evident such as perforation, pneumatosis or septic thrombosis (IMBRIACO and BALTHAZAR 2001).

19.2.2
Crohn's Colitis

The acute phase of Crohn's disease is characterized by focal inflammation with superficial aphthoid ulcers. This progresses to a cobblestone pattern produced by intersecting deep transverse and longitudinal ulcerations and transmural inflammation with lymphoid aggregates and granuloma formation. Subsequently, fistula and sinus tracts may develop. With further progression of disease, fibrosis and strictures ensue. Crohn's disease most commonly involves the right side of the colon and often there is associated terminal ileum involvement.

Barium studies and colonoscopy are better than CT for demonstrating superficial changes in the mucosa. CT usually misses the early and superficial mucosal inflammatory changes of Crohn's disease. However, full thickness transmural changes are well shown by CT with wall thickening usually measuring between 1–2 cm (PHILPIOTTS et al. 1994). Such thickening is most frequently found in the terminal ileum but may be present throughout the gastrointestinal tract (RAPTOPOULOS et al. 1997). In the acute phase and in the absence of cicatrizing changes, the small bowel and colon demonstrate a target or double-halo sign. As with ulcerative colitis, the inner most ring represents mucosal enhancement. The low-density intermediate ring has an attenuation near to that of water or fat corresponding to submucosal edema or fat infiltration. The outer ring is of higher density and represents the muscularis propria. Both mucosa and serosa may demonstrate increased enhancement after an intravenous bolus of contrast material. The degree of enhancement correlates with the severity of the disease. Diffuse colonic edema can thicken haustral folds to produce the "accordion" sign. However, this is not specific for Crohn's colitis and was originally described in Clostridium difficile colitis (MOUTANOS and MANOLAKAKIS 2001). In one small series of five patients, virtual colonoscopy was able to successfully depict both intraluminal and transmural disease (TARJAN et al. 2000).

When CT clearly visualizes mural stratification, transmural fibrosis has not yet occurred and medical therapy may improve luminal narrowing and decrease wall thickness. Once transmural fibrosis has developed, mural stratification is no longer seen and the changes are irreversible (Fig. 19.2). In such cases,

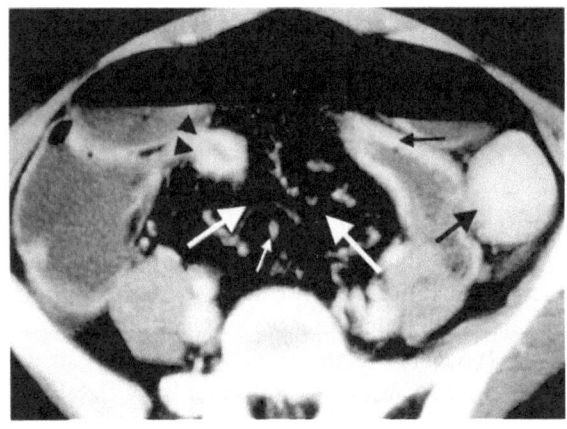

Fig. 19.2. Patient with Crohn's disease of the terminal ileum and skip area in colon. The terminal ileum near the ileocecal valve (*arrowheads*) is markedly thickened and no mural stratification can be seen indicative of an irreversible stricture. The ileum proximal to the stenosed area is thick-walled and dilated (*small black arrow*). Fibrofatty proliferation (*large white arrows*) and adenopathy (*white small arrow*) is present in the mesentery. Mild wall thickening also is present in the left colon (*large black arrow*)

surgical intervention is needed to relieve obstructive symptoms (RAPTOPOULOS et al. 1997). CT can demonstrate loss of stratification reliably when a good intravenous bolus of contrast material is used and thin sections are obtained with a multidetector CT.

Additional benefits of CT are that axial imaging helps separate bowel loops, as this can be difficult by small bowel examination and CT has the ability to readily demonstrate phlegmon, abscess, fibrofatty proliferation of the mesentery, enlarged nodes and bowel wall thickening. CT is also particularly well suited to the assessment of the extraluminal manifestations of inflammatory bowel disease; the accurate identification of complications is important as they influence treatment and prognosis (FISHMAN et al. 1987; GOSSIOS and TSIANOS 1997).

"Creeping fat" or fibrofatty proliferation is an attempt by the body to contain the inflammatory process and results in separation of bowel loops. CT demonstrates an increase in fat in the mesentery that is of a higher density (20–60 HU) than subcutaneous fat because of edema and an inflammatory cell infiltrate (GORE et al. 1996). The sharp interface between the bowel wall and the mesentery is lost and usually mesenteric lymph nodes measuring <1 cm (range 3–8 mm) are present. Because the risk of carcinoma and lymphoma is increased in patients with Crohn's disease, lymph nodes measuring over 1 cm should be viewed with suspicion and malignancy needs to be excluded.

Mesenteric vessels appear engorged, dilated, widely spaced and at times tortuous as a result of hyperemia from the inflammatory process. The appearance of the mesenteric vessels in Crohn's disease has been described as the "comb sign", but this sign is not specific for active Crohn's disease and can be seen in any moderate to severe acute inflammatory condition of the small or large bowel. The presence of the comb sign may be used to differentiate active inflammatory bowel disease from lymphoma or metastatic carcinoma, which tend to be hypovascular (Low et al. 2000).

In Crohn's disease, a phlegmon may develop in the mesentery or omentum and is another common cause of separation of bowel loops. This is an ill-defined inflammatory mass that either resolves completely with antibiotic treatment or progresses to an abscess. When a phlegmon is present, CT shows a soft tissue mass with surrounding "streaky" densities extending into the mesentery or omentum and the definition of surrounding organs is lost.

Abscesses are most frequently associated with small bowel disease or ileocolitis and occur in 15%–20% of patients with Crohn's disease (HERLINGER et al. 1998; RIBEIRO et al. 1991). An abscess may extend into adjacent tissues or perforate and drain spontaneously into other bowel loops or organs. Abscesses usually are a result of a sinus tract, fistula, perforation or surgical intervention in Crohn's disease. At times, an abscess can be difficult to diagnose clinically as it may be masked by steroid therapy or misdiagnosed as an exacerbation of the underlying inflammatory bowel disease. CT demonstrates the exact location and extent of an abscess and in the pelvis can determine whether a perianal abscess extends to or through the levator ani muscles (FUNAYAMA et al. 1997; DENTON et al. 1996). While barium studies can show indirect signs of an abscess based on mass effect, spiculation or demonstration of a fistula tract, unlike CT they cannot demonstrate the extent of the disease. CT permits appropriate planning of therapy including the percutaneous drainage of collections (CASOLA et al. 1987).

Behçet's syndrome is characterized by a nonspecific vasculitis involving multiple organs with vaginal and oral ulceration. In 10%–50% the terminal ileum and cecum are involved and the inflammatory features are similar to those of Crohn's disease. Behçet's syndrome has a high rate of gastrointestinal complications such as perforation, fistula formation, hemorrhage and peritonitis. CT can demonstrate the extent of disease and its complications (CHUNG et al. 2001).

19.3
Infectious Colitis

Infectious colitis may be caused by bacterial, viral, fungal or parasitic organisms. While in Western countries bacterial colitis is most commonly encountered, in underdeveloped countries, parasitic infections are more common. In patients with bacterial colitis, imaging usually is not performed once the patient presents with dysenteric symptoms as the diagnosis is readily established with stool culture. These types of colitis are usually self-limited.

19.3.1
Bacterial Colitis

Patients with bacterial colitis present with an acute onset of dysenteric symptoms consisting of fever, cramp-like abdominal pain and tenderness, nausea and vomiting and diarrhea of small volume that may be bloody. Specialized cultures are often needed to isolate specific organisms. In most instances, only anecdotal imaging reports on bacterial colitis are available.

19.3.1.1
Campylobacteriosis

Campylobacteriosis is caused by *Campylobacter fetus*, subspecies jejuni, and is the commonest cause for bacterial colitis. The disease usually is self-limiting, lasting less than seven days, but if not treated with antibiotics, the infection may recur in 25% of cases. While both small and large bowel may be involved, colitis is more common. On CT, the disease can mimic ulcerative colitis or Crohn's disease (LAMBERT et al. 1979; BRODEY et al. 1982; KOLLITZ et al. 1981; BROWN et al. 2000). Hemorrhage, perforation and toxic megacolon have all been reported as complications. The diagnosis is made with serologic studies or stool culture.

19.3.1.2
Escherichia coli colitis

Colitis caused by the various strains of *Escherichia coli* is a common cause of traveler's diarrhea. It often is self-limited. A subtype (O157:H7) is noteworthy as it is often encountered in nursing home patients who develop watery diarrhea that may progress to a hemorrhagic colitis. The toxin produced by the infection may in some cases cause hemolytic-uremic syndrome. The infection is associated with a high morbidity and mortality. On CT, a thickened colonic wall of low-density from submucosal edema is identified. The transverse colon is predominantly involved but contiguous extension to the ascending and descending colon may occur and so the disease may resemble pseudomembranous or ischemic colitis (SHORTSLEEVE et al. 1989; MILLER et al. 2001). Patients should be isolated and treatment is supportive with fluid replacement.

19.3.1.3
Salmonellosis

Salmonella are gram-negative rods that are ingested with contaminated food or water. Salmonellosis may present as acute dysentery or typhoid fever (RUTGEERTS et al. 1982; TEDESCO et al. 1983; GRIFFITHS 1993). Salmonella typhi and paratyphi cause typhoid fever. The organisms are usually found in the spleen, mesenteric lymph nodes and Peyer's patches of the terminal ileum. When the colon is involved, the cecal wall is thickened and the lumen narrowed and there is associated wall thickening and ulceration of the terminal ileum. Colonic inflammatory change may extend beyond the cecum.

A wide variety of Salmonella serotypes, of which Salmonella enteritis is the commonest, cause food poisoning with sudden onset of diarrhea, fever and abdominal pain. Often there are outbreaks, particularly in the summer season when food tends to spoil. CT may show changes that mimic those of ulcerative colitis, although in most instances, imaging is unnecessary (FARMAN et al. 1973; SAFFOURI et al. 1979; BALTHAZAR et al. 1996).

19.3.1.4
Shigellosis

Shigellosis is an infection with a gram-negative rod. In the USA, *Shigella sonnei* is the most common organism whereas in Asia and Mexico, *Shigella dysenteriae* is more frequent. Carriers of the disease are common and infection is from contamination of food or the water supply. Symptoms are similar to those seen with salmonella infections and infections may also occur in outbreaks. Shigellosis produces a toxin that causes increased bowel secretion and watery diarrhea. Systemic absorption of the toxin can lead to secondary symptoms including seizures, peripheral neuropathy, arthritis, and hemolytic-uremic syndrome. On CT, shigellosis has similar features to ulcerative colitis. Inflammatory changes in the colon

are initially diffuse and continuous and there may be terminal ileum involvement (BALTHAZAR et al. 1996). Ulceration predominates in the rectosigmoid and occasionally inflammatory polyps develop (FARMAN et al. 1973; ZALEV and WARREN 1989). The diagnosis is made by stool culture. The disease is self-limiting, lasting 7–10 days, but inflammation persisting for up to 1 month has been encountered. In patients who are immunosuppressed the disease may prove fatal.

19.3.1.5
Yersinia colitis

Yersinia enterocolitica is a gram-negative bacillus that produces acute diarrhea and pain that can last for up to 6 weeks. This gastrointestinal infection is most common in Japan, Scandinavia and Canada (RUTGEERTS et al. 1982; GRIFFITHS 1993). It generally affects infants and children up to the age of 5 who often present with right lower quadrant pain that mimics appendicitis. The terminal ileum and right colon are most commonly involved but occasionally the left colon is also inflamed (LACHMAN et al. 1977; ATKINSON et al. 1983; MATSUMOTO et al. 1990). On CT, ileocolitis due to Yersinia closely resembles mild Crohn's disease with marked ileocecal edema and mesenteric adenopathy but without stenosis (LACHMAN et al. 1977; TUOHY et al. 1999). Hepatic abscess and septicemia may complicate. Diagnosis is by serological testing or stool culture. Resolution of the inflammatory changes may take several months.

19.3.1.6
Tuberculosis

Tuberculosis of the gastrointestinal tract has been seen with increasing frequency in Western countries and patients with AIDS are particularly at risk (BALTHAZAR et al. 1990). Most cases in the United States are secondary to pulmonary infection but in areas of Asia where tuberculosis is endemic, ingestion of the bovine bacillus is often the cause. Patients usually present with fever, pain, weight loss and diarrhea but diarrhea is not as prominent a feature as in bacillary dysentery. Tuberculosis in the gastrointestinal tract mimics most of the features seen in Crohn's disease (CHATZICOSTAS et al. 2002; AKHAN and PRINGOT 2002; ANDRONIKOU et al. 2002). Thickening of the wall of the colon and terminal ileum may be more prominent than in Crohn's disease (Fig. 19.3). On CT, lymph nodes are markedly enlarged and often of low density or calcified. Fistula and sinus tracts can be seen but are less common than in Crohn's disease.

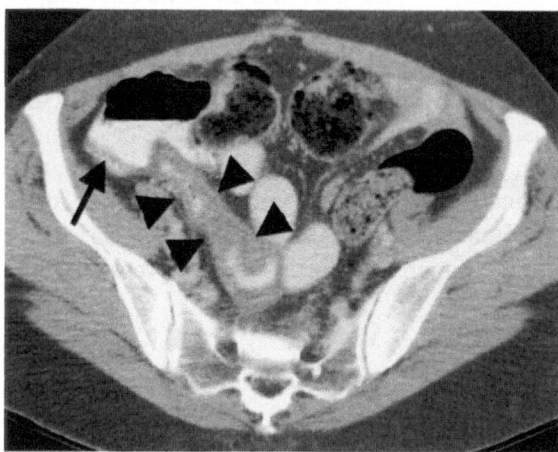

Fig. 19.3. Patient with tuberculosis of the terminal ileum. The terminal ileum is markedly thickened (*arrowheads*) and there is minimal thickening of the cecal wall (*arrow*). This appearance is indistinguishable from Crohn's disease

Diffuse colitis, segmental colitis and short strictures that mimic carcinoma may also be seen (THOENI and MARGULIS 1979; McDONALD and MIDDLETON 1976). In developing countries, if CT shows peritoneal thickening, ascites, abdominal lymphadenopathy and thickened intestinal walls, a diagnosis of abdominal tuberculosis should be considered (YILMAZ et al. 2002). Endoscopic and sometimes laparoscopic specimens are needed for a definitive diagnosis, which is based on caseating granulomas or positive cultures for the acid-fast bacillus. Correct identification of gastrointestinal tuberculosis is important as inadvertent administration of steroids, related to a mistaken diagnosis of idiopathic inflammatory bowel disease, can have disastrous consequences.

19.3.2
Viral Colitis

19.3.2.1
Cytomegalovirus (CMV) Colitis

Patients with CD4 counts of 200 mm³ or less are at risk for developing this infection. It is typically seen in severely immunosuppressed patients such as patients with AIDS. Positive cultures from the colon are diagnostic. In its typical presentation, the cecum and proximal ascending colon is involved but a diffuse colitis may develop and on occasions, extension to the terminal ileum is seen. CMV colitis produces marked thickening of the bowel wall with the target sign clearly visualized on cross-sections (BALTHAZAR et al. 1985;

KNOLLMAN et al. 1997), but these findings are not specific and can be seen in other types of infectious colitis (MONKEMULLER and WILCOX 1998). Often pericolonic inflammation and fluid is present and even some ascites and pneumatosis is described in this disease (WU et al. 1999). In very severe cases, increased attenuation within the bowel wall may be seen which represents hemorrhage and hemorrhagic colitis is often fatal in patients with AIDS (Fig. 19.4).

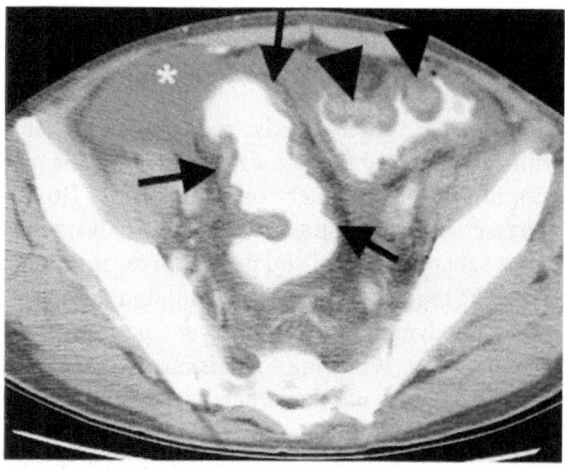

Fig. 19.4. Patient with AIDS and CMV colitis. The wall of the sigmoid colon is markedly thickened (*arrows*) and ascites (*asterisk*) is present. Hemorrhagic colitis is identified in the anterior sigmoid loop (*arrowheads*) as areas of increased density in the bowel wall

19.3.3
Parasitic Colitis

19.3.3.1
Cryptosporidiosis

Acute colitis due to cryptosporidium parvum is frequently encountered in patients with AIDS. While it causes a severe and lengthy illness in young children and immunocompromised adults, in patients with normal immune systems it either causes no symptoms or symptoms that resolve within 30 days. Patients present with diarrhea and cramping abdominal pain that is often localizing to the right side. The diarrhea is frequently profuse and watery.

Prior to 1976, this disease was considered a veterinary problem but the increase in HIV infection has brought with it an increase in cryptosporidiosis. Diagnosis is based on the identification of the parasite in fecal smears or intestinal biopsies. Infection is acquired by the fecal-oral route, close contact with an infected patient or from contamination of the water supply. As with CMV colitis, the disease usually involves the right colon but a pancolitis may develop and diffuse wall thickening with pericolonic inflammation is seen in the acute stage (Fig. 19.5) (Greyson-Fleg et al. 1986; Wall and Jones 1992).

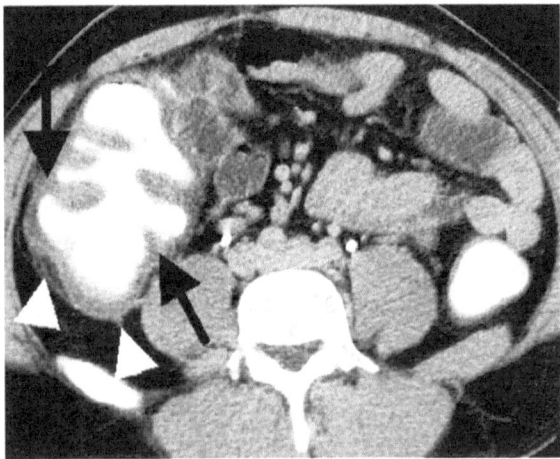

Fig. 19.5. Patient with AIDS and cryptosporidium colitis. Diffuse wall thickening of the right colon (*arrows*) with pericolonic inflammation (*arrowheads*) is seen in the acute stage. The findings are similar to those that can be observed in a patient with CMV colitis

19.3.3.2
Amebiasis

Amebiasis of the colon is rare in the United States. It is found most commonly in developing countries that have poor sanitary conditions. A total of 480 million people in the world carry amoeba in their colon, but only 50 million (about 10%) have symptoms. In the United States, it is usually found in immigrants or people who have traveled to developing countries. Infection results from ingesting the cysts of entamoeba histolytica as a result of poor hygiene from contaminated food or drinking water. The cyst wall is digested in the small bowel to release trophozoites that burrow into the wall of the colon.

The diagnosis of amebiasis is usually established by demonstrating the trophozoites in feces or rectal smear. Serologic studies may also be useful with *E. histolytica* antibodies appearing about 7 days after the onset of symptoms. Patients may be asymptomatic carriers, have mild symptoms or develop a fulminant colitis. Amoeba may enter the blood stream to produce abscesses in the liver, lungs or brain. Radiographically, amebiasis presents as an acute colitis that mimics ulcerative colitis. Skip areas may be seen with intervening colon usually involved to a lesser degree (Wagner-Manslau

et al. 1985; Matsui et al. 1989; Gulek and Onel 1999). Fulminant colitis may progress to toxic megacolon and perforation. In 10% of cases, amebomas develop, consisting of focal areas of pronounced granulation tissue formation (Cevallos and Farthing 1993). They are most common in the right colon. Diffuse colitis can occur, but the right colon and rectum tend to be most severely affected. With disease progression the cecum may become cone shaped. Even after treatment residual deformity or stricturing may remain. The terminal ileum is usually spared although occasionally the last few cm. may be involved. Focal involvement of the appendix is rare but may cause a patient to present with acute appendicitis.

19.3.4
Fungal Colitis

Colitis caused by a fungal infection can be seen with histoplasmosis, mucormycosis and candidiasis (Kirk et al. 1971). Histoplasmosis affects the lungs and skin but if the disease disseminates, multiple sites including the gastrointestinal tract may be involved. It occurs in patients who are immunosuppressed or severely debilitated (Fredericks et al. 1997). Patients with gastrointestinal histoplasmosis have fever, abdominal pain and diarrhea, but may present with hemorrhage, perforation or obstruction. The diagnosis is made by identifying or culturing histoplasma capsulatum from mucosal biopsy.

The ileocecal region is most commonly involved although in some cases the colitis is diffuse. There is associated mesenteric adenopathy, hepatosplenomegaly and an abnormal chest x-ray (Fig. 19.6). Polyps, structures and fistula may develop. CT demonstrates the wall thickening, mesenteric adenopathy and hepatosplenomegaly (Suh et al. 2001).

Mucormycosis occurs in immunosuppressed patients and is often fatal. Generally, the right colon is involved and CT shows focal thickening of the colonic wall and sometimes sinus tracts (Agha et al. 1985; Mariano et al. 1996). The lungs, sinuses and central nervous system usually are also affected.

19.4
Noninfectious Colitis

Among the noninfectious types of colitis, typhlitis, eosinophilic colitis and graft-versus-host-disease are important. Ischemic colitis has many features

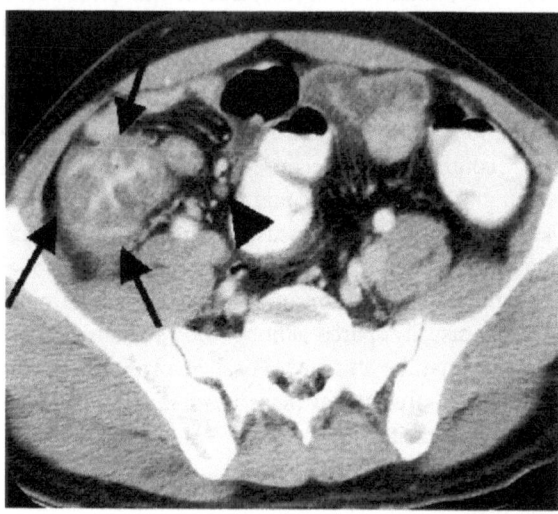

Fig. 19.6. Patient with histoplasmosis colitis. The ileocecal region is thick-walled (*arrows*) and the inflammatory changes in the colon and ileum are associated with mesenteric adenopathy (*arrowhead*). On sections through the upper abdomen (not shown), hepatosplenomegaly was also identified

that are shared with idiopathic or infectious colitis and so is included in this chapter but other entities such as collagenous or microscopic colitis, retractile mesenteritis and reactive inflammation of the colon are rare or involve the colon in a secondary fashion and so have not been included.

19.4.1
Typhlitis

Typhlitis or neutropenic colitis is a pronounced and potentially lethal infection of the cecum and ascending colon produced by enteric pathogens in patients with severe immunosuppression. It is frequently encountered in patients with acute leukemia and in patients undergoing chemotherapy (D'SOUZA and LINDBERG 2000). It also may be seen in patients who suffer from AIDS, aplastic anemia, multiple myeloma, cyclic neutropenia or who have had bone marrow transplantation (BAVARO 2002).

Clostridia infection is the commonest cause but a variety of bacteria, viruses and fungi may be responsible. The infectious agent penetrates the damaged mucosa and proliferates unimpeded due to the profound neutropenia. Patients with typhlitis present with fever, right lower quadrant pain and diarrhea.

On plain film there may be ileo-cecal dilatation and on CT there is marked thickening of the cecum and ascending colon and frequently, the terminal ileum is

also involved (Fig. 19.7) (ADAMS et al. 1985; McNAMARA et al. 1986). Pneumatosis also may be identified. The wall of the colon and small bowel is circumferentially thickened and there is pericolonic stranding and fluid. Prompt diagnosis and supportive therapy with intensive broad spectrum (including fungal) antibiotics and supplemental nutrition is necessary to prevent transmural necrosis and perforation (OTAIBI et al. 2002; SCHLATTER et al. 2002). CT often can suggest the correct diagnosis (MERINE et al. 1987; SCHLATTER et al. 2002). In severe cases, sepsis, abscess formation, intramural perforation, intestinal necrosis and/or hemorrhage may occur (GAYER et al. 2002). In the patients with these complications, surgical resection is often needed. CT also can be used to monitor the success of treatment by showing a decrease in thickness of the colon wall or by detecting complications such as pneumatosis when there is bowel wall necrosis or pneumoperitoneum when there is a silent perforation.

19.4.2
Eosinophilic Colitis

Eosinophilic gastroenteritis is a disease of unknown etiology that invariably involves the stomach and small bowel. Usually, peripheral eosinophilia is present and ascites is common (VAN HOE et al. 1994; MIYAMOTO et al. 1996). Occasionally, the right side of the colon is involved or there is a diffuse colitis. The colonic findings on CT mimic those seen in typhlitis or graft-versus-host disease. Narrowing of the intestinal lumen is a prominent feature (MACCARTY and TALLEY 1990) and the intestinal changes usually disappear with steroid therapy.

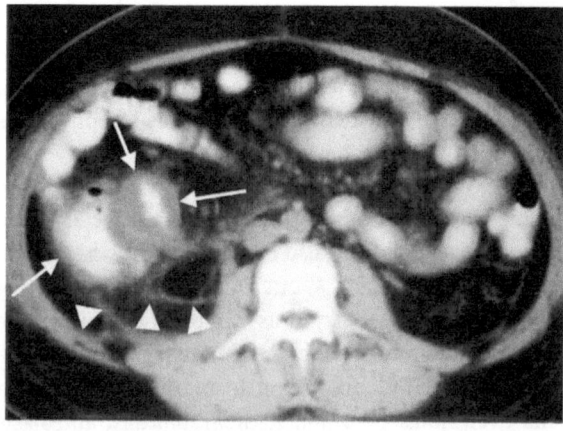

Fig. 19.7. Patient with acute leukemia and typhlitis. The cecum and terminal ileum (*arrows*) are thick-walled and associated with pericolonic stranding (*arrowheads*).

19.4.3
Graft-Versus-Host Disease

Colonic changes are common in graft-versus-host (GVHD) disease. In this disease mature donor lymphocytes attack the recipient tissues after bone marrow transplantation (BENYA et al. 1993; SCHETELIG et al. 2002). Patients with acute disease have symptoms of profuse diarrhea, nausea, vomiting, cramping abdominal pain and intestinal hemorrhage. Often there is a diffuse colitis but occasionally, only the right side of the colon is involved (JONES et al. 1988) and invariably there are inflammatory changes in the small bowel (Fig. 19.8).

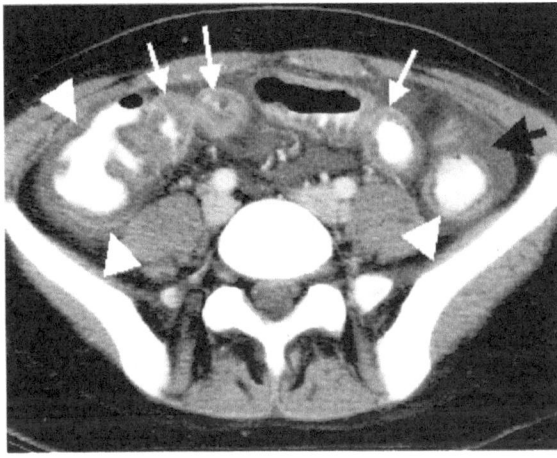

Fig. 19.8. Patient with graft-versus-host disease after bone marrow transplant. Diffuse thickening of the large (*arrowheads*) and small bowel is (*arrows*) present. Some ascites (*black arrow*) also is noted

In the acute stage, the colon appears markedly thickened on CT, as seen in viral colitis, and intraluminal secretions are increased. Wall thickening is from submucosal edema but in the chronic stage, edema is replaced by fat, which is readily seen on CT (MULDOWNEY et al. 1995). In some patients, an abnormally enhancing, thin mucosa and fluid-filled, dilated bowel loops are seen extending from the duodenum to the rectum (DONNELLY and MORRIS 1996). This appearance corresponds histologically to mucosal destruction and replacement, by a thin layer of highly vascular granulation tissue. Infiltration of mesenteric fat is seen in 91% of patients with GVHD (DONNELLY and MORRIS 1996).

19.4.4
Ischemic Colitis

Ischemic changes of the colon or small bowel with extensive wall thickening can mimic Crohn's disease, acute ulcerative colitis, infectious types of colitis, and pseudomembranous colitis. Distinction between ischemic and inflammatory etiology of bowel wall thickening can only be made if a typical vascular distribution pattern is detected or if the clinical history strongly suggests vascular compromise (Fig. 19.9). The most commonly involved arteries are the ileocolic branch of the SMA feeding the terminal ileum and cecum and the IMA with the watershed area in the transverse colon.

In patients with ischemia, cramp-like abdominal pain, abdominal distention, acidosis and occasionally melena or rectal bleeding are seen. Often co-morbidity exists such as cardiovascular disease, diabetes and renal failure. The most common cause is nonocclusive disease from a low-flow state and/or atherosclerosis. Ischemia from embolism or thrombosis is seen in only 9% and may occur as a complication of systemic disorders like systemic lupus erythematosus, lymphocytic phlebitis, Behçet's disease or Churg-Strauss syndrome (RADEMAKER 1998). Uncommon causes include vasculitis and the use of oral contraceptives, phenobarbital and nasal decongestants. Bowel ischemia also can occur with cocaine and amphetamine abuse (LINDER et al. 2000; DIRKX and GERSOVICH 1998). Cocaine is a potentially life-threatening cause of ischemic colitis and should be considered in any young adult or middle-aged patient with abdominal pain and bloody diarrhea, especially in the absence of oral contraceptive use or systemic disorders that can cause thromboembolic events, such as atrial fibrillation. Ischemic changes may also develop in markedly distended colon proximal to an obstruction and are

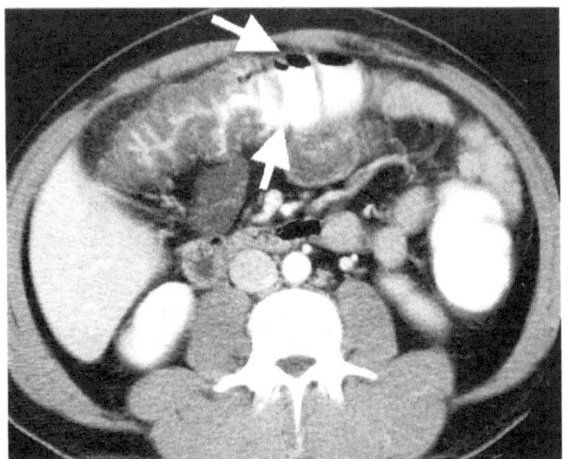

Fig. 19.9. Patient with ischemic colitis. The vascular distribution pattern of the colonic wall thickening is well shown. The transition from abnormal to normal colon occurs in the mid-transverse colon corresponding to the watershed area (*arrows*)

related to compression of arteries that feed the over-distended segment of large bowel (Ko et al. 1997).

Initially, marked bowel wall thickening, thumb printing and pericolonic stranding can be seen on CT (Horton and Fishman 2001). In the later stage, strictures may form if the ischemia is transmural. Involvement of the colon follows a vascular distribution pattern that is diagnostic and can be readily recognized on CT. In elderly patients or patients with known cardiovascular risk factors, the diagnosis of ischemic proctosigmoiditis should be considered when there is wall thickening confined to the rectum and sigmoid colon that is associated with perirectal fat stranding (Wiesner et al. 2002). Colonic wall density changes cannot be used on CT to diagnose or predict infarction (Balthazar et al. 1999). However, pneumatosis and/or portal venous gas are ominous signs when associated with bowel wall thickening.

Pneumatosis coli or intestinalis can be diagnosed by demonstrating air bubbles within the colonic or intestinal wall. The gas bubbles are arranged in a linear fashion and best visualized with the window setting for bone or lung. While pneumatosis can be a benign condition when it is often associated with chronic obstructive pulmonary disease, steroid treatment or scleroderma it may be associated with ischemia, severe colitis or GVHD. Pneumatosis coli or intestinalis can also be seen in patients with infectious colitis or following radiation or chemotherapy. When the wall of the colon and/or small bowel is compromised by ischemia soft tissue stranding may be present in the tissue surrounding the involved bowel. If hemorrhage into the bowel wall occurs in patients with intestinal ischemia, the hematoma may produce localized wall thickening or a mass. Such findings may also be encountered in patients on anticoagulation therapy or in patients with hemophilia when sometimes long segments of bowel may be involved.

19.5
Exogenous Causes of Colitis

Exogenous causes of colitis include antibiotics, chemotherapeutic agents, vasoconstrictive drugs, antihypertensive medications, nonsteroidal anti-inflammatory drugs and oral contraceptives. Other exogenous causes of colitis are substances that are introduced per rectum and produce a caustic colitis. Some of these agents lead to pseudomembranous colitis whereas others produce ischemia-related inflammation.

19.5.1
Pseudomembranous Colitis

Pseudomembranous colitis is encountered with increasing frequency as a complication of the use of antibiotics and chemotherapy. Overgrowth of Clostridium difficile and the subsequent release of a cytotoxic enterotoxin cause this potentially life-threatening disease (Klingler et al. 2000). The cytotoxin causes mucosal ulcerations and membranes that consist of sloughed epithelial cells, leukocytes, fibrin and mucus (Brar and Surawicz 2000). Pseudomembranous colitis should be suspected in patients receiving antibiotics who develop sudden onset of watery, foul smelling diarrhea often combined with fever, abdominal tenderness and leukocytosis. Patients are usually hospitalized or have had recent surgery. While many patients develop the disease within two days to two weeks of the start of antibiotic therapy, some develop symptoms as late as eight weeks after the antibiotic medication has been discontinued. Diagnosis involves identification of the enterotoxin in stool or by stool culture which is more sensitive but takes several days.

Mild cases may demonstrate changes on CT that are barely detectable but severe cases show a markedly thickened colonic wall with thumb printing, low attenuation from mucosal and submucosal edema, irregular mucosal contour with polypoid protrusions, pericolonic stranding and even a small amount of ascites (Fishman et al. 1991; Kawamoto et al. 1999; Ros et al. 1996). The appearance of the colon may resemble that of an accordion (Boland et al. 1995). Following administration of intravenous contrast material, the target sign may be seen with enhancement of mucosa and serosa. The average wall thickness is 14.7 mm (range 3 to 32 mm) (Fig. 19.10) (Fishman et al. 1991). Complications of untreated pseudomembranous colitis include toxic megacolon and intestinal perforation. CT has a positive predictive value of 88% for the diagnosis of Clostridium difficile colitis and can be used to initiate treatment (Kirkpatrick and Greenberg 2001) and to monitor the response to medical treatment with vancomycin and metronidazole (Klingler et al. 2000).

19.5.2
Drug-Induced Colitis

Chemotherapeutic agents for cancer treatment may produce inflammatory changes in the large bowel related to their inhibitory action on mucosal epithelium. Such patients may also develop typhlitis (see

Patients with caustic colitis often present with bloody diarrhea. CT demonstrates thumbprinting and thickening of the wall of the large bowel in the areas that came in contact with the caustic agent. Caustic changes are most commonly seen in the distal colon close to the entry site (Fig. 19.11), but prolonged contact or spasm can induce changes in the transverse or even right-sided colon, often associated with skip areas. Severe cases may require colectomy or defunctioning colostomy.

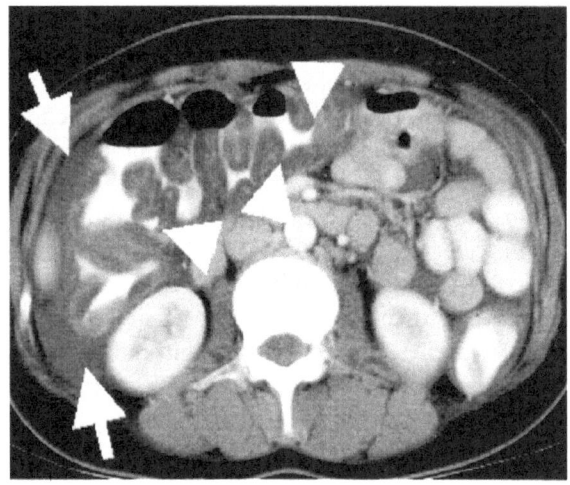

Fig. 19.10. Patient with pseudomembranous colitis. At 5 days following antibiotic treatment, this patient developed pronounced wall thickening in the right colon and thumb printing (*arrowheads*) and pericolonic stranding and fluid (*arrows*)

Sect. 19.4.1) because they develop neutropenia following treatment. Pseudomembranous colitis due to antibiotics has been discussed. Antibiotics, such as penicillin, ampicillin, erythromycin and amoxicillin, may cause a hypersensitivity reaction with a right-sided colitis. There is a mosaic pattern of "blisters" on barium enema and wall thickening on CT. This type of colitis subsides when the offending agent is withdrawn (FORTSON and TEDESCO 1984). Nonsteroidal anti-inflammatory drugs may result in diffuse or segmental colitis with discrete ulcers; the cecum being most commonly involved (GIBSON et al. 1992). Vasoconstrictive medications, antihypertensive drugs and oral contraceptives may all produce ischemic changes in the bowel wall.

19.5.3
Caustic Colitis

Depending on the corrosive substance introduced, the rectal mucosa may show changes ranging from transient mild inflammation to complete sloughing of the mucosa with subsequent stricture formation. In some third world countries, herbal enemas can produce a caustic colitis but in the western world soapsuds or detergent enemas are a more common cause (KIRCHNER et al. 1977; KIM et al. 1980; DA FONESCA et al. 1998). Colitis may also result from introducing fluid enemas whose temperature is too high (JACKSON et al. 1981) or following colonoscopy if the colonoscope has been inadequately cleansed following sterilization with glutaraldehyde (BERNBAUM et al. 1995).

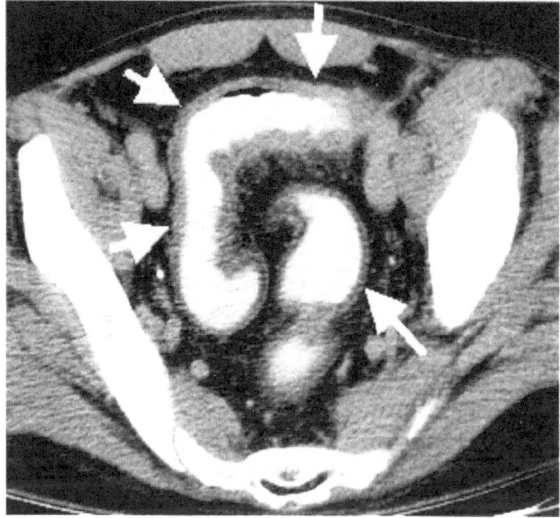

Fig. 19.11. Patient with caustic colitis after soapsuds enemas. Diffuse thickening of the rectum and sigmoid colon (*arrows*) was caused by rectal administration of the detergent with subsequent sloughing of the mucosa

19.6
Epiploic Appendagitis

Epiploic appendagitis represents an acute inflammation of the appendices epiploicae and can be confused with focal inflammation of the colon. Torsion or infarction of these appendices causes appendagitis. It can mimic appendicitis if located in the right colon and diverticulitis if located in the sigmoid colon. In patients with epiploic appendagitis, well-localized tenderness without peritoneal irritation is usually the only physical finding and blood tests are normal. In acute diverticulitis, the pain is more evenly distributed throughout the lower abdomen and nausea, fever, and leukocytosis are more frequent (SON et al. 2002). Appendagitis is a self-limited disease that resolves after a few days. Usually only supportive therapy with analgesia is needed (BOULANGER et al. 2002; MCCLURE et al. 2001).

CT reveals a well-defined oval or round area of fat with an enhancing rim located immediately adjacent to the colon (Fig. 19.12) (RIOUX and LANGIS 1994; RAO et al. 1997; MOLLA et al. 1998; VAN BREDA VRIESMAN and PUYLAERT 2002; SIRVANCI et al. 2000). The colon wall usually is not thickened but there may be some pericolonic stranding. The density of the fat within the enhancing rim is slightly increased. The CT appearance is characteristic so epiploic appendagitis can be readily diagnosed. Over time, the abnormal appendage shrinks in size, and disappears or calcifies.

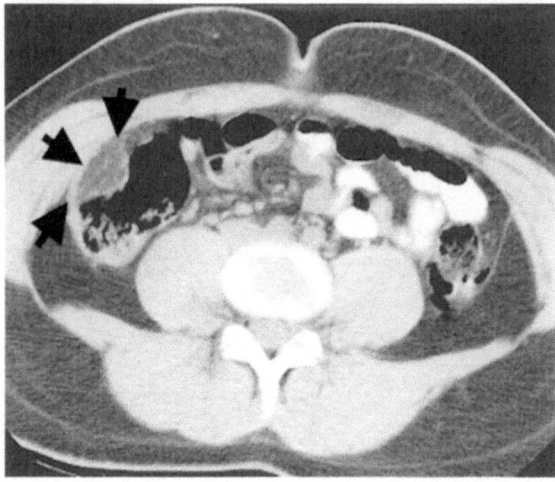

Fig. 19.12. Patient with right lower quadrant pain and appendagitis. An ovoid area with a well-defined and slightly enhancing rim (*arrows*) is closely associated with the ascending colon. The density of the fat within this oval-shaped region is slightly increased representing the infarcted or torsed appendix epiploicum

19.7
Differential Diagnosis and Summary

CT is a valuable imaging technique for detecting and characterizing many inflammatory conditions of the colon. The extent and appearance of wall thickening and the location of the involved segment may help distinguish Crohn's disease from ulcerative colitis. In ulcerative colitis, the diagnosis is based on the CT findings of thickening of the colon wall with a mean of 7.8 mm, inhomogeneous attenuation, a "target" appearance to the rectum, proliferation of perirectal fat (GORE et al. 1984) and dilatation of the terminal ileum (backwash ileitis). In Crohn's disease, the CT features are of bowel wall thickening with a mean of 13 mm, homogeneous attenuation, skip lesions, fistula and abscess formation, and fibrofatty proliferation in the mesentery. Often the small bowel is also involved. Patients with indetermi-

nate colitis usually show colonic changes on CT that are observed in both disorders. CT can often but not always differentiate patients with well established ulcerative and Crohn's colitis (GORE et al. 1984).

A considerable overlap exists between infectious and idiopathic inflammatory changes of the colon. Infectious types of colitis can mimic idiopathic inflammatory bowel disease, usually of the ulcerative type, but in acute infectious colitis ascites is more frequently seen. Pseudomembranous, ischemic and acute infectious types of colitis often show evidence of ascites whereas ascites is rare in idiopathic inflammatory bowel disease, even if its acute. In infectious colitis, the site and thickness of the involved colon may suggest a specific organism. The amount of wall thickening in pseudomembranous colitis and CMV colitis is typically greater than that in any other inflammatory disease of the colon except Crohn's disease. Deposition of fat in the submucosa may occur in subacute and chronic colitis, most commonly with ulcerative colitis. Submucosal fat deposition also has been seen after chemotherapy when it can develop in a relatively short period of time (range 12–185 days) (MULDOWNEY et al. 1995). Sinus tracts are commonly seen in both Crohn's disease and ulcerative colitis, but may occur in patients with fungal infections and gastrointestinal tuberculosis. Fistula, while most common with Crohn's disease may also be seen in patients with tuberculosis, actinomycosis, blastomycosis and strongyloidiasis.

In ischemic colitis, CT typically demonstrates circumferential, symmetric wall thickening with fold enlargement in a vascular distribution pattern. In radiation colitis, clinical history and the location of the abnormalities in the radiation port are key to the diagnosis as the CT findings can be nonspecific. In typhlitis, CT demonstrates cecal distention and circumferential thickening of the cecal wall, which may have low attenuation from edema. The terminal ileum may or may not be involved. CT findings of graft-versus-host disease usually include both small bowel and colonic wall thickening and there may be luminal narrowing and separation of bowel loops. On CT, a dilated, thickened appendix with fat stranding is suggestive of appendicitis and contiguous inflammation of terminal ileum and cecum may mimic typhlitis. The key to distinguishing diverticulitis from other inflammatory conditions of the colon is the focal nature of the disease and the presence of diverticula in the involved segment. A one to four centimeter, oval, fatty pericolonic lesion with surrounding mesenteric inflammation is diagnostic of epiploic appendagitis. Often, the infarcted or torsed epiploic appendix appears as a well defined, rim-enhancing area of fat.

References

Adams GW, Rauch RF, Kelvin FM et al (1985) CT detection of typhlitis. J Comput Assist Tomogr 9:363–365

Agha FP, Lee HH, Boland CR et al (1985) Mucormycoma of the colon: early diagnosis and successful management. AJR 86:86–90

Akhan O, Pringot J (2002) Imaging of abdominal tuberculosis. Eur Radiol 12:312–323. Am Surg 68:1022–1025

Andronikou S, Welman CJ, Kader E (2002) The CT features of abdominal tuberculosis in children. Pediatr Radiol 32:75–81

Atkinson GO, Gay BB, Ball TI et al (1983) Yersinia enterocolitica enterocolitis in infants. Radiographic changes Radiology 148:113–116

Balthazar EJ, Megibow AJ, Fazzini E et al (1985) Cytomegalovirus colitis in AIDS: radiographic findings in 11 patients. Radiology 155:585–589

Balthazar EJ, Gordon R, Hulnick D (1990) Ileocecal tuberculosis: CT and radiologic evaluation. AJR 154:499–503

Balthazar EJ, Charles HW, Megibow AJ (1996) Salmonella- and Shigella-induced ileitis: CT findings in four patients. J Comput Assist Tomogr 20:375–378

Balthazar EJ, Yen BC, Gordon RB (1999) Ischemic colitis: CT evaluation of 54 cases. Radiology 211:381–388

Bavaro MF (2002) Neutropenic enterocolitis. Curr Gastroenterol Rep 4:297–301

Benya EC, Sivit CJ, Quinones RR (1993) Abdominal complications after bone marrow transplantation in children: sonographic and CT findings. AJR Am J Roentgenol 161:1023–1027

Bernbaum BA, Gordon RB, Jacobs JE (1995) Glutaraldehyde colitis: radiologic findings. Radiology 195:131–134

Boland GW, Lee MJ, Cats AM et al (1995) Clostridium difficile colitis: correlation of CT findings with severity of clinical disease. Clin Radiol 50:153–156

Boulanger BR, Barnes S, Bernard AC (2002) Epiploic appendagitis: an emerging diagnosis for general surgeons. Am Surg 68:1022–1025

Brar HS, Surawicz C (2000) Pseudomembranous colitis: an update. Can J Gastroenterol 14:51–56

Brodey PA, Fertig S, Aron JM (1982) Campylobacter enterocolitis: radiographic features. AJR 139:1199–1201

Brown G, Bui A, Vrazas J (2000) Florid computed tomographic appearance of acute Campylobacter enterocolitis. Australas Radiol 44:204–205

Casola G, von Sonnenberg E, Neff CC et al (1987) Abscess in Crohn's disease: Percutaneous drainage. Radiology 163:19–22

Cevallos AM, Farthing MJG (1993) Parasitic infections of the gastrointestinal tract. Curr Opin Gastroenterol 9:96–102

Chatzicostas C, Koutroubakis IE, Tzardi M et al (2002) Colonic tuberculosis mimicking Crohn's disease: case report. BMC Gastroenterol 2:10

Chung SY, Ha HK, Kim JH et al (2001) Radiologic findings of Behcet syndrome involving the gastrointestinal tract. Radiographics 21:911–924

Da Fonseca J, Brito MJ, Freitas J et al (1998) Acute colitis caused by caustic products. Am J Gastroenterol 93:2601–2612

Denton ERE, Jamieson CP, Rankin SC (1996) Abscess of the adductor muscles of the thigh – an unusual complication of Crohn's disease. Br J Radiol 69:865–866

Dirkx CA, Gerscovich EO (1998) Sonographic findings in methamphetamine-induced ischemic colitis. J Clin Ultrasound 26:479–482

Donnelly LF, Morris CL (1996) Acute graft-versus-host disease in children: abdominal CT findings. Radiology 199:265–268

D'Souza S, Lindberg M (2000) Typhlitis as a presenting manifestation of acute myelogenous leukemia. South Med J 93:218–220

Duran JC, Beidle TR, Perpet R et al (1997) CT imaging of acute right lower quadrant disease. AJR Am J Roentgenol 168:411–416

Farman J, Rabinowitz JG, Meyers MA (1973) Roentgenology of infectious colitis. AJR 119:375–381

Fishman EK, Wolf EJ, Jones B et al (1987) CT evaluation of Crohn's disease: effect on patient management. AJR 148:537–541

Fishman EK, Kavuru M, Jones B et al (1991) Pseudomembranous colitis: CT evaluation of 26 cases. Radiology 180:57–60

Fortson WC, Tedesco FJ (1984) Drug-induced colitis: a review. Am J Gastroenterol 79:878–883

Fredricks DN, Rojanasthien N, Jacobson MA (1997) AIDS-related disseminated histoplasmosis in San Francisco, California. West J Med 167:315–321

Funayama Y, Sasaki I, Naito H et al (1997) Psoas abscess complicating Crohn's disease: a pictorial essay. Radiographics 17:101–107

Gayer G, Apter S, Zissin R (2002) Typhlitis as a rare cause of a psoas abscess. Abdom Imaging 27:600–602

Gibson GR, Whiteacre EB, Ricotti CA (1992) Colitis induced by nonsteroidal anti-inflammatory drugs. Arch Intern Med 152:625–632

Gore RM, Marn CS, Kirby DF et al (1984) CT findings in ulcerative, granulomatous, and indeterminate colitis. AJR Am J Roentgenol 143:279–284

Gore RM, Gharemani GG, Miller FH (1996) Cross-sectional imaging in the evaluation of Crohn's disease. In: Prantera C, Koreltiz (eds) Crohn's disease. Dekker, New York, pp 145 185

Gossios KJ, Tsianos EV (1997) Crohn's disease: CT findings after treatment. Abdom Imaging 22:160–163

Greyson-Fleg RT, Jones B, Fishman EK et al (1986) Computed tomography findings in gastrointestinal involvement by opportunistic organisms in acquired immune deficiency syndrome. J Comput Tomogr 10:175–181

Griffiths JK (1993) Colonic infections. Curr Opin Gastroenterol 9:83–87

Gulek B, Onel S (1999) US and CT findings of rectal amebian abscess. Eur Radiol 9:719–720

Herlinger H, Furth EE, Rubesin SE (1998) Fibrofatty proliferation of the mesentery in Crohn's disease. Abdom Imaging 23:446–448

Horton KM, Fishman EK (2001) Computed tomography evaluation of intestinal ischemia. Semin Roentgenol 36:118–125

Horton KM, Corl FM, Fishman EK (2000) CT evaluation of the colon: inflammatory disease. Radiographics 20:399–418

Imbriaco M, Balthazar EJ (2001) Toxic megacolon: role of CT in evaluation and detection of complications. Clin Imaging 25:349–354

Jackson KR, Ott DJ, Gelfand DW (1981) Thermal innjury of the colon due to colostomy irrigation. Gastrointest Radiol 6:231–233

Jones B, Kramer SS, Saral R et al (1988) Gastrointestinal inflammation after bone marrow transplantation: graft-versus-host disease or opportunistic infection? AJR 150:277–281

Kawamoto S, Horton KM, Fishman EK (1999) Pseudomembranous colitis: spectrum of imaging findings with clinical and pathologic correlation. Radiographics 19:887–897

Kim SK, Cho C, Levinsohn EM (1980) Caustic colitis due to detergent enema. AJR Am J Roentgenol 134:397–398

Kirchner SG, Buckspan GS, O'Neill JA et al (1977) Detergent enema: a cause of caustic colitis. Pediatr Radiol 6:141–146

Kirk ME, Lough J, Warner HA (1971) Histoplasma colitis: an electron microscopic study. Gastroenterology 61:46–54

Kirkpatrick ID, Greenberg HM (2001) Evaluating the CT diagnosis of Clostridium difficile colitis: should CT guide therapy? AJR Am J Roentgenol 176:635–639

Klingler PJ, Metzger PP, Seelig MH et al (2000) Clostridium difficile infection: risk factors, medical and surgical management. Dig Dis 18:147–160

Knollmann FD, Grunewald T, Adler A et al (1997) Intestinal disease in acquired immunodeficiency: evaluation by CT. Eur Radiol 7:1419–1429

Ko GY, Ha HK, Lee HJ et al (1997) Usefulness of CT in patients with ischemic colitis proximal to colonic cancer. AJR Am J Roentgenol 168:951–956

Kollitz JPM, Davis GB, Berk RN (1981) Campylobacter colitis: a common infectious form of acute colitis. Gastrointest Radiol 6:227–229

Lachman R, Soong J, Wishon G et al (1977) Yersinia colitis. Gastrointest Radiol 2:133–135

Lambert JR, Tischler ME, Karmali MA et al (1979) campylobacter ileocolitis: an inflammatory bowel disease. Can Med Assoc J 121:1377–1379

Latella G, Vernia P, Viscido A et al (2002) GI distension in severe ulcerative colitis. Am J Gastroenterol 97:1169–1175

Linder JD, Monkemuller KE, Raijman I et al (2000) Cocaine-associated ischemic colitis. South Med J 93:909–913

Low RN, Francis IR, Politosre D et al (2000) Crohn's disease evaluation: comparison of contrast-enhanced MR imaging and single-pase helical CT scanning. J Magn Reson Imaging 11:127–135

Macari M, Balthazar EJ (2001) CT of bowel thickening: significance and pitfalls of interpretation. AJR Am J Roentgenol 176:1105–1116

MacCarty RL, Talley NJ (1990) Barium studies in diffuse eosinophilic gastroenteritis. Gastrointest Radiol 15:183–187

Mariano F, Rossano C, Goia F et al (1996) Systemic mucormycosis in dialysis: computed tomography picture and histologic lesions. Minerva Urol Nefrol 48:51–54

Matsui T, Iida M, Tada S et al (1989) The value of double-contrast barium enema in amebic colitis. Gastrointest Radiol 14:73–78

Matsumoto T, Iida M, Matsui T et al (1990) Endoscopic findings in Yersinia enterocolitica enterocolitis. Gastrointest Endosc 36:583–587

McClure MJ, Khalili K, Sarrazin J et al (2001) Radiological features of epiploic appendagitis and segmental omental infarction. Clin Radiol 56:819–827

McDonald JB, Middleton PJ (1976) Tuberculosis of the colon simulating carcinoma. Radiology 118:293–294

McNamara MJ, Chalmers AG, Morgan M, Smith SE (1986) Typhlitis in acute childhood leukaemia:radiological features. Clin Radiol 37:83–86

Merine DS, Fishman EK, Jones B et al (1987) Right lower quadrant pain in the immunocompromised patient: CT findings in 10 cases. AJR Am J Roentgenol 149:1177–1179

Miller FH, Ma JJ, Scholz FJ (2001) Imaging features of enterohemorrhagic Escherichia coli colitis. AJR 177:619–623

Miyamoto T, Shibata T, Matsuura S et al (1996) Eosinophilic gastroenteritis with ileus and ascites. Intern Med 35:779–782

Molla E, Ripolles T, Martinez MJ et al (1998) Primary epiploic appendagitis: US and CT findings. Eur Radiol 8:435–438

Monkemuller KE, Wilcox CM (1998) Diagnosis and treatment of colonic disease in AIDS. Gastrointest Endosc Clin North Am 8:889–911

Mountanos GI, Manolakakis IS (2001) The accordion sign at CT: report of a case of Crohn's disease with diffuse colonic involvement. Eur Radiol 11:1433–1434

Muldowney SM, Balfe DM, Hammerman A et al (1995) "Acute" fat deposition in bowel wall submucosa: CT appearance. J Comput Assist Tomogr 199:390–393

Otaibi AA, Barker C, Anderson R et al (2002) Neutropenic enterocolitis (typhlitis) after pediatric bone marrow transplant. J Pediatr Surg 37:770–772

Philpotts LE, Heiken JP, Westcott MA, Gore RM (1994) Colitis: use of CT findings in differential diagnosis. Radiology 190:445–449

Rademaker J (1998) Veno-occlusive disease of the colon -- CT findings. Eur Radiol 8:1420–1421

Rao PM, Wittenberg J, Lawrason JN (1997) Primary epiploic appendagitis: evolutionary changes in CT appearance. Radiology 204:713–717

Raptopoulos V, Schwartz RK, McNicholas MM et al (1997) Multiplanar helical CT enterography in patients with Crohn's disease. AJR Am J Roentgenol 169:1545–1550

Ribeiro MB, Greenstein AJ, Yamazaki Y et al (1991) Intraabdominal abscess in regional enteritis. Ann Surg 213:32–36

Rioux M, Langis P (1994) Primary epiploic appendagitis: clinical, US, and CT findings in 14 cases. Radiology 191:523–526

Ros PR, Buetow PC, Pantograg-Brown L et al (1996) Pseudomembranous colitis. Radiology 198:1–9

Rutgeerts P, Geboes K, Ponette E et al (1982) Colitis caused by endemic pathogens in Western Europe; endoscopic features. Endoscopy 14:212–219

Saffouri B, Bartolomeo RS, Fuchs B (1979) Colonic involvement in salmonellosis. Dig Dis Sci 24:203–208

Schetelig J, Kroger N, Held TK et al (2002) Allogeneic transplantation after reduced conditioning in high risk patients is complicated by a high incidence of acute and chronic graft-versus-host disease. Haematologica 87:299–305

Schlatter M, Snyder K, Freyer D (2002) Successful nonoperative management of typhlitis in pediatric oncology patients. J Pediatr Surg 37:1151–1155

Shortsleeve MJ Wilson ME, Finkelstein M et al (1989) Radiologic findings in hemorrhagic colitis due to Escherichia coli O157:H7. Gastroiintest Radiol 14:341–344

Sirvanci M, Tekelioglu MH, Duran C et al (2000) Primary epiploic appendagitis: CT manifestations. Clin Imaging 24:357–361

Son HJ, Lee SJ, Lee JH et al (2002) Clinical diagnosis of primary epiploic appendagitis: differentiation from acute diverticulitis. J Clin Gastroenterol 34:435–438

Suh KN, Anekthananon T, Mariuz PR (2001) Gastrointestinal histoplasmosis in patients with AIDS: case report and review. Clin Infect Dis 32:483–491

Tarjan Z, Zagoni T, Gyorke T et al (2000) Spiral CT colongraph-yin inflammatory bowel disease. Eur J Radiol 35:193–198

Tedesco FJ, Moore S (1982) Infectious diseases mimicking inflammatory bowel disease. Am Surg 6:243–249

Tedesco FJ, Hardin RD, Harper RN et al (1983) Infectious colitis endoscopically simulating inflammatory bowel disease: a prospective evaluation. Gastrointest Endosc 29:195–197

Thoeni RF, Margulis AR (1979) Gastrointestinal tuberculosis. Semin Roentgenol 14:283–294

Tuohy AM, O'Gorman M, Byington C et al (1999) Yersinia enterocolitis mimicking Crohn's disease in a toddler. Pediatrics 104:e36

Van Breda Vriesman AC, Puylaert JB (2002) Epiploic appendagitis and omental infarction: pitfalls and look-alikes. Abdom Imaging 27:20–28

Van Hoe L, Vanghillewe K, Baert AL et al (1994) CT findings in nonmucosal eosinophilic gastroenteritis. J Comput Assist Tomogr 18:818–820

Wagner-Manslau C, Reiser M, Lukas P (1985) Computed tomographic findings in amebiasis. Radiologe 25:597–598

Wall SD, Jones B (1992) Gastrointestinal tract in the immunocompromised host: opportunistic infections and other complications. Radiology 185:327–335

Wiesner W, Mortele KJ, Glickman JN et al (2002) CT findings in isolated ischemic proctosigmoiditis. Eur Radiol 12: 1762–1767

Wu CM, Davis F, Fishman EK (1999) Radiologic evaluation of the acute abdomen in patients with acquired immunodeficiency syndrome (AIDS): the role of CT scanning. Semin Ultrasound CT MR 19:190–200

Yilmaz T, Sever A, Gur S et al (2002) CT findings of abdominal tuberculosis in 12 patients. Comput Med Imaging Graph 26:321–325

Zalev AH, Warren RE (1989) Shigella colitis with radiologic

20 MRI of Colitis

Francesca Maccioni

CONTENTS

20.1   Introduction *201*
20.2   Classification and General Features of Colitis *201*
20.3   MRI of Inflammatory Bowel Disease:
        General Technical Considerations *202*
20.4   MRI Findings in Crohn's Colitis *204*
20.4.1. Wall Characterization *204*
20.4.2 Detection of CD Complications *204*
20.4.3 Assessment of Crohn's Disease Activity *209*
20.5   MRI Findings in Ulcerative Colitis *209*
20.6   Differential Diagnosis Between CD
        and UC with MRI *210*
20.7   Conclusions: Role of MRI
        in the Management of Colitis *212*
        References *212*

20.1
Introduction

Until recently the role of MRI in the evaluation of bowel diseases has been limited to the assessment of ano-rectal abnormalities, as long acquisition times resulted in motion artifacts from breathing and intestinal peristalsis. Recent technological advances have greatly improved the quality of abdominal MRI so as to allow it to be used for the evaluation of the bowel wall in inflammatory bowel disease (IBD). Rapid acquisition sequences have resulted in a significant reduction in motion artifacts and can now provide excellent dynamic contrast-enhanced studies of the bowel wall. Spatial resolution can be increased by using phased array coils. The contrast of the image can be modulated and improved by suppressing the signal of fat in either T1 or T2 weighted images, or through the administration of positive or negative oral contrast agents, both of which are now commercially available (GIOVAGNONI et al. 2002). Three-dimensional post-processing can be used in

MRI as well as CT, to produce maximum intensity projection (MIP) or volume rendered images that are comparable to barium contrast studies and to conventional endoscopic views, respectively (WILDERSMUTH and DEBATIN 1999) and in the future, real time MRI (fluoro-MRI) will become available. These advances, together with the inherent high soft tissue contrast, the lack of ionizing radiation and the ability to acquire images in multiple planes with different imaging parameters (such as T1-T2 weighting), make MRI a valuable diagnostic tool for the evaluation of bowel disease (DEBATIN and PATAK 1999; LOMAS 1999; MACCIONI 2002). The disadvantages of MRI are its high cost and limited availability. Compared to spiral CT, MRI has higher tissue contrast, greater contrast enhancement, multiple imaging parameters, safer contrast agents and avoids ionizing radiation, whereas CT has higher spatial resolution, fewer artifacts, shorter examination time and lower costs.

Thanks to recent technological advances, interest in the use of MRI in IBD has increased significantly over the last few years, particularly for Crohn's disease, and to a lesser extent for ulcerative colitis (SHOENUT et al. 1993; KETTRITZ et al. 1995; ERNST et al. 1998; MADSEN et al. 1998; MACCIONI et al. 2000; RIEBER et al. 2000; GOURTSOYIANNIS et al. 2001; KOH et al. 2001; LOW et al. 2002). However, the role of MRI in the evaluation of the bowel pathology, and in particular IBD, has yet to be fully investigated and defined.

20.2
Classification and General Features of Colitis

The term idiopathic IBD refers to Crohn's disease (CD) and ulcerative colitis (UC), both having an unknown etiology and a chronic relapsing and remitting course that may last all of a patient's life.

UC is a contiguous, confluent, circumferential and symmetric disease that begins in the rectum

F. MACCIONI, MD
Istituto di Radiologia, Policlinico Umberto I, Università La Sapienza, Viale Regina Elena 324, 00161 Roma, Italy

and extends proximally to involve a varying proportion of the colon (ulcerative proctitis, sigmoiditis,
left-sided colitis or pancolitis). Haustration is often
lost in the late phase (JEWELL 1993). Histologically,
exacerbation are characterized by an acute inflammatory process that is usually confined to the inner
layers of the bowel wall with disruption of the
mucosa (RIDDELL 1998). In 10%–20% of patients
with a pancolitis there is associated mucosal inflammation of the distal 5–25 cm of ileum (backwash
ileitis). Most patients develop mild to moderate
disease but occasionally, the disease is severe and
does not respond to pharmacological therapy and
requires urgent colectomy. The main complications
of an acute relapse are toxic megacolon, perforation
and hemorrhage, whereas strictures, carcinoma of
the colon, sclerosing cholangitis and cholangiocarcinoma are late developments (MINER 2000). The
diagnosis of UC is based on clinical and laboratory
findings, endoscopic evaluation of the colon and histology from endoscopic biopsies.

CD is a chronic granulomatous disease that may
involve any portion of the gastrointestinal tract. It is
characterized by a transmural inflammation of the
bowel wall, with a tendency to extend to the serosa,
frequently leading to sinus tracts and fistula formation (RIDDELL 1998). Fibro-fatty proliferation of the
mesentery, or creeping fat, is frequently observed
in long-standing CD and is associated with lymphadenopathy and dilation of feeding blood vessels.
Local intestinal complications include phlegmon,
abscesses, entero-enteric, entero-cutaneous and
entero-vesical fistulas and strictures (LASHNER
2000). The affected bowel frequently shows a typical
patchy discontinuous involvement. Ileocolic, small
intestinal and upper gastrointestinal CD occurs in
approximately 30%–55%, 25%–35% and 5%–10% of
patients respectively, whereas disease limited to the
colon accounts for 15%–25% (FARMER et al. 1975;
TRUELOVE and PENA 1976). Indications for surgery
include strictures causing obstructive symptoms, fistulas, abscesses, bleeding and rarely carcinoma.

The diagnosis of CD rests upon a constellation of
clinical, radiologic, endoscopic and microscopic features, any of which may strongly suggest the diagnosis. Barium studies, although not useful in assessing
the clinical activity of CD or UC, can be indispensable
in distinguishing between the two diseases (GOLD-
BERG et al. 1979; WILLS et al. 1997; GORE et al. 1997).
Small bowel contrast studies are usually normal in
UC, although backwash ileitis can be appreciated
in approximately 10% of patients. Because 75% of
patients with CD have some small bowel disease

and only 20% have disease confined to the colon, a
normal small bowel series favors UC.

Cross sectional imaging (sonography, CT and
MRI) can be useful for characterizing the extra-
intestinal and suppurative complications of CD, such
as hydronephrosis and abscess and perirectal sinus
formation. The cross sectional imaging characteristics of the bowel wall may help in making a diagnosis.
The mean value for wall thickening in UC is 7.8 mm
as opposed to 11 mm (up to 20 mm) for CD. The outer
contour of the bowel wall is smooth and regular in
95% of patients with UC, whereas serosal and outer
wall irregularity are found in 80% of the patients with
CD (KLEIN et al. 1995; GORE et al. 1997).

Differentiation between these two diseases can be
made on radiological grounds in 90%–95% of cases
(GORE et al. 1996, 1997) but, in 10%–20% of patients
with chronic colitis, a precise diagnosis may not be
possible, resulting in the colitis being designated
"*indeterminate*". Careful observation over time can
reduce the proportion of patients with indeterminate
colitis to 8%–13% (PRICE 1978; KANGAS et al. 1994).
Differentiation between an initial attack of IBD and
an infectious colitis can be difficult and rests on the
bacteriology and histology.

Infectious colitides may simulate acute IBD.
Yersinia enterocolitis, tuberculosis, salmonellosis
and typhlitis may simulate ileocolic or colonic CD,
and shigellosis, salmonellosis, amebiasis, *E. coli* and
Clostridium difficile infection may simulate UC.

Non-infectious colitides such as diverticulitis, ischemic and radiation colitis may show similar findings
to CD and UC.

20.3
MRI of Inflammatory Bowel Disease: General Technical Considerations
(T1- and T2-Weighted Imaging and Intestinal Contrast Agents)

MRI should be performed with high field magnets
(1–1.5 T) using either a body or phased array coil,
depending on the MR system.

The majority of MR studies of IBD are based
on the preferential use of T1-weighted sequences
(SEMELKA et al. 1991; ERNST et al. 1998; KOH et al.
2001; LOW et al. 2002).

The MRI examination for IBD should always
include T1-weighted pre- and post-gadolinium
images, as they demonstrate the abnormal features of
the disease in a similar way to that seen on contrast-

enhanced CT. In particular, after i.v. gadolinium, the degree of wall enhancement of the inflamed bowel is directly proportional to the inflammatory activity of the disease (SHOENUT et al. 1994; MACCIONI et al. 2000; KOH et al. 2001; LOW et al. 2002).

To obtain good quality T1-weighted images and satisfactory dynamic contrast enhancement during gadolinium injection, the use of fast breath-hold gradient echo sequences is recommended. These sequences are labeled in different ways by different MR manufacturers, so FSPGR (fast spoiled gradient echo), TFE (turbo field echo) and FLASH (fast low angle single shot) are all characterized by an acquisition time of 1 s or less per slice and usually 20 slices are acquired during an 18- to 27-s breath-hold time. A delay time of 60 s after gadolinium injection is usually adequate to obtain a good assessment of the wall and the mesenteric vascularization.

Suppression of the signal of the mesenteric fat can be helpful in the evaluation of the wall enhancement after gadolinium injection, although it may obscure mesenteric lymph nodes. We suggest obtaining pre-contrast non-suppressed and post-contrast fat-suppressed T1-weighted images.

To distend the lumen and homogenize the luminal content on T1-weighted images it is preferable to use a negative oral contrast agent, as the use of a positive contrast agent can appear to reduce wall enhancement after the intravenous injection of gadolinium.

A negative luminal signal on T1-weighted images can be obtained by rectal insufflation of air, or by oral or rectal administration of a *negative contrast agent*. Superparamagnetic contrast agents (suspension of iron oxide particles) given orally produce a negative signal on both T1- and T2-weighted images, and *biphasic contrast agents* [usually iso-osmolar water solutions such as polyethylene glycol (PEG)] produce a negative signal on T1- but a positive signal on T2-weighted images.

The passage of the contrast agent through the small bowel is usually extremely rapid in CD and UC and often less than 1 h is needed to obtain homogeneous opacification of the small and large bowel but for adequate opacification of the entire colon we recommend waiting 60–90 min. Distension of the colon and improved negative contrast can be achieved by rectal insufflation of air or the additional rectal administration of a superparamagnetic contrast agent prior to starting the examination.

In CD it is important to image both the small and large bowel, but if the examination is to be focused solely on the colon then the administration of the contrast agent can be exclusively rectal.

The use of *positive intraluminal contrast agents* is not recommended with i.v. gadolinium. Positive contrast agents can be used on T1-weighted imaging to produce a sort of MR colon enema, with the purpose of studying the lumen rather than the colonic wall. Approximately 1000 cc of a gadolinium water solution (1 ml Gd/100 cc water) can be rectally administered to obtain complete distension and opacification of the colonic lumen. Fast 3D T1-weighted sequences are usually suggested to study the opacified colon and subsequently a MIP reconstruction can be performed to obtain a barium enema-like effect.

T2-weighted sequences are very sensitive for detecting inflammation, but only if imaging conditions and parameters are optimized and intestinal contrast agents used.

T2-weighted sequences have low contrast resolution when performed without the use of an adequate intestinal contrast agent as bowel content gives an inhomogeneous signal, ranging from very bright (fluid) to gray to very dark (air). Moreover, mesenteric fat is very bright and the wall signal varies, according to the pathologic condition.

To overcome the problem of the poor contrast resolution, the signal of the bowel can be reduced through the oral administration of a superparamagnetic negative contrast agent (iron oxide particles) or through the rectal insufflation of air. In this way, the lumen becomes homogenously dark and the bowel loops can be easily distinguished from the bright mesenteric fat. In addition, the signal of the perivisceral fat can be darkened by using a fat-suppression technique, thus the high T2 signal of the inflamed bowel wall is maximally enhanced between the dark lumen and the dark perivisceral fat. Furthermore, in the presence of active disease, the perivisceral fat may show a persistent bright signal after fat-suppression, suggestive of edema (mesenteritis) or minimal amounts of free fluid, not otherwise detectable on MR images (see Sect. 20.4.3).

The use of a biphasic oral contrast agent, such as PEG, with T1- and T2-weighted sequences has been suggested as it is readily available and inexpensive (LAGHI et al. 2001). The effect of a biphasic agent, which is negative in T1 and positive in T2, is extremely valuable for T1-weighted imaging but less effective with T2-weighting as it is less effective at homogenizing the content of the bowel than the superparamagnetic contrast agents and it does not allow an accurate evaluation of the inflamed bowel wall whose thickening and T2 signal can be underestimated.

The use of *fat-suppression* is mandatory with T2-weighted TFE images to detect inflammation of the bowel wall and perivisceral mesenteric fat.

Conversely, the use of fat suppression with T1-weighted TFE images is optional. Some use it as it improves contrast between bowel wall and perivisceral fat, particularly after gadolinium injection (KOH et al. 2001; Low et al. 2002), whereas others (RIEBER et al. 2000) avoid fat suppression with T1-weighted images, as it results in complete cancellation of lymph nodes. A good compromise is to avoid fat suppression before, but to use it after, the gadolinium injection.

20.4
MRI Findings in Crohn's Colitis

In CD, the colon is involved in over 60% of patients. Crohn's colitis is frequently associated with a distal ileitis (30%–55% of cases) and the disease is limited to the colon in only 15%–25% of cases (RIDDEL 1998). In Crohn's colitis the rectum is involved in approximately 50% of patients.

The typical features of the disease, such as segmental bowel involvement, wall thickening, wall enhancement, fibrofatty proliferation, dilation of mesenteric vessels, mild enlargement of local mesenteric lymph nodes, abscesses, phlegmon, fissures and fistulas can be observed in both small and large bowel disease (MACCIONI 2002).

20.4.1.
Wall Characterization

Bowel *wall thickening* is the most common morphological change of CD and usually indicates active disease. This finding can be observed in axial and coronal planes, on T1- and T2-weighted images. The thickening ranges from 4 to 20 mm and is usually more pronounced in the colon than the small bowel. Sometimes, in active ileocolic disease, wall thickening exceeds 20 mm, and inflammatory tissue fills the entire lumen of the cecum (Fig. 20.1). Elsewhere in the colon wall involvement is usually more regular and circumferential (Fig. 20.2).

Wall enhancement is a characteristic finding of active CD. It was first described with contrast-enhanced CT but is clearly observed on post-gadolinium T1-weighted MR images (Fig. 20.3). Gadolinium enhancement on T1-weighted images is greater than the enhancement of iodinated contrast agents in CT thanks to the higher intrinsic contrast resolution of MRI. Wall enhancement with gadolinium can be pronounced in active disease, and can be further

improved by using fat-suppression. Sometimes, marked wall thickening can be observed in inactive disease but, in such cases, the wall shows neither significant gadolinium enhancement nor significant T2 signal, probably as a consequence of wall fibrosis.

The T2 signal of the wall, only recently investigated, is another MR parameter that is strongly related to disease activity. It is clearly observed only on T2-weighted fat-suppressed images after oral administration of a superparamagnetic contrast agent, but in non-suppressed images it is less evident (Fig. 20.1).

Fibrofatty proliferation of the mesentery is another typical feature of CD. MRI can evaluate the amount of fibrofatty tissue and its signal on T2-weighted fat suppressed images, which can be an expression of the mesenteric inflammation (Fig. 20.4).

Fibrofatty tissue proliferation can be present in both active and inactive disease, although with long-standing CD the amount of fatty proliferation is greater than with recent disease. The amount of fibrofatty tissue is easily evaluated on both T1- and T2-weighted MR images, without fat suppression. However, the T2 signal of mesenteric fat can be assessed only after fat suppression as if the signal of the fat persists, it can be related to local edema or free fluid and can be considered an expression of local inflammation. The T2 signal of mesenteric fat can probably be related to a local "mesenteritis" (edema and dilation of local vessels) associated with minimal amounts of free fluid (MACCIONI et al. 2000), similar to the increased density of the mesenteric fat observed on CT imaging in active disease (GORE et al. 1997) (Fig. 20.5).

In inactive disease a marked fibrofatty proliferation is frequently observed, but in this case the T2 signal on fat suppressed images is low or absent.

Local enlarged *lymph nodes* can be detected using either T1 or T2 weighted plain non-suppressed sequences. It is necessary, however, to use a high matrix size and to have good spatial resolution, as inflamed lymph nodes are usually small and are frequently missed if the spatial resolution is low (Fig. 20.1).

20.4.2
Detection of CD Complications

The value of MRI in the assessment of *intestinal and extraintestinal complications of CD* has recently been investigated (MACCIONI et al. 2002). In clinical practice complications are frequently assessed by barium studies, US and CT.

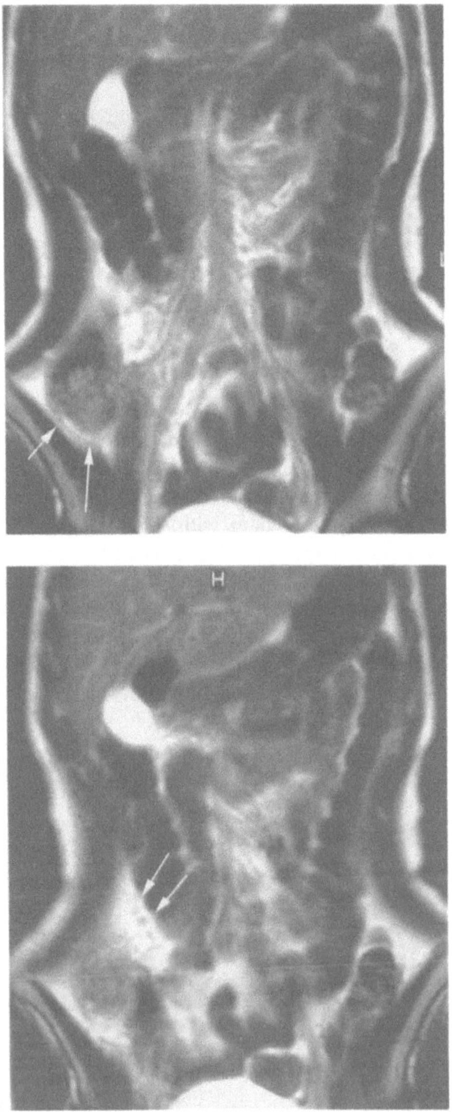

Fig. 20.1a,b. Clinically active ileocecal Crohn's disease in a 23-year-old patient. **a** Coronal T2-weighted TSE image obtained at 1.5 T after oral administration of a negative superparamagnetic contrast agent. An inflammatory mass is evident within the caecum, filling most of the lumen *(arrows)*. **b** Outside the caecum several small mesenteric lymph nodes are seen *(arrows)*. The distal ileum is also inflamed. **c** Axial T2-weighted image shows marked and irregular thickening of the cecal wall. **d** Fat suppressed T2-weighted axial image, obtained at the same level, shows high wall signal, suggestive of high grade wall inflammation. Endoscopy confirmed the presence of severe CD of the caecum

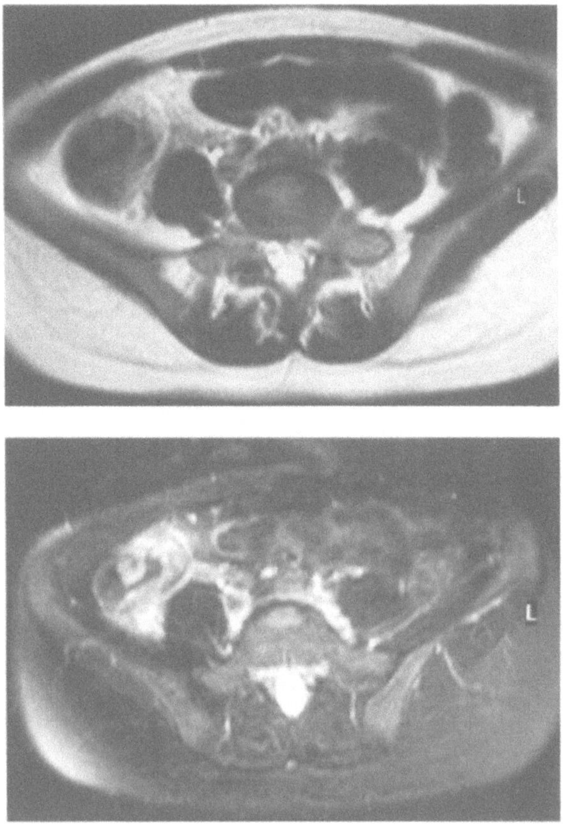

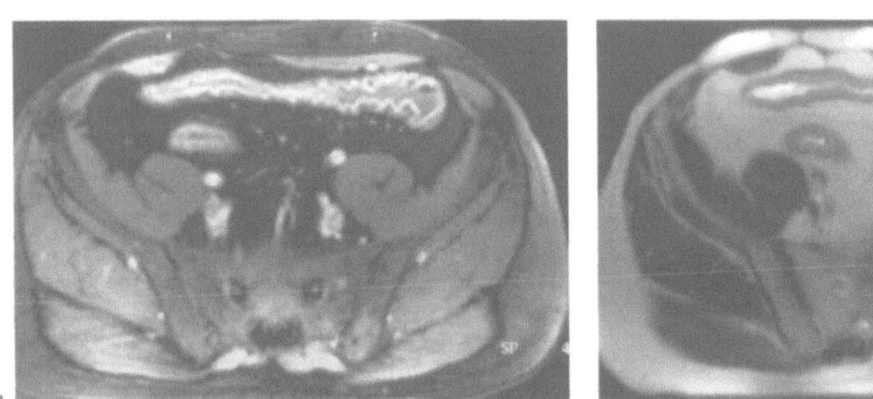

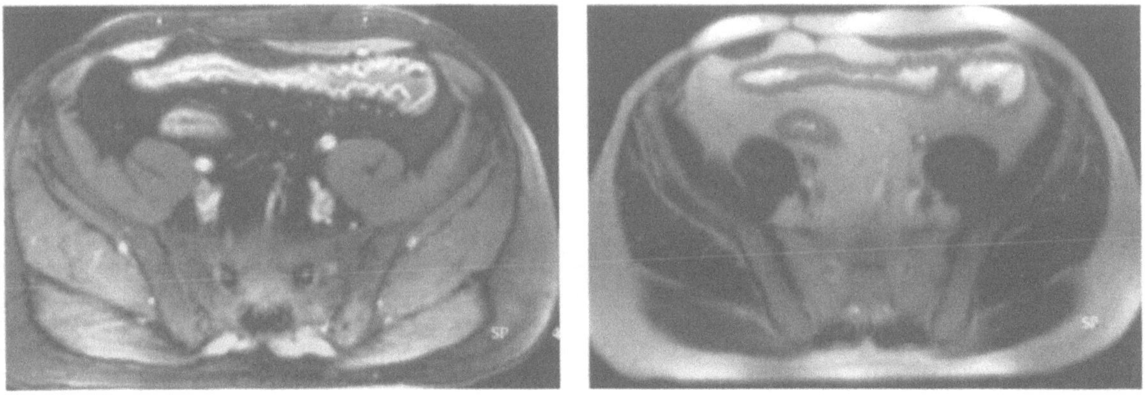

Fig. 20.2a,b. Active Crohn's disease of the sigmoid colon. **a** T1-weighted fat-suppressed post-gadolinium FLASH axial image shows marked wall enhancement and thickening. Dilation of local mesenteric vessels can be observed. **b** T2-weighted axial image shows diffuse wall thickening. The lumen is hyperintense due to the presence of intestinal fluid. Fibrofatty proliferation is evident outside the colon

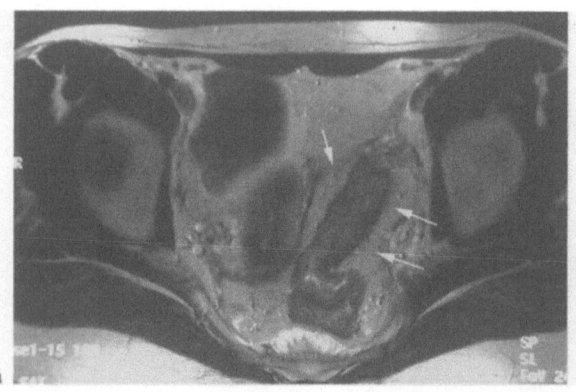
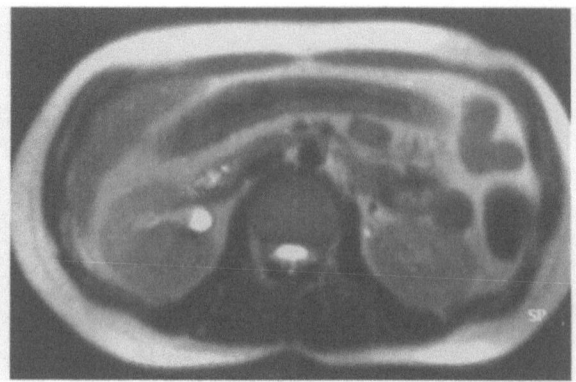

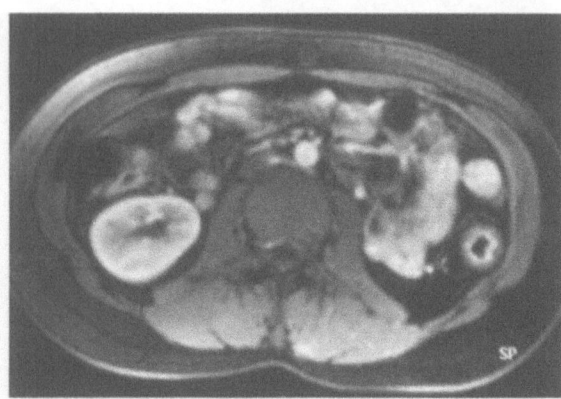

Fig. 20.3a–c. Crohn's colitis, with continuous involvement of the colon from the recto-sigmoid to the hepatic flexure. a High resolution breath-hold axial TSE T2-weighted image of the pelvis at 1.5 T showing marked wall thickening (more than 10 mm) of the entire sigmoid colon, with slight irregularity of the outer margin (*arrows*); signs suggestive of transmural involvement of CD. b HASTE T2-weighted breath-hold image (lower resolution) shows diffuse and marked wall thickening of the transverse and descending colon. c T1-weighted FLASH post-gadolinium axial image showing marked wall enhancement of the descending colon with dilation of the mesenteric vessels, suggesting active disease

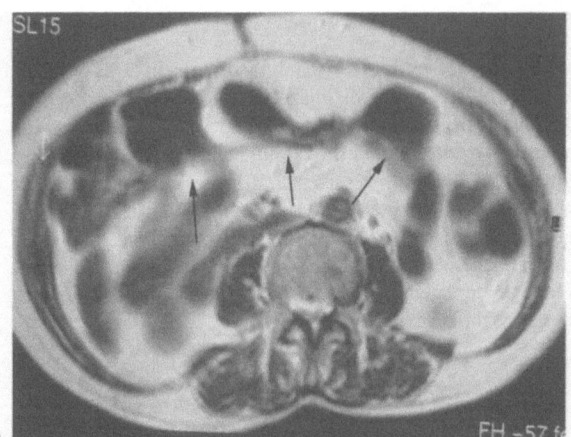
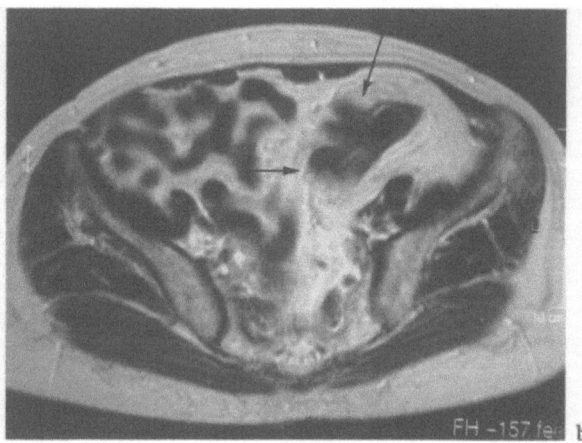

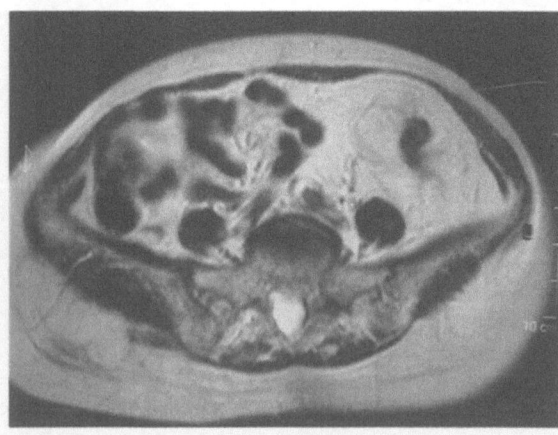

Fig. 20.4a–c. An 81-year-old female patient, with a long history of Crohn's pancolitis treated with corticosteroids. a Axial image obtained at the level of the transverse colon shows multiple sacculations of the anti-mesenteric border opposite a scarred mesenteric border (*arrows*). b Axial T2-weighted TSE image shows similar findings at the level of the sigmoid colon: marked wall thickening, pseudo-diverticular (*arrows*) of the antemesenteric border, and marked surrounding fibro-fatty proliferation. c An adjacent axial section better shows the large amount of fibrofatty proliferation with "mass effect" and displacement of adjacent ileal loops

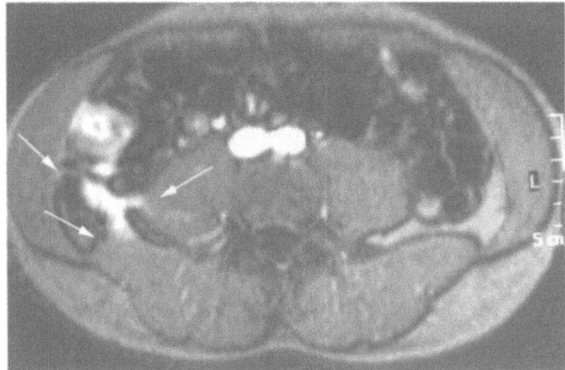

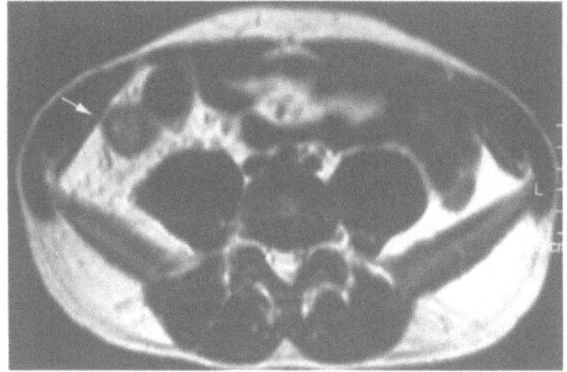

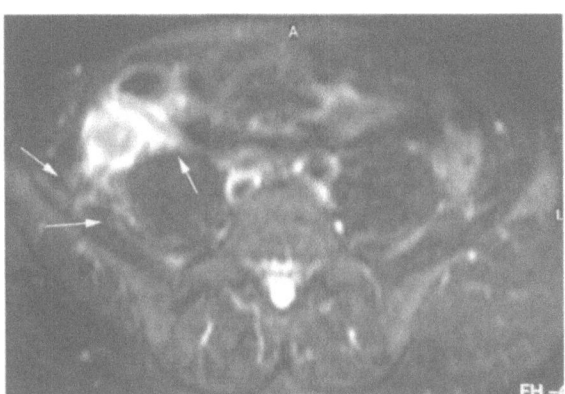

Fig. 20.5a–c. Crohn's disease of the right colon, complicated by a sinus that is involving the right psoas muscle. **a** Axial T1-weighted post-gadolinium image showing thickening and enhancement of the wall of the right colon from transmural inflammation and an inflammatory sinus tract directed towards the right psoas and quadratus lumborum muscles (*arrows*). **b** T2-weighted axial image, showing wall thickening of the right colon and surrounding hypertrophic mesenteric fat. **c** T2-weighted fat-suppressed axial image at a similar level showing transmural inflammation of the right colon and severe inflammation of the mesenteric fat (*arrows*) that was undetected on the non-suppressed image

The *site and severity of strictures* can be easily assessed by MRI on coronal T2-weighted images (Figs. 20.6). The evaluation of post-gadolinium T1-weighted images can be useful if there is significant wall enhancement at the site of the stricture, otherwise strictures are better appreciated on T2-weighted images.

The degree of stricturing can be evaluated on the basis of the pre-stenotic dilation, particularly if the examination is performed without anti-peristaltic agents (Fig. 20.7).

Adhesions are frequent in Crohn's disease and can be detected by MRI. Two adjacent thickened bowel loops that do not change position during the examination are associated with increased gadolinium enhancement and T2 signal at the level of contact, frequently with inhomogeneous perivisceral fat or free fluid, are typical findings of adhesions.

Adhesions frequently precede fistulation. *Fistulas* can be difficult to detect with MRI using negative contrast agents, as the tract can be missed or it can be impossible to differentiate between a fistula and an adhesion. Nevertheless fistulas are frequently detected in both axial and coronal planes on T1-weighted post-Gd and T2-weighted images (Figs. 20.7).

Abscesses can also be detected with MRI by using T1-post-contrast or T2-weighted sequences. MRI will also detect the other *main extraintestinal complications* of CD, including hydronephrosis, biliary and pancreatic disease.

Hydronephrosis due to ureteric obstruction may be caused by stones or by adjacent bowel inflammation or abscess. The left ureter can be involved by extensive sigmoid inflammation, whereas the right can be obstructed by severe inflammation of the distal ileum. A dilated renal pelvis and ureter has a hyperintense signal on T2-weighted axial and coronal images and the site and cause of obstruction can usually be recognized, particularly when using MIP reconstructions.

Biliary complications of CD include cholelithiasis, sclerosing cholangitis and cholangiocarcinoma. MRI is widely used to diagnose these complications. T2-weighted images and cholangio-MRI are used to evaluate obstructive disease, whereas gadolinium enhanced images are essential for the diagnosis of cholangiocarcinoma.

Pancreatic diseases associated with CD include pancreatitis (frequently related to immunosuppressive drugs) and pancreatic duct dilation, due to stones. Pancreatic duct dilation can be detected by using a cholangio-MRI technique.

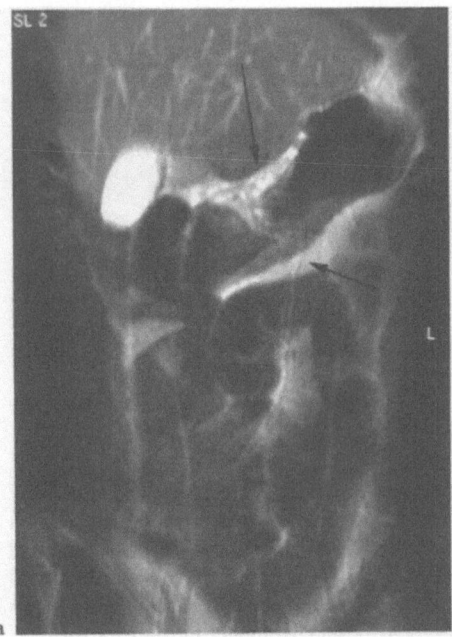

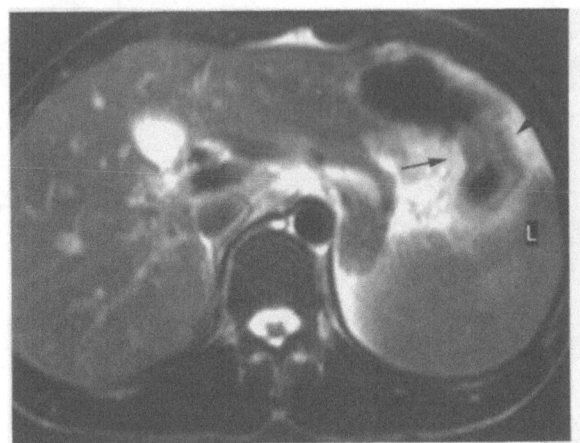

Fig. 20.6a,b. Long-standing Crohn's colitis, with multiple strictures. **a** Coronal T2-weighted image shows a marked focal wall thickening of the transverse colon, causing a stricture (*arrows*). **b** The axial image shows another stricture at the splenic flexure with wall thickening and surrounding fibrofatty proliferation (*arrows*)

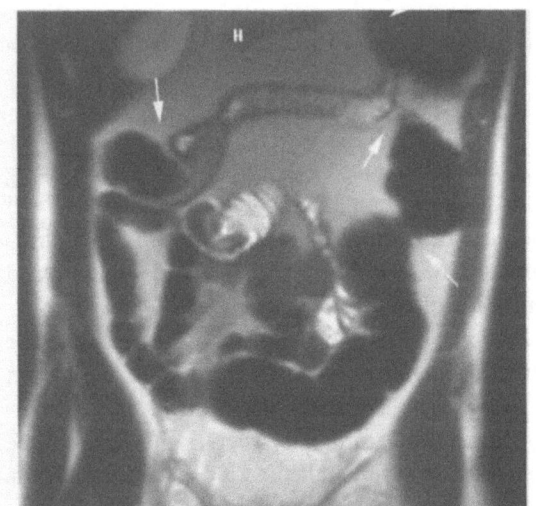

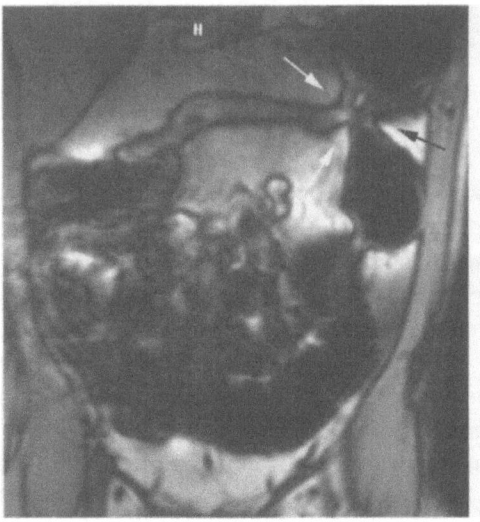

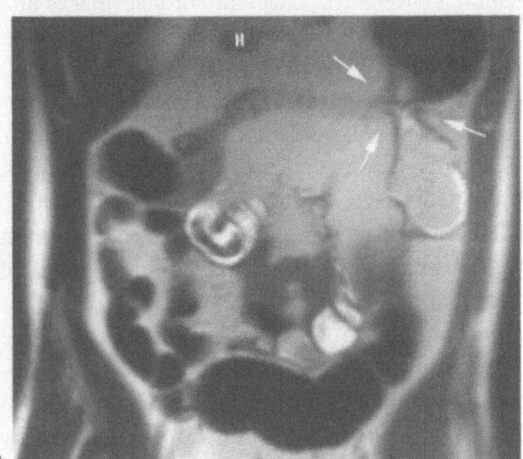

Fig. 20.7a–c. Long-standing Crohn's disease of the transverse and left colon with fistulation. **a** Coronal HASTE T2-weighted image, obtained after rectal insufflation of air. A long stricture of the transverse colon is evident, starting at the hepatic flexure where there is pre-stenotic dilation and mural thickening (*arrow*). Another short tight stricture is evident in the mid descending colon (*arrow*). The splenic flexure is distorted (*arrow*). **b** Adjacent coronal section clearly shows a fistula (*three arrows*) which by-passes the splenic flexure (distended by gas). **c** The fistula is also clearly seen, between the distal transverse colon and the proximal descending colon, on this coronal T1-weighted FLASH image

20.4.3
Assessment of Crohn's Disease Activity

Periodic assessment of the inflammatory activity predicts outcome and so determines pharmacological and surgical planning. The recent classification of CD into three sub-groups with increasing local inflammatory activity (fibro-stenosing, inflammatory and perforating disease), reflects the need of both gastroenterologists and gastrointestinal surgeons to distinguish between these three groups on the basis of local inflammatory activity (LASNER 2000). The first group usually benefits from surgical therapy, the second from pharmacological treatment, whereas the third usually requires both.

Assessment of inflammatory activity is also vital for monitoring the effects of drugs. So far, an effective and definitive pharmacological therapy does not exist, and each individual patient needs to be studied and monitored to assess which of the various drug regimes proves most effective. New drugs also continuously need to be assessed. Inflammation is currently evaluated by a combination of clinical symptoms, physical findings, laboratory parameters, endoscopy and barium studies.

Recent preliminary studies have shown MRI to be accurate in the evaluation of inflammation of the bowel wall and perivisceral fat. A significant statistical correlation has been found between all the main MRI signs of inflammation (wall enhancement/T2 wall signal/T2 mesenteric fat signal) and active disease (Figs. 20.1d, 20.5c), whereas in inactive lesions these signs were absent (Figs. 20.4). A significant statistical correlation ($p<0.0001$, correlation values ranging from 0.847 to 0.927) has been found between gadolinium wall enhancement and biological activity of the disease (KOH et al. 2001; LOW et al. 2002; MACCIONI 2002); a similar statistical correlation was also found for the high T2 signal of the wall and the T2 hyperintensity of the mesenteric fat (MACCIONI et al. 2000; MACCIONI 2002).

Monitoring disease activity with MRI without exposing patients to radiation is attractive to researchers conducting clinical trials on new drugs for UC and CD. In a recent trial of the new drug anti-TNF-alpha (infliximab) in severe CD, it was found, that after 4 weeks of treatment, MRI showed a marked decrease in wall thickening, T2 signal and gadolinium enhancement in those patients who showed clinical and biological signs of response to the new treatment.

20.5
MRI Findings in Ulcerative Colitis

Classically, UC involves the rectosigmoid (95% of patients at endoscopy) and extends proximally, involving the colon continuously; only rarely does the disease just involve the right colon. The distal ileum can be inflamed in the presence of a pancolitis.

Thickening of the bowel wall can be easily visualized on axial and coronal T1- and T2-weighted images. The thickening is less pronounced than in CD, with a mean of 7.8 mm as compared to 13 mm for CD (PHILPOTTS et al. 1994). However, a marked thickening of the rectal wall, exceeding 10 mm, can frequently be observed in active UC (Figs. 20.8). The inner profile of the wall may have a wavy configuration (Fig. 20.9) in both UC and CD but as the inflammation is intramural in UC the outer wall is sharper and smoother as compared to CD where there is transmural extension of the inflammation (Fig. 20.3).

Increased thickness of the submucosal layer from edema or proliferation of submucosal fat, is a typical feature of UC observed on CT (JONES et al. 1986; MULDOWNEY et al. 1995; GORE et al. 1996). This feature is also observed with MRI but with T2-weighted fat-suppressed images, it is possible to distinguish between submucosal fat and edema, thus characterizing the wall inflammation and grading the activity of the disease (Fig. 20.8).

Wall enhancement following gadolinium on T1-weighted images is usually observed in active UC and CD and associated with wall thickening. The degree of wall enhancement can be related to the inflammatory activity (Figs. 20.8, 20.9).

Mesenteric fibrofatty proliferation is a finding associated with CD rather than UC. However, prominent perirectal fibrofatty proliferation and widening of the presacral space has frequently been reported in UC and this may extend to the mesentery of the sigmoid colon (Figs. 20.8, 20.9).

Although *signs of perivisceral inflammation* are typical of CD, it is not uncommon to observe on T2-weighted images minimal amounts of fluid around diseased bowel in UC indicative of local serosal inflammation (Fig. 20.9). Adhesions can also be observed in UC but are less frequent than in CD.

Finally, in patients with UC who have had a total colectomy and an ileo-anal pouch constructed, inflammation of the wall of the pouch can be observed ("*pouchitis*"). MRI can not only assess the inflammation of the walls of the pouch but can also detect complications, such as strictures, adhesions and phlegmon.

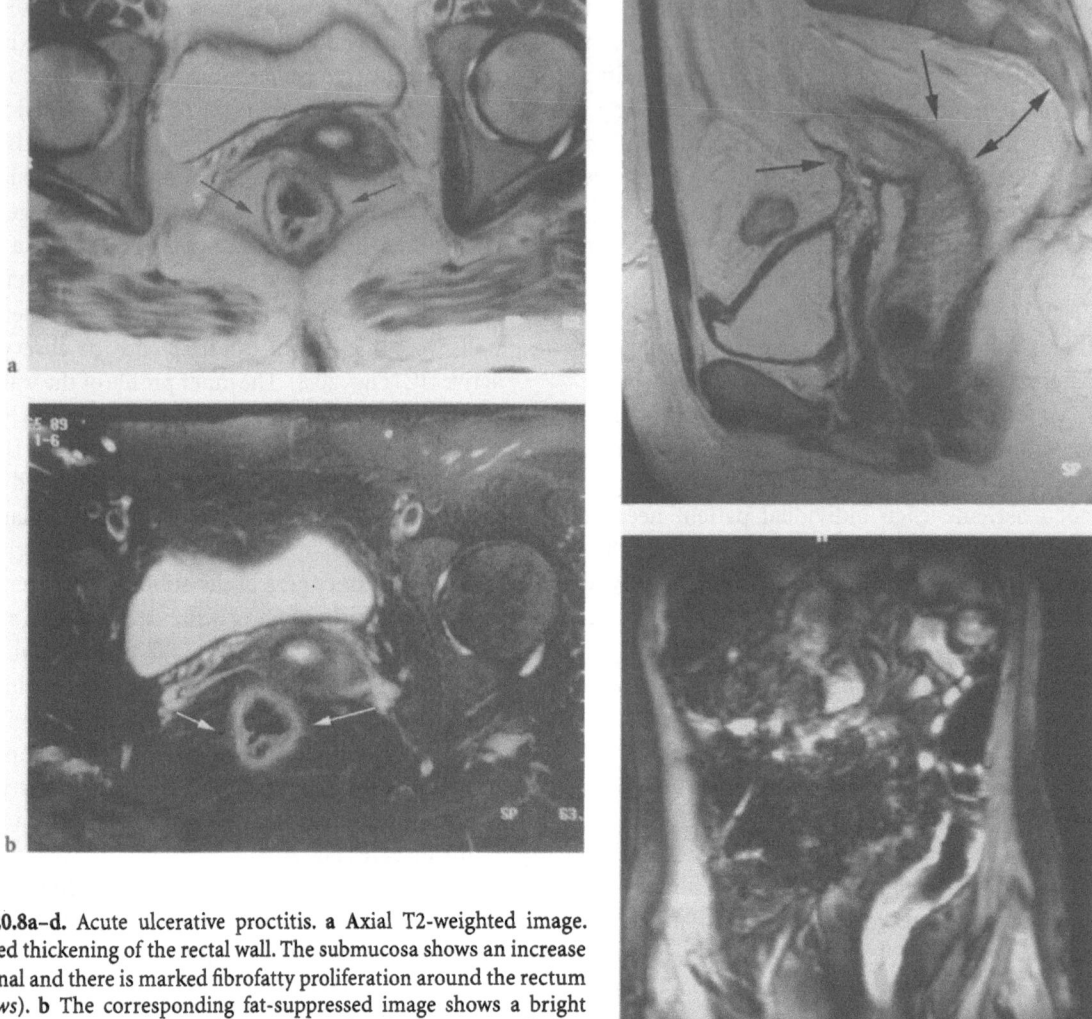

Fig. 20.8a–d. Acute ulcerative proctitis. **a** Axial T2-weighted image. Marked thickening of the rectal wall. The submucosa shows an increase in signal and there is marked fibrofatty proliferation around the rectum (*arrows*). **b** The corresponding fat-suppressed image shows a bright signal from the submucosa of the rectal wall, indicating active disease with submucosal edema. **c** The same findings are well displayed in the sagittal plane. There is diffuse rectal wall thickening (*arrows*), as well as thickening of the pre-sacral fat (*arrows*). A balloon catheter is present at the ano-rectal junction for colonic insufflation. **d** The T1-weighted post-gadolinium image shows cranial extension of the ulcerative colitis to the mid descending colon. The involved colon shows wall thickening and gadolinium enhancement

The diagnosis of *infectious colitis* is made by bacteriology and so far, there is no experience of the role of MRI in the evaluation of infectious acute colitis. The ability to detect bowel wall and mesenteric inflammation predicts a potential role for MRI for evaluating the extent and severity of these diseases (Fig. 20.10). Nevertheless, the definitive diagnosis of infectious or idiopathic inflammatory bowel disease ultimately depends on histology and bacteriology (GORE et al. 1997).

20.6
Differential Diagnosis Between CD and UC with MRI

As MRI can demonstrate inflammation of both the small and large bowel it can be useful for differentiating between CD and UC. However, although inflammation of both the small and large bowel strongly suggest CD, mild inflammation of the distal ileum can be observed in UC (backwash ileitis).

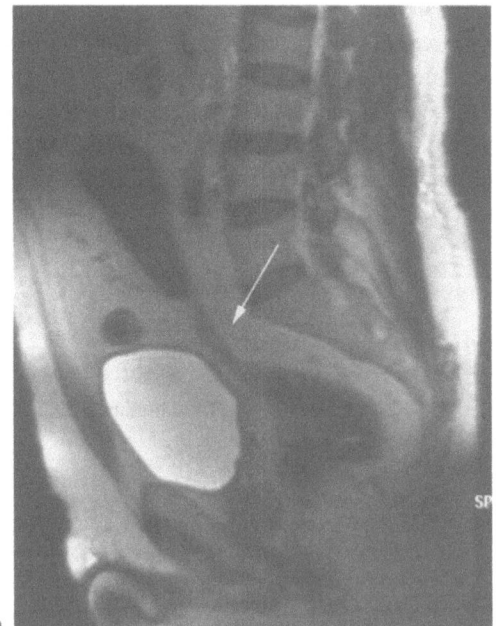

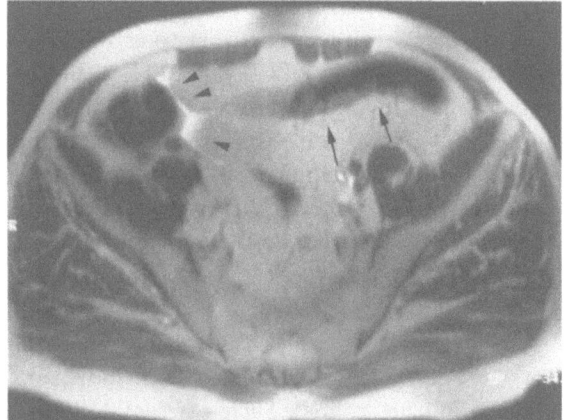

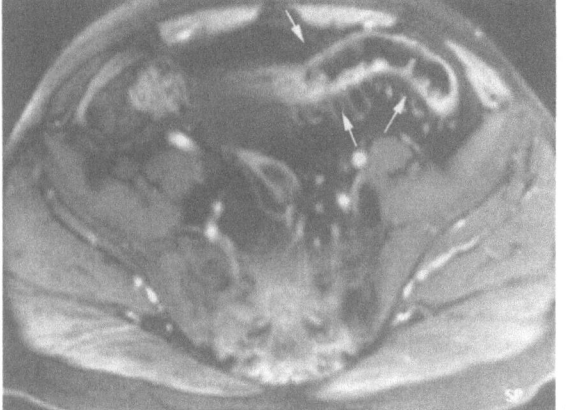

Fig. 20.9a–c. Active ulcerative proctosigmoiditis with a stricture at the recto-sigmoid junction. **a** Sagittal T2-weighted HASTE image shows a tight stricture above the rectum that prevented the passage of an endoscope. Thickening of the pre-sacral fat is also evident. **b** The axial T2-weighted HASTE image shows wall thickening of the sigmoid colon, with a regular outer margin and an irregular inner margin (*arrows*); signs characteristic of ulcerative colitis. A minimal amount of free fluid is evident (*arrowheads*) and there is a possible adhesion to the cecal wall. Active disease of the entire sigmoid colon was diagnosed. c Axial T1-weighted FLASH post-gadolinium image shows diffuse wall enhancement at the level of the sigmoid colon, suggesting active disease

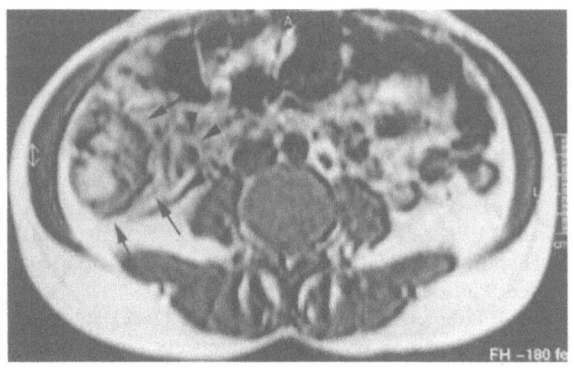

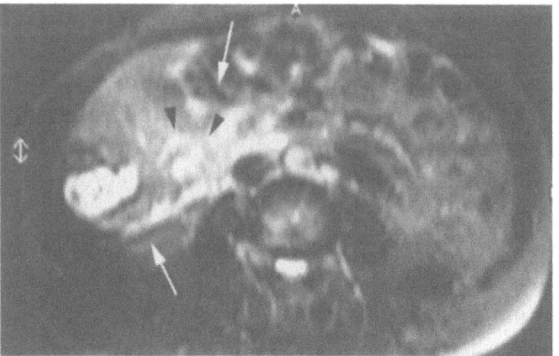

Fig. 20.10a,b. *Yersinia enterocolitis* in a patient affected by thalassemia minor. **a** The examination was performed with a 0.5-T magnet. Thickening of the cecal wall (*arrows*) is evident on this T1-weighted axial image and there is proliferation and inhomogeneity of the perivisceral fat, with local lymph node enlargement (*arrowheads*). **b** On the T2-weighted fat suppressed image there is a diffuse hyperintensity to the perivisceral fat suggesting mesenteric inflammation (between *arrows*)

The differential diagnosis can be more difficult when inflammation is confined to the colon. Segmental involvement or the evidence of trans-mural disease favors a diagnosis of CD (Figs. 20.5, 20.6, 20.7). There is usually less bowel wall thickening in UC and the outer wall profile is sharper and smoother. (Figs. 20.3, 20.9). Inflammatory involvement of the mesenteric fat is more frequently observed in CD and fistulas, sinus tracts, adhesions and abscesses are hallmarks of CD. However, in some patients with chronic colitis, a precise diagnosis may not initially be possible either clinically, histologically or by using any of the other diagnostic modalities, including MRI ("indeterminate" colitis). Such cases at MRI have a mixture of features of CD and UC (PRICE 1978; KANGAS et al. 1994).

20.7
Conclusions: Role of MRI
in the Management of Colitis

The intrinsic proprieties of MRI, such as its high contrast resolution, the availability of multiple imaging parameters, the sensitivity of T2-weighted sequences for inflammation, the possibility of modulating the signal by using fat-suppression, the enhancement obtained after gadolinium injection, make it an excellent imaging modality for the investigation of the entire bowel. For this reason it is likely that MRI will play an increasing role in the evaluation of IBD.

In CD and UC, MRI, when performed with attention to technique, has been shown to be a reliable diagnostic tool, capable of detecting most of the typical features of these diseases and their complications.

As UC is an inflammatory disease limited to the inner layers of the wall, with rare extra-intestinal complications, a predictable course which progresses proximally and continuously through the colon, and rare involvement of the distal ileum, it can be easily and completely assessed by colonoscopy. The role of imaging, and particularly of MRI, can be to distinguish between CD and UC in uncertain cases; to assess ileal involvement; to assess the extent of disease in the presence of tight strictures that prevent endoscopic evaluation of the entire colon; to evaluate the degree of wall inflammation by considering gadolinium enhancement and the T2 signal.

Finally MRI can assess the ileo-anal pouch after total colectomy.

MRI is at present the only imaging modality able to produce excellent images of affected bowel in any spatial plane using different imaging parameters and without radiation exposure. Preliminary studies have shown MRI to be a powerful diagnostic tool for detecting the main morphological abnormalities, degree of inflammation, and complications of CD in both the small and large bowel, and thus MRI will probably become a primary imaging modality for the global assessment of CD.

References

Debatin JF, Patak MA (1999) MRI of the small and large bowel. Eur Radiol 9:1523–1534

Ernst O, Asselah T, Cablan X et al (1998) Breath-hold fast spin-echo MR imaging of Crohn's disease. AJR 170:127–128

Farmer RG, Hawk WA, Turnbull RB (1975) Clinical patterns in Crohn's disease: a statistical study of 615 cases. Gastroenterology 68:627–635

Giovagnoni A, Fabbri F, Maccioni F (2002) Oral contrast agent in MRI of the gastrointestinal tract. Abdom Imaging 27: 367–375

Goldberg HI, Caruthers SB Jr, Nelson JA et al (1979) Radiographic findings of the National Cooperative Crohn's Disease Study. Gastroenterology 77:925–933

Gore RM (1994) Cross sectional imaging of the colon. In: Gore RM, Levine MS, Laufer I (eds) Textbook of gastrointestinal radiology. Saunders, Philadelphia, pp 1052–1063

Gore RM, Balthazar EJ, Ghahremani GG et al (1996) CT features of ulcerative colitis and Crohn's disease. AJR 167:3–15

Gore RM, Ghahremani GG, Miller FH (1997) Inflammatory bowel disease: radiologic diagnosis. In: Balfe DM, Levine MS (eds) Syllabus of Radiological Society of North America Categorical Course in Gastrointestinal Radiology. RSNA, pp 95–110

Gourtsoyiannis N, Papanikolaou N, Grammatikakis J et al (2001) MR enteroclysis protocol optimization: comparison between 3D FLASH with fat saturation after intravenous gadolinium injection and true FISP sequences. Eur Radiol 11:908–913

Hann PF, Stark DD , Lewis JM et al (1990) First clinical trial of a new superparamagnetic iron oxide for use as an oral gastrointestinal contrast agent in MR imaging. Radiology 175:695–700

Jewell DP (1993) Ulcerative colitis. In: Sleisenger MH, Foerdtran JS (eds) Gastrointestinal disease, 4th edn. Saunders, Philadelphia, pp 1305–1330

Jones B, Fishman EK, Hamilton SR et al (1986) Submucosal accumulation of fat in inflammatory bowel disease: CT/pathologic correlation J Comput Assist Tomogr 10: 759–763

Kangas E, Matikainen M, Mattila J (1994) Is "indeterminate colitis" Crohn's disease in the long-term follow-up? Int Surg 79:120–125

Kettritz U, Isaaks K, Warshauer DM et al (1995) Crohn disease. Pilot study comparing MRI of the abdomen with clinical evaluation. J Clin Gastroenterol 21:249–253

Klein VHM, Wein B, Adam G et al (1995) Computed tomography of Crohn's disease and ulcerative colitis. Fortschr Roentgenstr 163:9–15

Koh DM, Miao Y, Chinn RJ et al (2001) MR imaging evaluation of the activity of Crohn's disease. AJR 117:1325–1332

Laghi A, Carbone I, Catalano C et al (2001) Polyethyline glycol solution as an oral contrast agent for MR Imaging of the small bowel. Am J Roentgenol 177:1333–1334

Lasner BH (2000) Clinical Features, course, laboratory findings, and complications in ulcerative colitis. In: Kirsner JB (ed) Inflammatory bowel disease, 5th edn. Saunders, Philadelphia, pp 305–314

Lee JK, Semelka RC (1998) MR imaging of the small bowel using the HASTE sequence. AJR 170:1457–1463

Lomas DJ (1999) The potential of MR for small bowel imaging. Imaging 11:161–169

Low RN, Sebrechts CP, Politoske DA et al (2002) Crohn disease with endoscopic correlation: single shot fast spin echo and gadolinium enhanced fat-suppressed spoiled gradient-echo MR imaging. Radiology 222:652–660

Maccioni F (2002) Current status of gastrointestinal MRI. Abdom Imaging 27:384–393

Maccioni F, Viscido A, Broglia L et al (2000) Evaluation of Crohn disease activity with MRI. Abdom Imaging 25:219–228

Maccioni F, Viscido A, Marini M et al (2002) MRI evaluation of Crohn's disease of the small and large bowel with the use of negative superparamagnetic oral contrast agents. Abdom Imaging 27:384–393

Madsen SM, Thomsen HS, Munkholm P et al (1998) Active Crohn's disease and ulcerative colitis evaluated by low-field magnetic resonance imaging. Scand J Gastroenterol 33:1193–1200

Madsen SM, Thomsen HS, Schlichting P et al (1999) Evaluation of treatment response in active Crohn's disease by low-field magnetic resonance imaging. Abdom Imaging 24:232–239

Miner PB (2000) Clinical features, course, laboratory findings, and complications in ulcerative colitis. In: Kirsner JB (ed) Inflammatory bowel disease, 5th edn. Saunders, Philadelphia, pp 299–304

Muldowney SM, Balfe DM, Hammerman A et al (1995) "Acute" fat deposition in bowel wall submucosa: CT appearance. J Comput Assist Tomogr 19:390–393

Philpotts LE, Heiken JP, Westcott MA et al (1994) Colitis: use of CT findings in differential diagnosis. Radiology 190:445–449

Price AB (1978) Overlap in the spectrum of non-specific inflammatory bowel disease "colitis indeterminate". J Clin Pathol 31:567–574

Rieber A, Aschoff A, Nussle K et al (2000) MRI in the diagnosis of small bowel disease: use of positive and negative oral contrast media in combination with enteroclysis. Eur Radiol 10:1377–1382

Riddell RH (1998) Pathology of idiopathic inflammatory bowel disease. In: Kirsner JB (ed) Inflammatory bowel disease, 5th edn. Saunders, Philadelphia, pp 427–447

Rioux M, Gagnon J (1997) Imaging modalities in the puzzling world of inflammatory bowel disease. Abdom Imaging 22:173–174

Semelka RC, Shoenut RP, Silverman R et al (1991) Bowel disease: prospective comparison of CT and 1.5 T pre- and post-contrast MR imaging with T1-weighted fat-suppressed and breath-hold FLASH sequences. J Magn Res Imag 1:625–632

Shoenut JP, Semelka RC, Silverman R et al (1993) Magnetic resonance imaging in inflammatory bowel disease. J Clin Gastroenterol 17:73–78

Shoenut JP, Semelka RC, Magro CM et al (1994) Comparison of magnetic resonance imaging and endoscopy in distinguishing the type and severity of inflammatory bowel disease. J Clin Gastroenterol 19:31–35

Truelove SC, Pena AS (1976) Course and prognosis of Crohn's disease. Gut 17:192–198

Wildersmuth S, Debatin JF (1999) Virtual endoscopy in abdominal MR imaging. Magn Reson Imaging Clin North Am 7:349–364

Wills JS, Lobis IF, Denstman FJ (1997) Crohn disease: state of the art. Radiology 202:597–610

21 Colonic Scintigraphy

PHILIP J. A. ROBINSON

CONTENTS

21.1   Introduction 215
21.2   Scintigraphic Investigation of Colonic Bleeding 215
21.2.1 The Clinical Problem 215
21.2.2 Technique using Labelled Autologous
        Red Blood Cells 216
21.2.3 Interpretation of Labelled RBC Images 216
21.2.4 Labelled Colloid Technique and Interpretation 217
21.2.5 Results of Scintigraphic Methods 218
21.3   Radionuclide Imaging of Colitis 218
21.3.1 Techniques 218
21.3.2 Interpretation 219
21.3.3 Clinical Applications 219
21.4   Colonic Transit Studies Using Radionuclides 220
21.4.1 Techniques 220
21.4.2 Interpretation 221
21.4.3 Clinical Applications 222
21.5   Immuno-scintigraphy for Colonic Cancer 222
21.5.1 Techniques 223
21.5.2 Interpretation 224
21.5.3 Results in Colon Cancer 224
21.5.4 Radio-immuno-Guided Surgery (RIGS) 224
        References 225

21.1
Introduction

First-line investigation of colonic pathology requires anatomic imaging. The use of scintigraphic studies is limited to specific clinical situations in which the physiologic disturbances caused by disease are recognised most effectively by functional imaging. These include intestinal bleeding, inflammatory bowel disease, motility disturbances, and malignancy.

P. J. A. ROBINSON, MD
Professor of Radiology, Clinical Radiology Department, St. James's University Hospital, Leeds, LS9 7TF, UK

21.2
Scintigraphic Investigation of Colonic Bleeding

21.2.1
The Clinical Problem

A steady decline in the incidence of peptic ulcer disease over the last few decades has changed the spectrum of patients presenting with gastrointestinal bleeding. There is still a majority of patients in whom the source is in the oesophagus, stomach or duodenum and in most of these cases early endoscopy identifies the site of bleeding and provides access for direct local treatment of the lesion. Bleeding sites in the remainder of the patients are most often in the large bowel, with the small intestine and Meckel's diverticulum accounting for a lesser proportion of cases.

Colonoscopy is less successful than upper GI endoscopy for several reasons. Colonic contents may obscure the endoscopic view, whilst bleeding may stop if time is allowed for full bowel preparation. Blood in the colonic lumen may move retrogradely, so the distribution of blood at colonoscopy is an unreliable indicator of the site of bleeding. Adherent thrombus and other stigmata of recent or active bleeding are less often found with colonic pathology than in the upper GI tract. Even when colonoscopy or barium enema shows large bowel pathology, there is no certainty that the lesion found is the site of bleeding, particularly with diverticular disease which is commonly present in asymptomatic patients.

In the majority of cases, colonic bleeding stops spontaneously so supportive treatment is usually adequate and colonoscopy or barium enema examination can follow after full bowel preparation, in order to seek structural abnormalities. It is in those patients in whom bleeding continues or recurs that identification of the bleeding site becomes urgent. Morbidity and mortality are greatest in those patients whose bleeding site is not found, so the use of scintigraphic techniques to localise the bleeding lesion allows suitably focused surgical or angiographic treatment. In relation to angiography, scintigraphy has advantages in that it is a little more sensitive in detecting low rates of bleeding, it can detect venous extravasation as well as arterial bleeding, it can detect intermittent bleeding over a period of several hours, and it is less invasive. Finally, there has been a recent increase in the proportion of patients presenting with GI haemorrhage who have co-morbidities, in many cases unrelated to the gastrointestinal tract (GOSTOUT et al. 1992). In these patients the GI bleeding is a complication of severe illness arising from other pathologies (for example advanced malignancy, severe renal or hepatic insufficiency, haematological disorders) and this factor increases the risk of exploratory surgical intervention and emphasises the need for non-invasive localisation techniques.

Although the scintigraphic methods described below have been shown to detect very slow bleeding rates in experimental models (ALAVI et al. 1977), in clinical practice the amount of intestinal bleeding required to produce a positive scintigraphic result is approximately the same as that required to produce melena. GI bleeding which is of such a slow rate that it does not produce melena and can only be detected by chemical tests for blood in the stool, will rarely if ever be detected by scintigraphic methods.

In summary, the appropriate indicators for selecting patients for scintigraphic investigation of GI bleeding are:

1. At least enough bleeding to cause melena
2. Continuing or recurrent episodes of bleeding
3. Colonoscopy negative, inconclusive, or contra-indicated
4. The presence of co-morbidities which increase the risks of invasive investigation and treatment

21.2.2
Technique using Labelled Autologous Red Blood Cells

The most widely used technique involves labelling a sample of the patient's own red cells with ^{99m}Tc-pertechnetate, then re-injecting them into the patient (FORD et al. 2001). Labelling is best carried out in vitro, which allows free pertechnetate to be washed off the cell sample before re-injection. An in vivo technique can be performed by first tagging the cells with a reducing agent (e.g. stannous chloride), then subsequently injecting sodium pertechnetate. This is quicker and simpler, but produces less effective

binding and the small proportion of free pertechnetate which remains in the circulation may make interpretation of the images more difficult. A compromise technique involves withdrawing blood into a heparinized syringe containing the pertechnetate and reducing agent, mixing the blood in the syringe (still attached to the patient) for several minutes, then re-injecting.

A fast dynamic sequence of abdominal images, obtained immediately after a bolus injection of red cells labelled with up to 400 MBq of ^{99m}Tc pertechnetate, is used to detect major vascular abnormalities. Subsequently, images are obtained at 5 min intervals up to about 1 h and if no abnormality has been shown, at further intervals up to 24 h. With effective labelling, the tracer remains in the circulation with only a small amount of free pertechnetate being gradually excreted via the urinary tract.

21.2.3
Interpretation of Labelled RBC Images

Intestinal bleeding produces an accumulation of labelled red cells adjacent to the bleeding point which can then be detected by gamma camera imaging. With this method the blood background remains high, so the volume of extravasation needed for detection is in the region of 50–70 ml of blood, which is about the same amount required to produce melena. Because the tracer remains stable within the circulation, sequential imaging up to 24 h gives an opportunity to detect intermittent or very slow rates of bleeding.

The initial vascular phase indicates the relative blood flow to the main abdominal organs and later images show persistent blood pool activity in the liver, spleen, kidneys and often also the proximal small bowel. The aorta, IVC, iliac vessels and portal vein are usually visible. A bleeding site is recognised as a focus of extravasated activity outside the normal vascular landmarks. With small bowel bleeding, the extravasated activity usually moves along the lumen quite quickly, changing its location between consecutive images at 5-min intervals. With colonic bleeding, the movement of extravasated blood is slower and it is important to remember that blood in the colon can move proximally as well as distally. It may be helpful, particularly in patients who have undergone previous bowel resection, to compare the scintigraphic images with a recent abdominal radiograph or barium study in order to delineate the anatomic layout of the large bowel. Visible extravasation within the first hour or so after injection of the labelled cells is usually a reliable indicator of the location of bleeding (Fig. 21.1). When extravasation is only visualised on delayed images, consideration needs to be given to the likelihood of movement of blood along the bowel lumen. For example, extravasation which is first seen in the caecum on late images could result from bleeding within the caecum but might also arise from slow or intermittent small bowel haemorrhage. In general, the earlier the detection of extravasation, the more reliable is the localisation of the bleeding lesion. Studies which are positive only on delayed images are less accurate in predicting subsequent surgical or angiographic findings, but also indicate less rapid blood loss.

Replay of sequential images as a cine-loop gives a helpful demonstration of the movement of extravasated activity along the bowel, and may assist localisation in difficult cases. Pitfalls in interpretation include the presence of free pertechnetate in the circulation which is excreted by the urinary tract.

Bladder activity is usually easy to recognise, but activity in a dilated renal pelvis could simulate bowel haemorrhage. Free pertechnetate is also secreted by the normal colonic mucosa, producing a faint visualisation of the colon which is a normal finding on 24 h images. In female patients, particularly in the younger age group, the uterus can produce a fairly intense and persistent vascular blush.

21.2.4
Labelled Colloid Technique and Interpretation

An alternative technique which is less widely used involves the intravenous injection of ^{99m}Tc labelled colloid. Particles in the size range 30–1000 nm are rapidly removed from the circulation by reticuloendothelial cells in the liver, spleen and bone marrow. In patients who are actively bleeding at the time of injection, a

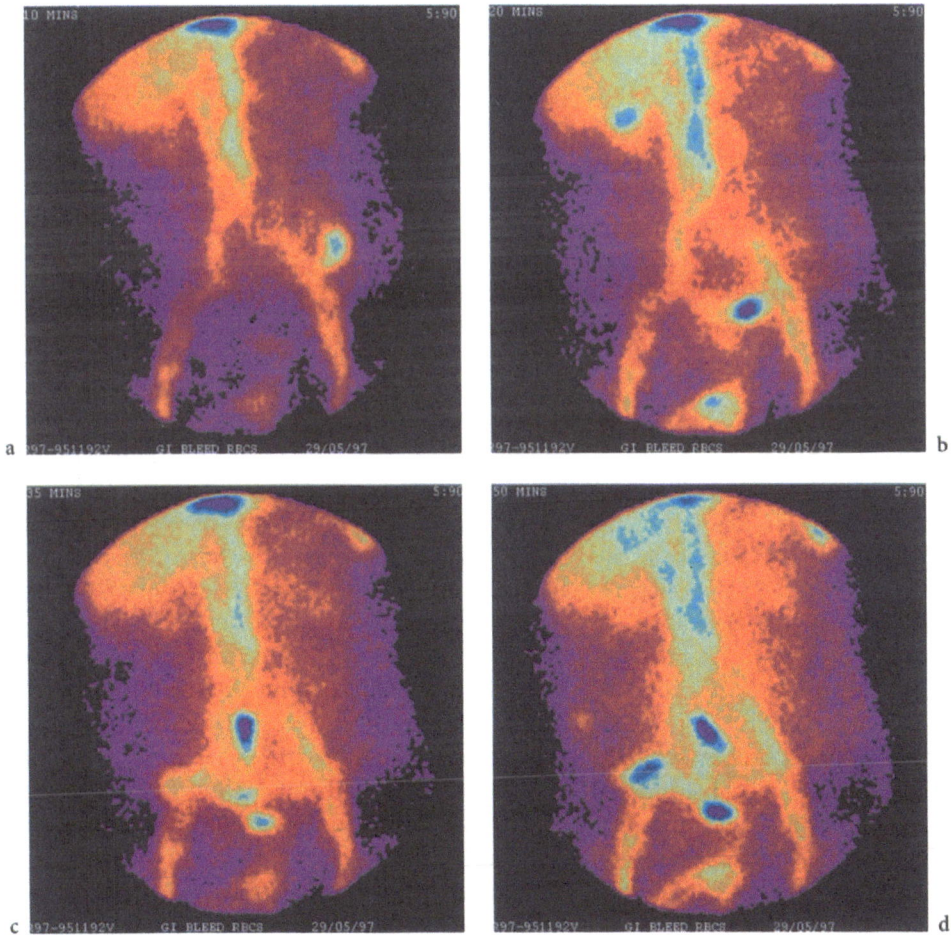

Fig. 21.1a–d. Tc^{99m} labelled red blood cell scintigraphy in a patient with colonic bleeding. Images at 10 min (**a**), 20 min (**b**), 35 min (**c**) and 50 min (**d**) after re-injection of autologous labelled red cells showing extravasation into distal descending colon (**a**) and subsequent onward movement of the extravasated blood into the pelvic colon

focus of extravasated tracer accumulates adjacent to the bleeding point and because the blood background is cleared within a few minutes, even a small focus of bleeding can be visualised. In animal models, this technique is more sensitive than the labelled red cell method both in detecting low rates of bleeding (down to 0.1–0.2 ml/min) and in the accuracy of localisation. These advantages arise from the short blood half-life of the labelled colloid (2–3 min) which enables small volumes of extravasation to be detected, but this factor is also responsible for the main disadvantage of the colloid method – success requires the patient to be bleeding actively. Since bleeding is often intermittent, a spurious negative result may be obtained if the patient has stopped bleeding at the time of the investigation. The major advantage of the colloid method is that when it is positive, the result is obtained within a few minutes and the localisation is accurate. The technique is relatively simple – up to 400 MBq of ^{99m}Tc-colloid (proprietary kits are suitable) is injected and sequential images obtained during the first pass phase, then at 1-min intervals up to 5 min, then at 5-min intervals up to 30 min. Oblique views are often helpful to assist in localisation. After the initial vascular phase, the tracer is rapidly taken up by the liver, spleen and bone marrow. A bleeding site is indicated by a focus of activity outside the normal anatomic landmarks. Because uptake in the liver and spleen obscures the upper abdomen, it is important to continue imaging up to 30 min in order to detect movement of blood along the colonic lumen which might indicate a bleeding point in the splenic or hepatic flexures.

21.2.5
Results of Scintigraphic Methods

Since their introduction about 25 years ago, the scintigraphic techniques have been compared with angiography, endoscopy, surgery and follow up. Using autologous red cells labelled with ^{99m}Tc pertechnetate, numerous reports indicate that the presence and approximate site of bleeding is detected correctly in 75%–90% of patients in whom later invasive methods confirm a source of bleeding (Suzman et al. 1996; Rantis et al. 1995; Sommer et al. 1996). Although the colloid technique, when positive, is quicker, more sensitive and more precise than the red cell method, the intermittent nature of bleeding in many patients reduces the value of this approach, and direct comparison of the two methods in the same population of patients has favoured using the red cell method. Numerous surgical reports have confirmed a role for scintigraphic imaging in those

patients with intestinal bleeding in whom endoscopy is inconclusive or negative. Positive scintigraphy helps to direct the subsequent angiographic or surgical treatment with a consequent reduction in morbidity and mortality. Negative scintigraphy is also helpful since it is associated with a better prognosis, reduced likelihood of subsequent surgery, and a shorter stay in hospital.

21.3
Radionuclide Imaging of Colitis

Several different radiopharmaceuticals have been used to localise infection. Initially promising results with labelled colloids, human immunoglobulin, porphyrins, dextran, and polyethylene glycol-liposomes remain unconfirmed. A labelled antibody fragment (^{99m}Tc-sulesomab) has been used, but appears less accurate than ^{99m}Tc-labelled leukocytes (Stokkel et al. 2002). Some success has been achieved with ^{99m}Tc-labelled ciprofloxacin (Infecton) but more development is needed before this agent can be brought into routine clinical use. The techniques which are most widely used, and with which most experience has been obtained, involve labelling of autologous leukocytes with either ^{111}In or ^{99m}Tc.

21.3.1
Techniques

Initial experience with leukocyte imaging used a combination of ^{111}In (half-life 68 h) with one of several chelating agents, of which tropolone is the most widely employed. The technique requires harvesting the leukocytes from 30–50 ml of the patient's blood, labelling the cells in vitro, and re-injecting them into the patient. Gamma camera images are then obtained at about 4 and 24 h later. Careful technique is needed to avoid damaging the leukocytes during the labelling process. The accuracy of imaging is probably improved by labelling the granulocyte fraction rather than the mixed leukocyte population, but this marginal advantage may be outweighed by the technical difficulty of fractionating the cells.

Although the early clinical work which validated the accuracy of leukocyte imaging in inflammatory bowel disease used indium labelled cells, most centres are now using ^{99m}Tc-labelled hexamethylpropyleneamine oxime (HMPAO). This agent also requires in-vitro labelling of the patient's leukocytes, but it has a number of technical and logistic advantages. The ^{99m}Tc labelling procedure is simpler than the ^{111}In technique, image quality is better because of the superior physical characteristics of ^{99m}Tc compared with ^{111}In, the radiation dose to the patient is much less with ^{99m}Tc and the preparation is available in kit form with a long shelf life. Because images are typically obtained at 1 and 4 h after reinjection of the ^{99m}Tc-labelled cells, the procedure can be completed in a single visit to the department, whist the ^{111}In technique normally requires images up to 24 h.

21.3.2
Interpretation

Labelled leukocytes accumulate in the liver and bone marrow, and particularly in the spleen which typically shows the maximum intensity of uptake on the images. With ^{99m}Tc-HMPAO, the cell preparation may contain a small proportion of unbound tracer which is excreted by glomerular filtration so that a low level of activity in the kidneys and bladder may be seen on early images. Transient retention of the labelled cells in the lung is also a normal feature of early images, but this normally clears by 4 h. Persistent lung activity suggests either a faulty labelling procedure or the presence of lung disease. Gradual migration of the tracer into the bowel lumen is also a normal feature of ^{99m}Tc HMPAO studies, so faint uptake in the colon may be a normal finding on 4 h images, although no

bowel uptake should be visualised at 1 h. Active bowel disease is indicated by colonic activity which is visible at 1 h, but typically becomes more intense at 4 h. The distribution and intensity of abnormal activity may be taken as an indicator of the extent and severity of inflammatory bowel disease (Figs. 21.2, 21.3).

Localisation of disease on leukocyte images is easier if a plain abdominal radiograph, barium enema, or CT study is available for anatomic correlation, particularly in patients who have undergone previous bowel resection. Increased colonic activity is seen not only in Crohn's disease and ulcerative colitis, but also in acute infective or ischemic colitis, in bowel infarction, haemorrhage, and occasionally in tumours which have an inflammatory component. Results are more likely to be positive in patients with a high leukocyte count in the peripheral blood and false negatives may occur in patients undergoing prolonged steroid therapy or those who are immunosuppressed.

21.3.3
Clinical Applications

In the detection of both Crohn's disease (MOLNAR et al. 2001) and ulcerative colitis (BENNINK et al. 2001), leukocyte scintigraphy is at least as sensitive as colonoscopy and barium studies, and may be the only abnormal finding in early disease. Because the technique is non-invasive and relatively simple for

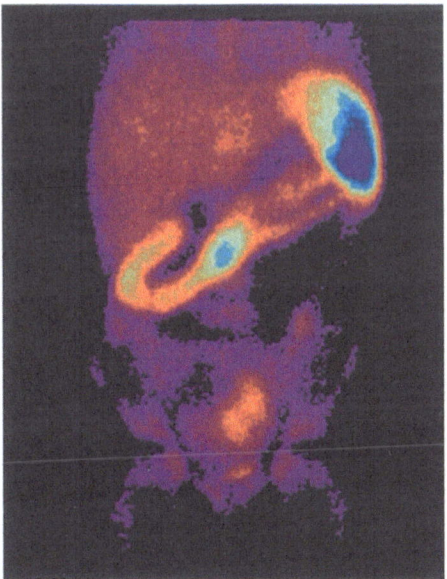
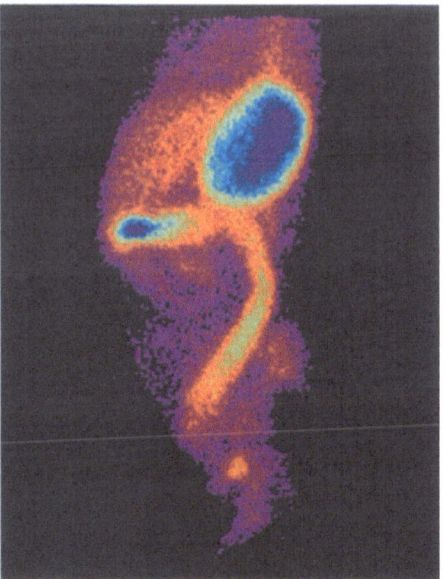

Fig. 21.2a,b. Tc[99m] HMPAO labelled white cell scintigraphy in Crohn's disease. Images obtained at 3 h in anterior (**a**) and left lateral (**b**) views showing diffuse involvement of the transverse and descending colon with active inflammatory disease. The intense uptake in spleen is normal

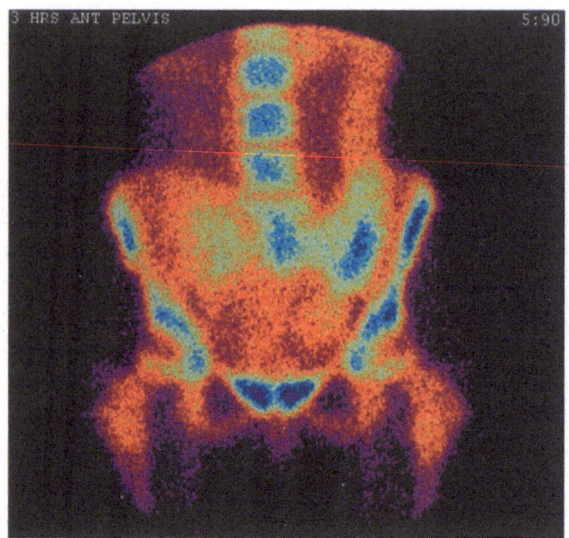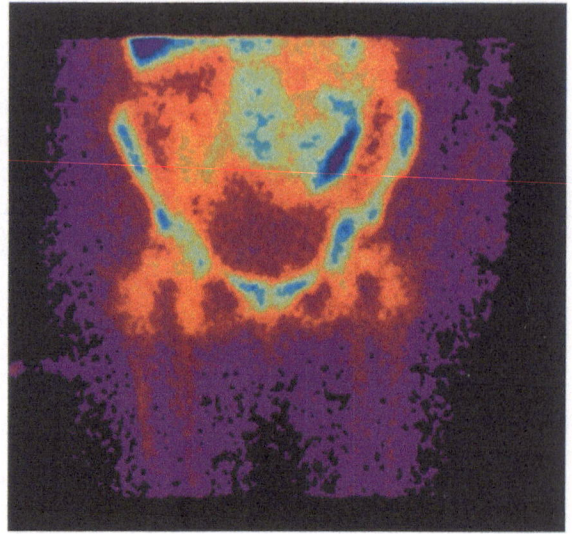

Fig 21.3a,b. Tc[99m] HMPAO labelled white cell scintigraphy in two different patients (**a, b**), both with Crohn's disease localised to the left colon. Uptake in bone marrow of the spine and pelvis is normal

the patients, it may be preferable as the initial test, particularly in children (CHARRON et al. 1999).

In patients with an established diagnosis of inflammatory colitis, WBC scintigraphy may be used to assess the extent and location of the disease (WELDON et al. 1995). This may assist in the distinction between Crohn's disease and ulcerative colitis – predominance of right-sided disease, discontinuity of colonic involvement, and rectal sparing all favouring Crohn's disease (CHARRON et al. 1998).

Scintigraphy may be used to assess the response to therapy in patients with established disease, and also to screen for suspected recurrences. The surgical complications of inflammatory bowel disease will often require endoscopy, barium studies or CT for diagnosis. However, leukocyte scintigraphy may be helpful in differentiating between infected collections and pockets of sterile fluid or isolated loops of bowel which may be confusing on anatomic imaging. In assessing strictures, those which show leukocyte uptake indicating an inflammatory component are more likely to respond to medical therapy whilst those which are quiescent on scintigraphy are more likely to need surgical treatment.

21.4
Colonic Transit Studies Using Radionuclides

Colonic motor physiology is still incompletely understood. Manometric studies show that colonic contrac-

tions generate areas of high pressure which may be either stationary or propagated along the bowel. The movement of bowel contents along the lumen depends on propagating contractions. Studies of normal colonic motility have shown that there is considerable variation between individuals, and at different times in the same individual. The colon is more active during waking hours than during sleep, and transit is faster in male volunteers than in females, in whom cyclical hormonal changes may cause additional variation. It is against this background that non-invasive scintigraphic techniques have been developed to detect the presence and severity of transit abnormalities in the colon, and to distinguish different patterns of abnormality which may help to select the most appropriate form of treatment.

21.4.1
Techniques

Visualising colonic transit requires a tracer which is not absorbed in the gastrointestinal tract and which has a suitable half-life for imaging over several days. The agent most widely used is [111]In (half-life 68 h) although good results have also been obtained using ^{67}Ga-citrate (half-life 78 h) which may be given orally and is also not absorbed (BELLEN et al. 1995). With both of these nuclides, the gamma emissions are suitable for imaging, and using as little as 2–3 MBq of activity, the radiation dose to the patient is small compared with that delivered by abdominal radiographs or computed tomography. The preferred method (NOTGHI et al. 1994) involves absorption of ^{111}In on to an ion-exchange resin which is then incorporated in a pH-sensitive enteric-coated capsule designed to liberate the labelled resin in the distal ileum. The tracer is given in the morning, and the patient allowed to eat and drink normally from midday. It is recommended that during the procedure patients avoid spicy food, excessive alcohol, laxatives and other drugs with gastrointestinal effects.

Serial images of the abdomen and pelvis are obtained for up to three days. Early images (up to 6 h) are rarely contributory, but a view at 8–10 h is useful to detect those patients with abnormally rapid transit. Progression of the tracer through the colonic lumen is assessed both visually and quantitatively. Methods for quantitation vary in detail but all involve dividing the large bowel into anatomic regions and measuring the proportion of ingested activity located in each of the regions. NOTGHI et al. (1993) also use a diagrammatic representation of the distribution of activity at different times after ingestion to provide a more user-friendly display (Figs. 21.4–21.6). In order to compare results amongst groups of patients, the distribution of colonic activity at specified times after ingestion can be represented as the geometric centre of activity. This is a figure calculated by allocating a numerical value to each of the anatomic regions of the large bowel, and determining the weighted average of the counts in each region.

21.4.2
Interpretation

In the normal subject (Fig. 21.4), most of the activity is located within the right colon at 8 h. Predominance of activity in the left colon at 8 h indicates abnormally rapid transit. One day after ingestion, much of the activity has normally moved to the transverse colon and splenic flexure with a little in the left colon. Two days after ingestion, most of the activity has been evacuated with a little remaining in the descending colon and rectum. Patients with slow transit constipation typically show either prolonged hold-up in the right side of the colon (Fig. 21.5) or a more

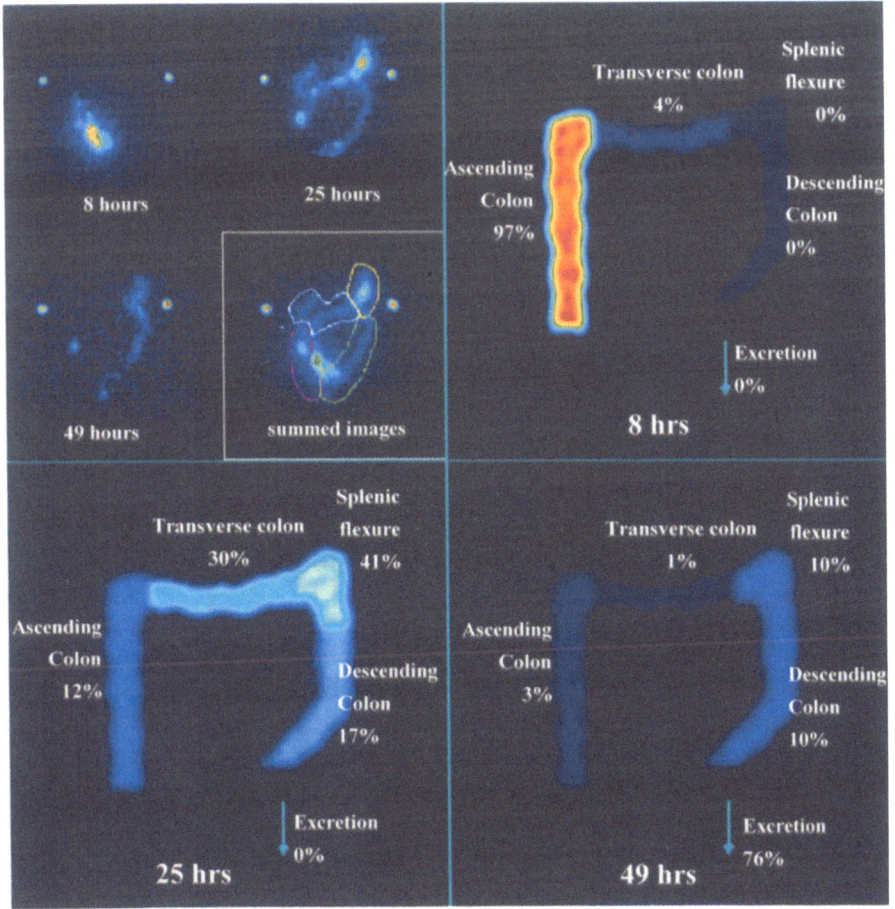

Fig. 21.4. Radionuclide colonic transit study – normal; activity is mostly in the right colon at 8 h, is spread through the transverse and left colon by 25 h, and a high proportion is evacuated by 49 h. [Courtesy of Dr A. NOTGHI]

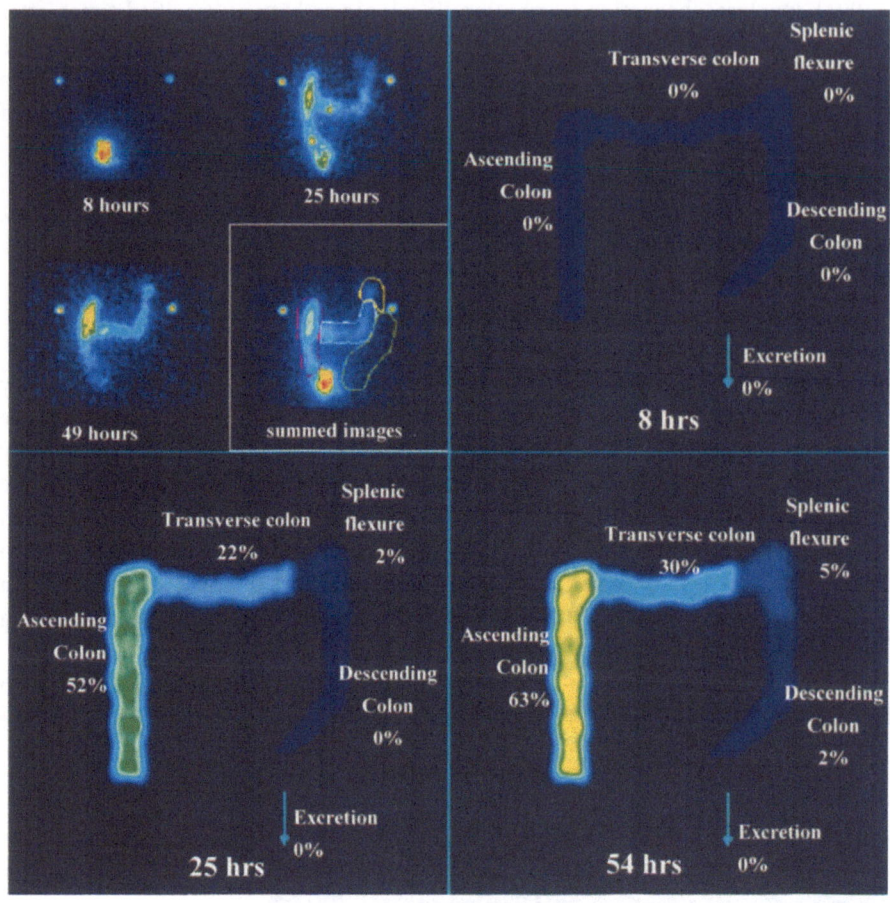

Fig. 21.5. Radionuclide colonic transit study – proximal delay; activity is slow to reach the ascending and transverse colon and shows little onward movement at 54 h. [Courtesy of Dr A. Notghi]

generalised slow transit throughout the whole of the large bowel (Fig. 21.6). Where transit appears normal in the right side of the colon, but pronounced delay occurs in the descending colon and recto-sigmoid, a disorder of evacuation with dysfunction of the pelvic floor may be diagnosed.

21.4.3
Clinical Applications

In the investigation of constipation, scintigraphic studies distinguish between those patients whose transit is normal, those who have abnormal evacuation due to pelvic floor dysfunction, and those who have right-sided or generalised colonic dysmotility (HUTCHINSON et al. 1995; GATTUSO et al. 1996). Scintigraphy may be used to confirm the presence of abnormal motility in patients with onset of constipation following childbirth or spinal cord injury. Diabetic patients and those with systemic sclerosis (WANG et al. 2001) have a significant incidence of delayed colonic transit, whilst accelerated transit may be a feature of portal hypertension (MADSEN et al. 2000). In patients with established colonic dysfunction, scintigraphy may help to decide the appropriate location for a colostomy and transit studies may also be used to determine the functional effects of surgical reconstructions or drug treatment for bowel disorders.

21.5
Immuno-scintigraphy for Colonic Cancer

The possibility of detecting malignant lesions non-invasively using tumour-specific radionuclides has been explored extensively over the last 20 years. Immuno-scintigraphy uses radio-labelled antibodies or antibody fragments to localise antigens which are either specific to tumours or found in abnormally high concentrations in tumour cells. Both human and murine antibodies take the form of a Y-shaped polypeptide structure comprising two light chains

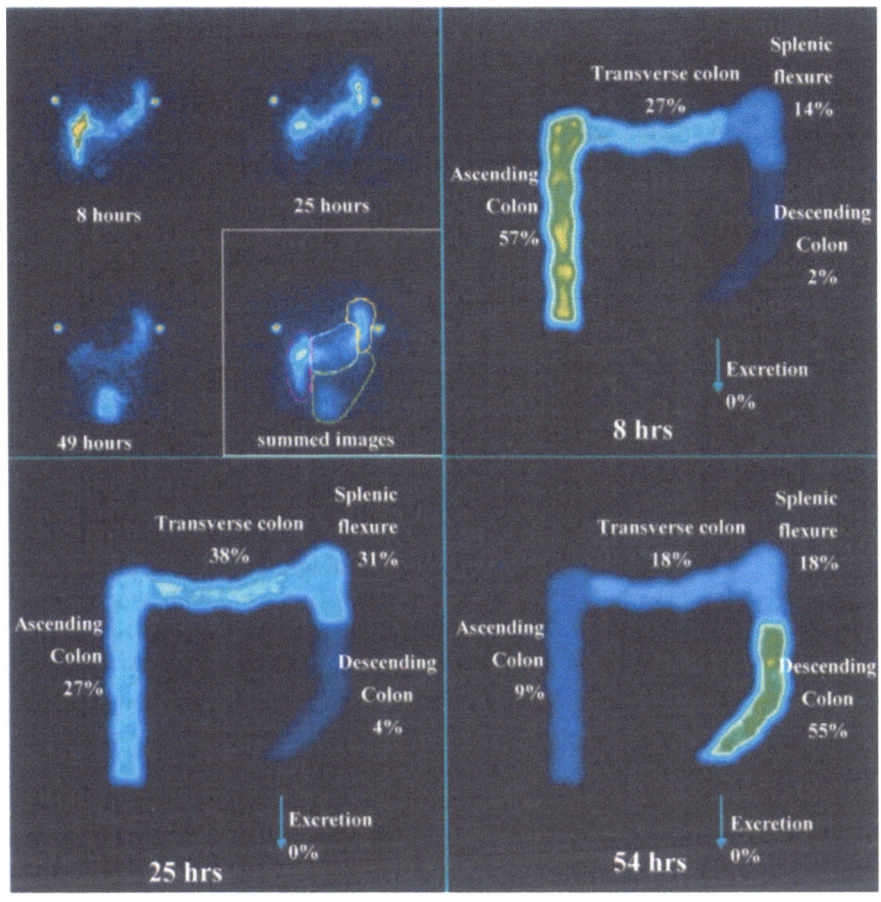

Fig. 21.6. Radionuclide colonic transit study – generalised delay; activity reaches the right and transverse colon but onward movement to the left colon and subsequent evacuation are delayed. [Courtesy of Dr A. NOTGHI]

and two heavy chains. The arms of the "Y" – the F(ab) fragments – contain the antibody binding sites. Antibodies for clinical use are biosynthesised in tissue culture from single clones of mouse cells, selected for their high specificity against the target antigen. In the context of colorectal cancer, two main types of antibody have been used, targeted either against carcinoembryonic antigen (CEA) or against tumour-associated glycoproteins. Early studies used radio-iodine (initially ^{131}I, later ^{123}I) as the tracer, but more stable labelling can be achieved by using either indium (^{111}In) with a suitable chelating agent, or ^{99m}Tc-pertechnetate. Antibodies themselves can be antigenic, so the clinical use of whole monoclonal antibodies entails a risk of adverse reactions at the time of the study, or the later development of antibodies against the agent used (human anti-mouse antibodies, HAMA). The F(ab) fragments are much less likely to provoke antibody formation or allergic reactions and several large studies using these molecules have found adverse effects to be rare, even with repeated administrations over months and years.

21.5.1
Techniques

So far the most widely used agents have been the anti-CEA agent arcitumomab, an F(ab) fragment which is labelled with 750–1000 MBq of ^{99m}Tc, and satumomab, a whole antibody which is labelled with 150–200 MBq of [111]In. In either case, the protein content of the preparation is about 1 mg.

Although only a minority of the administered activity is excreted by the urinary tract, it is important to minimise bladder activity at the time of imaging by keeping the patients well hydrated, emptying the bladder immediately before imaging, and obtaining the pelvic views first. SPECT images of pelvis, abdomen and thorax, as well as planar views of the whole body, are acquired at about 3–4 h after injection using the ^{99m}Tc-labelled agent, or at 48–72 h with ^{111}In labelling. With either agent, if initial images are equivocal it may help to obtain delayed views on the following day.

21.5.2
Interpretation

In the first few hours after injection, a considerable proportion of the tracer remains within the circulation, so early images outline the heart and major vessels. Clearance takes place into liver, spleen and bone marrow and early excretion is via the urinary tract, so kidneys and bladder are normally visualised. Other areas of normal uptake include the genitalia, breasts, recent surgical scars, and stoma sites. Bowel activity typically increases over time but also shows movement on interval images, and may be removed by administration of cathartics. Foci of tumour typically show localised uptake equal to or greater than the intensity of liver activity, in sites which are anatomically distinguishable from normal structures. Careful review of SPECT images, and correlation with CT or other anatomic imaging, is helpful in interpretation. Large tumours may show a rim of increased activity around a necrotic or poorly vascularized centre with little or no tracer uptake.

21.5.3
Results in Colon Cancer

Numerous studies have correlated the imaging findings using labelled antibodies with CT, surgery, histology, and follow up (WINZELBERG et al. 1992; MOFFAT et al. 1996; PINKAS et al. 1999). Immuno-scintigraphy has been highly successful in detecting the presence and location of primary colorectal cancers. However, since virtually all colon cancers are detectable by a combination of colonoscopy, barium enema, and CT methods, the added value of immuno-scintigraphy is not established. Detection of liver metastases by immuno-scintigraphy is also fairly successful, in spite of the normal accumulation of the agent in healthy liver tissue, since metastatic nodules show a visibly greater concentration of the agent. However, with its limited spatial resolution, liver scintigraphy, even with these targeted agents, is unlikely to improve on anatomic imaging methods.

The major role for immuno-scintigraphy is in those patients in whom the results of CT are less effective, i.e. the early detection of local tumour recurrence, and recognition of lymph node metastases. Immuno-scintigraphy has been shown to improve on CT in distinguishing between fibrosis and recurrent tumour at the site of previous surgery, and the use of routine anti-CEA imaging as a surveillance procedure following surgery for primary colorectal cancer has been shown to influence long-term survival by correctly detecting early recurrence (LECHNER et al. 2000). Probably the most useful application of immuno-scintigraphy currently is in the differentiation of post-operative or post-radiation fibrosis in patients with equivocal CT findings. Immuno-scintigraphy may also resolve uncertainties about lymph node involvement when CT studies are suspicious but not conclusive.

21.5.4
Radio-immuno-Guided Surgery (RIGS)

Recent techniques have been developed for the intra-operative localisation of tumour foci using a hand-held gamma probe to detect abnormal accumulations of labelled anti-tumour antibodies. As with gamma camera immuno-scintigraphy, early work with RIGS has used several different antibodies or antibody fragments. Several different nuclides have been used, but the best results so far have been obtained using ^{125}I-iodine, which has a much longer half-life but lower gamma energy than the nuclides used for gamma camera imaging. The tracer is injected a few days or even weeks before surgery, allowing time for background activity to clear whilst tumour binding remains high. Because of the low energy of the tracer, the radiation dose to the surgical team is minimal, whilst the hand-held gamma probe is highly sensitive for detection of local fluctuations in tracer concentration.

Clinical studies with RIGS have shown that this approach improves on conventional CT and surgical assessment by detecting occult sites of recurrent or metastatic disease in a significant proportion of patients (MANAYAN et al. 1997; SCHNEEBAUM et al. 1997). In vitro testing of the sensitivity of the gamma probe using preparations of tumour cells labelled with ^{125}I-monoclonal fragments showed that tumour foci of less than 1 mm^3 could be detected (OREDIPE et al. 1988). In a further study, lymph nodes of normal size which appeared uninvolved at surgery, but showed high count rates with the gamma probe, were subsequently found to contain microscopic metastases at careful histologic examination (COTE et al. 1996). The potential applications for RIGS remain to be explored more thoroughly, but the method promises improvements in the surgical staging of disease and the detection of occult tumour foci.

References

Alavi A, Dann RW, Baum S et al (1977) Scintigraphic detection of acute gastrointestinal bleeding. Radiology 124:753–756

Bellen JC, Chatterton BE, Penglis S et al (1995) Gallium-67 complexes as radioactive markers to assess gastric and colonic transit. J Nucl Med 36:513–551

Bennink R, Peeters M, D'Haens et al (2001) Tc-99m HMPAO white blood cell scintigraphy in the assessment of the extent and severity of an acute exacerbation of ulcerative colitis. Clin Nucl Med 26:99–104

Charron M, del Rosario JF, Kocoshis S (1998) Use of technetium-tagged white blood cells in patients with Crohn's disease and ulcerative colitis: is differential diagnosis possible? Pediatr Radiol 28:871–877

Charron M, del Rosario FJ, Kocoshis S (1999) Pediatric inflammatory bowel disease: assessment with scintigraphy with 99mTc white blood cells. Radiology 212:507–513

Cote RJ, Houchens DP, Hitchcock CL et al (1996) Intraoperative detection of occult colon cancer micrometastases using 125I-radiolabeled monoclonal antibody CC49. Cancer 77:613–620

Ford PV, Bartold SP (2001) Procedure guideline for gastrointestinal bleeding and Meckel's diverticulum scintigraphy 1.0: Society of Nuclear Medicine Procedure Guidelines Manual 2001-2002. Society of Nuclear Medicine, Reston, Va, pp 41–48

Gattuso JM, Kamm MA, Morris G et al (1996) Gastrointestinal transit in patients with idiopathic megarectum. Dis Colon Rectum 39:1044–1050

Gostout CJ, Wang KK, Ahlquist DA et al (1992) Acute gastrointestinal bleeding – experience of a specialised management team. J Clin Gastroenterol 14:260–267

Hutchinson R, Notghi A, Smith NB et al (1995) Scintigraphic measurement of ileocaecal transit in irritable bowel syndrome and chronic idiopathic constipation. Gut 36: 585–589

Lechner P, Lind P, Goldenberg DM (2000) Can postoperative surveillance with serial CEA immunoscintigraphy detect resectable rectal cancer recurrence and potentially improve tumor-free survival? J Am Coll Surg 191:511–518

Madsen JL, Brinch K, Hansen EF et al (2000) Gastrointestinal motor function in patients with portal hypertension. Scan J Gastroenterol 35:490–493

Manayan RC, Hart MJ, Friend WG (1997) Radioimmunoguided surgery for colorectal cancer. Am J Surg 173:386–389

Moffat FL Jr, Pinsky CM, Hammershaimb L et al (1996) Clinical utility of external immunoscintigraphy with the IMMU-4 technetium-99m Fab antibody fragment in patients undergoing surgery for carcinoma of the colon and rectum: results of a pivotal, phase III trial. The Immunomedics Study Group. J Clin Oncol 14:2295–2305

Molnar T, Papos M, Gyulai C et al (2001) Clinical value of technetium-99m-HMPAO-labelled leukocyte scintigraphy and spiral computed tomography in active Crohn's disease. Am J Gastroenterol 96:1517–1521

Notghi A, Kumar D, Panagamuwa B et al (1993) Measurement of colonic transit time using radionuclide imaging: analysis by condensed images. Nucl Med Commun 14:204–211

Notghi A, Hutchinson R, Kumar D et al (1994) Simplified method for the measurement of segmental colonic transit time. Gut 35:976–981

Oredipe OA, Barth RF, Tuttle SE et al (1988) Limits of sensitivity for the radioimmunodetection of colon cancer by means of a hand held gamma probe. Int J Rad Appl Instrum 15:595–603

Pinkas L, Robins PD, Forstrom LA et al (1999) clinical experience with radiolabelled monoclonal antibodies in the detection of colorectal and ovarian carcinoma recurrence and review of the literature. Nucl Med Commun 20: 689–696

Rantis PC Jr, Harford FJ, Wagner RH et al (1995) Technetium-labelled red blood cell scintigraphy: is it useful in acute lower gastrointestinal bleeding? Int J Colorectal Dis 10: 210–215

Schneebaum S, Papo J, Graif M et al (1997) Radioimmunoguided surgery benefits for recurrent colorectal cancer. Ann Surg Oncol 4:371–376

Sommer A, Wetzel E, Loose R et al (1996) The role of colloid and labelled red blood cell scintigraphy in the investigation of acute or intermittent gastrointestinal bleeding. Rofo Fortschr Geb Rontgenstr Neuen Bildgebenden Verfahren 16:64–69

Stokkel MPM, Reigman HIE, Pauwels EKJ (2002) Scintigraphic head-tohead comparison between ^{99m}Tc-WBCs and ^{99m}Tc-Leukoscan in the evaluation of inflammatory bowel disease: a pilot study. Eur J Nucl Med 29:251–254

Suzman MS, Talmor M, Jennis R et al (1996) Accurate localization and surgical management of active lower gastrointestinal hemorrhage with technetium-labelled erythrocyte scintigraphy. Ann Surg 224:29–36

Wang SJ, Lan JL, Chen DY et al (2001) Colonic transit disorders in systemic sclerosis. Clin Rheumatol 20:251–254

Weldon MJ, Masoomi AM, Britten AJ et al (1995) Quantification of inflammatory bowel disease activity using technetium-99m HMPAO labelled leukocyte single photon emission computerised tomography (SPECT). Gut 36:243–250

Winzelberg GG, Grossman SJ, Rizk S et al (1992) Indium-111 monoclonal antibody B72.3 scintigraphy in colorectal cancer. Correlation with computed tomography, surgery, histopathology, immunohistology, and human immune response. Cancer 69:1656–1663

22 CT Angiography of Splanchnic Vessels

Andrea Laghi, Riccardo Ferrari, Filippo Mangiapane, Simona Trenna,
Daniele Marin, Roberto Passariello

CONTENTS

22.1 Introduction 227
22.2 Technique 227
22.2.1 Image Acquisition 227
22.2.2 Image Analysis and 3D Reconstructions 228
22.3 Arterial Vascular System 230
22.4 Venous Vascular System 231
22.5 Conclusions 232
References 232

22.1
Introduction

Computed tomographic angiography (CTA) is a powerful tool for a minimally-invasive, safe, relatively comfortable and low-cost evaluation of the vascular system (Rubin et al. 1999). Using dedicated scanning protocols, low-dose acquisitions can also be obtained, minimizing radiation exposure (van Gelder et al. 2002). As a result, CTA has now the potential to be a diagnostic alternative to conventional angiography.

The development of multislice spiral CT technology is a significant advance for CTA (Rubin et al. 2000), particularly as it allows the splanchnic vessels to be evaluated (Horton and Fishman 2000; Laghi et al. 2001). Acquisition time is faster with multislice spiral CT scanners than with conventional single-slice spiral CT scanners, thus enabling larger anatomic cover with no misregistration or respiratory motion artifacts (McCollough and Zink 1999). Using thin-slice collimation protocols increases the spatial resolution along the longitudinal axis, providing virtually isotropic three-dimensional voxels; consequently, image quality is improved with better diagnostic evaluation of small

A. Laghi, MD; R. Ferrari, MD; F. Mangiapane, MD;
S. Trenna, MD; D. Marin, MD
Department of Radiology, University of Rome "La Sapienza", Policlinico Umberto I, Viale Regina Elena 324, 00161 Rome, Italy
R. Passariello, MD
Professor and Director, Department of Radiology, University of Rome "La Sapienza", Policlinico Umberto I, Viale Regina Elena 324, 00161 Rome, Italy

peripheral vascular branches (Hu et al. 2000). Finally, contrast enhancement is improved by more accurate injection timing and better separation between arterial and venous phases.

However, in order to exploit the benefits of using multislice CT, it is important to optimize study protocols and to improve image display (Rubin 2000). Three-dimensional datasets are reconstructed and interactively evaluated on dedicated workstations using axial and two-dimensional multiplanar images, as well as more complex rendering techniques, such as maximum intensity projections (MIP), surface shaded displays (SSD), and volume rendering (Heath et al. 1995; Kuszky et al. 1995).

22.2
Technique

22.2.1
Image Acquisition

To acquire three-dimensional datasets of high quality attention must be paid to the longitudinal spatial resolution (dependent on slice collimation, effective slice thickness and pitch) and optimal timing of the contrast medium injection (in order to acquire pure arterial and portal venous phases).

Before the study, patients receive 800 ml of water as an oral contrast agent to produce negative contrast in the stomach and small bowel; the use of a positive oral contrast agent might create difficulties when generating the three-dimensional reconstructions.

Intravenous contrast medium is delivered using an automatic injector. Adequate venous access is required, as a fast flow rate is necessary to obtain separation between arterial and portal venous phases, as well as a good peak arterial enhancement. A lower flow rate might also impair opacification of smaller arterial vessels due to inadequate intra-vessel concentration of contrast medium. Usually, 120–140 ml of nonionic iodinated contrast medium is infused intravenously at a flow rate of 4–5 ml/s into a peripheral vein; usually the antecubital vein. Following a bolus injection of 20 ml of contrast medium, sequential dynamic slices are acquired at the level of the origin of the superior mesenteric artery in order to determine the optimal delay that should be applied before scanning.

Spiral CT scans of the abdomen and pelvis are obtained in both the arterial (delay calculated on bolus test injection) and portal venous phase (delay, 60–70 s). Imaging parameters need to be optimized for different scanners. In our personal experience (LAGHI et al. 2001), using a four-slice multislice spiral CT scanner (Somatom Plus 4 Volume Zoom; Siemens, Erlangen, Germany) equipped with flying spot, adaptive array matrix, and a gantry rotation time of 0.5 s, images should be acquired using 1-mm slice collimation, 1–1.25-mm slice thickness, 6-mm/s table feed, 120 mAs, and 120 kVp. Breath-hold time ranges between 30 and 35 s, depending on the size of the patient. Patients are instructed to hyperventilate before scanning and to exhale slowly if they cannot suspend respiration for the entire examination. Image reconstruction interval is another important factor affecting the quality of three-dimensional images. In principle, in order to obtain optimal image quality, 20%–40% overlap should be implemented; this means using a reconstruction index of 0.6–0.8 mm. A 1-mm slice collimation protocol produces 300–400 images/scan per patient and so to reduce workload on the workstation, it is sometimes advisable to limit the image reconstruction interval to 1 mm, with no image overlap.

22.2.2
Image Analysis and 3D Reconstructions

Once acquired, images are downloaded to an offline dedicated workstation in order to generate 3D reconstructions. 3D data sets can be examined using different reconstruction techniques, starting with multiplanar reformations along three orthogonal axes and oblique planes. 3D reconstructions can be obtained by using either maximum intensity projection (MIP), surface rendering or volume rendering algorithms (JOHNSON et al. 1996; HONG and FREENY 1999) (Fig. 22.1). For better anatomic representation and evaluation of spatial relationships, as well as for a faster and easier interaction with 3D datasets, volume rendering is the preferred reconstruction algorithm, although diagnosis is made from a combined evaluation of source and reconstructed images (WINTER et al. 1996; HORTON and FISHMAN 2002). With volume rendering, selective vessel representation is obtained using different rendering curves. A panoramic overview of the entire main abdominal branches can be obtained using a preset opacity curve showing only the vascular surface (Fig. 22.2). The evaluation of minor vessels (i.e., second, third, and more distal orders) requires the analysis of 3D data sets by using interactive multiplanar cut planes ("oblique trim") (Fig. 22.3) and by modulating the opacity of the anatomical structures under evaluation and window/level parameters in order to see vessels "through" abdomi-

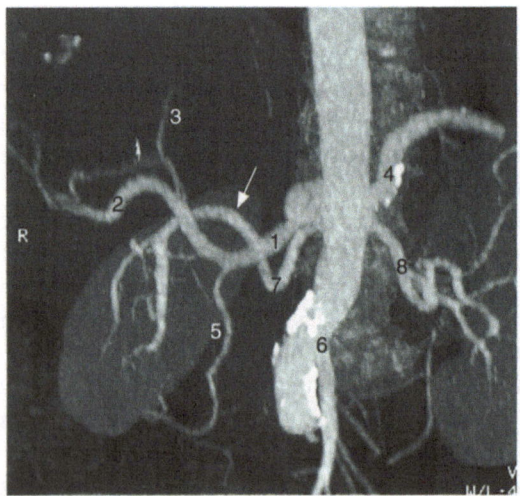
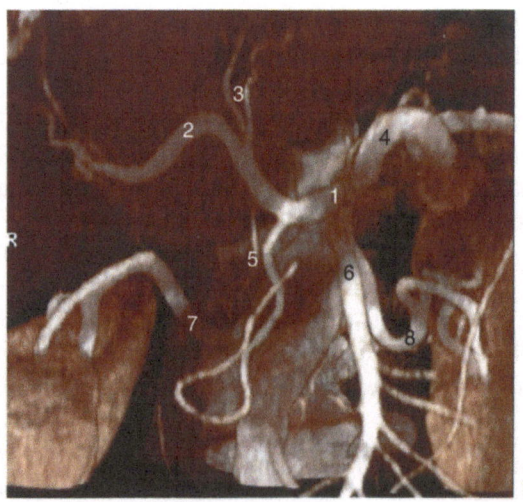

Fig. 22.1a,b. Maximum intensity projection (MIP) and volume rendered reconstruction for the evaluation of the celiac trunk and the proximal superior mesenteric artery (SMA). **a** The MIP image provides a panoramic overview of the arteries but 3D spatial relationships are missing. In this coronal projection, the hepatic artery (*arrow*) is superimposed on the right renal artery; the origin of the SMA is not clearly depicted due to the overlapping density of the abdominal aorta. **b** With volume-rendered 3D reconstruction, using intermediate opacity, vessels and parenchyma can both be evaluated. The use of virtual lighting and shading provides better 3D evaluation of the spatial relationships between the arteries. Hepatic artery (*1*); right hepatic artery (*2*); left hepatic artery (*3*); splenic artery (*4*); gastroduodenal artery (*5*); superior mesenteric artery (*6*); right renal artery (*7*); left renal artery (*8*)

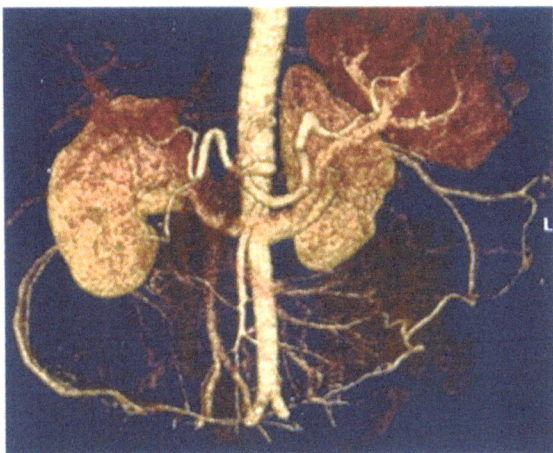
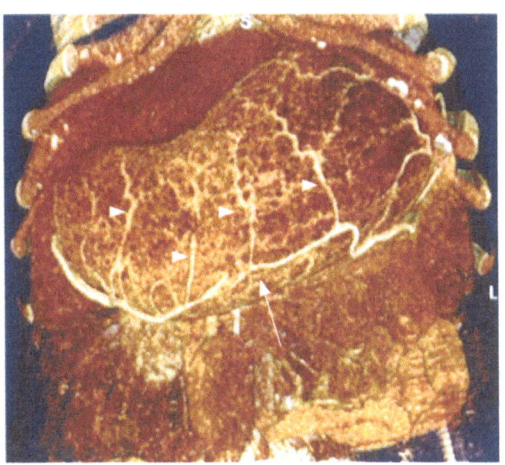

Fig. 22.2a,b. Modulation of the opacity values provides selective visualization of different anatomical structures. **a** Opacity curve selectively showing the arteries; in this particular case a panoramic evaluation of the gastroepiploic arcade (*arrows*) is obtained. **b** Using different opacity values, the gastric surface is seen together with the gastroepiploic arcade (*arrows*) and the short gastric vessels (*arrowheads*)

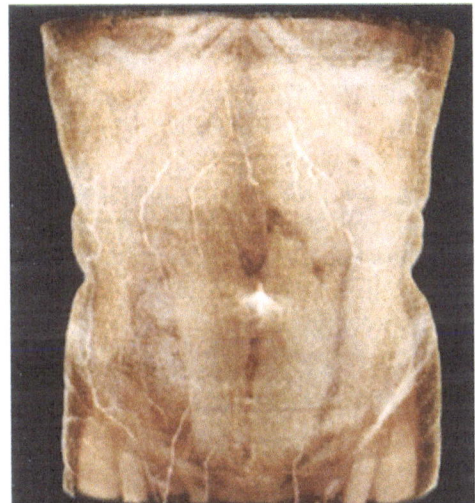

Fig. 22.3a–c. The use of interactive "cut planes" permits virtually dissection of the abdominal volume. **a** Surface view of the body. **b,c** Oblique cut planes show the interior of the abdominal volume

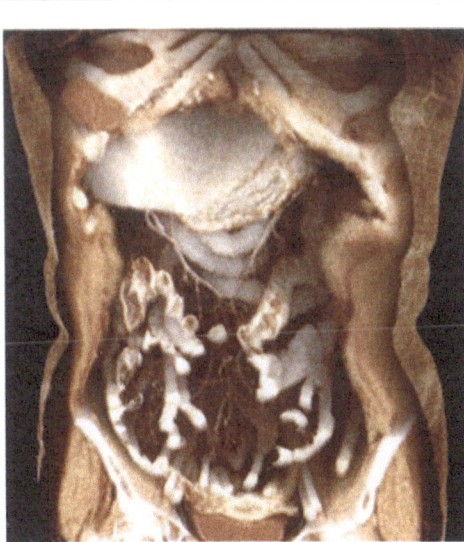
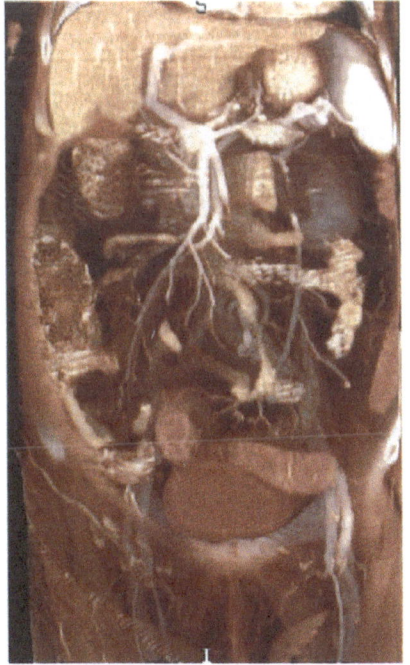

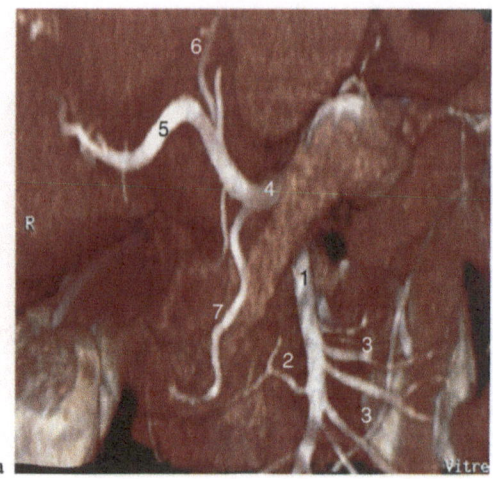

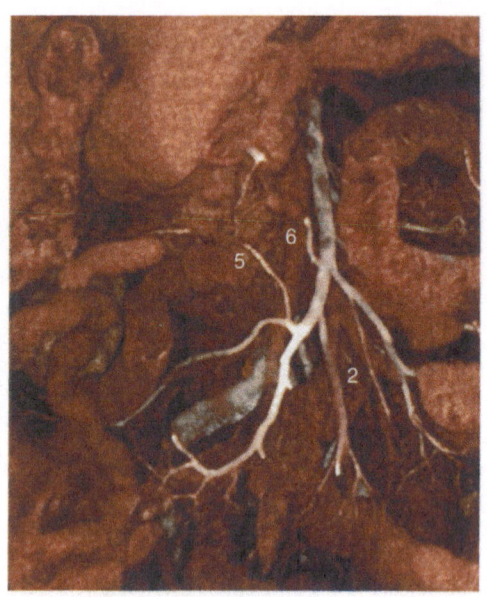

Fig 22.4a,b. Superior mesenteric artery (*1*). **a** Magnified view showing the inferior pancreaticoduodenal artery (*2*) and jejunal branches (*3*). Hepatic artery (*4*); right hepatic artery (*5*); left hepatic artery (*6*); gastroduodenal artery (*7*). **b** Magnified view showing the ileal branches (*2*), the terminal artery (*3*), the ileocolic artery (*4*) and the right colic artery (*5*). The origin of the middle colic artery (*6*) is also noted

nal organs. Image analysis requires direct operator interpretation at the workstation, where 2D axial and multiplanar reconstructions and 3D images are simultaneously available. A complete analysis of arterial and venous vessels involves a mean interpretation time of 20 min.

22.3
Arterial Vascular System

The superior mesenteric artery (SMA) can be identified, including its major and distal branches (Fig. 22.4). The SMA usually arises less than 1.5 cm below the origin of the celiac trunk. Major collateral branches are the inferior pancreaticoduodenal artery, which has an oblique course, anastomosing superiorly with the superior pancreaticoduodenal artery, a branch of the gastroduodenal artery; the right and middle colic arteries, with the latter absent in up to 80% of normal individuals, supplying blood to the right colon; the jejunal branches, arising from the left side of the SMA above the level of the middle colic artery and the ileal branches arising from the left side of the SMA below the level of the middle colic artery and the terminal ileo-colic artery supplying blood to the distal ileum and caecum.

The inferior mesenteric artery (IMA) arises from the aorta about 7 cm below the origin of the SMA. The IMA divides into the left colic artery, which has a straight superior course, supplying the transverse

and descending colon, the sigmoid arteries, two to four vessels supplying the sigmoid colon and the superior hemorrhoidal artery, a terminal branch that supplies the upper rectum (Fig. 22.5).

The high spatial resolution of multislice CTA allows detailed evaluation of small distal vessels including the anastomotic arcades along the mesenteric and mesocolic sides of small and large bowel as well as the vasa recta (Fig. 22.6).

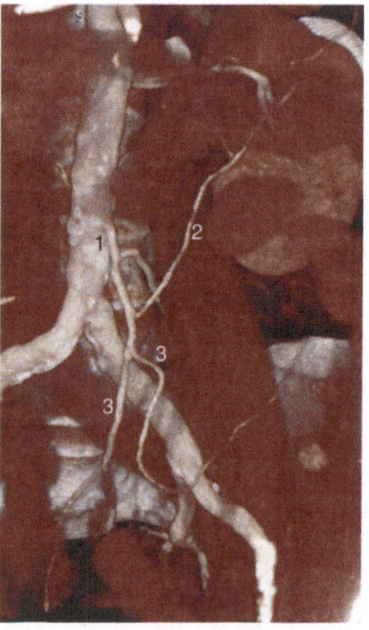

Fig. 22.5. Inferior mesenteric artery (*1*) arising from the left side of the aorta. Left colic artery (*2*) and sigmoid arteries (*3*)

22.4
Venous Vascular System

All major veins of the portal venous systems (portal vein, splenic vein, superior mesenteric and inferior mesenteric vein) can be depicted as well as the collateral branches. The portal vein is demonstrated along its entire course together with the intra-hepatic segmental branches (Fig. 22.7). Portal cavernous transformation, following occlusion of the main portal trunk, is demonstrated in cirrhotic patients as well as esophagogastric, omental and splenorenal collateral vessels.

The superior mesenteric vein (Fig. 22.8) is usually a single trunk, receiving blood from the middle and right colic veins, the ileocolic vein, the gastrocolic vein and from jejunal and ileal branches. The inferior mesenteric vein (Fig. 22.9) receives blood from the left colic vein, the sigmoid veins (Fig. 22.10) and the superior hemorrhoidal vein.

A major problem when evaluating the venous system is discerning small arteries from veins, both of which are opacified on delayed images. Correct image analysis is time consuming and involves the use of all the available software tools on the workstation.

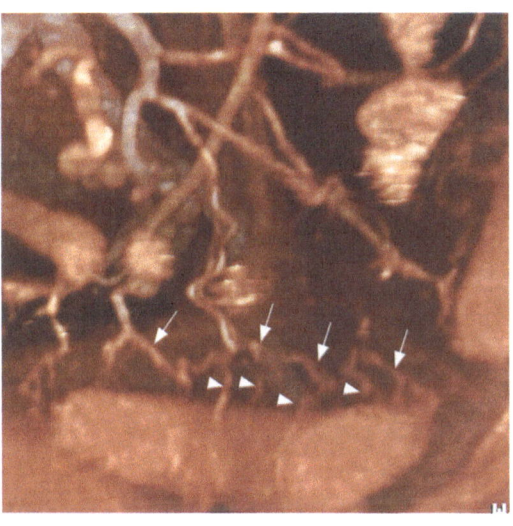

Fig. 22.6. Sigmoid arterial vascular arcade (*arrowheads*) with vasa recta (*small arrows*) feeding the bowel wall

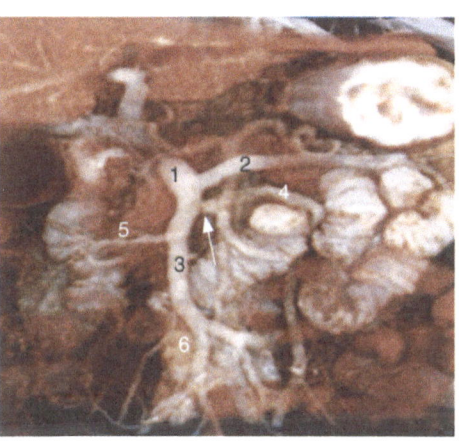

Fig. 22.7. Volume-rendered image showing portal (*1*), splenic (*2*), superior (*3*) and inferior (*4*) mesenteric veins. Branches of the superior mesenteric vein (SMV), including the right colic (*5*) and ileocolic (*6*) vessels, are also depicted. In this patient the inferior mesenteric vein joins the SMV (*arrow*)

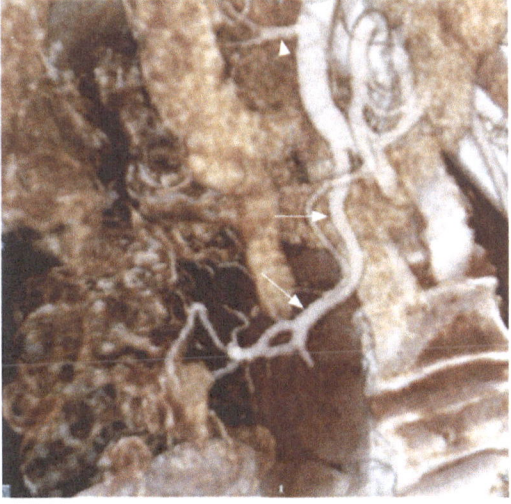

Fig. 22.8. Magnified view of the ileocolic vein (*arrows*) with terminal branches draining the caecum. The right colic vein is also noted (*arrowhead*)

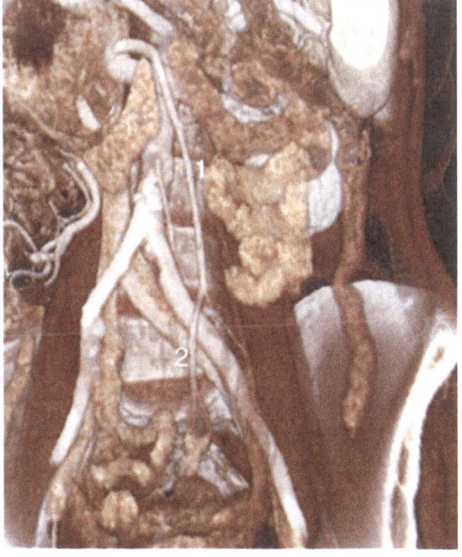

Fig.22.9. Inferior mesenteric vein (*1*) with sigmoid branches (*2*)

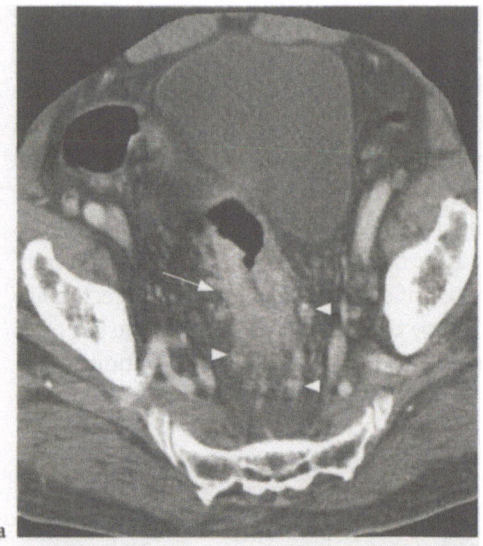

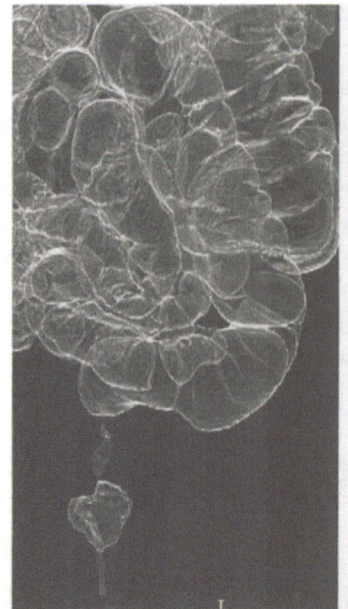

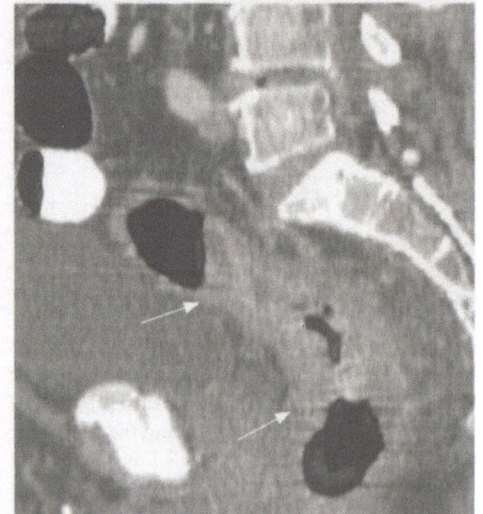

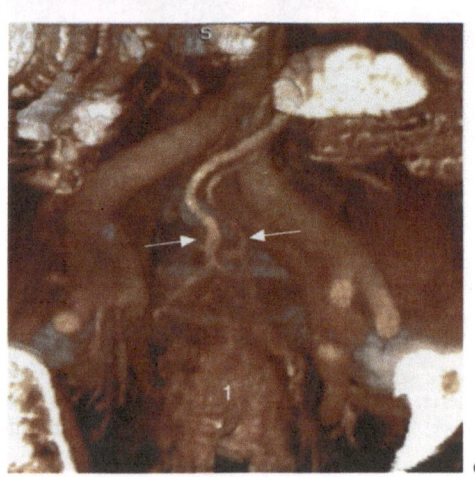

Fig. 22.10a–d. a Stenosing carcinoma of the sigmoid colon (*arrow*) with infiltration of the peri-colonic fat and loco-regional lymphadenopathy (*arrowheads*) (TNM: T3, N1). **b** On volume-rendered sagittal reconstruction, the longitudinal extension of the tumor (*arrows*) is shown as is the infiltration of the presacral fat plane. **c** Volume-rendered "virtual double-contrast enema" shows the luminal stricture (*arrow*). **d** A 3D volume-rendered vascular map shows both sigmoid artery and vein (*arrows*); sigmoid carcinoma (*1*)

22.5
Conclusions

Multislice CTA, thanks to enhanced image resolution, is able to overcome the technical challenge of depicting small mesenteric vessels, providing a detailed anatomical view similar to digital subtraction angiography, with the advantages of being less expensive, safer, and better tolerated by patients; moreover, multislice CTA offers a panoramic view of the entire abdominal vessels within a single injection of contrast medium. The technique involves using dedicated reconstruction algorithms on a workstation with volume-rendering, by virtue of its ability to display the 3D spatial relationships between vessels and surrounding organs, representing the most suitable algorithm. The widespread application of this technique can be expected in the near future as multislice CT scanners become more readily available, workstation design and performance is improved, and radiologists become familiar with 3D software. A cost–benefit analysis needs to be performed in order to better understand the impact of this new imaging modality on patients outcome.

References

Heath DG, Soyer PA, Kuszyk BS et al (1995) Three-dimensional spiral CT during arterial portography: comparison of 3D rendering techniques. Radiographics 15:1001–1011

Hong KC, Freeny PC (1999) Pancreaticoduodenal arcades and dorsal pancreatic artery: comparison of CT angiography with three-dimensional volume rendering, maximum intensity projection, and shaded-surface display. AJR 172: 925–931

Horton KM, Fishman EK (2000) 3D CT angiography of the celiac and superior mesenteric arteries with multidetector CT data sets: preliminary observations. Abdom Imaging 25:523–525

Horton KM, Fishman EK (2002) Volume-rendered 3D CT of the mesenteric vasculature: normal anatomy, anatomic variants and pathologic conditions. Radiographics 22: 161–172

Hu H, He HD, Foley WD et al (2000) Four multidetector-row helical CT: image quality and volume coverage speed. Radiology 215:55–62

Johnson PT, Heath DG, Kuszyk BS et al (1996) CT angiography with volume rendering: advantages and applications in splanchnic vascular imaging. Radiology 200:564–568

Kuszyk BS, Heath DG, Ney DR et al (1995) CT angiography with volume rendering: imaging findings. AJR 165: 445–448

Laghi A, Iannaccone R, Catalano C et al (2001) Multislice spiral computed tomography angiography of mesenteric arteries. Lancet 358:638–639

McCollough CH, Zink FE (1999) Performance evaluation of a multi-slice CT system. Med Phys 26:2223–2230

Rubin GD (2000) Data explosion: the challenge of multi detector-row CT. Eur J Radiol 36:74–80

Rubin GD, Shiau MA, Schmidt AJ et al (1999) Computed tomographic angiography: historical perspective and new state-of-the-art using multi detector-row helical computed tomography. J Comput Assist Tomogr 23:S83–S90

Rubin GD, Shiau MC, Kee ST et al (2000) Aorta and iliac arteries: single versus multiple detector-row helical CT angiography. Radiology 215:670–676

Van Gelder RE, Venema HW, Serlie IW et al (2002) CT colonography at different radiation dose levels: feasibility of dose reduction. Radiology 224:25–33

Winter TC III, Nghiem HV, Schmiedl UP et al (1996) CT angiography of the visceral vessels. Semin US CT MRI 17:339–351

23 Diagnosis and Management of Acute Colonic Bleeding

Iain Robertson and Richard Edwards

CONTENTS

23.1   Introduction *235*
23.2   Aetiology *235*
23.3   Investigation of Colonic Bleeding *236*
23.4   Provocation Angiography *237*
23.5   Therapeutic Angiography *238*
23.5.1 Embolization *238*
23.5.2 Vasopressin *239*
23.6   Conclusion *240*
        References *241*

23.1 Introduction

The majority of patients who present with acute colonic haemorrhage will stop bleeding spontaneously with conservative management. Patients who have severe blood loss associated with hypotension or persistent significant blood loss require emergent investigation. Localization of the source of gastrointestinal (GI) bleeding prior to surgery is important as "blind" segmental colonic resection is associated with higher mortality, a higher incidence of rebleeding, and substantially increased morbidity (PARKES et al. 1993).

23.2 Aetiology

The true aetiology of lower GI bleeding is more complex than has been appreciated previously as many studies record potential sources of bleeding rather than a proven source. A further complicating factor is that patients may have more than one potential lesion within the colon (CAOS et al. 1986). Diverticular disease is the most frequent cause of lower gastrointestinal bleeding and accounts for 20%–50% of cases of colonic bleeding depending on the diagnostic criteria. Angiodysplasia is the next commonest source of acute bleeding. However, angiodysplastic lesions are present in 1%–2% of normal subjects at autopsy and therefore caution is advised before attributing an angiodysplastic lesion as the source of bleeding unless active extravasation is seen. The classical angiographic appearances of angiodysplasia are a vascular blush associated with early filling of a prominent draining vein (Fig. 23.1). Small areas of angiodysplasia are better seen at colonoscopy where they are seen as red, flat lesions occasionally with a prominent adjacent vessel. Although primary colonic neoplasia rarely causes acute GI blood loss, this diagnosis must be borne in mind as significant bleeding can occasionally occur at presentation. Inflammatory and infectious conditions are usually recognised during clinical examination and rarely cause the degree of haemorrhage that requires emergent investigation.

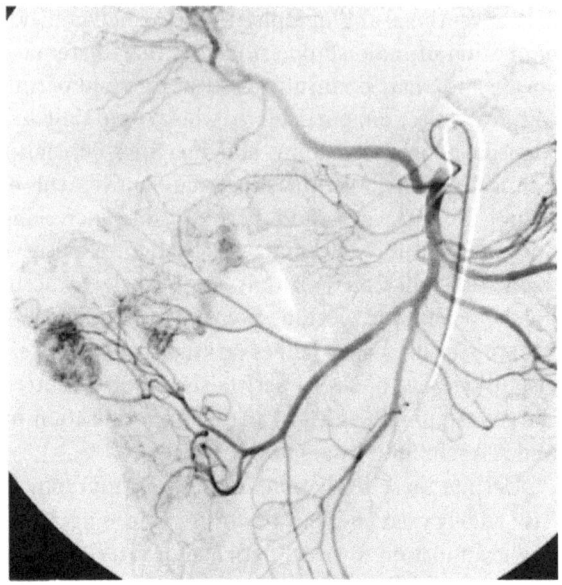

Fig. 23.1. Mid arterial SMA angiogram demonstrating hyperaemic area consistent with angiodysplasia in the ascending colon. An incidental finding is a replaced right hepatic artery

I. ROBERTSON, MD; R. EDWARDS, MD
Consultant Interventional Radiologist, Gartnavel General Hospital, North Glasgow University Hospitals Trust, 1053 Great Western Road, Glasgow G12 0YN, United Kingdom

23.3
Investigation of Colonic Bleeding

A thorough clinical assessment is the key to appropriate diagnosis and therapy and a carefully elicited clinical history often helps to identify the aetiology of bleeding and guide further management. Proctoscopy is an important part of the initial assessment as haemorrhoidal bleeding accounts for 2%–9% of cases and may be readily treated by simple measures such as endoscopic banding. Ideally, initial assessment should also include gastroduodenoscopy, as a proximal source of bleeding will be identified in 10%–15% of patients presenting with lower GI blood loss and endoscopic therapy is successful in the majority of these patients (FARRELL and FREIDMAN 2001).

Further investigations depend on the availability of equipment and personnel. In most centres the next investigation is either Technetium-labelled red cell scintigraphy or arteriography. Elderly patients with significant co-morbidities are at particularly high risk if emergency laparotomy is performed without prior anatomical localization of the source of bleeding.

The technique and interpretation of nuclear medicine studies for GI bleeding is discussed in detail in Chap. 21. Red cell scintigraphy offers several advantages as it is non-invasive and theoretically delayed imaging for up to 24 h is possible. Furthermore, it is more sensitive than diagnostic arteriography. Bleeding rates as low as 0.1–0.5 ml/min can be detected on scintigraphy compared with 0.5–1.0 ml/min required by conventional angiography. Unfortunately, a major limitation of radioisotope studies is that anatomical localisation may be insufficiently accurate to permit surgical resection, particularly when some time has elapsed between bleeding and imaging. Peristalsis can cause antegrade or retrograde movement of radioisotope tracer within the bowel, thus increasing the potential for inaccurate localisation. A positive early red cell scan (<2 h) is more likely to accurately localise the bleeding point (GUPTA et al. 1984; DUSOLD et al. 1995), whereas delayed scans are rarely useful because of bowel peristalsis. In most centres, surgeons are reluctant to operate on localisation by red cell scintigraphy alone.

Despite these limitations red cell scintigraphy is still widely used and may perform a role as a screening examination to select patients for arteriography. The basis of this approach is to perform a red cell scan and only proceed to angiography if the radioisotope scan is positive. There is evidence that this strategy increases the positive diagnostic yield of angiogra-

phy by effectively restricting its use to patients who are actively bleeding (GUNDERMAN et al. 1998).

Diagnostic visceral angiography is an invasive examination with potential risks but offers superior anatomical localisation and in some patients will also determine the cause of blood loss. Arteriography also offers the potential therapeutic options of vasopressin infusion and colonic embolization to control or arrest haemorrhage.

The positive yield from mesenteric angiography is greatest when the patient is actively bleeding and varies between 43%–87% (FIORITO et al. 1989; ALLISON et al. 1982). If patients are not actively bleeding at the time of angiography the diagnostic return drops considerably (GUNDERMAN et al. 1998). Angiography should therefore be performed as rapidly as possible while the patient is being resuscitated with intravenous fluids but is still showing evidence of haemodynamic compromise, i.e. hypotension and tachycardia. Waiting for the patient to be "stabilised" while normotension is restored will reduce the diagnostic yield of the examination.

A visceral arteriogram can represent a considerable challenge in the elderly patient with lower GI bleeding. Patients are frequently restless, breathless and have wide-spread vascular disease. Meticulous attention to angiographic technique is usually rewarded by diagnostic angiograms. The goal of the examination is to identify extravasation indicating the definite source of active bleeding (Fig. 23.2). Identification of a structural lesion such as angiodysplasia may not indicate the current source of blood loss as such lesions are commonly seen in the elderly.

Vigorous bowel peristalsis, often precipitated by the insufflated air from recent endoscopic examinations, will readily obscure bleeding on digital subtraction angiograms and it is essential that Buscopan or a similar agent is utilised to paralyse the bowel. It is rare that the patient can breath-hold for the duration of the angiographic run and "multi-masking" can minimise the effect of breathing artefacts. The patient is instructed to breathe gently throughout the angiogram and approximately two respiratory phases of mask images are acquired prior to the injection of contrast, this provides a bank of mask images that can usually be matched to any phase of the angiographic run.

Non-selective aortic injections are rarely useful. Selective catheterization of the IMA is usually the first step as contrast in the bladder will later obscure this territory. AP and oblique views of the IMA are required to open out the sigmoid colon and splenic flexure. In a patient with active bleeding it is important not to spend too long trying to catheterize a

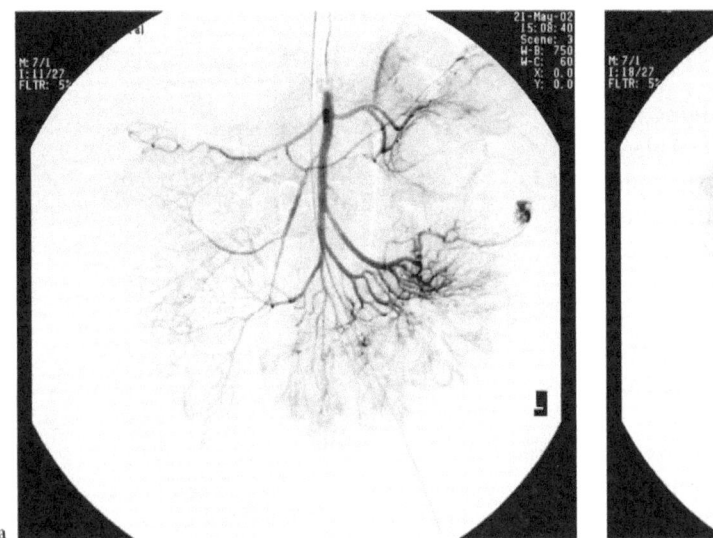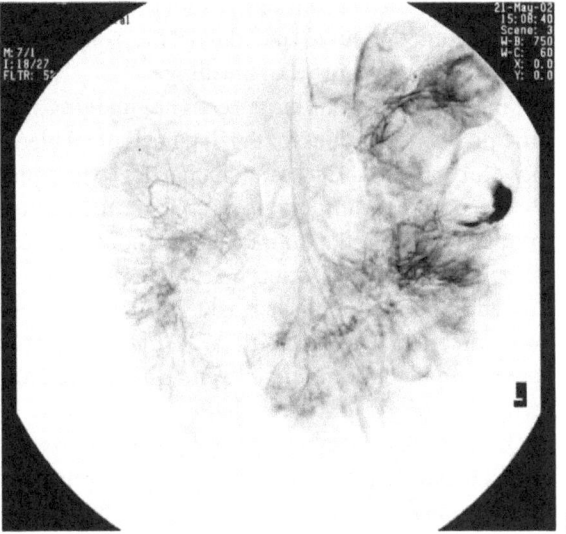

Fig. 23.2a,b. a Mid arterial SMA phase image demonstrating an irregular dense contrast stain indicating extravasation. **b** Early venous phase image shows a change in shape of the stain, typical of extravasation

small IMA. If unsuccessful within a few minutes the operator should perform SMA angiography and return to the IMA if the SMA arteriogram is negative. Ensure that the whole of the SMA territory is imaged. This is often not possible on a single angiographic field of view and overlapping views are frequently required.

Examine the overview SMA runs carefully looking for definite evidence of extravasation. Particular care must be applied if there are any areas of peristalsis as these will readily obscure bleeding. Examination of the unsubtracted images are helpful in distinguishing between peristalsis artefact and true extravasation. Take time to go through the whole run considering the arterial, capillary and venous phase. Potential structural lesions require further more localised views with selective catheterization. If the overview angiogram is completely negative, most angiographers will precede to more selective views of the ileocolic, right colic and middle colic arteries. If these studies are negative, bilateral selective internal iliac angiography should be performed to exclude bleeding from an inferior rectal arterial source.

23.4
Provocation Angiography

In reality, the intermittent nature of colonic bleeding means that a number of patients will have stopped bleeding during the time taken to organise the angio-

gram. This group of patients poses a difficult management problem. Ideally, the angiogram should be deferred until the next bleed. However there is often considerable pressure to perform angiography particularly if there has been a number of intermittent haemodynamically significant bleeds. Provocation angiography may be a potentially useful diagnostic intervention in this group of patients. Unfortunately, there is no uniform technique or dosage schedule for provocation arteriography. Either anticoagulant or thrombolytic agents are injected into the suspected arterial territory to provoke bleeding during angiography and thus identify the source of blood loss. Clearly, preparations and facilities must be appropriate to permit vigourous resuscitation if necessary.

RYAN et al. (2001) reported their experiences of provocation angiography in 17 patients with occult lower GI bleeding using a combination of heparin, vasodilator and tissue plasminogen activator. All patients had previous extensive investigation with negative endoscopic and angiographic studies. In 37.5% of patients a site of bleeding was identified. In a further two patients a vascular abnormality was identified which did not bleed at the time of angiography, therefore an abnormality was identified in 50% of patients. There were no significant procedural complications during provocation. A number of reported series with smaller numbers record a similar increase in bleeding site detection rates varying from 29%–65% (KOVAL et al. 1987; GLICKERMAN et al. 1988; MALDEN et al. 1998). Currently, it seems that provocation angiography may have a role to play in the diagnosis of occult lower gastrointestinal haemorrhage but further work is required to determine the optimum protocol and define the role of this technique in acute lower GI bleeding.

Finally, advances in cross-sectional imaging may provide new techniques for the diagnosis of GI bleeding. Modern spiral CT scanners, particularly multislice technology, can provide a rapid contrast-sensitive assessment of the entire colon without the need for selective catheterization or colonic preparation. Currently limited published data is available. However, detection rates as high as 72% for a source of active colonic bleeding have been reported in small series (Fig. 23.3) (ETTORE et al. 1997).

On balance, the increasing role of embolization means that if facilities and technical expertise permit, then angiography with the recourse to embolization is frequently the most appropriate option.

23.5
Therapeutic Angiography

A major advance in the management of patients with acute lower GI bleeding has been the refinement in the techniques of colonic embolization over the last 10 years. Most bleeding sites can now be successfully and safely embolized using modern coaxial catheters and microcoils. Embolization provides a rapid, more durable control of bleeding than vasopressin therapy and should be the first line therapeutic option. In a minority of cases, due to failure of subselective catheterization or the presence of an extensive angiographic abnormality, embolization may not be appropriate and vasopressin infusion can be of value.

23.5.1
Embolization

Embolization of colonic haemorrhage was first described in 1977 by GOLDBERGER and BOOKSTEIN. Initial enthusiasm for the technique was dampened by reports of colonic infarction in as many as 20% of treated patients; secondary to the combination of the limited collateral supply of the large bowel and the relatively proximal embolization achievable with 7-F catheters (ROSENKRANZ et al. 1982). Advances in catheter and guidewire technology over the last 20 years has permitted a resurgence in embolization as a safe and in some cases definitive treatment option for patients with colonic haemorrhage.

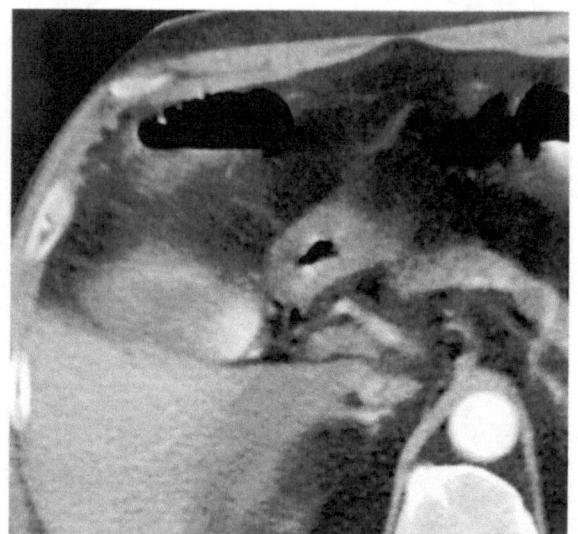

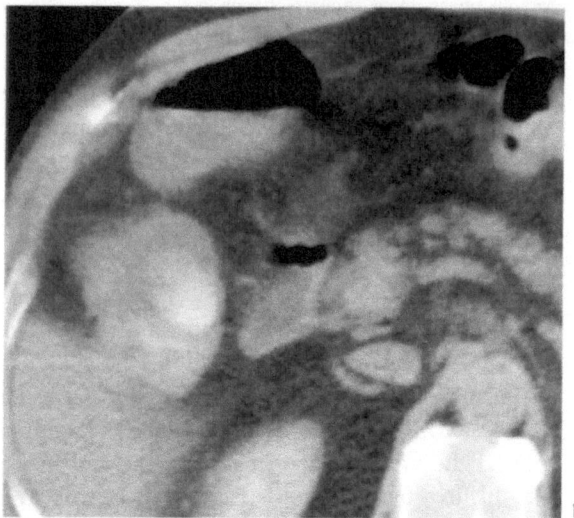

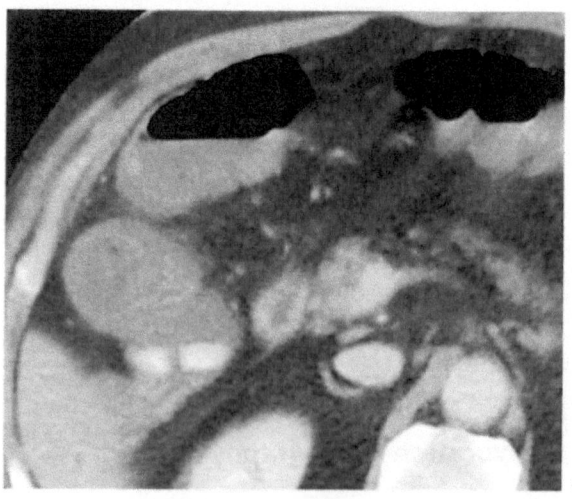

Fig. 23.3a–c. Spiral dynamic CT scan with acquisition at 30 s (a), 70 s (b) and 180 s (c) demonstrating a focal area of extravasation at the hepatic flexure

Modern hydrophilic 4- and 5-F catheters allow subselective catheterization and when used in combination with coaxial microcatheters, very distal embolization of the vasa recta can be achieved. Contemporary case series record technical success rates varying between 76%–100% (Table 23.1).

The aim of the angiographer must be to achieve embolization as close as possible to the bleeding source and in most series this is achieved at the level of the vasa recta (Fig. 23.4). Particular care must be taken to limit devascularization around the watershed areas of the colon, such as the splenic flexure.

There are reports of successful embolization with a number of different agents including Gelfoam, polyvinyl alcohol particles and coils but increasingly, microcoils are recognised as the agent of choice. (Table 23.1). Microcoils measuring 2 or 3 mm offer a readily controllable embolic agent that will occlude the feeding vessel with minimal danger to the collateral supply of the colon.

Even with the use of distal embolization there remains a small risk of intestinal ischaemia or infarction. Bowel ischaemia and infarction requiring operative intervention is a rare event in most series but must be considered during the consent process and aftercare (Table 23.1). While clinical symptoms of colonic ischaemia are uncommon, a significant proportion of patients develop asymptomatic mucosal ischaemia most often demonstrated on colonoscopic examination. BANDI et al. reported their long-term follow-up, extending to a number of years, of 25 of 35 patients treated by subselective embolization for acute colonic haemorrhage. In this series no patient developed symptomatic stricturing or ischaemia in the embolized territory.

The balance between limiting embolization to ensure enough blood supply remains to maintain bowel integrity and arresting haemorrhage can be difficult. The need to limit embolization in colonic haem-

orrhage may account for the significant rebleeding rate recorded in most studies which can be as high as 25% (Table 23.1). Clearly, if a patient rebleeds further coil embolization is usually possible if a distal embolization was performed initially. Interestingly, BANDI et al. (2001) have described the phenomenon of rebleeding from previously embolized lesions some months after the initial treatment (mean 74 days).

Frequently, it is not possible to determine the cause of bleeding at angiography and while control of haemorrhage can be successfully achieved it is imperative to ensure that further investigation occurs to determine the source of haemorrhage and consider appropriate medical or surgical therapy.

23.5.2
Vasopressin

Vasopressin acts by direct action, causing constriction of smooth muscle of the GI tract and vasculature. The drug has a rapid onset of action and requires continuous infusion to control haemorrhage. Major complications are secondary to systemic vasoconstriction and include myocardial ischaemia, severe hypertension and pulmonary oedema which may occur in up to 20% of patients. Minor complications include fluid retention, transient arrhythmias and hyponatraemia.

Vasopressin is usually delivered as a direct intra-arterial infusion. After initial identification of the site of bleeding the catheter is either placed in the proximal SMA or IMA. Subselective catheterization is avoided as this increases the risk of bowel infarction. A vasopressin infusion is then commenced and the dose titrated to stop bleeding as seen on check angiography. A typical schedule will commence with a dose of 0.2 U/min with repeat arteriography after 30 min to ensure haemorrhage has ceased. If there is continuing

Table 23.1. Embolization for colonic haemorrhage

Author	No. of patients	Technical failures	Technical success	Haemostasis	Embolic material	Rebleeding	Complications (number of patients)
BANDI et al 2001	48	13	77%	37	PVA(28) Coils (11)	12	Asymptomatic mucosal ischaemai (6)
FUNAKI et al 2001	27	2	95%	26	Coils	2	Bowel infarction (1), asymptomatic ischaemia (1)
DEBARROS et al 2002	27	0	100%	27	Coils	6	Bowel infarction (1), asymptomatic ischaemia (1)
NICHOLSON et al 1998	14	0	100%	12	Coils	0	Bowel infarction (1), asymptomatic ischaemia (1)
GORDON et al 1997	17	4	76%	13	Coils	N/A	Bowel infarction (1), asymptomatic ischaemia (1)

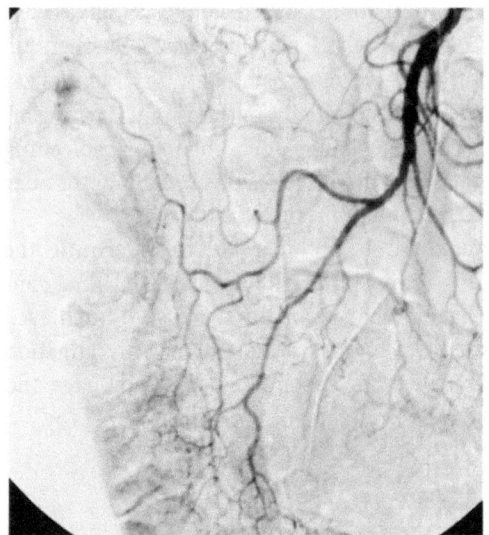

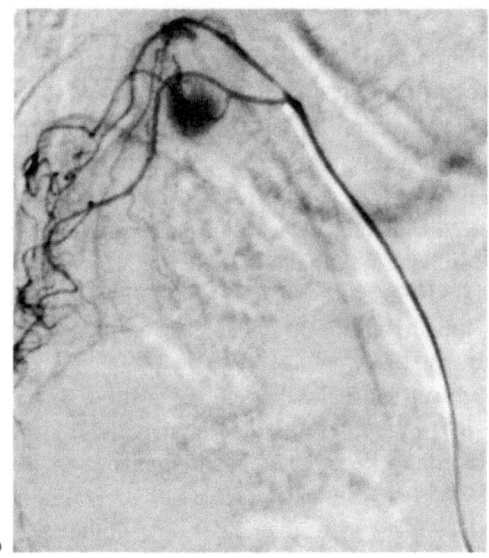

haemorrhage the dose may be increased to 0.4 U/min and again angiography is repeated after 30 min. If a dose of 0.4 U/min does not control haemorrhage then preparations are made for either an attempt at embolization or surgery. If the bleeding has been successfully controlled after 12–24 h the vasopressin infusion is progressively tapered down and the patient carefully observed for evidence of recurrent bleeding.

Vasopressin infusion achieves initial control of colonic bleeding in 80%–90% of cases of colonic haemorrhage (CLARK et al. 1981). Unfortunately rebleeding will recur acutely in up to 30% of patients.

Many elderly patients with colonic haemorrhage present relative if not absolute contraindications to vasopressin therapy because of coronary and peripheral vascular disease. In addition, even for patients in whom there is no direct contraindication there is a significant risk of a complication or rebleeding. Increasingly, vasopressin therapy is reserved for those patients in whom subselective embolization is not technically possible.

23.6
Conclusion

Diagnostic arteriography remains a cornerstone in the management of patients with acute colonic bleeding. Non-invasive techniques, particularly multi-slice CT, may offer anatomical localisation in the future and help provide a screening test that will allow selection of patients with ongoing blood loss for embolization. Distal coil embolization offers a safe and effective method to arrest acute colonic haemorrhage.

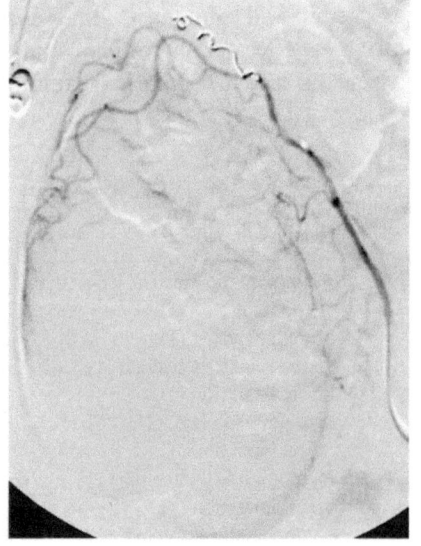

Fig. 23.4a–c. a Arterial phase SMA arteriogram demonstrating extravasation at the hepatic flexure. **b** Selective angiogram with the tip of the microcatheter at the level of the vasa recta. Extravasation is clearly seen. **c** Post embolization angiogram demonstrating feeding vessel occlusion after two 3-mm microcoils have been deployed. Note the distension of the ascending colon secondary to bleeding

References

Allison DJ, Hemmingway AP, Cunningham DA (1982) Angiography in gastrointestinal bleeding. Lancet 2:30–33

Bandi R, Shetty P, Sharma RP et al (2001) Superselective arterial embolization for the treatment of lower gastrointestinal hemorrhage. J Vasc Intervent Radiol 12:1399–1405

Caos A, Benner KG, Manier J et al (1986) Colonoscopy after Golytely preparation in acute rectal bleeding. J Clin Gastroenterol 8:46–49

Clark RA, Colley DP, Eggers FM (1981) Acute arterial gastrointestinal haemorrhage: efficacy of transcatheter control Am J Roentgenol 136:1185–1189

Debarros J, Rosas L, Cohen J et al (2002) The changing paradigm for the treatment of colonic hemorrhage: superselective angiographic embolization. Dis Colon Rectum 45:802–808

Dusold R, Burke K, Carpentier W et al (1995) The accuracy of technetium 99m labelled red cell scintigraphy in localizing gastrointestinal bleeding. Am J Gastroenterol 89:345–348

Ettore GC, Francioso G, Garribba AP et al (1997) Helical CT angiography in gastrointestinal bleeding of obscure origin. Am J Roentgenol 168:727–730

Farrell JJ, Freidman LS (2001) Gastrointestinal bleeding in the elderly Gastroenterol Clin North Am 30:377–407

Fiorito JJ, Brandt LJ, Kozicky et al (1989) The diagnostic yield of superior mesenteric angiography: correlation with the pattern of gastrointestinal bleeding. Am J Gastroenterol 84:878–881

Funaki B, Kostelic JK, Lorenz J et al (2001) Superselective microcoil embolization of colonic haemorrhage Am J Roentgenol 177:829–836

Glickerman DJ, Kowdley KV, Rosch J (1988) Urokinase in gastrointestinal tract bleeding. Radiology 168:375–376

Goldberger LE, Bookstein JJ (1977) Transcatheter embolization for treatment of diverticular haemorrhage. Radiology 122:613–617

Gordon RL, Ahl KL, Kerlan RK Jr et al (1997) Selective arterial embolization for the control of lower gastrointestinal bleeding. Am J Surg 174:24–28

Gunderman R, Leef J, Ong K et al (1998) Scinitigraphic screening prior to visceral arteriography in acute lower gastrointestinal bleeding J Nucl Med 39:1081–1083

Gupta S, Luna E, Kingsley S et al (1984) Detection of gastrointestinal bleeding by radionuclide scintigraphy. Am J Gastroenterol 79:26–31

Koval G, Benner KG, Rosch J et al (1987) Aggressive angiographic diagnosis in acute lower gastrointestinal haemorrhage. Dig Dis Sci 32:248–253

Malden ES, Hicks ME, Royal HD (1998) Recurrent gastrointestinal bleeding: use of thrombolysis with anticoagulation in diagnosis. Radiology 207:147–151

Nicholson AA, Ettles DF, Hartley JE et al (1998) Transcatheter coil emblotherapy: a safe and effective option for major colonic haemorrhage. Gut 43:79–84

Parkes PM, Obeid FN, Sorensen VJ et al (1993) The management of massive lower gastrointestinal bleeding. Am Surg 59:676–678

Rosenkranz H, Bookstein JJ, Roesn RJ et al (1982) Postembolic colonic infarction. Radiology 142:47–51

Ryan MJ, Key SM, Dumbleton SA et al (2001) Nonlocalized lower gastrointestinal bleeding: provocative bleeding studies with intra-arterial tpa, heparin and tolazoline. J Vasc Intervent Radiol 12:1273–1277

24 Colonic Lymphoma

Niklas Hennessy, Jenny Macpherson, Ken Tung

CONTENTS

24.1 Introduction *243*
24.2 Histological Types *243*
24.3 Clinical Features *244*
24.4 Radiological Appearances *244*
24.4.1 Intraluminal Mass *244*
24.4.2 Infiltrative Lesion *244*
24.4.3 Endo-exoenteric Mass *246*
24.4.4 Aneurysmal Dilatation *247*
24.4.5 Mesenteric Invasion *247*
24.4.6 Diffuse Mucosal Nodularity *248*
24.5 Conclusion *249*
References *249*

24.1
Introduction

Lymphoma involves the colon either as a primary neoplasm or as part of disseminated disease. Colorectal lymphoma accounts for between 7% and 15% of gastrointestinal lymphoma and the colon is the third commonest site after stomach and small bowel (Freeman et al. 1972; Herrman et al. 1980; Lewin et al. 1978; Meigbow et al. 1983; Weinsrad et al. 1982).

Dawson et al. originally defined the criteria for the diagnosis of primary colonic lymphoma in 1961: no palpable superficial lymph nodes; no lymphadenopathy on the chest radiograph; at laparotomy the alimentary lesion predominates and lymph node involvement is confined to the drainage area of the involved segment of gut; no liver or spleen involvement. Lewin et al. (1978) described alternative criteria, which are

N. Hennessy, FRCR
Specialist Registrar in Radiology, Southampton University Hospital, Tremona Road, Southampton SO16 6YD, United Kingdom
J. Macpherson, MRCP, FRCR
Fellow in Abdominal Radiology, Vancouver Hospital and Health Sciences Centre, 855 West 12th Avenue, Vancouver, British Columbia V5Z 1M9, Canada
K. Tung, FRCP, FRCR
Consultant Radiologist, Southampton University Hospital, Tremona Road, Southampton SO16 6YD, United Kingdom

now more often used. These criteria define primary colonic lymphoma as including those patients who have either obvious predominant alimentary tract signs or who present initially with gastrointestinal symptoms that prove to be caused by gastrointestinal involvement with lymphoma. Secondary lymphoma includes patients whose gastrointestinal involvement is detected following previously diagnosed extra-abdominal lymphoma.

Barium enema examinations and computed tomography are used as complimentary studies in the evaluation of primary colonic lymphoma. A barium enema examination is often the first investigation used in the investigation of a patient with bowel symptoms. Early descriptions and classifications of the radiological appearances of colonic lymphoma have been restricted to the barium enema appearances. Computed tomography is necessary for staging purposes but can also define the extent of endo-exoenteric tumour masses and suggest features to help differentiate primary lymphoma from adenocarcinoma. Barium enema examination is helpful in diagnosing complications such as fistula formation and the evaluation of subtle mucosal filling defects that could be missed on computed tomography. However, the advent of colonography, available with multislice computed tomography, may reduce the need for barium enema studies.

24.2
Histological Types

Primary colonic lymphoma is rare, accounting for less than 0.1% of primary colonic malignancies and less than 3% of extra-nodal lymphomas (Dodd 1990; Lewin et al. 1992). Secondary colonic involvement in patients with advanced lymphoma is not uncommon and microscopic evidence of tumour is found in up to 46% of cases at autopsy (Herrman et al. 1980). However, it is often undetected, as patients with disseminated lymphoma involving the colon usually do not have specific bowel symptoms.

These tumours are believed to arise from the lymphoid tissue of the lamina propria. Most lymphomas affecting the colon are B cell non-Hodgkin's lymphomas, of which diffuse large B cell lymphoma is the most common subtype. The other main subtypes are mantle cell lymphoma, Burkitt's lymphoma and Burkitt-like lymphoma. Primary Hodgkin's and T cell lymphomas have been reported but are rare (THOMAS et al. 1997; SON et al. 1997).

24.3
Clinical Features

Primary colonic lymphoma is usually seen in middle-aged or elderly people. Males are twice as likely to be affected as females (CORNES et al. 1961; WYCHULIS et al. 1966). The average duration of symptoms is 4–6 months (MARSHAK et al. 1979; WYCHULIS et al. 1966). Common presenting symptoms and signs include abdominal pain, abdominal mass, weight loss and changing bowel habit. Rectal bleeding and diarrhoea are less common and seen in 25% of patients.

Predisposing factors to the development of gastrointestinal lymphoma include acquired immunodeficiency syndrome and immunosuppression following solid organ transplantation. Recent studies question long-term inflammatory bowel disease as a predisposing factor although immune modifier therapy could be potentially implicated in a small percentage of cases of lymphoma occurring in the setting of inflammatory bowel disease (LEWIS et al. 2001; LOFTUS et al. 2000).

24.4
Radiological Appearances

The radiological appearances can be classified as focal or diffuse. The focal types can be subdivided into intraluminal mass, infiltrative lesion, endo-exoenteric mass, aneurysmal dilatation and mesenteric invasion. The most common sites of involvement are the caecum and rectum. There is no correlation between the histological subtype and the focal appearance. The diffuse pattern takes the form of mucosal nodularity and is seen predominantly in the mantle cell subtype (CALLAWAY et al. 1997; LAVERGNE et al. 1994).

Differentiating colonic lymphoma from adenocarcinoma can be helped by certain CT findings. The possibility of lymphoma should be considered when caecal tumours involve the terminal ileum, when tumours do not invade the pericolonic fat or adjacent structures, when tumours perforate in the absence of desmoplastic reaction and when there are secondary findings such as splenomegaly or bulky lymph node enlargement (BRUNETON et al. 1983; WYATT et al. 1993).

24.4.1
Intraluminal Mass

These bulky polypoid lesions are the most common focal type, usually presenting with a palpable abdominal mass associated with abdominal pain. The lesions are lobulated, broad-based, sessile lesions with or without central depressions or ulcerations. They vary in size from 4 cm to 20 cm and are commonly situated in the caecum, causing irregular enlargement of the ileocaecal valve. They rarely cause obstruction although colocolic intussusception has been reported (O'CONNELL and THOMPSON 1978). These polyps are often indistinguishable from adenomatous polyps and biopsy is required to make the diagnosis (Figs. 24.1, 24.2).

24.4.2
Infiltrative Lesion

On computed axial tomography the infiltrating form characteristically shows concentric bowel wall thickening over a long segment of colon (Figs. 24.2–24.4). The colonic lumen may be narrowed but obstruction is uncommon. The barium enema typically shows a

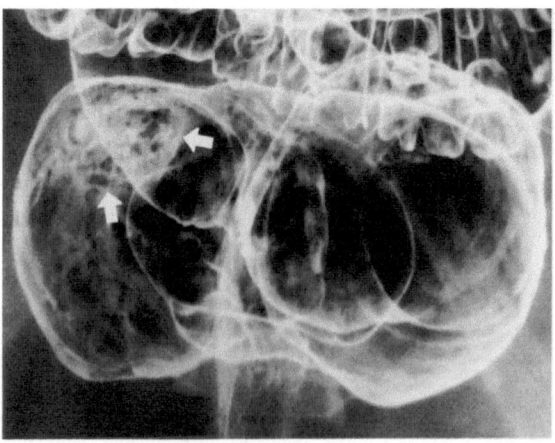

Fig. 24.1. A 71-year-old woman with diffuse large B cell lymphoma, who initially presented with cervical lymphadenopathy. She relapsed some time after chemotherapy and the barium enema shows an intraluminal rectal mass (*arrows*)

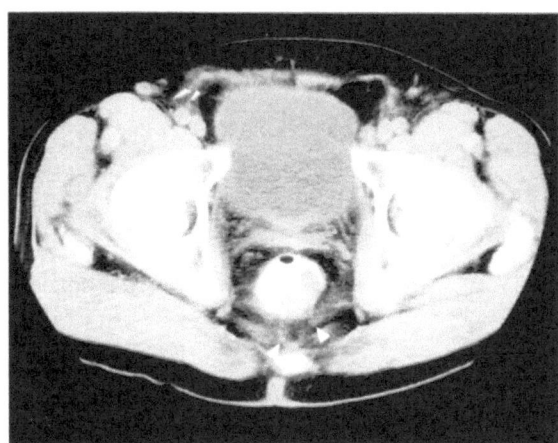
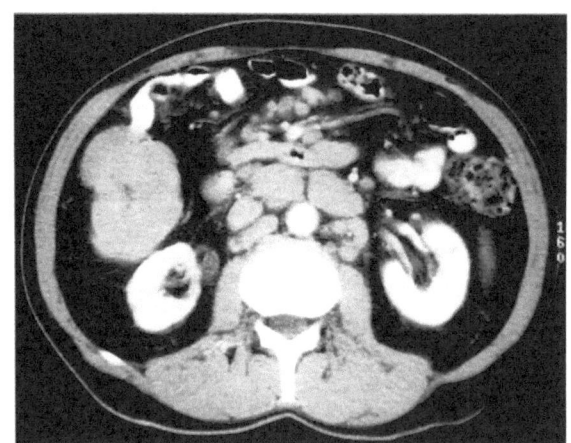

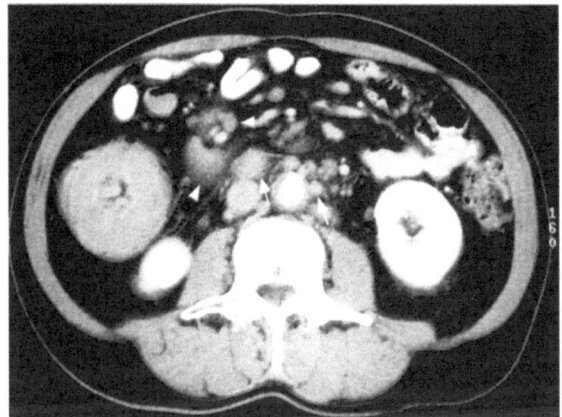

Fig. 24.2a–c. A 70-year-old man presented with rectal bleeding. CT with intravenous, oral and rectal contrast. **a** There is a mural-based, lobulated, posterior intraluminal rectal mass, with hazy nodularity in the peri-rectal fat (*arrowheads*). On biopsy this was found to be mantle cell lymphoma. The patient also had a large caecal mass (**b**), which extended to the ascending colon where there is concentric stratification (**c**) typical of an infiltrative lesion, and multiple mesenteric (*arrowheads*) and retroperitoneal lymph nodes (*arrows*)

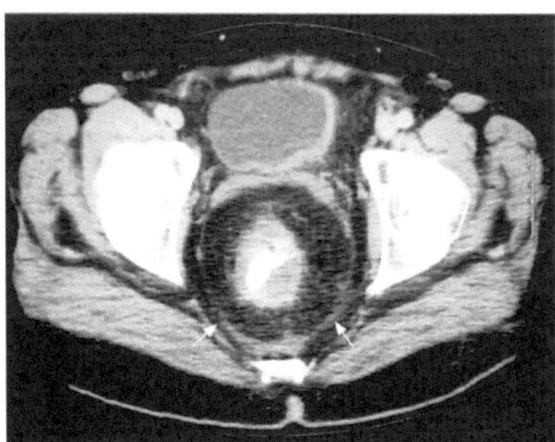
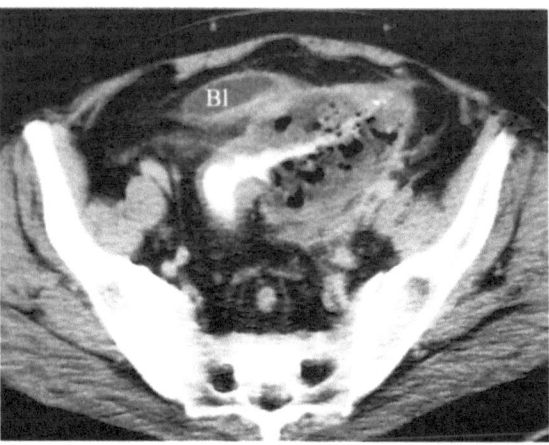

Fig. 24.3a,b. A 56-year-old man with a history of ulcerative colitis. **a** CT with intravenous, oral and rectal contrast shows diffuse thickening of the rectum. There is hazy nodularity in the peri-rectal fat and thickening of the peri-rectal fascia (*arrows*). **b** This is contiguous with a thick walled sigmoid colon (lying posterior to the bladder dome). There are gas locules within an intramural abscess. Infiltrative diffuse large B cell lymphoma. *Bl*, bladder

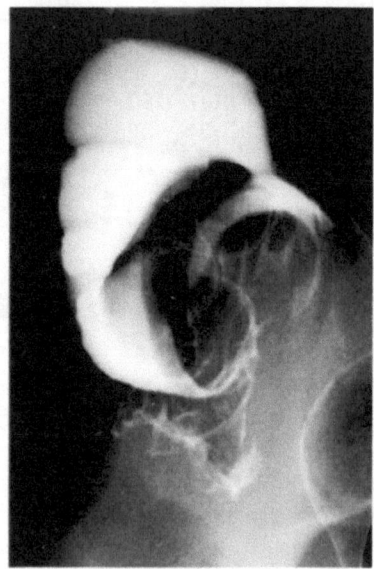

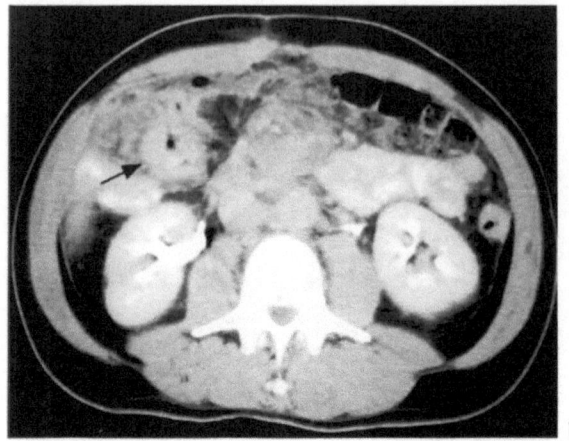

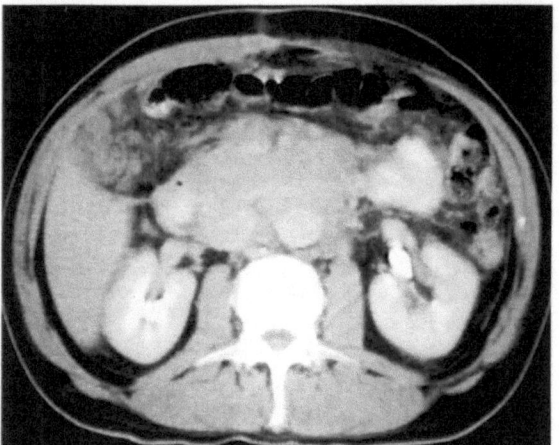

Fig. 24.4a-c. This 57-year-old man presented with a short history of colicky abdominal pain. **a** Barium enema showed a partially intussuscepted ileo-caecal mass. A right hemicolectomy was performed and Burkitt's lymphoma was confirmed. The patient relapsed after chemotherapy. CT showed recurrent tumour at the ileo-colonic anastamosis (*arrow*) (**b**), nodular omental thickening (**c**) and confluent retroperitoneal lymphadenopathy

rigid ahaustral segment with smooth mucosal nodularity, suggesting submucosal infiltration rather than ulceration. The appearances are not specific and the major considerations in the differential diagnosis are ischaemic stricture and colonic carcinoma.

24.4.3
Endo-exoenteric Mass

This form was defined by MARSHAK et al. (1961), with reference to the small bowel, as a large excavated mass with multiple fistulous communications to adjacent loops of intestines. In the colon the commonest site this bulky cavitating tumour is the rectum. Fistulae are not always present. On barium enema there is a perirectal mass with displacement, encasement and narrowing of the rectum with local mucosal destruction. Fistulae to ileum or bladder occur and local perforations produce perirectal abscesses (Figs. 24.5–24.7) (O'CONNELL and THOMPSON 1978). Elsewhere in the colon the tumour may extend into the mesentery.

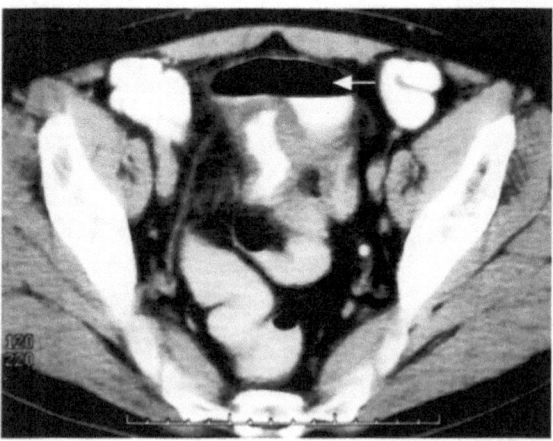

Fig. 24.5. A 49-year-old man presented with pneumaturia and fecaluria. CT with intravenous and oral contrast shows a complex mass involving small bowel, sigmoid colon and bladder. There is gas in the bladder (*arrow*) as a result of a colovesical fistula. Endo-exoenteric form of diffuse large B cell lymphoma

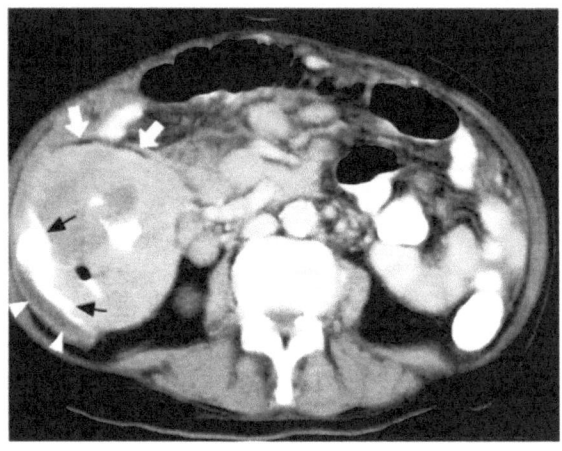 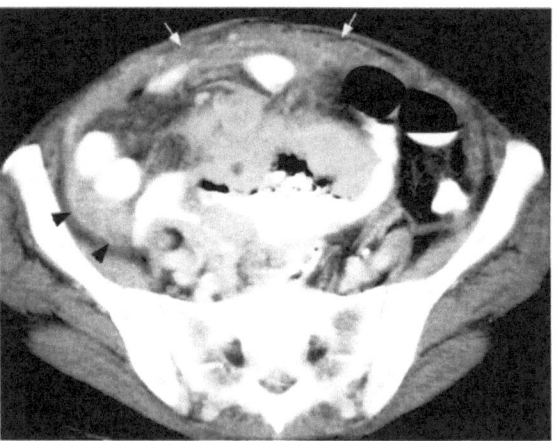

a b

Fig. 24.6a,b. A 78-year-old woman presented with fever and abdominal pain. CT with intravenous and oral contrast. **a** There is an endo-exoenteric mass involving the caecum and ascending colon and outlined anteriorly by a rim of fat (*thick white arrows*). There is a localised perforation with leakage of contrast into the lateral subserosal space (*black arrows*) with a small amount of ascites in the right paracolic gutter (*arrowheads*). **b** There is also a cavitating and thick walled mass arising from the sigmoid colon, with infiltrative change in omentum (*small arrows*). There are mesenteric and retroperitoneal lymph nodes and a small amount of ascites (*arrowheads*). Diffuse large B cell lymphoma

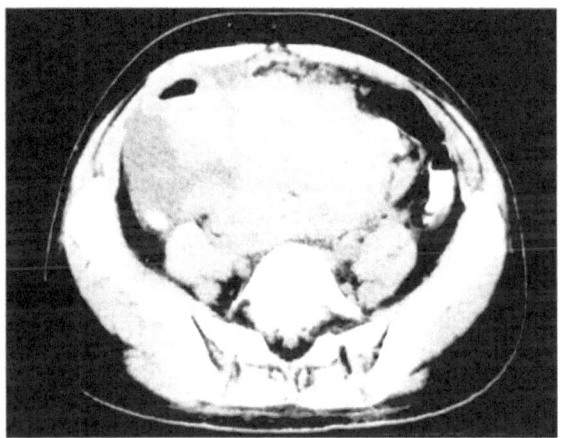 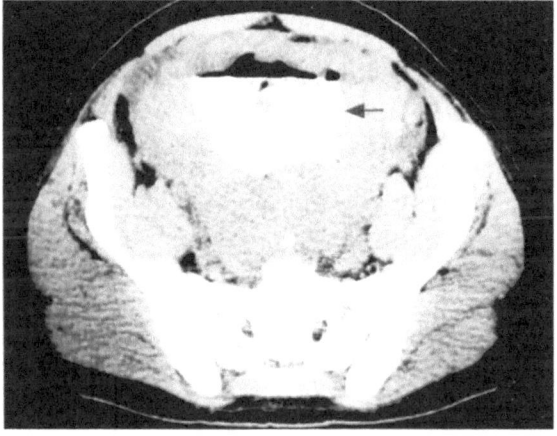

a b

Fig. 24.7a,b. This 20-year-old man presented with an abdominal mass and blood in the stools. **a,b** CT shows a large lobulated endo-exoenteric lymphoma mass involving the sigmoid and ascending colon. There is a large cavity containing gas and oral contrast (*arrow*). Variant of Burkitt's lymphoma

Obstruction is uncommon. The differential diagnosis includes perforated adenocarcinoma, stromal tumour (leiomyosarcoma), Crohn's disease, tuberculosis, Hodgkin's disease and actinomycosis.

24.4.4
Aneurysmal Dilatation

This is an uncommon appearance of colonic lymphoma and this radiological pattern is more often seen in small bowel lymphoma. Aneurysmal dilatation as the sole radiological feature has been described by

MONTGOMERY and CHEW (1997) and is the result of infiltration of the muscularis propria and the autonomic plexus (Fig. 24.8). More frequently, dilatation of the colonic wall is seen in association with other focal forms of colonic lymphoma.

24.4.5
Mesenteric Invasion

These tumours are entirely extraluminal. Radiologically they consist of a soft tissue mass causing extrinsic compression without mucosal infiltration. There

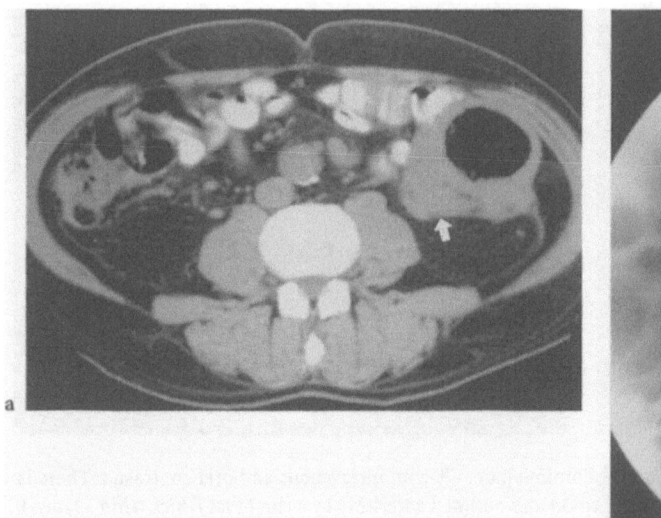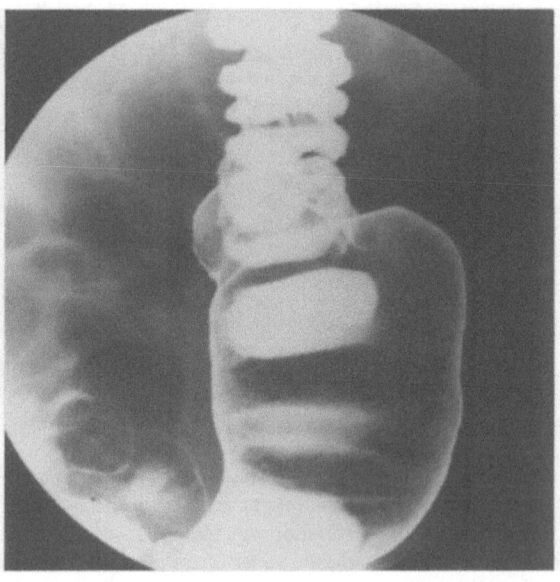

Fig. 24.8a,b. A 68-year-old man presented with recurrent abdominal pain and rectal bleeding. **a** CT showed mural thickening of a segment of descending colon, with aneurysmal dilatation and exophytic masses (*arrow*). **b** The aneurysmal dilatation is also shown on a barium enema examination. The histology was low-grade B-cell lymphoma with plasmacytic differentiation. (Courtesy of M. Montgomery MD and F. Chew MD)

may be a desmoplastic response causing tethering and retraction of the colon. On barium enema the haustral pattern may be absent due to serosal fibrous reaction (O'CONNELL and THOMPSON 1978).

24.4.6
Diffuse Mucosal Nodularity

This diffuse form is associated with primary mantle cell lymphoma or disseminated disease from a nodal primary lymphoma. The nodules are numerous and vary in size from 2 mm to 25 mm with an average diameter of 7 mm (O'CONNELL and THOMPSON 1978). The nodules are commonly smooth and sessile but can be irregular, elongated, pedunculated, umbilicated or filiform. A long segment or the entire colon may be involved. There is often a conglomerate, discrete caecal mass (WILLIAMS et al. 1984) and associated mesenteric lymph nodes are usually enlarged (Fig. 24.9). The primary lymphoma disseminates early in its course to the liver, spleen, peripheral lymph nodes and bone

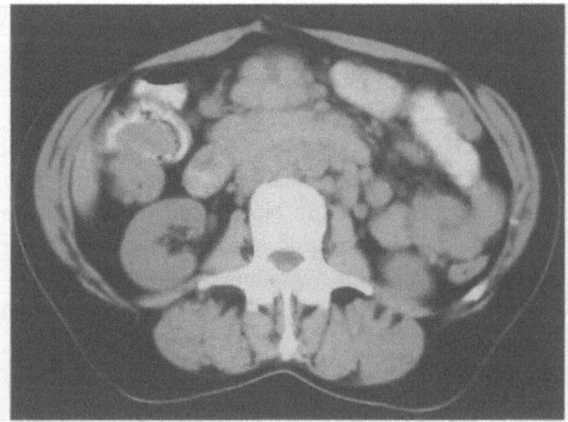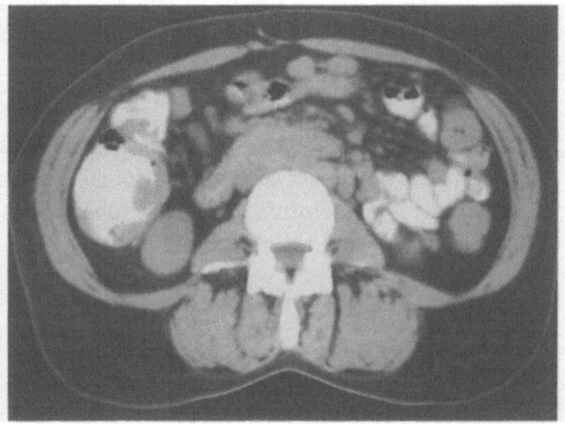

Fig. 24.9a,b. This 65-year-old woman presented initially with intussusception. **a** CT with oral contrast showed a caecal mass with mesenteric and retroperitoneal lymph nodes. The patient underwent limited surgery and chemotherapy but relapsed 6 years later when CT (**b**) showed numerous polypoid nodules projecting into the lumen of the caecum and ascending colon. Biopsy confirmed recurrent mantle cell lymphoma

marrow, and may involve the stomach and small bowel (Issacson and Wright 1995). Diffuse colonic lymphoma can be associated with acute toxic dilatation or pneumatosis coli but this is rare (Moya Sanz et al. 2000; O'Connell and Thompson 1978).

The nodular mucosal pattern resembles the pseudopolyposis of long standing ulcerative colitis. However, the haustral pattern is maintained in colonic lymphoma and ulceration is uncommon. Other conditions to be considered in the differential diagnosis include familial polyposis, lymphoid hyperplasia, cystic fibrosis, pseudomembranous colitis and schistosomiasis although the combination of features previously described should favour the diagnosis of lymphoma.

24.5
Conclusion

Primary colonic lymphoma is rare and most often due to B cell non-Hodgkin's lymphoma. Secondary involvement of the colon in disseminated lymphoma is more common but usually does not cause specific bowel symptoms. The radiological appearances can be classified as focal or diffuse, some of which have features that are characteristic of lymphoma. Other findings such as splenomegaly or bulky abdominal lymph node enlargement should also suggest the possibility of colonic lymphoma.

References

Bruneton JN, Thyss A, Bourry J, Bidoli R, Scneider M (1983) Colonic and rectal lymphomas. A report of six cases and a review of the literature. Fortschr Geb Rontgenstr Nuklearmed 138:283–287

Callaway MP, O'Donovan DG, Lee SH (1997) Case report: malignant lymphomatous polyposis of the colon. Clin Rad 52 :797–798

Cornes JS, Wallace MH, Morson BC (1961) Benign lymphomas of the rectum and anal canal. J Pathol Bacteriol 82: 371–382

Dawson IMP, Cornes JS, Morson BC (1961) Primary malignant tumours of the gastrointestinal tract. Br J Surg 49:80

Dodd GD (1990) Lymphoma of hollow abdominal viscera. Radiol Clin North Am 28:771–783

Freeman C, Berg JW, Cutler SJ (1972) Occurrence and prognosis of extranodal lymphomas. Cancer 29:252–260

Herrman RA, Panahon AM, Barcos MP (1980) Gastrointestinal involvement in non-Hodgkin's lymphoma. Cancer 46: 215–222

Issacson PG, Wright DH (1995) Gut associated lymphoid tumors. In: Whitehead R (ed) Gastrointestinal and oesophageal pathology. Churchill Livingstone, Edinburgh, pp 755–775

Lavergne A, Brouland JP, Launay E et al (1994) Multiple lymphomatous polyposis of the gastrointestinal tract. An extensive histopathologic and immunohistochemical study of 12 cases. Cancer 74:3042–3050

Lewin KJ, Ranchod M, Dorfman RF (1978) Lymphomas of the gastrointestinal tract. A study of 117 cases presenting with gastrointestinal disease. Cancer 42:693–705

Lewin KJ, Riddle R, Weinstein W (1992) Gastrointestinal pathology and its clinical implications. Igaku-Shoin, New York, pp 167–180

Lewis JD, Bilker WB, Brensinger C et al (2001) Inflammatory bowel disease is not associated with an increased risk of lymphoma. Gastroenterology 121:1080–1087

Loftus EV Jr, Tremaine WJ, Habermann TM et al (2000) Risk of lymphoma in inflammatory bowel disease. Am J Gastroenterol 95:2308–2312

Marshak RH, Wolf BS, Eliasoph J (1961) The roentgen findings in lymphosarcoma of the small intestine. Am J Roentgenol Radium Ther Nucl Med 86:682–692

Marshak RH, Lindner AE, Maklansky D (1979) Lymphoreticular disorders of the gastrointestinal tract: roentgenographic features. Gastrointest Radiol 4:103–120

Megibow AJ, Balthazar EJ, Naidich DP, Bosniak MA (1983) Computed tomography of gastrointestinal lymphoma. AJR 141:541–547

Montgomery M, Chew S (1997) Primary lymphoma of the colon. AJR 168:688

Moya Sanz A, Gomez Codina J, Prieto Rodriguez M et al (2000) Toxic megacolon: a rare presentation of primary lymphoma of the colon. Eur J Gastroenterol Hepatol 12:583–586

O'Connell DJ, Thompson AJ (1978) Lymphoma of the colon: the spectrum of radiologic changes. Gastrointest Radiol 2: 377–385

Son HJ, Rhee PL, Kim JJ et al (1997) Primary T-cell lymphoma of the colon. Korean J Inter Med 12:238–241

Thomas DB, Huston BM, Lamm KR, Maia DM (1997) Primary Hodgkin's disease of the sigmoid colon; a case report and review of the literature. Arch Pathol Lab Med 121:528–532

Weinsrad D, De Cosse JJ, Sherlock P et al (1982) Primary gastrointestinal lymphoma. Cancer 49:1258–1265

Williams SM, Berk RN, Harned RK (1984) Radiologic features of multinodular lymphoma of the colon. AJR 143:87–91

Wyatt SH, Fishman EK, Jones B (1993) Primary lymphoma of the colon and rectum: CT and barium enema correlation. Abdom Imaging 18:376–380

Wychulis AR, Beahrs OH, Wodner LB (1966) Malignant lymphoma of the colon. Arch Surg 93:215–225

25 Colorectal Trauma

DINA F. CAROLINE and ANTHONY H. CHAPMAN

CONTENTS

25.1   Iatrogenic Colorectal Complications *251*
25.1.1 Endoscopy *251*
25.1.2 Barium Enema *253*
25.2   Foreign Bodies *256*
25.3   Blunt Trauma *256*
25.4   Penetrating Trauma *259*
        References *260*

25.1
Iatrogenic Colorectal Complications

25.1.1
Endoscopy

Diagnostic and therapeutic endoscopic examinations of the colon have well understood risks. These range from small ulcerations at the site of mucosal biopsy or cauterization, to hematomas from traumatic manipulation of the endoscope, to frank perforation. Colorectal perforation is the most serious complication of colonoscopy, particularly if unrecognized at the time so that the patient re-presents with peritonitis. While perforation is a rare complication in the hands of experienced endoscopists, the risk of perforation and mortality is real. The incidence varies considerably, but most estimate the risk as 0.2% (1/500) with a mortality of 0.02% (1/5000) (VALLERA and BAILIE 1996; MUHLDORFER et al. 1992; CARPIO et al. 1989; GARBAY et al. 1996; HALL et al. 1991). Diagnostic colonoscopy carries a lower risk than therapeutic procedures (KAVIN et al. 1992; LO and BEATON 1994; MACRAE et al. 1983; WAYE et al. 1992) and perforation from flexible sigmoidoscopy is exceptionally rare. The mechanism of perforation during colonoscopy may be mechanical, pneumatic or thermal. Mechanical per-

foration occurs from maneuvers used to advance or withdraw the colonoscope. Tears are most often on the antimesenteric border of the sigmoid and tend to be longitudinal and long and often extend into the peritoneal cavity (VELEZ et al. 1997). Thermal injury is the usual mechanism of injury during therapeutic colonoscopy for biopsy or polypectomy. Such perforations are usually small and have a less serious morbidity than perforations from diagnostic procedures (LO and BEATON 1994).

Endoscopic perforation is invariably associated with a sizeable pneumoperitoneum (Fig.25.1) (MEYERS and GHAHREMANI 1975) because both insufflated air and intestinal gas escape into the peritoneal cavity and in such cases, the symptomatic patient is usually taken emergently to surgery without further diagnostic procedures.

D. F. CAROLINE, MD
Department of Diagnostic Imaging, Temple University Hospital, 3401 Broad and Ontario Streets, Philadelphia, PA 19140, USA
A. H. CHAPMAN, FRCP, FRCR
Head of Radiology, Leeds Teaching Hospitals Trust, St. James's University Hospital, Leeds, LS9 7TF, UK

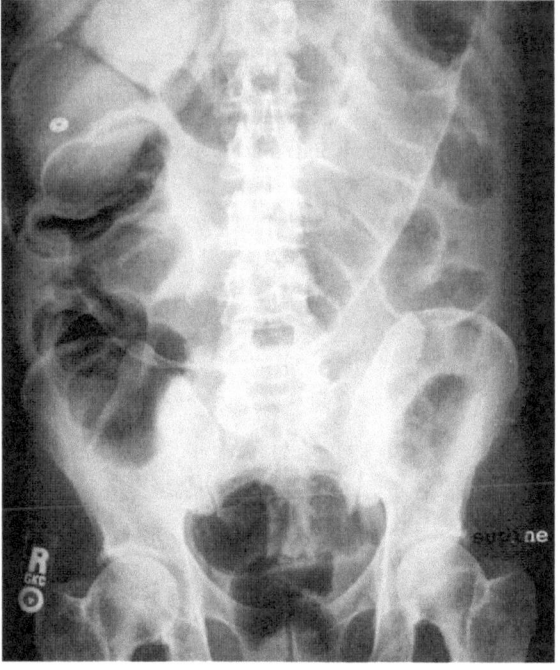

Fig. 25.1. Colonoscopic perforation. Supine abdominal film. Intraperitoneal perforation with massive pneumoperitoneum. Rigler sign is evident

Free peritoneal air may be diagnosed on supine abdominal films although erect abdominal or chest films are more sensitive as the air is easily recognized when subdiaphragmatic.

If the patient cannot stand or sit, a left lateral decubitus film of the abdomen is taken to show free air between the liver and the right hemidiaphragm. The patient should lie in this position for 10 min before taking this film, or before taking the standard standing or sitting erect film, so as to allow time for free air to move to a subdiaphragmatic location.

CT is more sensitive than plain films for the identification of intraperitoneal air (JEFFREY et al. 1983) as plain films may not identify the air if a perforation is very small, seals itself spontaneously or if the air is contained by adjacent structures (Fig. 25.2). Such perforations may only become clinically significant

some time after the inciting trauma and are more likely to become significant if complicated by another factor such as bowel distension or inflammation.

Extraperitoneal perforations may occur in the rectum and the posterior wall of the sigmoid, ascending and descending colon (Fig. 25.3) Rarely a perforation may occur into the mesentery of the associated bowel segment and not progress to the peritoneal cavity (CHO et al. 1990) and as such may remain clinically silent and be treated conservatively or only manifest clinically after a delay of hours or days (GHAHREMANI 1993).

Imaging, especially CT, may suggest the site of perforation from the distribution of extra-luminal air (GHAHREMANI 2000). A rectal perforation causes air to dissect into the perirectal tissues (MEYERS and GHAHREMANI 1981; NGUYEN and BECKMAN 1992) and this may extend bilaterally along the psoas mus-

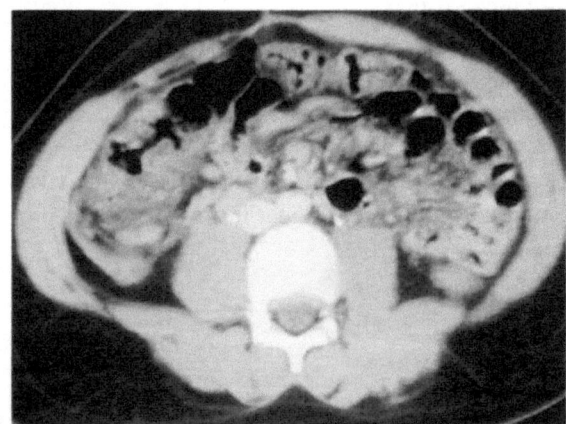
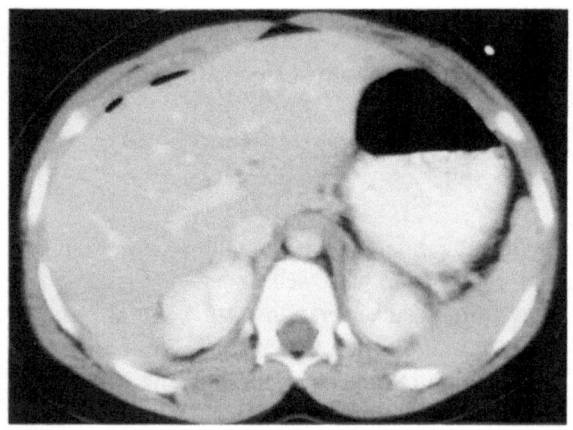

Fig. 25.2a,b. Child passenger in a car involved in a motor vehicle accident. Axial CT scans. **a** Hemoperitoneum is visible in the right paracolic gutter. **b** Small pneumoperitoneum over anterior surface of liver

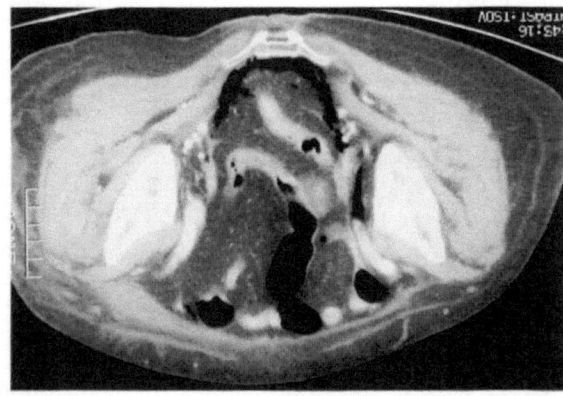

Fig. 25.3a,b. Retroperitoneal perforation of rectosigmoid from colonoscopy. **a** Prone CT showing presacral air. **b** Water soluble contrast enema spot film showing contrast leaking into the perirectal retroperitoneum. Note ring pessary

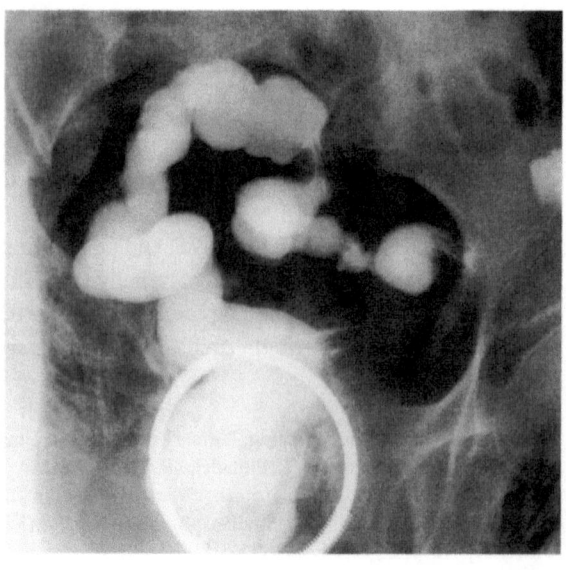

cles to the *posterior pararenal spaces* and even into the flank fat stripes and anterior abdominal wall.

Retroperitoneal perforations of the posterior wall of the sigmoid, ascending or descending colon usually manifest as a unilateral collection of air in the in the *anterior pararenal space* (Fig. 25.4). Such perforations rarely extend to the flank stripe or to the contralateral side (MEYERS and GHAHREMANI 1981).

Imaging plays a critical role in diagnosis of perforation enabling the initiation of prompt and appropriate treatment. Intraperitoneal perforations are likely to be treated surgically, whereas extra-peritoneal perforations may be treated conservatively. Treatment also depends on the condition of the patient; laparoscopy being increasingly used for the primary repair of intraperitoneal perforations in fit patients when the diagnosis is made early.

25.1.2
Barium Enema

The risk of perforation from barium enema is less than from colonoscopy. It is estimated as 0.01% (1/1000) with a resulting mortality of 0.002% (1/50,000) (GHAHREMANI 2000; MEYERS and GHAHRE-MANI 1981; OTT et al. 1985; WILLIAMS and HARNED 1991). The mechanism of injury is usually from traumatic insertion of the enema tip or inflation of a rectal balloon which usually leads to an extra-peritoneal perforation. Intraperitoneal perforation usually occurs in abnormal areas of the bowel weakened by inflammation, ischemia, neoplasia, or deep endoscopic biopsies (GHAHREMANI 2000) and is associated with a higher mortality than an extraperitoneal perforation.

The policy of waiting 5 days from the time of a rectal biopsy to allow healing before performing a barium enema should be observed when biopsies are performed through proctoscopes and rigid sigmoidoscopes as the biopsy forceps used are capable of taking a full thickness sample of the rectal wall (VELEZ et al. 1997). This precaution is unnecessary for biopsies taken through flexible sigmoidoscopes or colonoscopes where the biopsy forceps are smaller and can only take mucosal samples (Fig. 25.5). The risk of performing a barium enema after a polypectomy depends on the nature of the procedure and the likely damage to the colon wall but again the barium enema would normally be postponed for 5 days.

Intraperitoneal barium (Fig. 25.6) initially results in fluid loss into the peritoneal cavity and hypovolemia which must be rapidly corrected. Peritonitis develops which may become suppurative and lead to endotoxic shock. Even if infection is avoided barium produces a granulomatous reaction and a dense adhesive peritonitis. Management consists of giving antibiotics and proceeding to surgery without delay for peritoneal lavage. Surgery will usually involve resecting the site of the perforation.

Most retroperitoneal perforations are from tears of the rectum. They may be asymptomatic and only discovered coincidentally at subsequent radiology (Fig.25.7), but if infection develops then the dense granulomatous fibrotic reaction induced by the barium makes it difficult to eradicate. Fibrosis may lead to a stricture of the bowel and has even been known to cause ureteric obstruction (VAN-DENDRIS and GIANNAKOPOULOS 1981). It should be remembered that retroperitoneal perforations at barium enema may be caused by vaginal tears as a result of misplacement of the rectal tube. This usu-

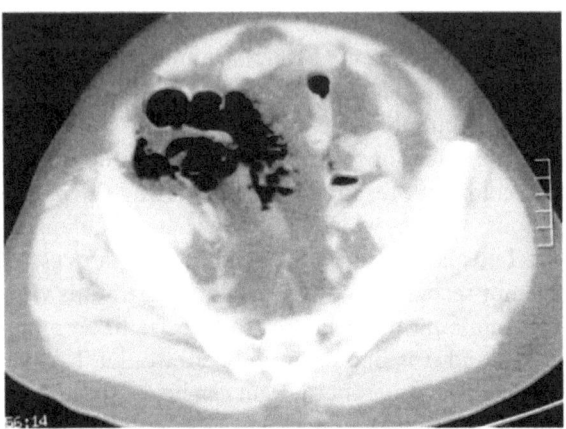 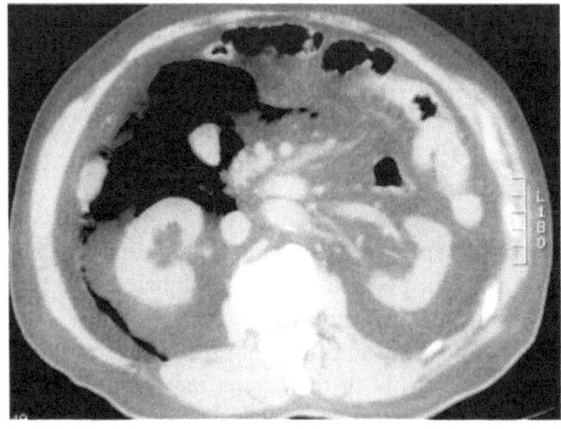

a   b

Fig. 25.4a,b. Retroperitoneal perforation of the posterior wall of the sigmoid during colonoscopy. Axial CT images. **a** Site of leak. **b** Gas in anterior pararenal and in perirenal space

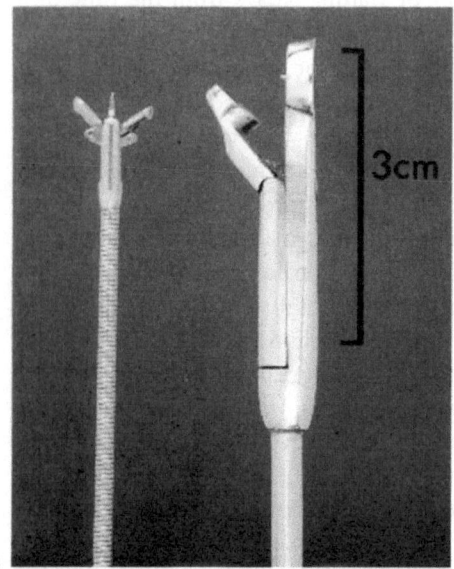

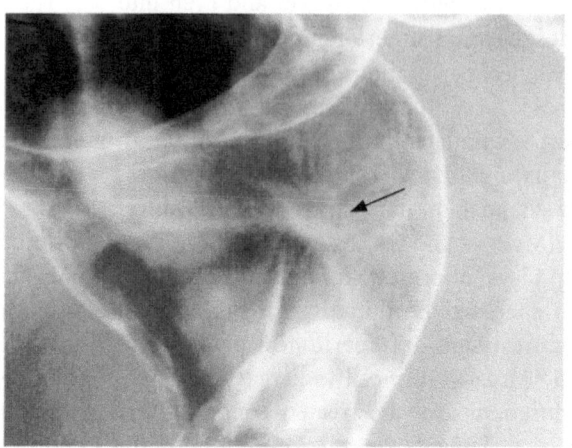

Fig. 25.5a,b. a The jaws of rigid biopsy forceps measure 13 mm whereas those of flexible biopsy forceps measure only 3 mm. **b** Scar (*arrow*) following a biopsy taken with rigid biopsy forceps

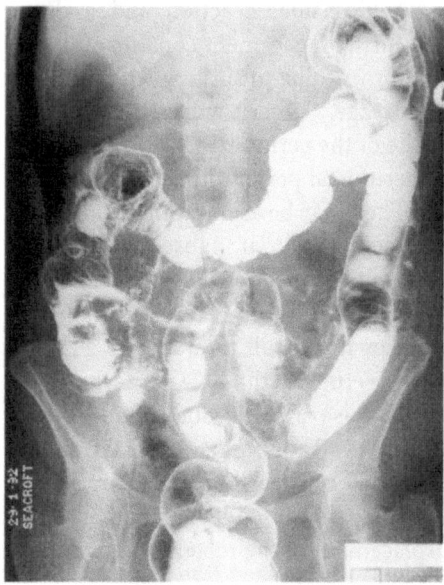

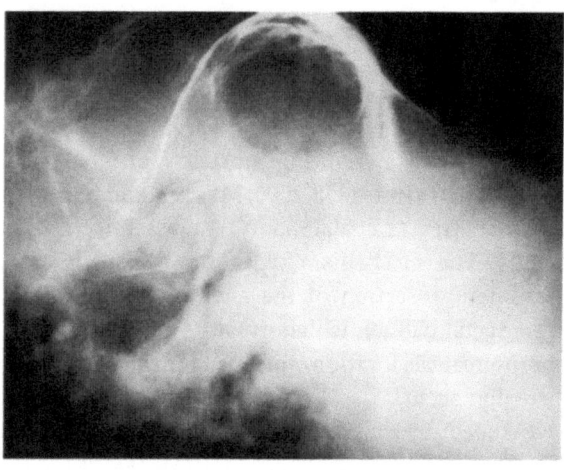

Fig. 25.7. Prone lateral film of pelvis. Extraperitoneal barium. Silent perforation at time of barium enema 3 years earlier

Fig. 25.6. Barium peritonitis. Perforation of a necrotic right-sided colonic carcinoid tumour during the course of a barium enema. There is subhepatic peritoneal air and barium lies between small bowel loops. The patient survived after prompt fluid replacement, antibiotics, and surgery

ally results from poor patient co-operation, obesity or a deficient perineum so that a lubricated rectal tube slips forward into the vagina as it is inserted. The use of a balloon catheter prevents incontinence and so the fornix of the vagina may rupture with extraperitoneal leakage of barium and sometimes venous intravasation (Fig. 25.8). Venous intravasation of barium is a feared complication (CHAPMAN and BLAKEBOROUGH 1998) and when it results from a low rectal or vaginal tear, barium enters the systemic venous circulation and can result in massive and fatal pulmonary embolism. Intravasation from a mucosal tear of the upper rectum or more proximal colon will result in barium entering the portal venous system which is somewhat less dangerous but may cause septicemia and liver abscesses. Prompt recognition of venous intravasation is vital if the amount of barium introduced is to be minimized and it is important to be aware that barium in the inferior mesenteric vein can be confused with contrast in the left ureter (Fig. 25.9).

Balloon catheters are used to prevent incontinence but their use increases the risk of extraperitoneal

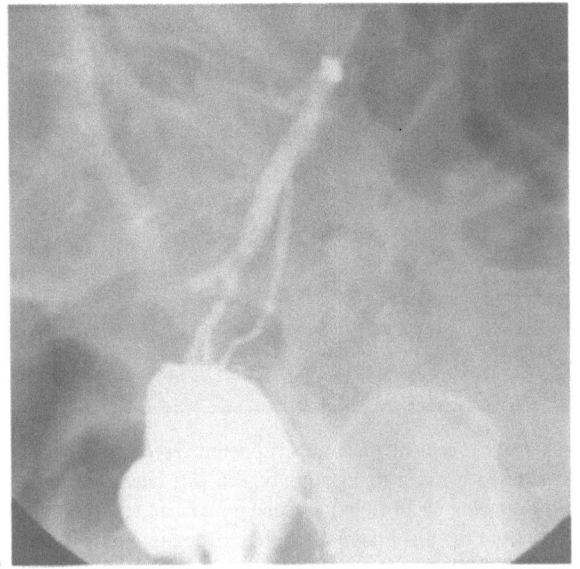

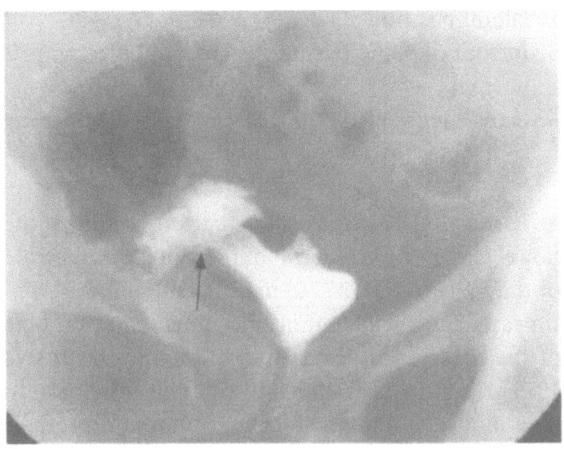

Fig. 25.8a,b. Vaginal intubation with a balloon catheter. **a** The fornix of the vagina has ruptured with venous intravasation. Later film showing fornix rupture (*arrow*) (**b**)

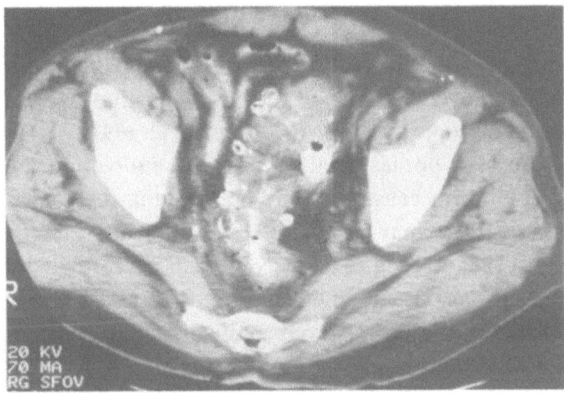

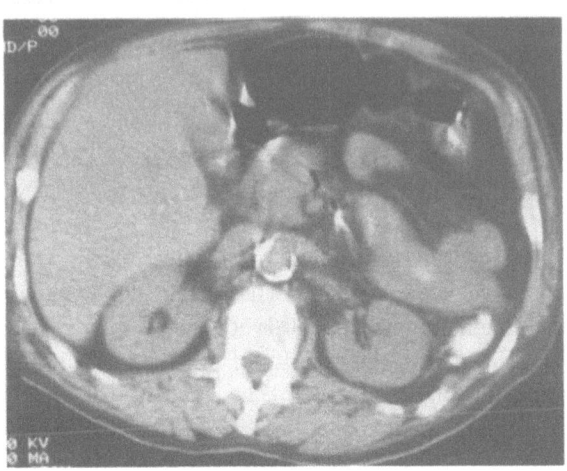

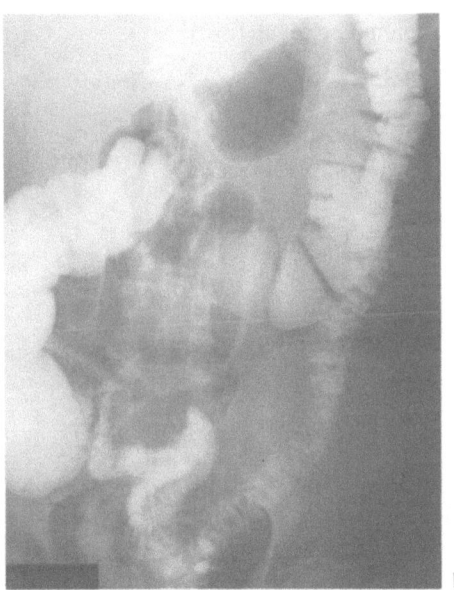

Fig. 25.9a–c. A patient with acute diverticulitis. **a** Axial CT scan shows a thick-walled sigmoid with diverticula and an adjacent pericolic abscess. **b** Barium enema. Barium has intravasated into the inferior mesenteric vein. At the time this was mistakenly thought to be the left ureter. **c** Axial CT scan shows barium and air in mesenteric veins (*arrows*) (KANEHANN et al. 1988, with permission)

rectal perforation by a factor of 2.5 (BLAKEBOROUGH et al. 1997). DODDS et al. (1980) made six recommendations to reduce the risks associated with the use of balloon catheters:

1. Determine if there is a clinical history of rectal disease
2. Perform a rectal examination
3. Inflate the balloon catheter oneself and do not

delegate the task to a radiographer or nurse
4. Introduce the tube with the patient in the left lateral position
5. Introduce some barium to ensure the rectum is normal
6. Only then inflate the balloon under screening control

A mucosal tear may allow barium to enter the bowel wall in which case both the outside and inside of the mucosa (Fig. 25.10) may be outlined or sometimes barium will outline the inner muscle fibres of the muscularis propria (CARNEY and STEPHENS 1973) resulting in transverse striations. The barium may induce a granulomatous reaction and produce a polypoid submucosal mass (granuloma), local inflammation or ulceration (ELLOWAY and DERIDDER 1991). Alternatively insufflated air may leak into the colon wall through a mucosal tear resulting in pneumatosis coli or air may dissect into the mesentery of the colon (CHO et al. 1990).

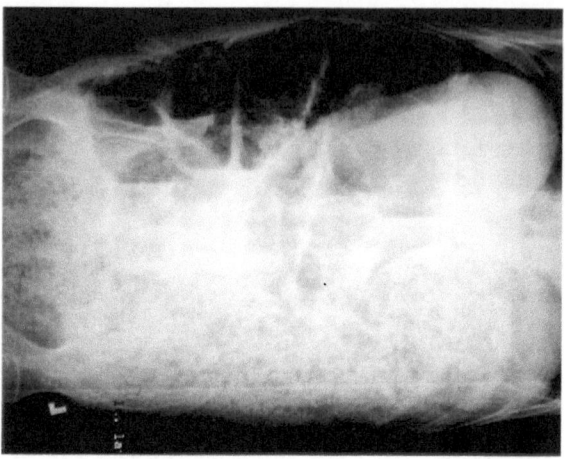

Fig. 25.11. Feculent pneumoperitoneum. Psychiatric patient swallowed a sharp nonopaque object. Left lateral decubitus film showing air in right paracolic gutter and separating the liver from the diaphragm. Feces has settled into a dependent position in the peritoneal cavity

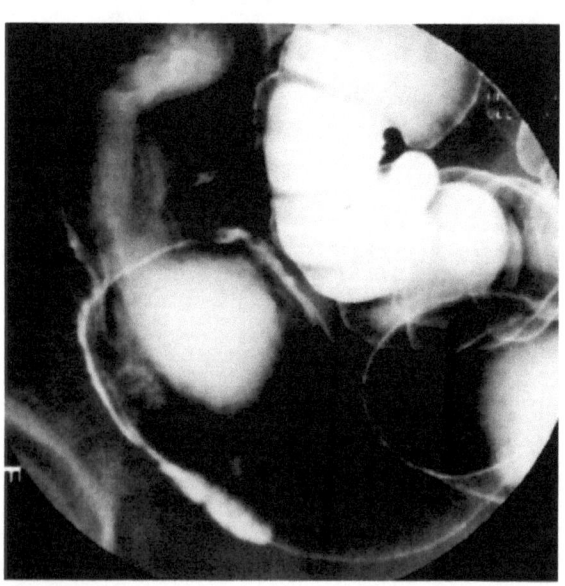

Fig. 25.10. Barium enema. Intramural dissection of barium

25.2
Foreign Bodies

Foreign bodies may reach the colon and rectum after being accidentally ingested. Most pass without complication but occasionally they may become impacted or perforate the bowel (Fig. 25.11).

Stents are used with increasing frequency to bridge strictured bowel segments. These may migrate, perforate, or cause colorectal bleeding. Stents which have migrated into the rectum and cannot be passed with bowel movement must be retrieved with fluoroscopic or endoscopic guidance (WHOLEY et al. 1997).

Foreign bodies inserted into the anorectum are a significant cause of colorectal trauma (OOI et al. 1998). They may be inserted too high for manual retrieval and require endoscopic removal, often with anesthesia. CT should be employed if a foreign body cannot easily be retrieved manually as penetration into the bowel wall or frank perforation may occur and in such cases a surgical approach may be necessary (Fig. 25.12).

25.3
Blunt Trauma

Blunt abdominal trauma most often results from motor vehicle accidents. Mortality from blunt abdominal trauma ranges from 10%–30% and is most closely associated with the severity of other injuries rather than the intestinal injury. The incidence of hollow viscus injury after blunt trauma is low at 0.7%–5% (WISNER et al. 1990; MALHOTRA et al. 2000), but delayed diagnosis of colonic perforation increases mortality by 25%–33% (DAUTERIVE et al. 1985). Injuries are equally distributed around the colon (BARDEN and MAULL 2000) although the rectum is less often involved. Bowel and mesenteric injuries are rarely isolated occurrences, but usually associated with

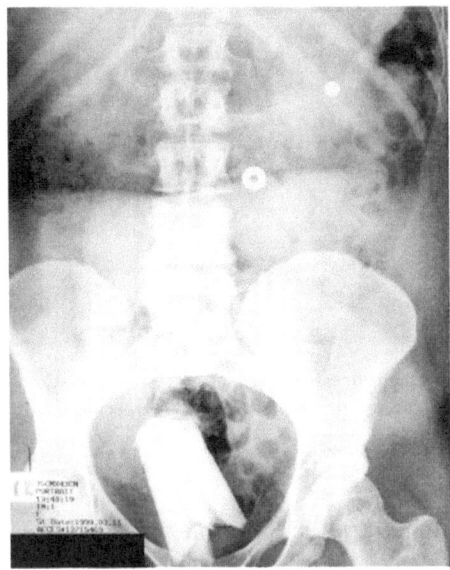

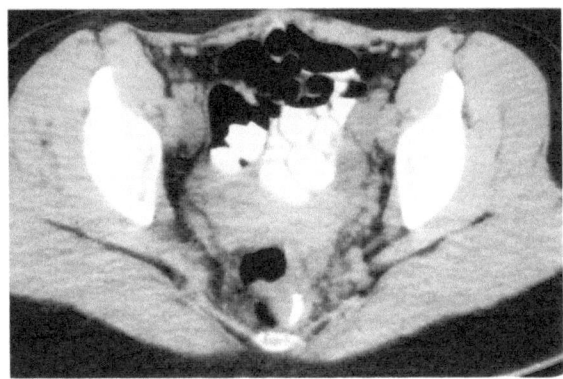

Fig. 25.12a,b. Glass bottle inserted and broken in rectum. a Plain film. b Axial CT scan showing glass within the bowel wall

other solid organ injuries and often extra-abdominal injuries (DAUTERIVE et al. 1985).

The mechanisms of injury include crushing of the viscera between the anterior abdominal wall and the spine, tangential tears at relatively fixed points along the bowel, and sudden increase in intra-abdominal pressure (CARILLO et al. 1996).

The transverse and sigmoid colon are prone to injury as a result of their impingement between the anterior abdominal wall and the spine (MAYS and NOER 1966). Intramural hematomas tend to occur in the ascending and descending colon and can be recognized by CT. (Fig. 25.13) (JEFFREY et al. 1982; DONOHUE et al. 1987). They usually resolve spontaneously but may progress to stenosis (MAYS and NOER 1966; ALTNER 1964).

Injury to abdominal vasculature from blunt trauma is either from shearing or compression. Shearing causes avulsion of vessels at points of mesenteric fixation. This type of shearing force occurs in deceleration injury as forward momentum remains in internal organs after the body has stopped moving. Compression injuries crush vessels as may occur between the abdominal wall and the spine from a seat belt injury. This type of injury may cause intimal tears and lead to thrombosis. The end result of either type of injury may be ischemia and necrosis of the affected bowel (Fig. 25.14). Compression injuries are often difficult to detect, unlike shearing injuries which present with free intraperitoneal hemorrhage (FELICIANO 1998).

CT is now the most widely used and reliable imaging modality for the evaluation of blunt abdominal

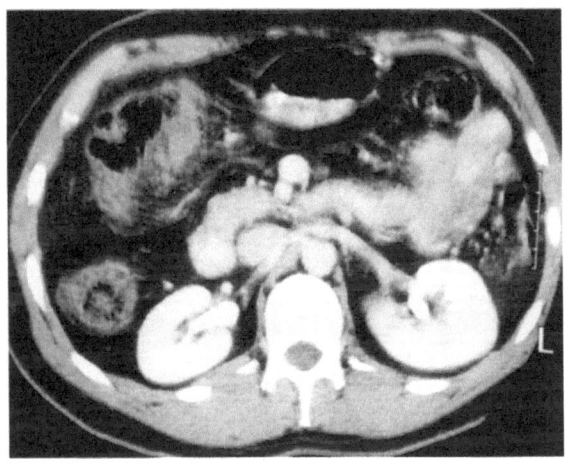

Fig. 25.13. Motor vehicle accident. Hematoma involving ascending colon and hepatic flexure

trauma. During the past decade, with the use of faster spiral CT scanners, the sensitivity and specificity of CT has increased for the diagnosis of bowel injury as a result of increased awareness of the findings in this type of injury (Fig. 25.15), improved scanning protocols, and increased use of bowel contrast (BECKER et al. 1998; SHERECK et al. 1994; RIZZO et al. 1989; DOWE et al. 1997).

CT scans should be viewed on "lung windows" to enhance the detectability of extra-luminal air. Extra-luminal air is considered a specific finding of perforation in blunt, but for obvious reasons not penetrating trauma. CT is sensitive for the detec-

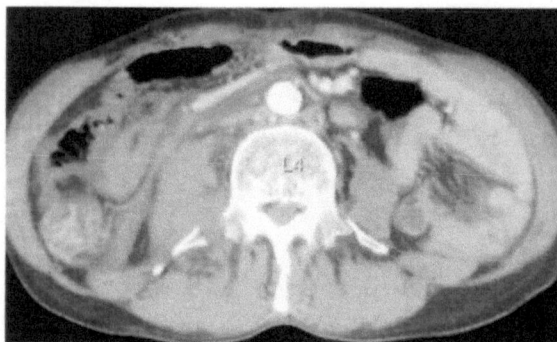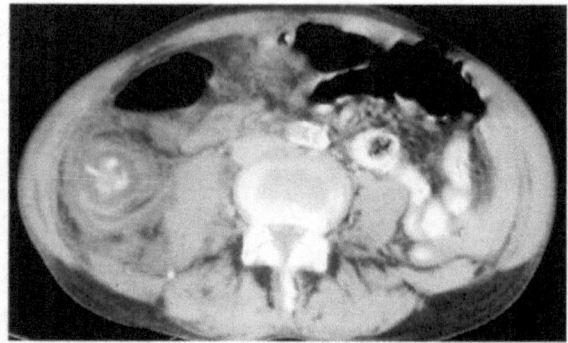

Fig. 25.14a,b. Blunt trauma from a motor vehicle accident. **a** Fracture (R) transverse process and associated psoas hematoma. Pericecal blood. Colon injury not detected. **b** Same patient 12 h later when clinical condition has deteriorated. Caecum is now thick-walled with submucosal edema. Colon was resected and found to be ischemic

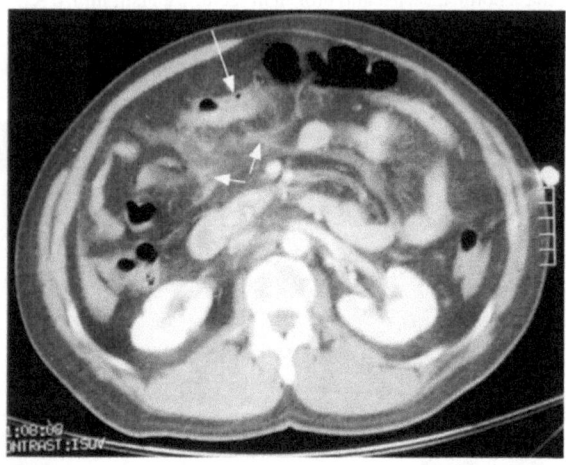

Fig. 25.15. Blunt trauma. Thickening of the wall of the transverse colon (*arrow*) and mesenteric infiltration (*small arrows*)

tion of free peritoneal air which may be diagnosed in only 50%–70% of cases with plain abdominal films (CHO and BAKER 1994). Free air is most often seen over the anterior peritoneal surface of the liver (Fig. 25.2b) but may be trapped between the mesenteric leaves close to the site of perforation.

Pneumothorax or pneumomediastinum may lead to pneumoperitoneum if air dissects through the diaphragm. Peritoneal lavage may also complicate CT interpretation by introducing air or fluid into the peritoneal cavity and so the value of these findings is diminished in this setting. CT has been found to be better than peritoneal lavage in the hemodynamically stable patient because of its accuracy in determining the specific site of injury (BECKER et al. 1998; PEVEC et al. 1991; NGHIEM et al. 1993).

On CT, sigmoid perforation may result in free air in the upper abdomen, although less often than with gastric or duodenal perforation, whereas free air in the pelvis is almost always due to colon perforation. Retropneumoperitoneum may be caused by colon or duodenal rupture but the combination of free air in the pelvis and retroperitoneal air around the liver is specific for sigmoid perforation (MANIATIS et al. 2000).

The most specific finding for perforation of the colon is the demonstration of extra-luminal contrast which has been administered orally, via NG tube or rectally. Ideally, the bowel should be completely opacified in order to be able to identify a leak. However, this is not always possible due to patient-related factors such as pain, nausea or vomiting, and bowel ileus may impede contrast filling. Small amounts of extravasated contrast may also potentially be resorbed prior to scanning. The availability of personnel to administer rectal contrast and time constraints in the scanning department are also important considerations.

Potential pitfalls in the diagnosis of perforation may result from extravasated opacified blood from vascular injury simulating leakage of intraluminal contrast medium (Fig. 25.16) (NGHIEM et al. 1993). Urine from bladder injury may simulate unopacified leaked bowel contents although if there is uncertainty a repeat delayed scan can be performed as this allows time for contrast to enter the bladder and leak from a bladder tear.

Other indirect CT signs of bowel injury include the presence of a "sentinel clot", focal bowel wall thickening and unexplained extra-luminal fluid adjacent to a bowel loop. The sentinel clot originates from bleeding from a mesenteric vessel and is a focal area of high signal (opacified blood) adja-

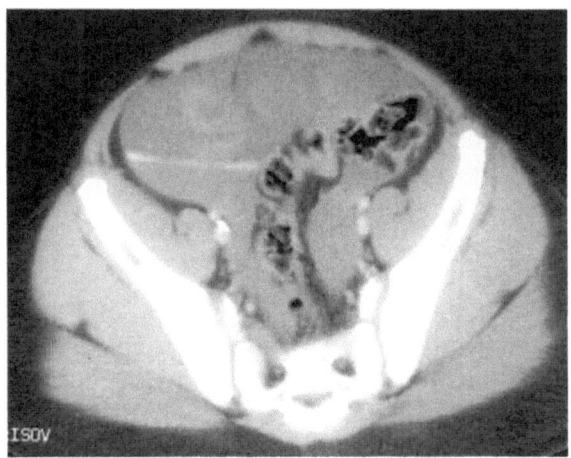

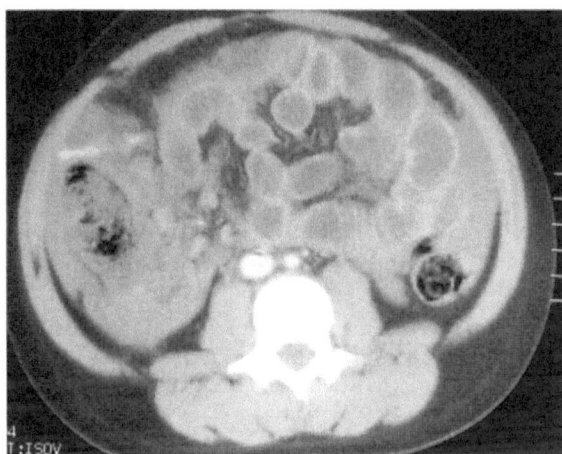

Fig. 25.16a,b. Blunt abdominal trauma in a child. **a** Axial CT scan showing a hemoperitoneum. Vascular contrast medium is seen mixing with the blood clot in the peritoneal cavity. This can be confused with leaked bowel contrast medium. **b** Higher slice showing hematoma involving and extending around the ascending colon and acute bleeding

cent to a mesenteric bowel loop (ORWIG and FEDERLE 1989). Focal bowel wall thickening (>3 mm in a distended loop), although not specific for bowel injury, should be considered with suspicion (SHERECK et al. 1994; RIZZO et al. 1989; CASEY et al. 1995). Focal streakiness of the mesenteric fat may result from bleeding or edema and is an indirect sign of injury in the setting of acute trauma (SHERECK et al. 1994; CASEY et al. 1995; HAGIWARA et al. 1995; MIRVIS et al. 1992; DOWE et al. 1997). Focal extraluminal fluid between loops of bowel may also be the only sign of injury to the adjacent bowel (LEVINE et al. 1995).

25.4
Penetrating Trauma

The incidence of penetrating trauma (from stab wounds and gunshot injury) in the US has been steadily increasing (FELICIANO and ROZYEK 1995). In 2000, 3042 US children and teenagers died from firearm injuries and homicide was the second leading cause of death for 15- to 24-year-olds (National Center for Injury Prevention and Control 2000).

Non-operative management for penetrating colonic injury was usually practiced until the time of the First World War when the defunctioning colostomy was introduced (OGILVIE 1944). Rapid evacuation from the field, availability of antibiotics and blood products, fluid replacement, and improvements in anesthesia have all played a part in reducing mortality so that by the time of the Vietnam war mortality had reduced from 60% to 13% (KARULF and FITZHARRIS 2003). In civilian trauma, penetrating colon injuries often results from handguns and stab wounds, whereas in traditional warfare they generally result from high velocity bullet wounds and shrapnel which impart more damage to the surrounding tissues. The trend is now towards primary colonic repair, particularly for civilian wounds, as this avoids the need to close a colostomy and shortens operating time and hospital stay (KAWENDO et al. 2002).

Plain films may be of value in diagnosing perforation and identifying radio-opaque fragments.

If a patient is unstable and therefore unfit for CT, plain films may be followed by focused abdominal sonography (FAST) or diagnostic peritoneal lavage, to determine if a patient should have immediate surgery, although in recent years there has been a trend towards replacing diagnostic peritoneal lavage by FAST. If stable, a patient may be evaluated by CT with both intravenous and oral contrast medium (Fig. 25.17). Windowing is necessary to distinguish between bone, bullet fragments, and contrast medium (Fig. 25.18).

Most abdominal vascular trauma (80%) is due to penetrating trauma (RAPAPORT et al. 1982). Patients who are hemodynamically stable often undergo diagnostic studies to determine whether laparotomy is required. CT performed after administration of oral, intravenous, and rectal contrast has been found to be highly accurate in excluding peritoneal violation and predicting the need for laparotomy in these patients (SHANMUGANTHAN et al. 2001). Wounds to the back or flank are not evaluated well with peritoneal lavage or FAST, whereas CT with oral, rectal, and IV contrast is effective in depicting retroperitoneal bowel injuries as well as injuries to solid viscera (PHILLIPS et al. 1986).

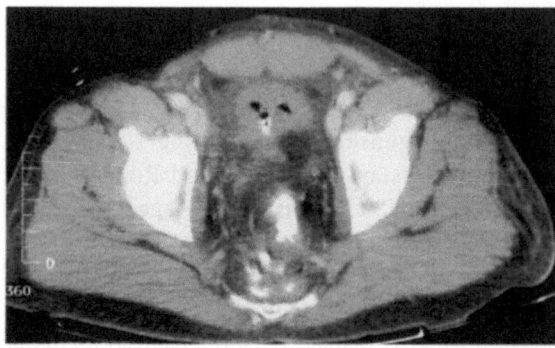

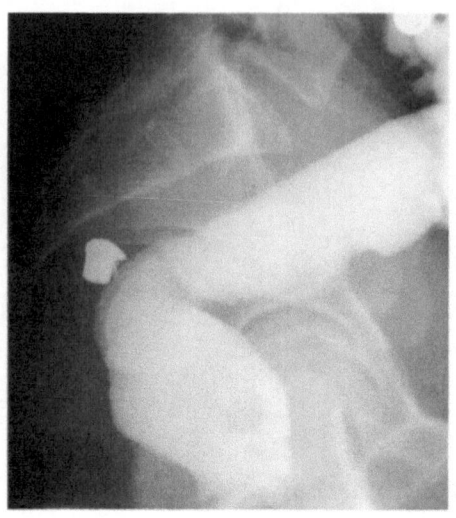

Fig. 25.17a,b. Gun shot wound to pelvis. **a** Axial CT scan showing presacral extravasation of rectal contrast. **b** Water soluble contrast enema prior to colostomy closure. Leak has closed. Bullet in presacral space

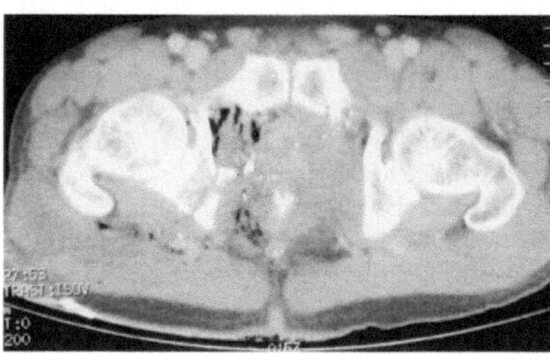

Fig. 25.18. Gun shot wound to right buttock. Perforated rectum. Bullet fragments lie in a diagonal tract. There is a comminuted fracture to the right ischium and perforation of the proximal urethra and prostate. Windowing will distinguish bone, bullet fragments and contrast medium

References

Altner PC (1964) Constrictive lesions of the colon due to blunt trauma to the abdomen. Surg Gynecol Obstet 118: 1257-1262

Barden BE, Maull KI (2000) Perforation of the colon after blunt trauma. S Med J 93:33-35

Becker CD, Mentha G, Schmidlin F et al (1998) Blunt abdominal trauma in adults: role of CT in the diagnosis and management of visceral injuries. Eur Radiol 8:772-780

Blakeborough A, Sheridan MB, Chapman AH (1997) Retention balloon catheters and barium enemas: attitudes, current practice and relative safety in the UK. Clin Radiol.52:62-64

Carney JA, Stephens DH (1973) Intramural barium (barium granuloma) of colon and rectum. Gastroenterology 65:316-320

Carpio G, Albu E, Gumbs MA et al (1989) Management of colonic perforation after colonoscopy. Dis Colon Rectum 32:624-626

Carrillo EH, Somberg LB, Ceballos CE et al (1996) Blunt traumatic injuries to the colon and rectum. J Am Col Surg 183: 548-552

Casey LR, Vu D, Cohen AJ (1995) Small bowel rupture after blunt trauma: CT signs and their sensitivity. Emerg Radiol 2:90-95

Chapman AH, Blakeborough A (1998) Complications from inflation of a retention rectal balloon catheter in the vagina at barium enema. Clin Radiol 53:768-770

Cho KC, Baker SR (1994) Extraluminal air. Diagnosis and significance. Radiol Clin North Am 32:829-844

Cho KC, Simmons MZ, Baker SR et al (1990) Spontaneous dissection of air into the mesocolon during double-contrast barium enema. Gastrointest Radiol 15:76-77

Dauterive AH, Flancbaum L, Cox EF (1985) Blunt intestinal trauma. Ann Surg 201:198-203

Dodds WJ, Stewart ET, Nelson JA (1980) Rectal balloon catheters and the barium enema examination. Gastrointest Radiol 5:277-284

Donohue JH, Federle MP, Griffiths BG et al (1987) Computed tomography in the diagnosis of blunt intestinal and mesenteric injuries. J Trauma 27:11-17

Dowe MF, Shanmuganathan K, Mirvis SE et al (1997) CT findings of mesenteric injury after blunt trauma: implications for surgical intervention. AJR 168:425-428

Elloway RS, DeRidder PH (1991) Barium granuloma of the rectum. Gastrointest Endosc 37:586-587

Feliciano DV (1988) Abdominal vascular injuries. Surg Clin North Am 68:741

Feliciano DV, Rozyek GS (1995) The management of penetrating abdominal trauma. Adv Surg 28:1-39

Garbay JR, Suc B, Rotman N et al (1996) Multicentre study of surgical complications of colonoscopy. Br J Surg 83: 42-44

Ghahremani GG (1993) Radiologic evaluation of suspected gastrointestinal perforations. Radiol Clin North Am 31: 1219-1234

Ghahremani G (2000) Iatrogenic gastrointestinal disorders. In: Gore RM, Levin MS (eds) Textbook of gastrointestinal radiology, 2nd edn. W.B. Saunders Co., Philadelphia, pp 2228-2242

Hagiwara A, Yukioka T, Satou M et al (1995) Early diagnosis of small intestine rupture from blunt abdominal trauma using computed-tomography: significance of the streaky density within the mesentery. J Trauma 38:630-633

Hall C, Dorricott NJ, Donovan IA et al (1991) Colon perforation during colonoscopy: surgical versus conservative management. Br J Surg 78:542-544

Jeffrey RB, Federle MP, Stein SM et al (1982) Intramural hematoma of the cecum following blunt trauma. J Comput Assist Tomogr 6:404-405

Jeffrey RB, Federle MP, Wall S (1983) Value of computed tomography in detecting occult gastrointestinal perforation. J Comput Assist Tomogr 7:825-827

Kanehann LB, Caroline DF, Friedman AC et al (1988) CT findings in venous intravasation complicating diverticulitis. J Comput Assist Tomogr 12:10147-1049

Karulf RE, Fitzharris G (2003) Colon Trauma. http:// www.fascrs.org/coresubjects/2002/karulf.html

Kavin H, Sinicrope F, Esker AH (1992) Management of perforation of the colon at colonoscopy. Am J Gastroenterol 87:161-167

Kawendo NY, Modiba MCM, Matlala NS et al (2002) Randomised clinical trial to determine if delay from time of penetrating colonic injury precludes primary repair. Br J Surg 89:993-998

Levine CD, Patel UJ, Wachsberg RH et al (1995) CT in patients with blunt abdominal trauma: clinical significance of intraperitoneal fluid detected on a scan with otherwise normal findings. AJR 164:1381-1385

Lo AY, Beaton Hl (1994) Selective management of colonoscopic perforations. J Am Coll Surg 179:333-337

Macrae FA, Tan KG, Williams CB (1983) Towards safer colonoscopy: a report on the complications of 5000 diagnostic or therapeutic colonoscopies. Gut 24:76-83

Malhotra AK, Fabian TC, Katsis SB et al (2000) Blunt bowel and mesenteric injuries: the role of screening computed tomography. J Trauma 48:991-1000

Maniatis V, Chryssikopoulos H, Roussaki A et al (2000) Perforation of the alimentary tract: evaluation with computed tomography. Abdom Imaging 25:373-379

Mays ET, Noer RJ (1966) Colonic stenosis after trauma. J Trauma 6:316-332

Meyers MA, Ghahremani GG (1975) Complications of fiberoptic endoscopy II. Colonoscopy. Radiology 115: 301-307

Meyers MA, Ghahremani GG (1981) Iatrogenic gastrointestinal complications. Springer, Berlin Heidelberg New York, pp 45-298

Mirvis SE, Gens DR, Shanmuganathan K (1992) Rupture of the bowel after blunt abdominal trauma: diagnosis with CT. AJR 159:1217-1221

Muhldorfer SM, Kekos G, Hahn EG et al (1992) Complications of therapeutic gastrointestinal endoscopy. Endoscopy 24:276-283

National Center for Injury Prevention and Control, Ten Leading Causes of Death, United States (2000) http:// www.cdc.gov/ncipc/wisqars

Nguyen BD, Beckman I (1992) Silent rectal perforation after endoscopic polypectomy: CT features. Gastrointest Radiol 17:271-273

Nghiem HV, Jeffrey RB, Mindelzun RE (1993) CT of blunt trauma to the bowel and mesentery. AJR 160:53-58

Ooi BS, Ho YH, Eu KW (1998) Management of anorectal foreign bodies: a cause of obscure anal pain. Aust J Surg 68(12):852-855

Ogilvie W (1944) Abdominal wounds in the western desert. Surg. Gynecol Obstet 78:225-238

Orwig D, Federle MP (1989) Localized clotted blood as evidence of visceral trauma on CT: the sentinel clot sign. AJR 153:747-749

Ott DJ, Gelfand DW, Chen YM et al (1985) Colonoscopy and the barium enema: a radiologic viewpoint. South Med J 78: 1033-1035

Pevec WC, Peitzman AB, Udekwu AO et al (1991) CT in the evaluation of blunt abdominal trauma. Surg Gynecol Obstet 173:262-267

Phillips T, Sclafani SJA, Goldstein A et al (1986) Use of the contrast-enhanced CT enema in the management of penetrating trauma to the flank and back. J Trauma 26:593-601

Rapaport A, Feliciano DV, Mattox KL (1982) An epidemiologic profile of urban trauma in America - Houston style. Tex Med 78:44-50

Rizzo MJ, Federle MP, Griffith BG (1989) Bowel and mesenteric injury following blunt abdominal trauma. Radiology 173:143

Shanmuganthan K, Mirvis SE, Chiu WC et al (2001) Triple-contrast helical CT in penetrating torso trauma: a prospective study to determine peritoneal violation and the need for laparotomy. AJR 177:1247-1256

Shereck J, Shatney C, Sensaki K et al (1994) The accuracy of computed tomography in the diagnosis of blunt small-bowel perforation. Am J Surg 168:670-675

Vallera R, Bailie J (1996) Complications of endoscopy. Endoscopy 28:187-204

Velez MA, Riff DS, Mule JM (1997) Laparoscopic repair of a colonoscopic perforation. Surg Endosc 11:387-389

Vandendris M, Giannakopoulos X (1981) Retroperitoneal barytoma. Urology 17:358-359

Waye JD, Lewis BS, Yessayan S (1992) Colonoscopy: a prospective report of complications. J Clin Gastroenterol 15:347-351

Wholey MH, Ferral H, Reyes R et al (1997) Retrieval of migrated colonic stents from the rectum. Cardiovasc Intervent Radiol 20:477-480

Williams SM, Harned RK (1991) Recognition and prevention of barium enema complications. Curr Probl Diagn Radiol 20:123-151

Wisner DH, Yong C, Blaisdell FW (1990) Blunt intestinal injury. Arch Surg 125:1319-1323

26 The Diagnosis and Management of Colonic Obstruction and Pseudo-Obstruction

Andrew Lowe and Anthony H. Chapman

CONTENTS

26.1   Obstruction   263
26.1.1   Introduction   263
26.1.2   Diagnosis   263
26.1.3   Complications   267
26.1.4   Management   267
26.2   Pseudo-obstruction   267
26.2.1   Definition   267
26.2.2   Clinical Features   268
26.2.3   Diagnosis   268
26.2.4   Aetiology   268
26.2.5   Complication   269
26.2.6   Treatment   269
26.2.7   Prognosis   270
26.3   Specific Colonic Obstructions   270
26.3.1   Intussusception   270
26.3.2   Volvulus   273
26.3.3   Adhesions   276
26.3.4   Hernias   276
26.3.5   Obturation Obstruction   276
26.3.6   Obstipation   276
26.3.7   Extrinsic Causes of Obstruction   276
         References   277

26.1
Obstruction

26.1.1
Introduction

Mechanical obstruction of the large bowel is four to five times less common than that of the small bowel, but whereas the majority of small bowel obstructions are due to adhesions, in over half the cases large bowel obstruction is the result of a carcinoma. Other causes include volvulus (11%), diverticulitis (9%) and extrinsic infiltration by malignant disease (8%). Adhesions, faecal impaction and hernias are rarer causes (Table 26.1).

A. Lowe, BSc, MB ChB (Hons), MRCP, FRCR
St. James's University Hospital, Leeds, LS9 7TF, United Kingdom
A. H. Chapman, FRCP, FRCR
Clinical Director of Radiology, Leeds Teaching Hospitals Trust, St. James's University Hospital, Leeds, LS9 7TF, United Kingdom

Table 26.1. The aetiology of colonic obstruction

Carcinoma	55%
Volvulus	11%
Diverticulitis	9%
Extrinsic malignant infiltration	8%
Adhesions	4%
Faecal impaction	3%
Hernia	2%

26.1.2
Diagnosis

26.1.2.1
Clinical Findings

As most colonic obstructions are due to cancer most patients are elderly and have symptoms related to the tumour location. Often, right sided lesions present insidiously as the colonic lumen is wide and the contents semi-liquid. Left sided lesions cause progressive constipation and ultimately obstipation, distension and pain. Vomiting may occur quite late as satisfactory absorption from the small intestine continues for some time after the onset of colonic obstruction. Pain is usually dull and lower abdominal and does not have such a clear rhythmic colicky nature as that seen in small bowel obstruction. Lesions at the ileocaecal valve may cause small bowel obstruction but the colonic response to more distal mechanical obstruction depends on the competence of the ileocaecal valve. With a competent valve, a closed loop obstruction develops as the colon cannot decompress and abdominal distension can be marked. Where the ileocaecal valve is incompetent, the small bowel serves to decompress the colon, distension is less pronounced and eventually feculent vomiting develops. Distension results in increased wall tension which is in proportion to the bowel diameter for a given intraluminal pressure (Laplace's Law: tension on wall = luminal calibre × intraluminal pressure). As the caecum has the greatest diameter in the colon, its walls are subjected to the greatest tension and therefore are the most likely to perforate (Welsh 1990). However, if the obstruction is due to a tumour, the most common site of perforation is adjacent to the tumour, rather than the caecum (WELSH 1990).

26.1.2.2
Plain Films

In the majority of patients with bowel obstruction the radiographic findings suggest that the obstruction is partial, as gas is frequently observed distal to the presumed site of obstruction (Fig. 26.1). In the colon the source of this gas may be attributed to prograde passage of gas, fermentation of stool, or endoscopic procedures. Contrary to popular belief, there is no evidence that digital rectal examination introduces radiographically visible quantities of air into the rectum (GOLDEN et al. 1981). In any event, the presence of rectal gas should not be regarded as evidence that obstruction is not present.

According to Laplace's law, in the absence of volvulus, the caecum should be the most distended segment of the obstructed colon, even in the presence of ileocaecal valve incompetence. If the colon is diffusely distended and the caecal diameter is less than that of other colonic segments then obstruction does not exist (WITTENBERG 1993).

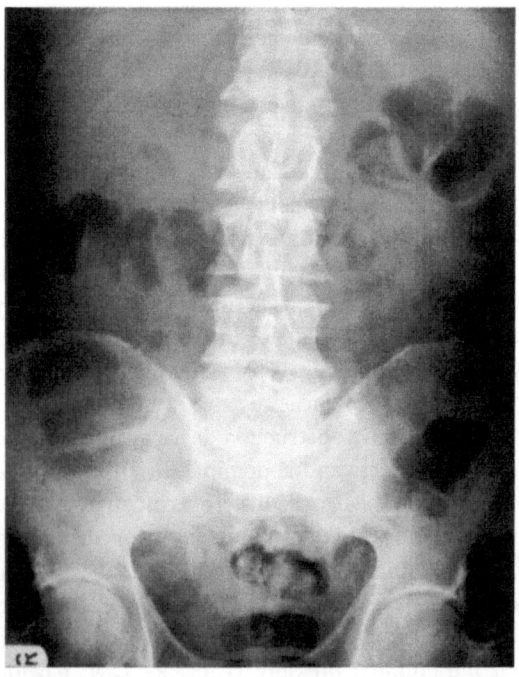

Fig. 26.1. Obstruction to the ascending colon. The caecum is distended with fluid and gas. Haustral markings in the caecum are thickened indicating ischaemia. Gas is observed in the colon distal to the site of complete obstruction. Diagnosis: carcinoma ascending colon

For diagnosing colonic obstruction calibre change is far less reliable than in the small bowel, as gas rises to the non-dependent segments (usually the transverse colon in a supine patient), whilst the dependant colon fills with fluid or in pseudo-obstruction may lie flaccid and collapsed. A left lateral decubitus film, by redistributing the gas, should discriminate between mechanical and functional problems in the descending colon or if the site of an obstruction is suspected at the sigmoid level, a prone film that includes the rectum should settle the issue (Fig. 26.2) (GOLDEN et al. 1981; BAKER 1990). However, turning elderly and sick patients for further radiography may be difficult or inappropriate.

Differentiating pseudo-obstruction from obstruction on plain films can be difficult. Whilst multiple fluid levels within the colon, and an abrupt cut of are typical features of obstruction, similar findings are reported in nearly half of patients with pseudo-obstruction. Typical features of pseudo-obstruction are gaseous colonic distension to the anal margin but a similar pattern is also seen in 9% of cases of colonic obstruction. This may be due to a low lying sigmoid, or rarely due to a combination of pseudo-obstruction and obstruction (Fig. 26.3 and 26.5). In addition, there are a significant number of indeterminate cases where colonic distension cannot be traced to the anal margin with confidence and there is no definite distal cut off point (ALWAN and VAN RIJ 1998). CHAPMAN et al. (1992) found plain films to have a sensitivity of only 84% and a specificity of 72% for colonic obstruction and they failed to identify the site of obstruction in 35% of cases. False proximal localization was caused by the presence of fluid or retained tone in the colon proximal to the site of obstruction. False distal localization was caused by redundant distended bowel falling into the pelvis.

In patients with suspected large bowel obstruction, or those in whom the level of obstruction is unknown and when turning the patient for further plain film radiology is difficult or poorly tolerated, a water soluble contrast enema or computed tomography (CT) is the next step. Barium is avoided as a contrast agent as its use may interfere with subsequent colonoscopy or CT and if a patient proves to have pseudo-obstruction or develops a post-operative ileus, residual barium may remain within the colon for days and inspissate.

26.1.2.3
Acute Contrast Enema

The technique for the performance of acute contrast enemas is discussed in detail elsewhere (CHAP-

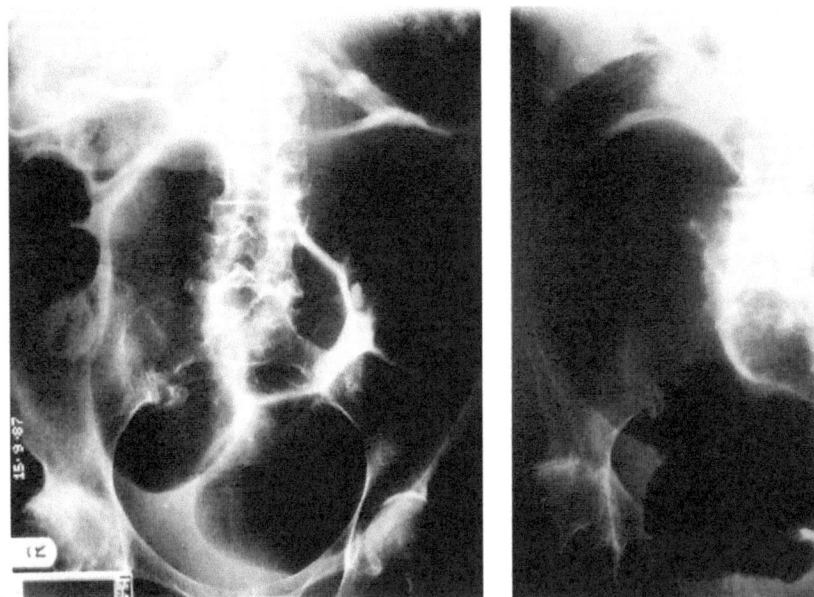

Fig. 26.2a,b. a Gaseous distension of the colon to the sigmoid. Clinician wished to exclude obstruction in this 75-year-old female with pneumonia. **b** Prone film. Gas is redistributed with distension to the anal margin and so obstruction is excluded. Diagnosis: Pseudo-obstruction

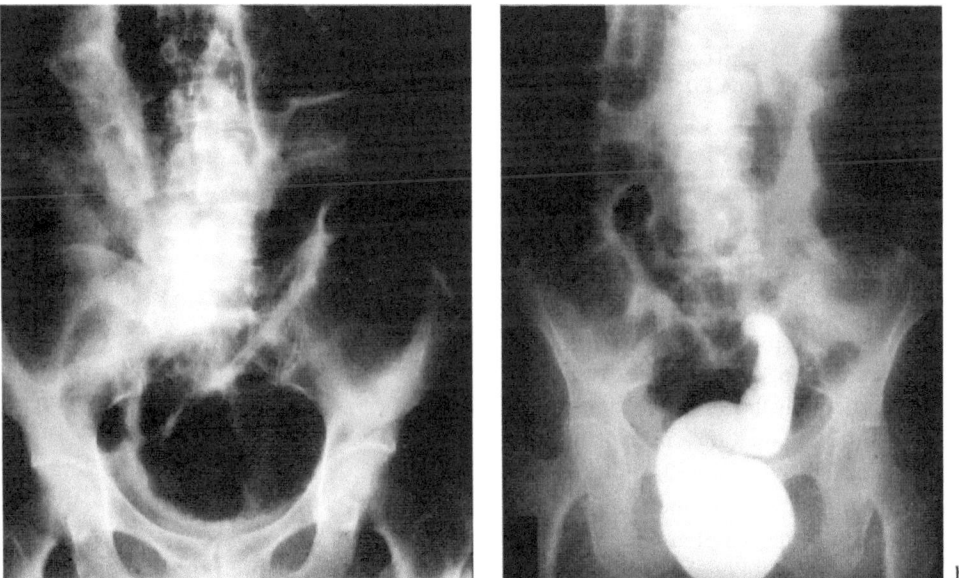

Fig. 26.3a,b. a Low-lying distended sigmoid simulating a colonic ileus. **b** Acute contrast enema shows the patient to have an obstructing sigmoid carcinoma

MAN et al. 1992). Urografin 150 (Schering, Berlin) is used and an antispasmodic, such as Buscopan (hyoscine butyl-bromide, Boehringer Ingelheim), is recommended to avoid false positive diagnoses from spasm. Oblique and angled prone views of the sigmoid should be obtained while filling the colon in an attempt to obtain unobscured views. Failure to do so can result in partially obstructing tumours being missed. Overall, the acute contrast enema has a sensitivity of 96% and a specificity of 98% for the diagnosis of colonic obstruction. Furthermore, in contrast to plain films, the level of obstruction can be accurately identified (Fig. 26.4) (CHAPMAN et al. 1992).

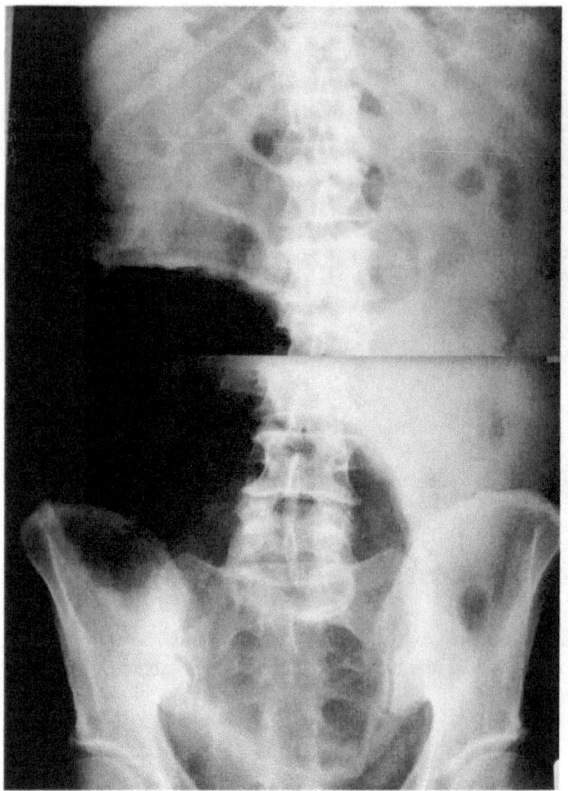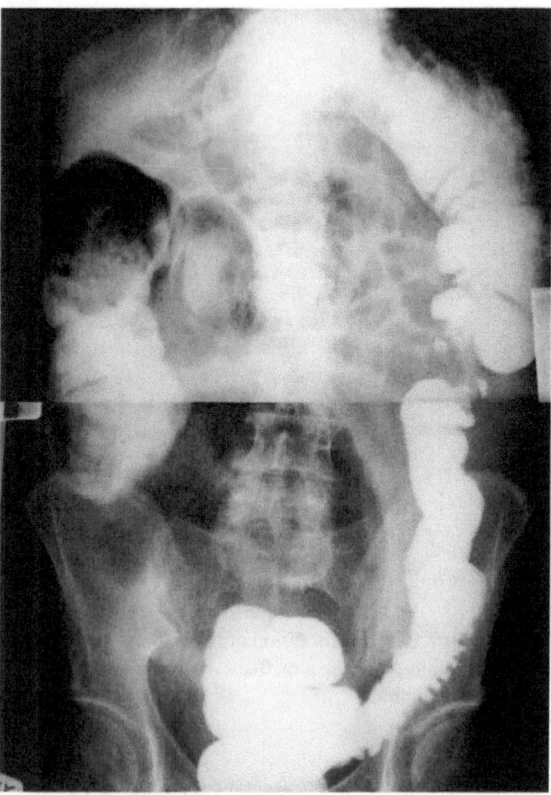

a   b

Fig. 26.4a,b. a Plain film suggests a right-sided colonic obstruction. **b** Acute contrast enema using Urografin shows an obstructing carcinoma in the upper descending colon. Size of patient necessitated two films

26.1.2.4
Computed Tomography

CT is a less invasive examination that is better tolerated by elderly patients and so is increasingly used to differentiate between obstruction and pseudo-obstruction (Fig. 26.5). It has the advantage of diagnosing extra-colonic disease, and is particularly useful where there is a history of abdominal malignancy, or a mass has been palpated clinically (MEGIBOW et al. 1991). CT is also a useful primary imaging technique where there are signs suggesting infection or bowel infarction, since appendicitis, diverticulitis and bowel infarction can all be diagnosed (MEGIBOW et al. 1991).

26.1.2.5
Ultrasound

Ultrasound has been used to differentiate intestinal obstruction from ileus in post-operative patients (WILSON 1992). In acute obstruction, peristalsis is characteristically vigorous, although it must be remembered that peristalsis decreases with time. Ultrasound is particularly useful in the assessment

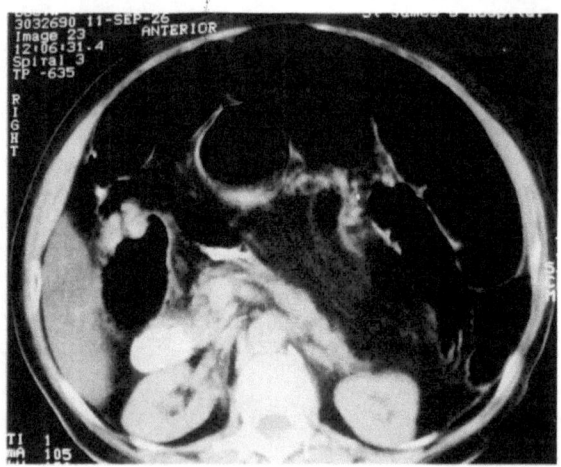

Fig. 26.5. CT in an elderly patient with obstructive symptoms. The CT shows an obstructing carcinoma at the hepatic flexure with colonic distension both proximal and distal to the tumour. This is an unusual combination of obstruction and pseudo-obstruction. The pseudo-obstruction was thought to be caused by associated hypokalemia

of patients with gasless abdomens on plain film in which there is a clinical suspicion of colonic obstruction and where tumour or hernia may be visualized as the cause of the obstruction (CARROLL 1989).

26.1.3
Complications

Perforation occurs in 2% of all patients with colonic obstruction, but in 12%–18% of those with malignant obstruction (Fig. 26.6) (UMPLEBY et al. 1984).

26.1.4
Management

26.1.4.1
Surgery

Initial management should include fluid resuscitation to restore normal blood volume and adequate gastrointestinal decompression by naso-gastric tube in order to prevent aspiration during anaesthesia. Suction applied through a naso-gastric tube will frequently empty the small bowel for a considerable distance.

Following midline incision, tense distended colon with an imminent risk of rupture may be dealt with immediately by needle decompression, preferably through the transverse colon, although this is not routinely performed. Surgery may involve a one or a two step procedure depending on individual patient circumstances.

26.1.4.1.1
Immediate Resection

In the absence of peritonitis, an extended right hemi-colectomy with ileocolic anastomosis is performed if the tumour is within the right colon or proximal transverse colon. If the tumour is within the distal transverse colon, then either an extended right hemi-colectomy or a left hemicolectomy may be performed. For sigmoid lesions an anterior resection may be feasible following orthograde lavage of the proximal bowel but if conditions for immediate anastomosis do not apply the proximal bowel may be brought out as a colostomy, after resection of the tumour, and the distal rectum oversewn (Hartmann procedure).

26.1.4.1.2
Delayed Resection

If the obstruction is at or distal to the splenic flexure but resection cannot be performed a transverse colostomy can be fashioned. This has become a more popular option where tumour is considered fixed when examined under anaesthetic or unresectable at

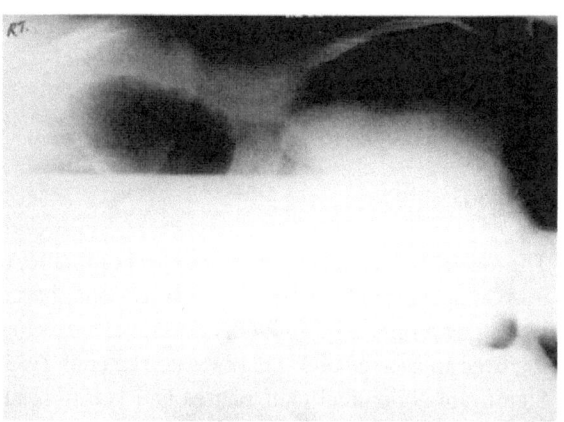

Fig. 26.6. Left lateral decubitus film. Obstructed colon with perforation. Subphrenic gas has collected between the liver and the lower rib cage

laparotomy. In such circumstances a defunctioning transverse colostomy allows time for proper imaging of the tumour with a view to possible down staging by chemoradiotherapy. In the case of a right sided obstruction where immediate right hemicolectomy is not feasible, there are three options: ileotransverse bypass, which is reserved for fixed primary tumours or where there is widespread peritoneal disease, ileostomy and mucous fistula and caecostomy. The latter should only be considered as a temporizing measure and is associated with significant complications, although it may be appropriate in very frail elderly patients.

26.1.4.2
Metal Stents

The use of metal stents (see Chap. 9) allows time to prepare the patient for a definitive one stage operation after staging examinations and evaluation of the rest of the colon. There is an obvious role in the palliation of inoperable or metastatic disease. Stent migration and perforation are complications.

26.2
Pseudo-obstruction

26.2.1
Definition

Adynamic ileus of the colon, pseudo-obstruction, non-obstructive colonic dilatation and Ogilvie's syndrome are all descriptive terms for a clinical entity in which the symptoms and signs of colonic obstruction are present in the absence of a mechanical obstruction. Patient's behave as though they are obstructed, but the problem is functional and not surgical.

26.2.2
Clinical Features

The mean age is 68 years, with a male predominance of 2:1 (GELLER et al. 1996). Pseudo-obstruction is characterized by pronounced abdominal distension developing over an average of 3–4 days (STRODEL et al. 1982). Significant abdominal pain, nausea and vomiting are variably reported in between 10% (GELLER et al. 1996) and 60%–80% (VANEK and AL-SALTI 1986) of patients. Bowel sound may be increased, normal, or decreased. A moderate increase in temperature and white cell count is not infrequent. Approximately 70% of patients continue to pass watery stool, but in 30% there is absolute constipation (STRODEL et al. 1982). The colonic dilatation may be chronic and relatively asymptomatic or acute, in which case symptoms are more likely, as well as the risk of caecal perforation, which has a mortality of 50% (WOJTALIK et al. 1973).

26.2.3
Diagnosis

The diagnosis of acute colonic pseudo-obstruction is one of exclusion. A definitive diagnosis can only be made after contrast enema, CT or colonoscopy has ruled out mechanical obstruction. All cases show colonic dilatation on plain radiographs. Whilst 30% show dilatation of the entire colon, dilatation is segmental in 70% (STRODEL et al. 1982) and of these the dilatation cut-off is at the splenic flexure in 50%, the hepatic flexure in 25% and at the sigmoid in 25% (Fig. 26.7). In the majority the transition from distended bowel to collapsed bowel is gradual, but a sudden cut off is seen in 23% (GILCHRIST et al. 1985). Air is present in the small bowel in 60% and small bowel distension results from an incompetent ileocaecal valve, air swallowing or peritoneal irritation. The caecal diameter ranges from 2 to13 cm (STRODEL et al. 1982). The upper limit of normal for the caecum is empirically taken to be 9 cm, calculated from a study of normal barium enema examinations. Caecal diameters above this are at risk of perforation, and perforated caeca at surgery have an average diameter of 10.9 cm (LOWMAN and DAVIS 1956).

26.2.4
Aetiology

Patients usually have other coexistent pathology (ALWAN and VAN RIJ 1998). A large number of associated conditions have been described but these can be divided into 'surgical' (two thirds of patients) and 'medical' (one third) (GELLER et al. 1996). Orthopaedic operations are most commonly implicated, followed by abdominal and thoracic surgery (WANEBOH et al.

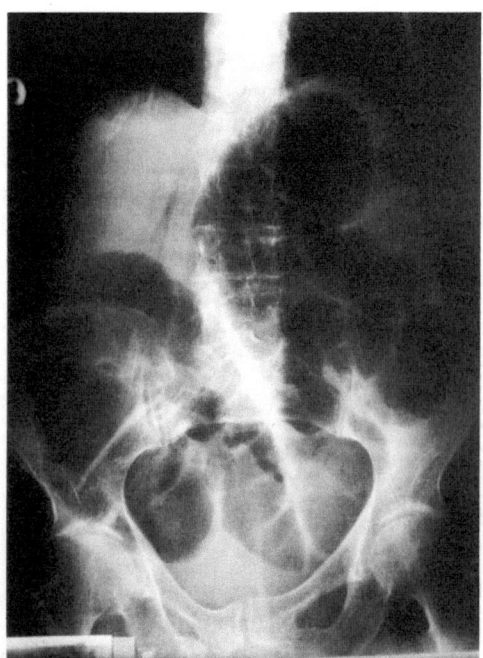
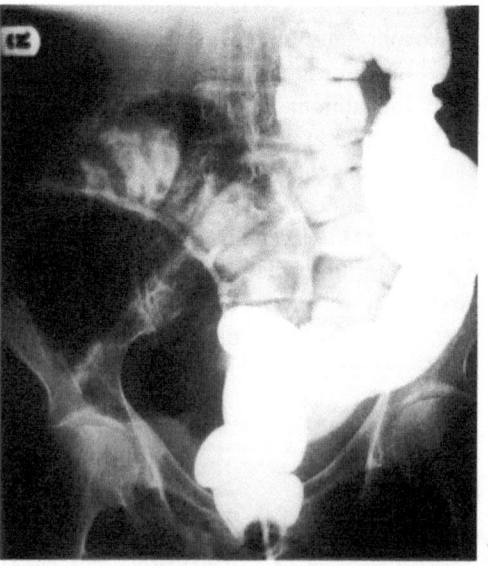

Fig. 26.7a,b. a Distended colon with cut-off at splenic flexure. **b** Acute contrast enema shows no evidence of obstruction. Diagnosis: Pseudo-obstruction secondary to poorly controlled diabetes

1971; Morton et al. 1960). Patients undergoing Caesarean section have also been sited as a major group (Hall 1985; Reece and Petrie 1982). Other conditions include heart disease and heart failure, chronic obstructive pulmonary disease and pneumonia, cirrhosis, sepsis, malignancy and metabolic disturbances, or following surgery or trauma.

Ogilvie speculated that inhibition of the sympathetic nerve supply to the colon is responsible, whilst others have theorised that it is an imbalance between the sympathetic and parasympathetic supply that causes a loss of normal spike and phasic motor activity in the colon (Ogilvie 1948; Sullivan et al. 1977). The result is a functional obstruction of the left colon leading to proximal dilatation. This is supported by the fact that a cut off at the splenic flexure is frequently present on plain abdominal x-ray (Vanek and Al-Salti 1986; Bachulis and Smith 1978; Spira et al. 1976).

More recently, 'gas locking' has been postulated as the mechanism by which pseudo-obstruction occurs (Lang et al. 1998). According to this theory, in which the Bernoulli equation for flow through a tube is applied, the accumulation of gas in non-dependent bowel loops, such as the hepatic and splenic flexures and the sigmoid colon, could result in a situation where the colon is no longer able to generate the pressures required to restore flow. Thus, the accumulated gas forms an effective blockage to intestinal transport and pseudo-obstruction ensues. Lang et al. (1998) report successful treatment of colonic pseudo-obstruction by active aspiration through a small bore catheter placed at the gas filled 'U' bend, rather than at the caecum. The observation that the level of gaseous dilatation often corresponds to sites of 'U' tube gas trapping, namely the flexures and sigmoid colon, also supports this theory (Bode et al. 1984).

26.2.5
Complication

Untreated pseudo-obstruction can lead to progressive dilatation and colonic perforation. As with mechanical obstruction the caecum dilates more than the rest of the colon (Laplace's Law) and increasing distension may result in progressive mural ischaemia, starting at the anti-mesenteric border (van Swalenburg 1907). With time the caecum may undergo infarction leading to perforation and peritonitis develops with significant associated mortality (Fig. 26.8) (Wojtalik et al. 1973; Gierson et al. 1975; Carrasquilla et al. 1970). Reported rates of perforation vary between 7%–10% (Fiorito et al. 1991).

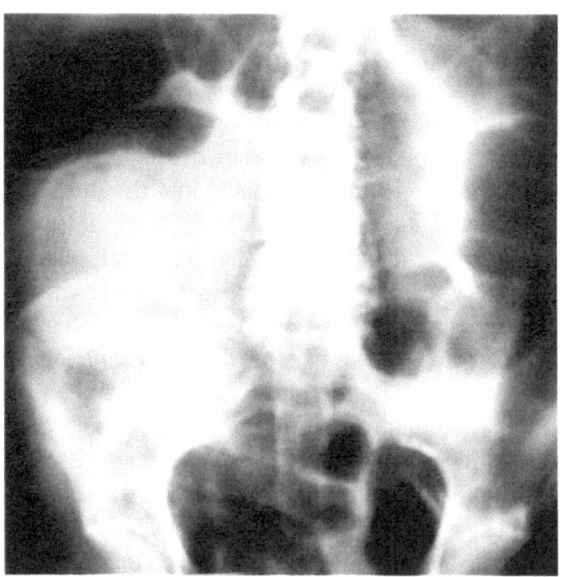

Fig. 26.8. Pseudo-obstruction following maxillary surgery. Fluid-filled caecum with gas in the bowel wall indicating caecal necrosis

26.2.6
Treatment

Despite anecdotal case reports of successful treatment with a wide variety of pharmacological agents including naloxone (Bianchi and Ubach 1994), epidural anaesthesia (Lee et al. 1988) and guanethidine with neostigmine (Hutchinson and Griffiths 1992), no controlled studies exist to confirm efficacy. Furthermore, pharmacological agents can be highly morbid and even associated with mortality. If the caecal diameter is less than 9 cm, initial management should include sitting the patient out, correction of fluid balance and electrolyte disturbances, cessation of any narcotic drugs and treatment of the underlying condition. Nasogastric tube placement to prevent further entry of air into the intestine is indicated if there is small bowel dilatation.

If a non-operative approach is employed, serial abdominal radiographs should be obtained to assess absolute caecal size as well as temporal changes in caecal diameter, and evidence of perforation. Unfortunately, such conservative measures are not always successful (Geller et al. 1996; Strodel et al. 1982; Lipton and Knauerb 1977; Lewis et al. 1978).

Colonoscopic decompression replaced surgery as the treatment of choice (Goshe et al. 1989; Martin et al. 1988; van Gossum et al. 1992) for patients with acute colonic pseudo-obstruction following its introduction by Kukora and Dent (1977). Clinical success can be expected in 95% of patients who respond to the first colonoscopic decompression (73%–100%), but this falls to 56% in those requiring multiple decompressions (10%–20%).

It is not always necessary to pass the colonoscope to the caecum to effect adequate decompression, but the colonoscope must be passed into the distended segment. Upon withdrawal of the scope intermittent suction should affect colonic luminal collapse. A guidewire can be introduced and a decompression tube can be placed over the guidewire after the colonoscope is withdrawn in order to effect prolonged decompression (BERNTON et al. 1982). Rather than simply decompressing the colon, there is some evidence that effective colonic decompression is more likely to occur if a decompression tube is left in situ (GELLER et al. 1996; HARIG et al. 1988). This appears to be particularly true for patients with serious systemic disease, where the underlying problem may not be rapidly reversible, such as those on mechanical ventilation or with sepsis (GELLER et al. 1996).

Colonoscopy has the added advantage of detecting impending perforation allowing emergency surgery to be performed before perforation occurs. In 7%–15%, a non-specific colitis is observed which is thought to be related to ischaemia (GELLER et al. 1996; VANEK and AL-SALTI 1986). Opinion varies as to whether the presence of a right sided colitis should prompt termination of colonoscopy and urgent laparotomy (VANEK and AL-SALTI 1986), or initial trial with colonoscopic decompression and tube placement which has been successful, even in the presence of ischaemia (GELLER et al. 1996; FIORITO et al. 1991). As a general rule, in the presence of caecal tenderness a decision will be made to progress to laparotomy.

Where colonoscopy has been unsuccessful, and caecal diameters remain above 12 cm, tube caecostomy should be considered.

Table 26.2. Causes of intussusceptions in adults. From literature review of 1048 cases (BEGOS et al. 1997)

Large bowel (36%)	Malignant (58%)	Adenocarcinoma Lymphoma Lymphosarcoma Leiomyosarcoma
	Benign (29%)	Previous anastomosis Lipoma Endometriosis Adenomatous polyp
Small bowel (64%)	Idiopathic (13%) Benign (63%) Malignant (14%) Idiopathic (23%)	

26.2.7
Prognosis

Overall, sustained colonic decompression can be achieved in 80%. Mortality is not usually the direct result of colonic pseudo-obstruction but results from the significant co-existing pathology (GELLER et al. 1996).

26.3
Specific Colonic Obstructions

26.3.1
Intussusception

26.3.1.1
Introduction

Intussusception is defined as the telescoping of one segment of the gastrointestinal tract into an adjacent segment.

A total of 95% of intussusceptions occur in children where 90% are spontaneous and only 10% are associated with an underlying abnormality of bowel. In adults, the reverse applies as 90% are associated with an underlying bowel abnormality and only 10% are spontaneous (Table 26.2). Intussusception accounts for up to 5% of all cases of adult bowel obstruction with approximately 30% occurring in the colon (BEGOS et al. 1997).

26.3.1.2
Clinical Features

Patients with colonic intussusception present with chronic or intermittent obstructive symptoms. Pain is experienced in the majority and is characteristically intermittent. Vomiting and the passage of red blood are the next most common symptoms. During the height of an attack, a palpable mass may be present, but this may resolve if the episode settles (ELLIS 1989).

26.3.1.3
Aetiology

In adults carcinoma is the commonest cause of colonic intussusception. SANDERS et al. (1958) reviewed over 350 cases of colonic intussusception and 68% had a malignant lead point. Adenocarcinoma is the most common histological diagnosis, but lymphomas and sarcomas can also be responsible (Table 26.2). Caeco-colic intussusception may have the appendix or a lipoma of the ileocaecal valve as a lead point. Causes of appendiceal intussusception include villous adenoma, mucinous cystadenoma, endometriosis and adenocarcinoma, but often no cause is identified (JEVON et al. 1992; CHETTY and DANIEL 1992). Intussusception secondary to adhesions, leiomyomas, benign polyps or a recent surgical anastomoses are also recognised (BEGOS et al. 1997).

26.3.1.4
Diagnosis

26.3.1.4.1
Plain Film

If the intussusception is ileocolic or colocolic, the pathognomonic 'crescent' sign may be seen caused by the trapping of intraluminal gas between the intussusceptum and the intussuscipiens. This gas may appear as a semi-lunar lucency, which is wider than normal bowel diameter and may be associated with a soft tissue density representing the mass created by the intussusception (Fig. 26.9) (BAKER 1990).

26.3.1.4.2
Barium Enema

The intussusceptum shows as a cup-shaped filling defect and the lead tumour may be seen as an additional filling defect. Barium in the peripheral sheath outlines circular bands which are crowded haustra of the intussuscipiens giving a spiral or 'coiled spring' appearance (Fig. 26.10) (WIOT and SPITZ 1970).

26.3.1.4.3
Ultrasound

Whilst ultrasound is well established for the diagnosis of intussusception in children, it has also been successfully used in adults. Typical features include the 'target' or 'doughnut' sign on transverse view. A hypoechoic halo is produced by the oedematous wall of the intussuscipiens. The hyperechoic centre is produced by the central interfaces of the compressed layers of the intussusceptum and to the side of this is the hypoechoic oedematous indrawn mesentery. In the longitudinal view a 'pseudo-kidney', or hay-fork' sign is produced by multiple thin parallel alternating hypoechoic and hyperechoic lines (Fig. 26.11) (WEISSBERG et al. 1977; ALESSI and SALERNO 1985). The major limitation of ultrasonography for evalu-

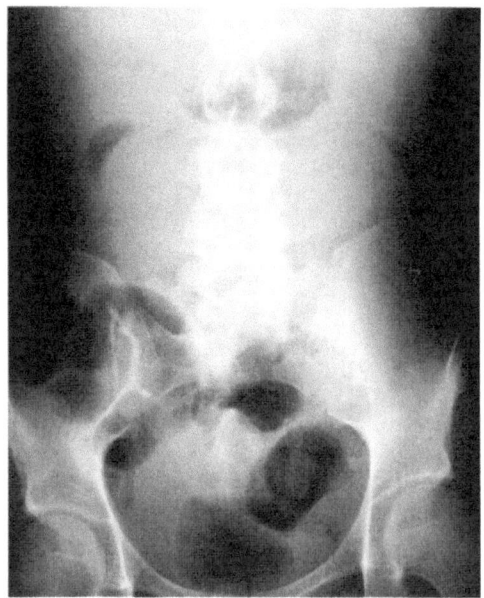

Fig. 26.9. Caecal intussusception extending to the left side of the transverse colon. Sausage-shaped central abdominal mass. Gas-filled small bowel loops in the right iliac fossa, but no caecal gas shadow. Diagnosis: Intussusception secondary to a caecal lipoma. (Courtesy of Dr D. Kessel, St James's University Hospital, Leeds, UK)

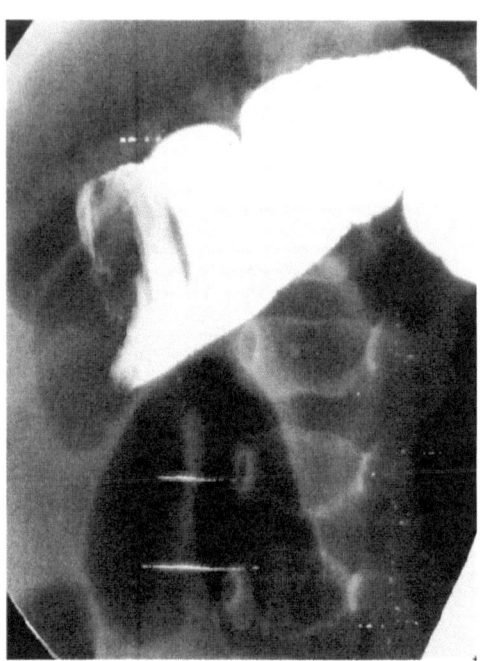

Fig. 26.10. Barium enema examination in intussusception. Barium caught between the intussusceptum and the intussuscipiens gives a spiral or 'coiled spring' appearance

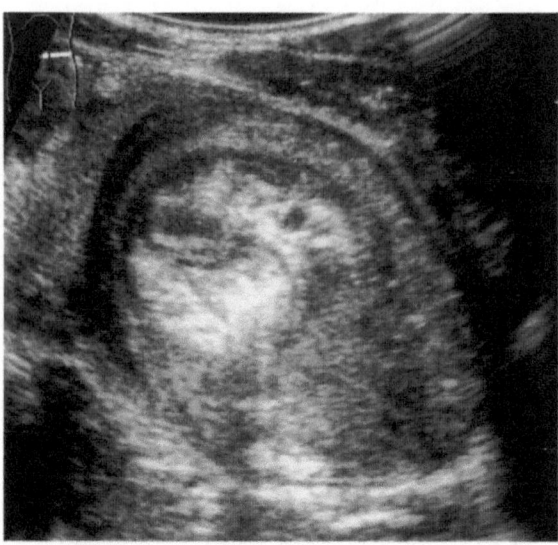
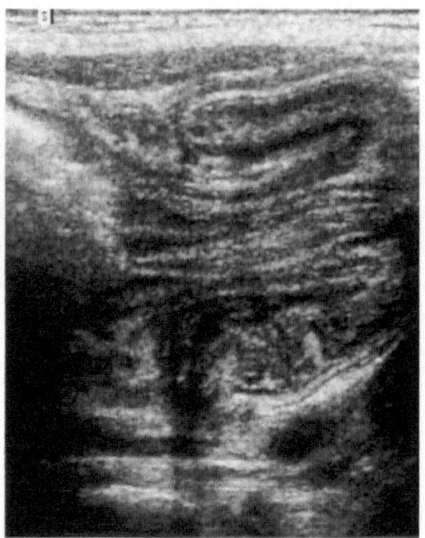

a   b

Fig. 26.11a,b. Ultrasound appearances of a caecal intussusception. **a** Transverse section shows an outer hypo-echoic halo produced by the oedematous wall of the intussuscipiens and a hyper-echoic centre produced by the central interfaces of the compressed layers of the intussusceptum. To the side of the hyper-echoic centre is the hypo-echoic oedematous indrawn mesentery (courtesy of Dr D Kessel, St James's University Hospital, Leeds, UK). **b** Longitudinal view of an intussusception showing the 'hay-fork' sign produced by multiple thin parallel alternating hypoechoic and hyperechoic lines

ating acute obstructive symptoms is the presence of air in the bowel which leads to poor sound wave transmission, and image quality.

26.1.4.4
Computed Tomography

The early CT features of intussusception are a target mass, encircling eccentric low density fat corresponding to the mesentery drawn into the intussuscipiens

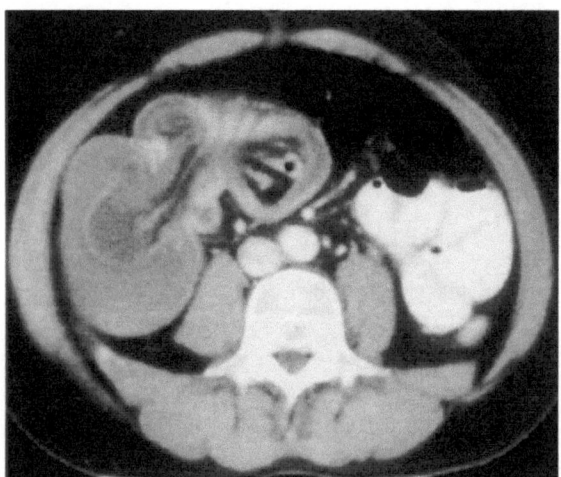

Fig. 26.12. CT scan showing caecal intussusception. The fat of the mesentery has been drawn into the intussusceptum

(Bar-Ziv and Soloman 1991). As time progresses, increasing mural congestion and oedema results in a sausage shaped mass with alternating layers of low and high attenuation (Fig. 26.12). If left untreated, a reniform mass develops resulting from severe mural oedema and vascular compromise which should be regarded as a surgical emergency. Other signs, such as proximal bowel distension, intra-peritoneal fluid and mesenteric oedema or haemorrhage secondary to traction or infarction may be present.

Colonoscopy and flexible sigmoidoscopy may also be used to evaluate an intussusception, especially when the patient presents with symptoms of large bowel obstruction. The findings are of a coiled spring polypoid mass. Biopsy is best avoided because of the risk of extended tissue necrosis in the vascularly compromised bowel (Hurwitz and Gertler 1986).

26.3.1.5
Complications

As the intussusceptum enters into the intussuscipiens, the mesentery is carried forward and trapped between the overlapping layers of bowel. The stretched and compressed mesentery results in vascular compression. The vascularly compromised bowel becomes oedematous, further compressing the vessels in the mesentery. Ischaemic necrosis of the bowel wall may ensue unless timely intervention is undertaken.

26.3.1.6
Treatment

Whilst surgical resection of the lesion is nearly always required, the extent of resection and whether or not the intussusception should be reduced before resection is a matter of debate (BEGOS et al. 1997).

Laparotomy is considered mandatory because of the likelihood of identifying a pathological lesion. In the case of ileocolic or colocolic intussusception, where the cause is likely to be an underlying malignancy, en bloc dissection of the mass should be performed as the primary operative manoeuvre. This theoretically reduces the chance of dissemination by transperitoneal seeding (SANDERS et al. 1958; REI-JNEN et al. 1989; NAGORNEY et al. 1981). In a patient with symptoms of partial or complete obstruction, but without clinical, laboratory or radiological evidence of bowel ischaemia, in which there is a history of recent trauma or bowel surgery, a cautious attempt at hydrostatic reduction may be considered. This would allow limited colonic cleansing prior to a one-step surgical procedure.

Successful treatment of ileocaecal intussusception caused by lipoma of the ileocaecal valve has been achieved by air insufflation followed by endoscopic resection (BEGOS et al. 1997).

26.3.2
Volvulus

26.3.2.1
Introduction

Volvulus refers to torsion or twist of an organ on a pedicle to a sufficient degree to cause symptoms secondary to bowel obstruction or strangulation of blood vessels or both. Volvulus can affect any part of the colon but most often involves the sigmoid, caecum, transverse colon and splenic flexure (WELSH 1990).

Sigmoid volvulus is the commonest type (50%–75%), followed by caecal (25%–40%) and transverse colon (0%–10%). Double volvulus, such as coexisting sigmoid and caecal volvulus, is also possible.

26.3.2.2
Clinical Features

Patients present with a slowly progressive obstruction of some days duration with increasing abdominal distension and failure to pass flatus. There may be a history of previous obstructive episodes, followed by diarrhoea and copious evacuation of flatus. These attacks are caused by twisting of the colonic mesentery followed by spontaneous reduction. Severe pain is not a feature and vomiting is a late event. With sigmoid volvulus in particular, there is considerably more abdominal distension than that seen is patients with large bowel obstruction caused by a tumour and this may even affect respiratory function by splinting the diaphragm.

26.3.2.3
Aetiology

Although volvulus may be idiopathic, there is an association with increasing age, chronic constipation, mental retardation, connective tissue disorders and Parkinson's disease. The condition is classically seen on care of the elderly or psychogeriatric wards, and in those on antipsychotic medication. Sigmoid volvulus is more common in Eastern Europe, Africa, India and the Middle East than in the UK, Australia and America reflecting an increased prevalence in regions where there is a high residue diet. Both a segment of redundant mobile colon and a relatively fixed point of mesenteric fixation are required for a volvulus to occur. Consequently, sigmoid colon, caecum, and transverse colon are the most common sites.

26.3.2.4
Sigmoid Volvulus

26.3.2.4.1
Diagnosis

26.3.2.4.1.1
Plain films

Plain films show a grossly distended sigmoid loop, which sometimes displays a coffee bean configuration with the axis pointing toward the left iliac fossa. The Friemann-Dahl radiographic sign consists of three dense lines converging towards the point of obstruction. This sign if often present and when seen is pathognomonic (Fig. 26.13). Haustral markings are absent due to the degree of distension of the twisted loop.

A single-contrast water-soluble enema is occasionally needed to differentiate volvulus from pseudo-obstruction. Features include 'beaking' at the site of obstruction, with the 'bird of prey' sign used to describe contrast outlining the distal side of the point of axial torsion (Fig. 26.14).

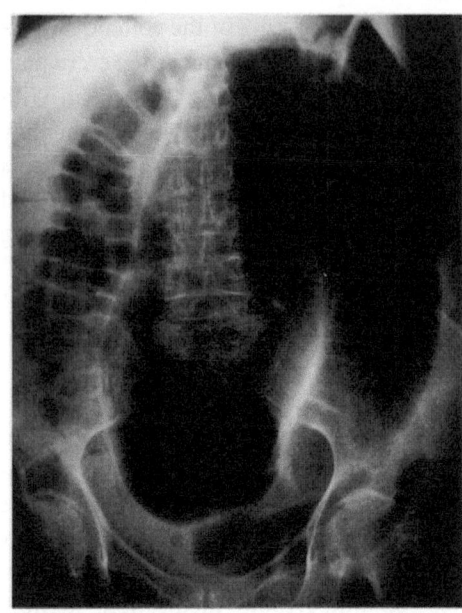

Fig. 26.13. Sigmoid volvulus. Three lines converge towards the point of obstruction in the pelvis. One line is produced by the interface between the inner margins of the twisted loop and a line is produced by each outer margin

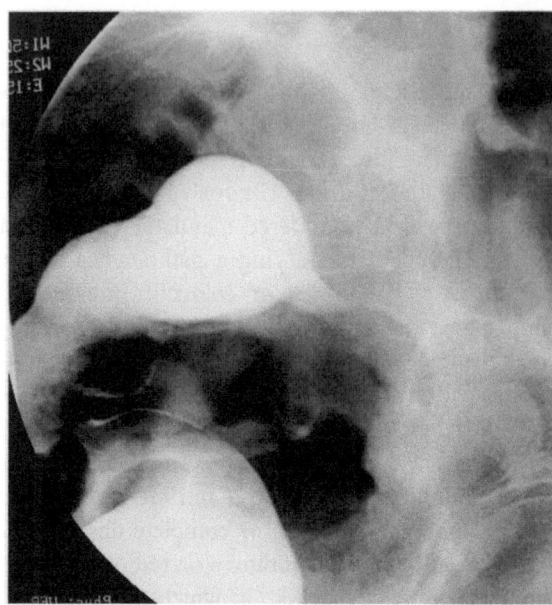

Fig. 26.14. Sigmoid volvulus. Acute contrast enema showing beaking at the site of volvulus

26.3.2.4.1.2
Computed Tomography

Occasionally, the diagnosis is made on CT where a 'whorl sign' has been used to describe the rotation of mesenteric vessels within a mesentery undergoing volvulus (Fig. 28.15) (SHAFF et al. 1985; FISHER 1981).

26.3.2.4.2
Complications

With decompression the bowel untwists but about 50% of patients represent within the subsequent 2 years with a recurrence. If the condition recurs, early elective sigmoid colectomy after bowel preparation is recommended as the treatment of choice. If decompression is unsuccessful or if there is blood stained contents suggesting colonic necrosis, urgent laparotomy is indicated.

26.3.2.4.3
Treatment

26.3.2.4.3.1
Non-surgical

Sigmoidoscopy should be performed with great caution and a flexible instrument is preferable. The

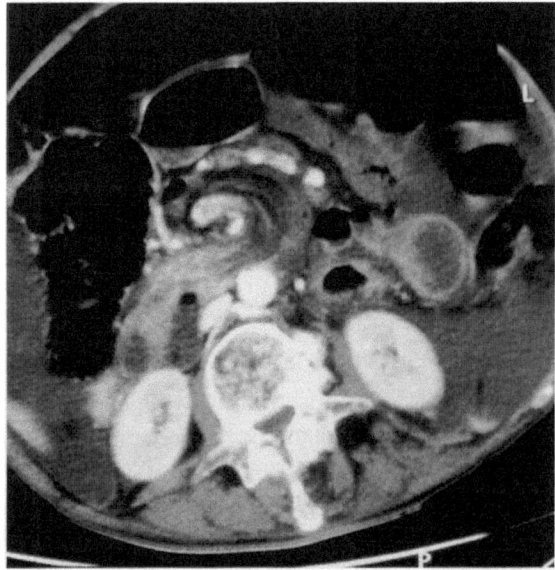

Fig. 26.15. Whorl sign describes the rotation of mesenteric vessels within the mesentery. CT of small bowel volvulus (courtesy of Dr. A Chalmers)

narrowing or twist is usually visible within 25 cm of the anus, and while the instrument may pass into the obstructed segment, more usually, it is necessary to introduce a well lubricated flatus tube. Successful decompression is marked by a sudden release of flatus and liquid faeces. The tube can be left in position to prevent early relapse, or removed straight away. Tubes left in should be fixed to the perianal skin.

26.3.2.4.3.2
Surgical

Because of the risk of recurrence, when the colon has been successfully decompressed by intubation, preparation should be made for elective resection with primary anastomosis. Also for recurrence following conservative treatment the patient should be fully decompressed by intubation, and full bowel preparation performed followed by sigmoid colectomy with primary anastomosis. There can be great disparity in size between the distended sigmoid colon and the upper rectum which makes anastomosis difficult. In such cases the safest procedure is to perform a sigmoid colectomy and bring out both ends as a common stoma (Paul Mikulicz procedure). It is possible for this kind of stoma to gradually heal, or the stoma can be reversed at a later date.

26.3.2.4.3.3
Percutaneous Sigmoidopexy

Under colonoscopic guidance PEG tubes have been used to fix the redundant sigmoid loop following decompression and untwisting of the colon. This technique is reserved for patients with recurrent volvulus who are unfit for surgery. Our approach is to use a combined percutaneous and endoscopic approach for maximum control and we prefer to use four T-fasteners to fix the distal vertical limb of the redundant sigmoid loop so as to reduce the risk of internal herniation (Fig. 26.16) (GALLAGHER et al. 2002).

26.3.2.5
Caecal Volvulus

26.3.2.5.1
Introduction

This is less common than sigmoid volvulus, patients usually present with a short history of intestinal obstruction, pain is severe and vomiting occurs early. Typically a palpable, tense and resonant mass occupies the central or left upper part of the abdomen, and is combined with a concavity in the right iliac fossa.

26.3.2.5.2
Aetiology

Some authors claim that a congenital abnormality of the mesentery is responsible for an increased likelihood of caecal volvulus. The caecum and ascending colon is generally on a free mesentery or a common

mesentery serves the whole of the intestine from the duodenojejunal flexure to the hepatic flexure .

26.3.2.5.3
Diagnosis

Plain films show an oval or hour-glass shaped gas-filled viscus occupying the central and upper part of the abdomen (Fig. 26.17). It may resemble a distended gas-filled stomach from which it must be distinguished by early gastric aspiration.

26.3.2.5.4
Surgery

The preferred surgery is a right hemicolectomy. The volvulus generally should not be untwisted as a sudden return of blood flow to infarcted tissue may cause profound hypotension and dysrhythmias. However, some surgeons will untwist a volvulus if there are no features of ischaemia and will fix the caecum by inserting a caecostomy tube.

26.3.2.6
Compound and Double Volvulus

Ileo-sigmoid knot is a compound volvulus in which the terminal ileum twists around the mesentery of a sigmoid volvulus. It is only common in certain tropical countries.

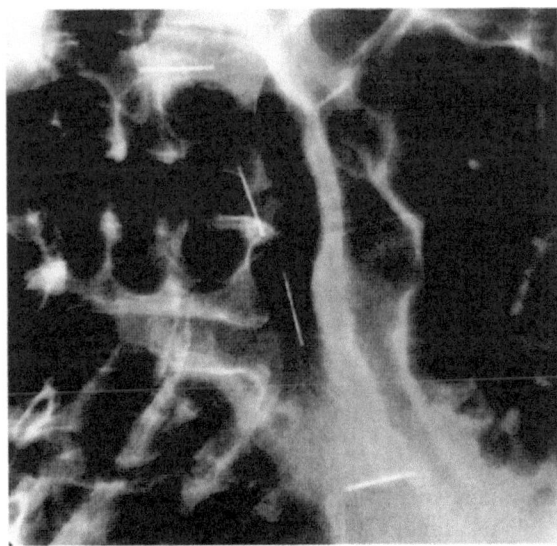

Fig. 26.16. Percutaneous sigmoidopexy. Four metal 'T-fasteners' have been used to fix the descending limb of the redundant sigmoid colon after the loop has been deflated and the volvulus has resolved

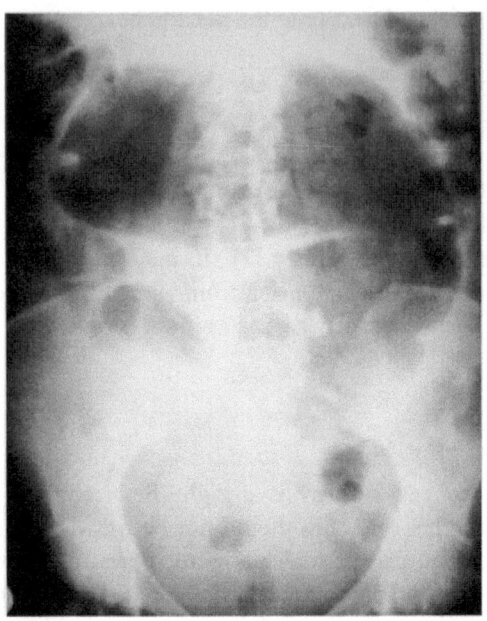

Fig. 26.17. Caecal volvulus with the caecal pole pointing up towards the liver

The plain film shows distended small bowel loops grouped to the left of an omega-shaped distended sigmoid, and there may be a suggestion of small bowel strangulation. The ascending, transverse and descending colon contain no gas, although faecal residue may be seen. Treatment involves resecting non-viable bowel en bloc as without treatment the patient's condition deteriorates quickly with onset of cardiovascular collapse.

Double volvulus is rare and its presence indicates multiple congenital or acquired abnormalities of the mesentery. The plain film appearance can be confusing but with a combined sigmoid and caecal volvulus the diagnosis may be made on a check film following the decompression of the sigmoid volvulus (Fig. 26.18).

26.3.3
Adhesions

Compared with the small bowel, the colon is remarkably resistant to adhesional obstruction. The mobile, redundant portions of the colon are the most vulnerable. Obstruction may be caused by congenital bands, or adhesions secondary to inflammatory or ischaemic change (HOLT and WAGNER 1984).

26.3.4
Hernias

Inguinal, femoral, umbilical, spigelian, incisional and diaphragmatic hernias can all contain colon and cause colonic obstruction, although less commonly than they cause small bowel obstruction (WELSH 1990). Internal hernias can also involve the colon (RICHARDSON and ANASTOPOULOS 1981).

26.3.5
Obturation Obstruction

The sigmoid colon is the narrowest part of the large bowel with a diameter of 2.5 cm. Between 3%–5% of patients with gallstone ileus have colonic obstruction. In these cases, the ileocaecal valve is bypassed by a cholecystocolic fistula with the gallstone usually impacting in the sigmoid colon, which may already be narrowed by previous episodes of diverticulitis. Other enteroliths, bezoars or food do not usually affect the colon unless there is a pre-existing stricture.

26.3.6
Obstipation

Faecal impaction (obstipation) may mimic an obstructing lesion of the rectosigmoid junction. It usually affects elderly or psychiatric patients who have neglected their diets and become progressively inactive. It is also seen in chronic laxative abuse.

The most common sites are the rectum (70%) and the sigmoid (20%). Diagnosis is usually made by digital rectal examination. These patients are managed by faecal disimpaction under sedation or general anaesthetic. There is anecdotal evidence of effective use of a Urografin enema for treatment of faecal impaction but there is no evidence it is more effective than a tap water or a soap suds enema.

26.3.7
Extrinsic Causes of Obstruction

The colon can be obstructed by disease arising in adjacent organs. The commonest sites affected are the sigmoid and transverse colon. Endometrial implants, cervical, uterine, renal, ovarian and prostatic tumours can all invade the colon directly, and gastric, ovarian and pancreatic neoplasms can invade by serosal metastases. Pancreatitis can obstruct by extrinsic compression

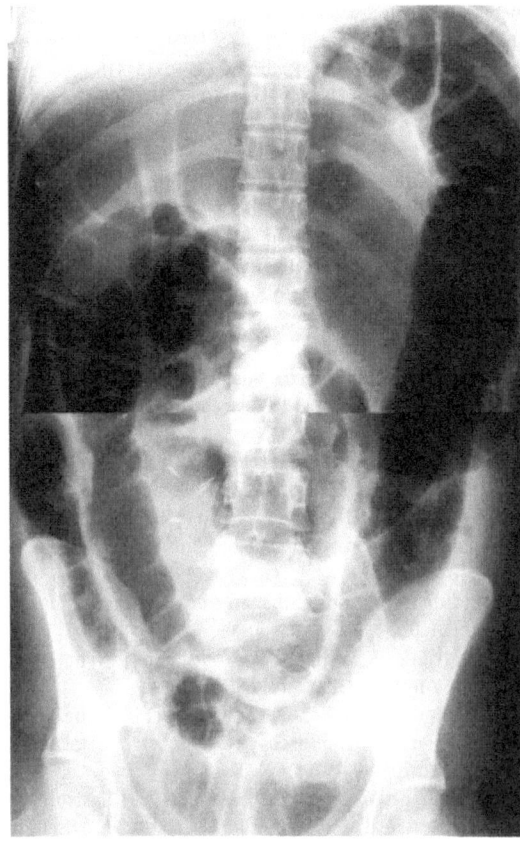
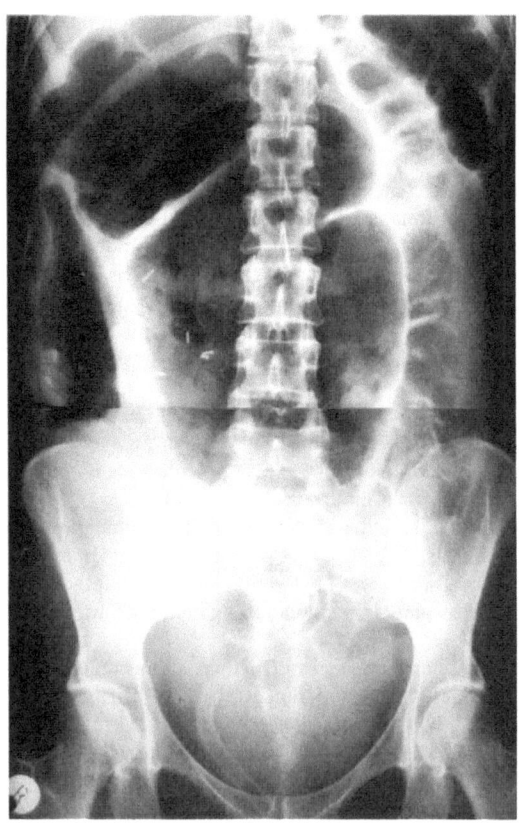

a   b

Fig. 26.18a,b. Caecal and sigmoid volvulus. **a** Confusing initial plain film in a young female patient with a short history of increasing abdominal distension. Sigmoid volvulus was demonstrated at sigmoidoscopy and a flatus tube placed. **b** Follow-up abdominal film shows the sigmoid volvulus to have decompressed with the flatus tube, but the caecal volvulus is now clearly seen. Size of patient necessitated two films

from phlegmon or pancreatic collection, or secondarily from oedema and necrosis caused by enzymes dissecting down the phrenocolic ligament or transverse mesocolon. Pelvic masses, lipomatosis, pregnancy, mesenteric panniculitis and retroperitoneal tumours are all rare causes of large bowel obstruction.

Acknowledgment
We would like to thank Mr. David J. Alexander MBBS, FRCS, MS, Consultant in General Surgery and Coloproctology, York District Hospital, for his invaluable help with the surgical aspects of this chapter.

References

Alessi V, Salerno G (1985) The 'hay fork' sign in the ultrasonic diagnosis of intussusception. Gastrointest Radiol 10:177-179

Alwan MH, van Rij AM (1998) Acute colonic pseudo-obstruction. Aust N Z J Surg 68:129-132

Bachulis BL, Smith PE (1978) Pseudo-obstruction of the colon. Am J Surg 136:66-72

Baker SR (1990) Plain film radiology of the intestines and appendix. In: The abdominal plain film, chap 5. Appleton and Lange, Norwalk, pp 155-242

Bar-ZivJ, Soloman A (1991) Computed tomography in adult intussusception. Gastrointest Radiol 16:264-266

Begos DG, Sandor A, Modlin IM (1997) The diagnosis and management of adult intussusception. Am J Surg 173:88-94

Bernton E, Myers R, Reyna T (1982) Pseudo-obstruction of the colon: case report including a new endoscopic treatment. Gastrointest Endosc 28:90-92

Bianchi A, Ubach M (1994) Acute colonic pseudo-obstruction caused by opiates treated with naloxone. Med Clin 103:78

Bode WE, Beart RW, Spencer RJ et al (1984) Colonoscopic decompression for acute pseudo-obstruction of the colon: report of 22 cases and review of the literature. Am J Surg 147:243-245

Carrasquilla C, Arbulu A, Fromm S et al (1970) Cecal perforation due to adynamic ileus. Dis Colon Rectum 13:252-254

Carroll BR (1989) US of the gastrointestinal tract. Radiology 172:605-608

Chapman AH, McNamara M, Porter G (1992) The acute contrast enema in suspected large bowel obstruction: value and technique. Clin Rad 46:273-278

Chetty R, Daniel WJ (1992) Mucinous cystadenoma of the appendix: an unusual cause of intussusception in an adult. Aust NZ J Surg 62:670-671

Ellis H (1989) Special forms of intestinal obstruction. In: Schwartz SI, Ellis H (eds) Maingot's abdominal operations. Appleton and Lange, East Norwalk, CT, pp 905-932

Fiorito JJ, Schoen RE, Brandt LJ (1991) Pseudo-obstruction associated with colonic ishaemia: successful management with colonoscopic decompression. Am J Gastroenterol 86: 1472-1476

Fisher JK (1981) Computed tomographic diagnosis of volvulus in intestinal malrotation. Radiology 140:145-146

Gallagher HJ, Aitken D, Chapman AH (2002) Additional experience of endoscopic T-bar Sigmoidopexy. Dis Colon Rectum 45:1565-1566

Geller A, Peterson BT, Gostout CJ (1996) Endoscopic decompression for acute pseudo-obstruction. Gastrointest Endosc 44:144-150

Gierson ED, Storm FK, Shaw W, Coyne SK (1975) Caecal rupture due to colonic ileus. Br J Surg 62:383-386

Gilchrist AM, Mills OM, Russell CFJ (1985) Acute large bowel pseudo-obstruction. Clin Rad 36:401-404

Golden DA, Warren B, Gefter MD (1981) Digital examination of the rectum as a source of rectal gas. Radiology 141:618

Goshe JR, Sharp JN, Larson GM (1989) Colonoscopic decompression for pseudo-obstruction of the colon. Am Surg 55: 111-115

Hall B (1985) Colonic pseudo-obstruction: an uncommon complication of caesarian section. Aust NZ J Obstet Gynaecol 25:121-123

Harig JM, Fumo DE, Loo FD at al (1988) Treatment of acute non toxic megacolon during colonoscopy: tube placement versus simple decompression. Gastrointest Endosc 34:23-27

Holt RW, Wagner RC (1984) Adhesional obstruction of the colon. Dis Colon Rectum 27:314-315

Hurwitz LM, Gertler SL (1986) Colonoscopic diagnosis of ileocolic intussusception. Gastrointest Endosc 32:217-218

Hutchinson R, Griffiths C (1992) Acute colonic pseudo-obstruction: a pharmacological approach. Ann R Coll Surg Engl 74:364-367

Jevon JP, Daya D Quizilbach AH (1992) Intussusception of the appendix. A report of four cases and review of the literature. Arch Pathol Lab Med 116:960-964

Kukora JS, Dent TL (1977) Colonic decompression of massive non-obsructive cecal dilatation. Arch Surg 112:512-517

Lang EV, Carson L, Gossler A (1998) Gas lock obstruction of the colon: Ogilvie's syndrome revisited. AJR 171:1014-1016

Lee JT, Taylor BM, Singleton BC (1988) Epidural anaesthesia for acute pseudo-obstruction of the colon (Ogilvie's syndrome). Dis Colon Rectum 31:686-691

Lewis TD, Daniel EE, Sarna SK et al (1978) Idiopathic intestinal pseudo-obstruction; report of a case with intraluminal studies of mechanical and electrical activity, and response to drugs. Gastroenterology 74:107-111

Lipton AB, Knauerb CM. (1977) Pseudo-obstruction of the bowel; therapeutic trial of metoclopramide. Am J Dig Dis 22:263-265

Lowman RM, Davis L (1956) An evaluation of cecal size in impending perforation of the cecum. Surg Gynaecol Obstet 103:711-718

Martin FM, Robinson AM Jr, Thompson WR (1988) Thera-peutic colonoscopy in the treatment of colonic pseudo-obstruction. Am Surg 54:519-22

MegibowAJ, Balthazar EJ, Cho KC et al (1991) Bowel Obstruction: evaluation with CT. Radiology 180:313-318

Morton JH, Schwartz SI, Gramiak R (1960) Ileus of the colon. Arch Surg 81:425-434

Nagorney DM, Sarr MG, McIlrath DC (1981) Surgical management of intussusception in the adult. Ann Surg 193: 230-236

Ogilvie H (1948) Large intestine colic due to sympathetic deprivation. A new clinical syndrome. BMJ 2:671-673

Reece EA, Petrie RH (1982) Colonic pseudo-obstruction following obstetric surgery. A review. Diagn Gynaecol Obstet 4:275-280

Reijnen HAM, Joosten HJM, de Boer HHM (1989) Diagnosis and treatment of adult intussusception. Am J Surg 158: 25-28

Richardson JB, Anastopoulos HA (1981) Hernia through the foramen of Winslow. MD State Med J 58:56-59

Sanders GB, Hagan WH, Kinnaird DW (1958) Adult intussusception and carcinoma of the colon. Ann Surg 147:796-803

Shaff MI, Himmelfarb E, Sacks GA et al (1985) The whirl sign: a CT finding in volvulus of the large bowel. J Comput Assist Tomogr 9:410

Spira IA, Rodrigues R, Wolff WI (1976) Pseudo-obstruction of the colon. Am J Gastroenterol 65:397-408

Strodel WE, Nostrant TT, Eckhauser FE et al (1982) Therapeutic and diagnostic colonoscopy in nonobstructive colonic dilatation. Ann Surg 197:416-421

Sullivan MA, Snape WJ, Matarazzo SA et al (1977) Gastrointestinal myoelectrical activity in idiopathic intestinal pseudo-obstruction. N Engl J Med 279:233-238

Umpleby HC, Williamson RCN, Chir M (1984) Survival in acute obstructing colorectal carcinoma. Dis Colon Rectum 27:299-304

Vanek VW, Al-Salti M (1986) Acute pseudo-obstruction of the colon (Ogilvie's syndrome). An analysis of 400 cases. Dis Colon Rectum 29:203-210

Van Gossum A, Bourgeois F, Gay F et al (1992) Operative colonoscopic endoscopy. Acta Gastroenterol Belg 55:314-326

Van Swalenburg CV (1907)Strangulation resulting from distention of hollow viscera. Ann Surg 46:780-786

Waneboh, Mathewson C, Conolly B (1971) Pseudo-obstruction of the colon. Surg Gynecol Obstet 133:44-48

WeissbergDL, Scheible W, Leopold GR (1977) Ultrasonic appearance of adult intussusception. Radiology 124:791-792

Welsh JP (1990) General considerations and mortality. In: Welsh JP (ed) Bowel obstruction. Saunders, Philadelphia, pp 59-95, 241-313 and 575-588

Wilson SR (1992) The gastrointestinal tract. In: Rumack CM, Wilson SR, Charboneau JW (eds) Diagnostic ultrasound. Mosby-Year Book, St Louis, pp 181-207

Wiot JF, Spitz HB (1970) Small bowel intussusception demonstrated by oral barium. Radiology 97:361-366

Wittenberg J (1993) The diagnosis of colonic obstruction on plain abdominal radiographs: Start with the caecum, leave the rectum to last. AJR 161:443-444

Wojtalik RS, Lindenauer SM, Kahn SS (1973) Perforation of the colon associated with adynamic ileus. Am J Surg 125:601-606

27 Barium Radiology of Unusual Colonic Morphology

Damian Tolan and Anthony H. Chapman

CONTENTS

27.1   Introduction   *279*
27.2   The Caecum   *279*
27.2.1 Mucosal and Submucosal Lesions   *279*
27.2.2 Extrinsic Infiltration   *282*
27.2.3 The Coned Caecum   *283*
27.3   The Rectum   *285*
27.3.1 Mucosal and Submucosal Lesions   *285*
27.3.2 Strictures   *287*
27.3.3 The Stretched Rectum   *288*
27.3.4 Anterior Indentation   *288*
27.3.5 Extrinsic Infiltration   *290*
27.4   The Colon   *291*
27.4.1 Mucosal and Submucosal Nodularity   *291*
27.4.2 Pseudodiverticula (Pseudosacculations)   *291*
27.4.3 Extrinsic Infiltration   *292*
27.4.4 Hematogenous Disease Spread   *294*
27.4.5 Mucosal Oedema   *295*
27.4.6 Fistulation   *296*
27.4.7 Diaphragm   *297*
        References   *297*

27.1
Introduction

The purpose of this chapter is to deal with pathology, demonstrated by barium enema, that has not been dealt with in other chapters of this book. We have concentrated on areas where diagnostic difficulties arise, rather than attempt to provide an exhaustive list of colonic diseases and their radiological appearances. A regional approach has been adopted and the various morphologies described so as to help the reader come to a diagnosis when confronted with a difficult case.

D. Tolan, MB, MRCP
St. James's University Hospital, Leeds, LS9 7TF, UK
A. H. Chapman, FRCP,FRCR
Head of Radiology, Leeds Teaching Hospitals Trust, St. James's University Hospital, Leeds, LS9 7TF, UK

27.2
The Caecum

27.2.1
Mucosal and Submucosal Lesions

Appreciation of normal and post-operative appearances is important particularly in respect of caecal imaging. The base of the normal appendix may be prominent but the *appendix stump* is formed by invagination of the appendix remnant after appendicectomy and can produce a smooth, lobular or irregular polypoidal mass at the caecal pole, easily confused with a polyp or a small carcinoma (Fig. 27.1) (Simpkins 1988). The size of the stump usually diminishes from the time of surgery but may remain up to 3 cm in size (Freedman et al. 1956).

Appendiceal pathology may also have a distinct appearance on barium enema. An *appendix abscess* may extrinsically compress the lumen of the caecum, ascending colon or more distant parts of the colon, depending on the position of the appendix (Fig. 27.2). Mucosal oedema produces crenulated mucosal folds in profile and multiple parallel folds enface (Fig. 27.2). In more severe cases the colon can be circumferentially involved in the inflammatory process and sometimes the abscess cavity may fill with barium (Chennels and Simpkins 1981). *A mucocoele* is a rare entity consisting of abnormal accumulation of mucus in the appendiceal lumen. There may be extrinsic compression of the caecum, terminal ileum or sigmoid according to size and position of the mass (Fig. 27.3) (Madwed et al. 1992) and the mucosa of the caecum at the insertion of the appendix may form a series of concentric rings, a vortical fold pattern, or a star pattern (Dackman et al. 1985). The protrusion formed by a mucocele may form the lead point for intussusception (Madwed et al. 1992). A rare subtype of the mucocele is *Myxoglobulosis*, where the accumulation of mucus is in discreet uniform sized globules, giving a characteristic 'frogs eggs' appearance (Dackman et al. 1985); these can be recognised as they may calcify and tend to shift with position.

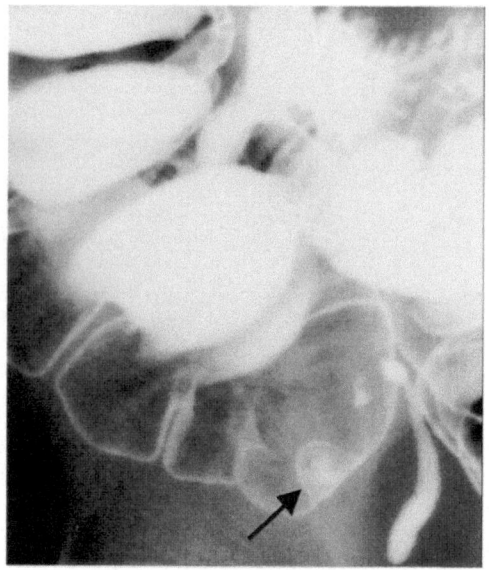

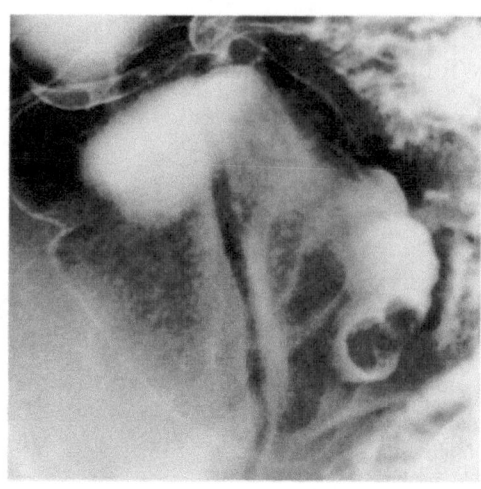

Fig. 27.1a,b. a Prominent base to a normal appendix (*arrow*). b Prominent oedematous appendix stump following appendicectomy

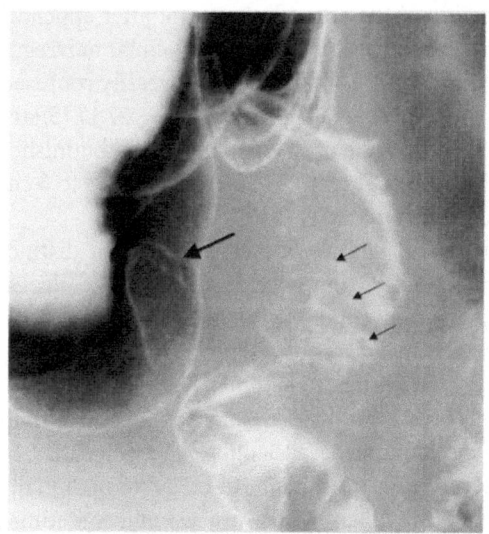

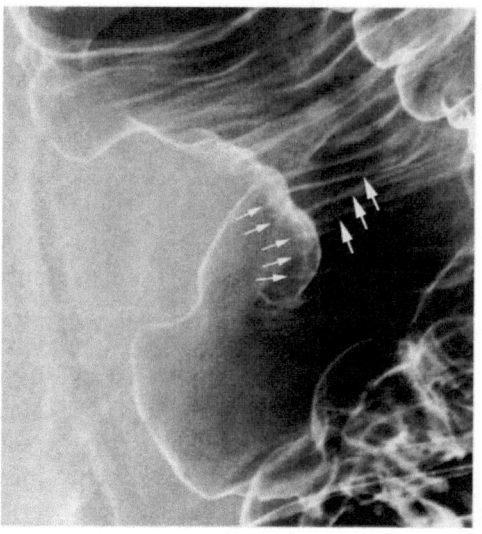

Fig. 27.2a,b. a Extrinsic impression on caecal pole and distal ileum from an appendix abscess. Neck of appendix has filled (*arrow*). Thickened ileal folds (*small arrows*) denote oedema. b Extrinsic compression on the lateral wall of the ascending colon from an abscess at the distal end of the appendix. The colonic mucosa is oedematous, with crenulated folds in profile (*small arrows*) and multiple parallel folds en face (*arrows*). (Courtesy of Dr T Blakeborough)

The *normal ileocaecal valve* demonstrates a range of normal appearances and can be round, ovoid or triangular (Fig. 27.4). The maximum accepted diameter for a normal valve is 4 cm. Asymmetry can be a normal finding (EL-AMIN et al. 2003), but surface irregularity should be regarded with suspicion (Fig. 27.5). A *lipomatous ileocaecal valve*, caused by fatty infiltration, is enlarged with intact surface mucosa (Fig. 27.6). The mucosa may appear lobulated and occasionally the valve may take on a polypoid appearance (BERK et al. 1973) in which case colonoscopic biopsy or CT scan-

ning will be necessary to confirm the benign nature of the condition. Swelling of the valve may also be seen with inflammatory conditions involving the caecum or when the distal ileum is inflamed by Crohn's disease, tuberculosis or *Yersinia enterocolitis*.

Solitary benign ulcer is a rare condition that may affect any part of the colon (Fig. 27.7) but has a predilection for the caecum and ascending colon (FELDMAN et al. 1998). The most common finding is a tapered or sometimes shelf-like stricture, with irregular mucosa and poor distensibility of the affected colonic segment

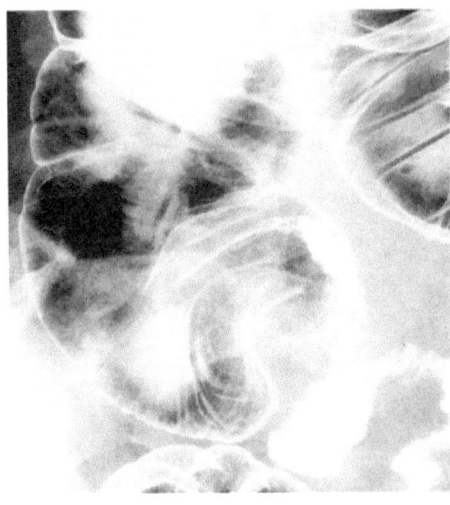

Fig. 27.3. Extrinsic impression on caecal pole and distal ileum but without inflammatory mucosal changes. Mucocele of appendix

(GARDINER and BIRD 1980; BRODLEY et al. 1977). There may be a submucosal mass causing luminal indentation with an identifiable collection of barium indicating the site of the ulcer (Fig. 27.7) (SHALLMAN et al. 1985). Other signs associated with the ulceration include mucosal oedema, spasm and perforation with intra-peritoneal contrast leak (GARDINER and BIRD 1980; SHALLMAN et al. 1985). Differentiation from colonic carcinoma is difficult, but if the diagnosis is confirmed endoscopically some cases can be managed successfully with a conservative approach (SHALLMAN et al. 1985).

Amebomata are discrete segmental lesions characteristically affecting the caecum and ascending colon, caused by infection with *Entamoeba histolytica* and are multiple in around 50% of cases. They appear as annular lesions with irregular mucosa and loss of haustration or as plaque-like or nodular filling defects (Fig. 27.8) (CARDOSO et al. 1977; KOLAWOLE and LEWIS 1974).

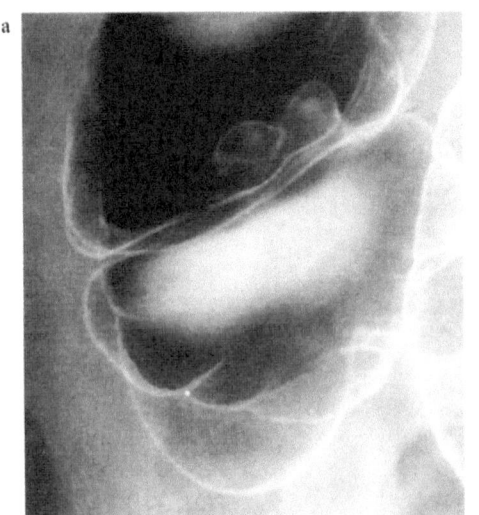

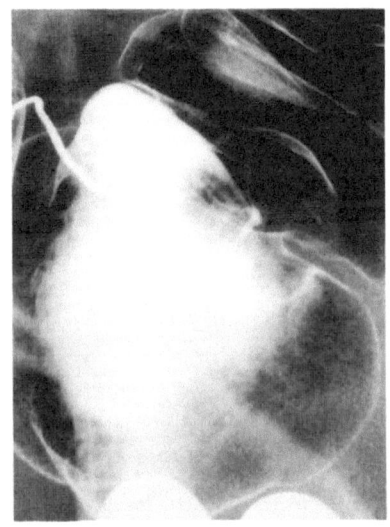

Fig. 27.4a,b. Ileocaecal valve. **a** In profile showing the lips of the valve. **b** En face showing central ostium and radiating folds

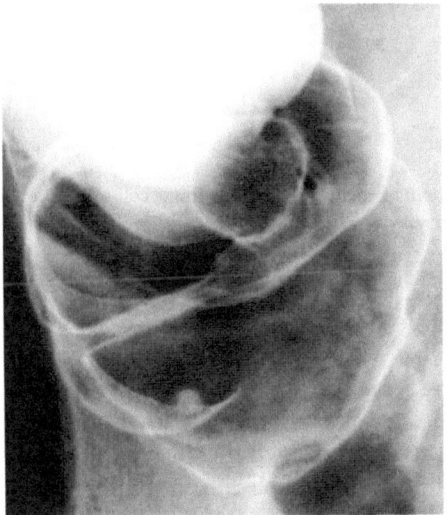

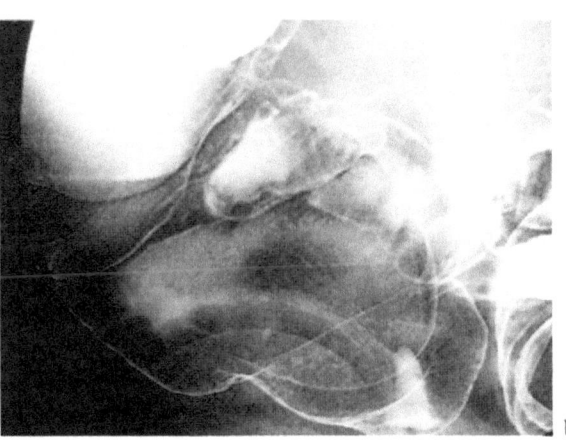

Fig. 27.5a,b. a Lipoma arising from the ileocaecal valve. **b** Carcinoma arising from the ileocaecal valve

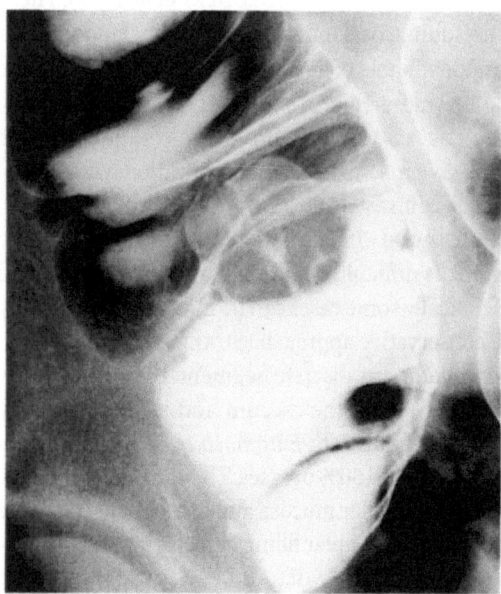

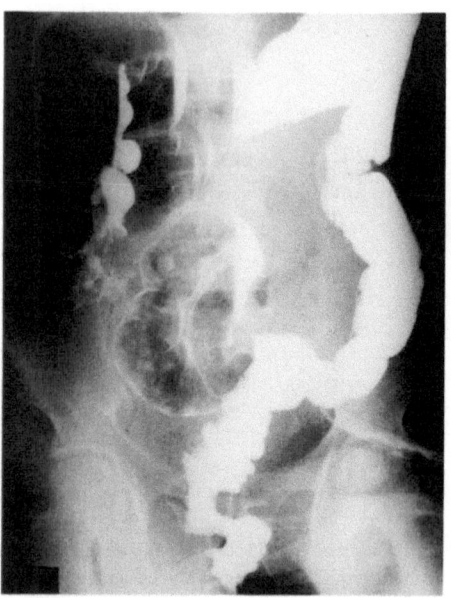

Fig. 27.6. Enlarged (lipomatous) ileocaecal valve caused by fatty infiltration

Fig. 27.8. Thickening of folds, narrowing and spasm in the rectum and sigmoid. Annular narrowed caecum with nodular filling defects. Amoebiasis

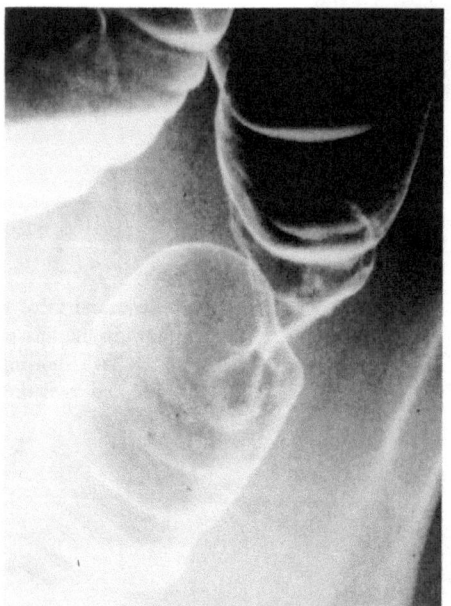
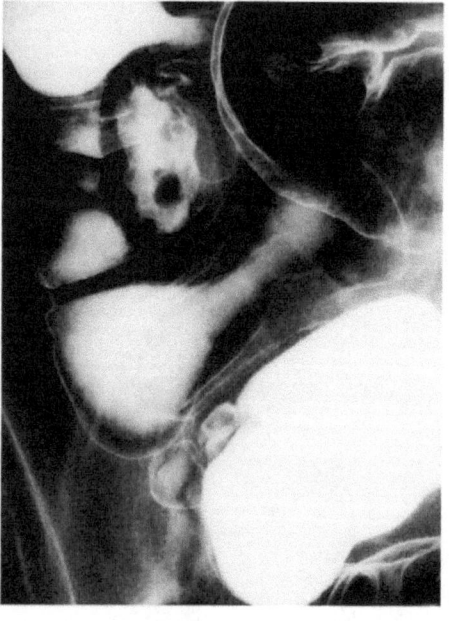

a   b

Fig. 27.7a,b. a Tapered 'benign' appearing stricture as a result of a solitary benign ulcer in the descending colon in a young female taking oral contraceptives **b** Large solitary benign ulcer in ascending colon

27.2.2
Extrinsic Infiltration

Endometriosis typically affects the anterior border of the upper rectum (Fig. 27.9), the inferior (antimesenteric) border of the sigmoid and the caecal pole. A broad based intramural mass develops and as with extrinsic neoplastic invasion, the associated desmoplastic reaction plicates the overlying mucosa to produce a crenulated margin when viewed in profile and multiple parallel folds when viewed en face (Fig. 27.9). Sometimes in the caecum a polypoid mass develops that resembles an appendiceal stump or carcinoid tumour (FAGAN 1974).

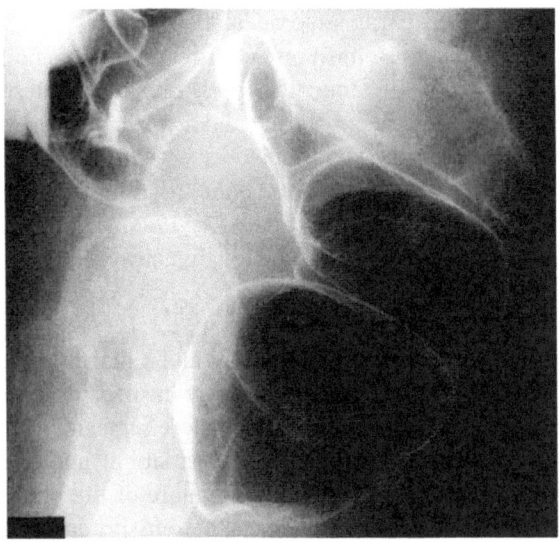
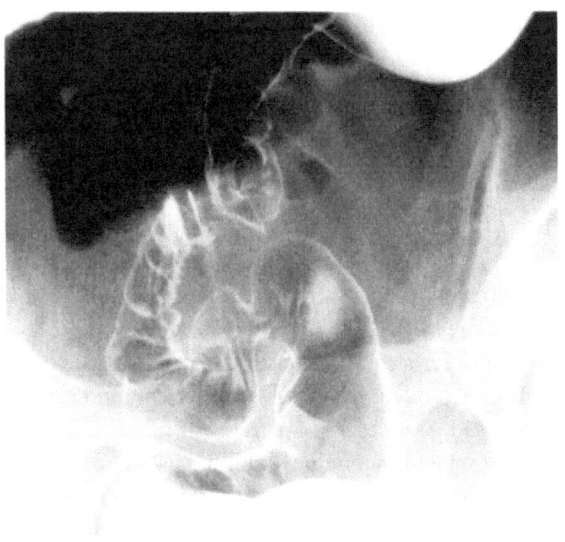

Fig. 27.9a,b. a Endometrioma in the rectovaginal recess impressing on the rectosigmoid junction. The associated desmoplastic reaction plicates the overlying mucosa to produce a crenulated margin and multiple parallel folds. b Endometriosis causing 'periodic' rectal bleeding. The disease is involving the anti-mesenteric border of the sigmoid

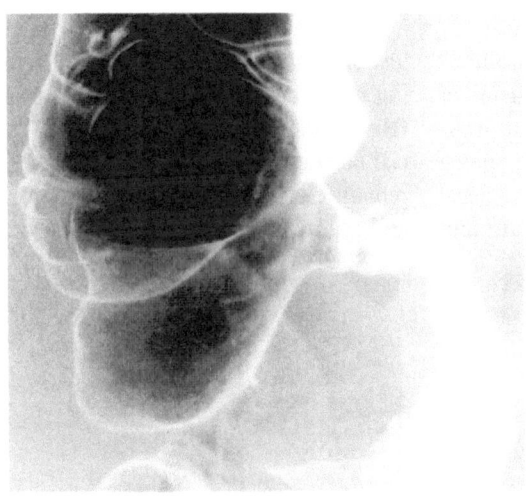
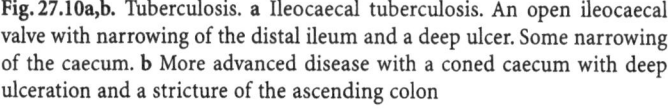
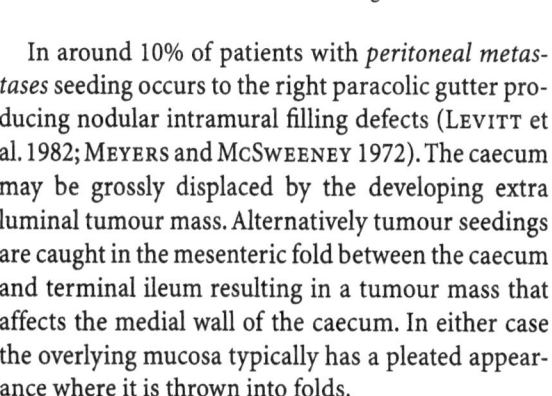
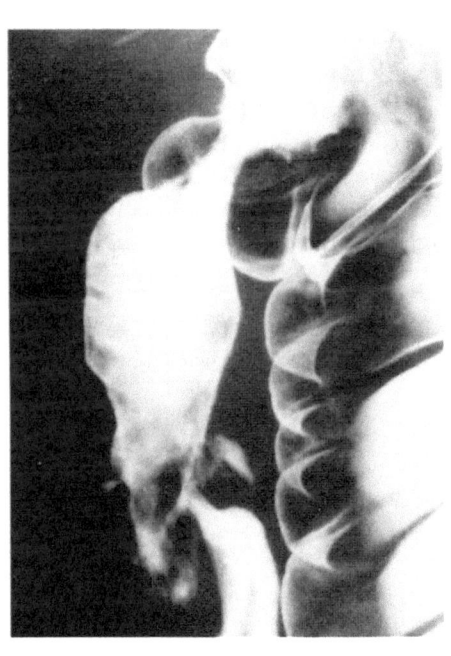

Fig. 27.10a,b. Tuberculosis. a Ileocaecal tuberculosis. An open ileocaecal valve with narrowing of the distal ileum and a deep ulcer. Some narrowing of the caecum. b More advanced disease with a coned caecum with deep ulceration and a stricture of the ascending colon

In around 10% of patients with *peritoneal metastases* seeding occurs to the right paracolic gutter producing nodular intramural filling defects (LEVITT et al. 1982; MEYERS and MCSWEENEY 1972). The caecum may be grossly displaced by the developing extra luminal tumour mass. Alternatively tumour seedings are caught in the mesenteric fold between the caecum and terminal ileum resulting in a tumour mass that affects the medial wall of the caecum. In either case the overlying mucosa typically has a pleated appearance where it is thrown into folds.

27.2.3
The Coned Caecum

Tuberculosis and Crohn's disease: tuberculosis of the colon most commonly affects the ileocaecal region (Fig. 27.10) (VAIDYA and SODHI 1978). Infection stimulates a dense fibrotic reaction causing shortening, narrowing and deformity of the caecum, sometimes producing a widened angle between the caecum and terminal ileum that gives rise to a 'Goose neck' deformity and leads to ileocaecal valve incompetence (Fig. 27.10) (KOLAWOLE and LEWIS 1975; VAIDYA and SODHI 1978). This is most commonly an isolated lesion, but there may be ulceration, fistulation or annular 'carcinoma-like' strictures present in other large bowel segments (KOLAWOLE and LEWIS 1975; WERDELOFF et al. 1973). Crohn's disease can produce identical appearances (Fig. 27.11) as the two diseases may be indistinguishable radiologically (SIMPKINS 1988), although on CT intra-abdominal lymphadenopathy is a much more prominent feature in tuberculosis.

Amoebiasis may produce an acute diffuse colitis but has a tendency to involve the rectum and caecum (Fig. 27.8). Skip lesions are frequent and the mucosal ulceration may manifest as aphthoid ulceration, a granular mucosa or deep ulceration. Amoeboma is a late manifestation of the disease seen after the acute dysentery has resolved. This consists of a mass of granulation tissue surrounding amoebae. In 90% the caecum is involved with concentric narrowing of the lumen and a coned appearance (BALIKIAN et al. 1974; CARDOSO et al. 1977). The terminal ileum is usually normal.

Typhlitis is an infection of the caecum caused by a variety of organisms and developing in immunocompromised patients. Initially there is distension of the caecum leading to circulatory compromise. Ischaemia results in oedema with thumb printing, spasm and sometimes a contracted caecal lumen. Pericaecal inflammation may displace the terminal ileum and

small bowel obstruction can ensue (DEL FAVA and CRONIN 1977; ABRAMSON et al. 1983).

Actinomycosis most often centres on the appendix producing an inflammatory mass that may infiltrate locally to encase the caecum and fistulate to adjacent bowel loops, the kidney, bladder or skin. The infection may spread to adjacent bones resulting in osteomyelitis (FOWLER and SIMPKINS 1983). The ileum may also be involved in the inflammatory mass with mucosal changes and deformity.

Cytomegalovirus produces mucosal granularity and ulceration, fold thickening and rigidity of the colon. The colon may be diffusely involved or there may be involvement of one or more segments with the caecum being the commonest site of infection (BALTHASAR et al. 1985). The calibre of the lumen diminishes as the colon wall thickens producing a coned appearance (TEIXIDOR et al. 1987).

Cathartic abuse, from bisacodyl, senna, phenolphthalein or cascara, produces a proximal colonic abnormality which progresses distally with continued laxative exposure. The caecum is always worst affected and becomes foreshortened and coned with eventual loss of the normal haustral pattern. In turn the ascending colon takes on a tubular appearance (Fig. 27.12) (HEILBRUN and BERNSTEIN 1955). There is superficial ulceration without fibrosis, allowing the colon to remain distensible but the affected colon is irritable and segments involved by prolonged spasm may be

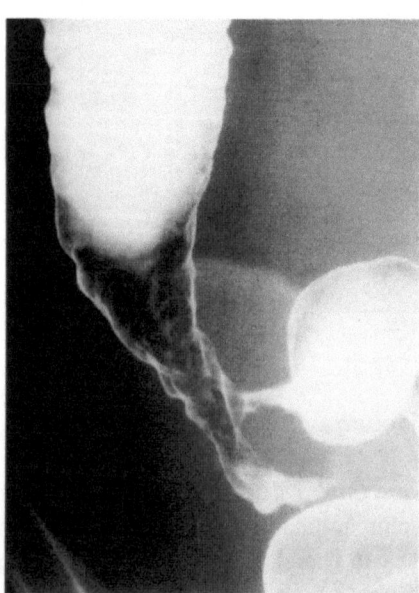

Fig. 27.11. Transmural fibrosis in Crohn's disease producing a coned caecum

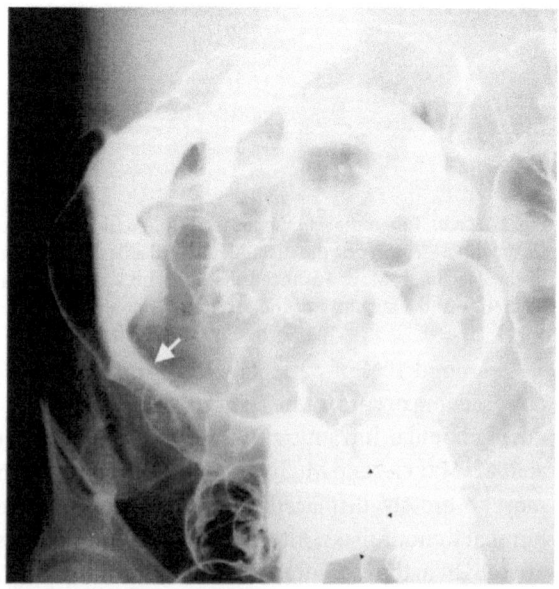

Fig. 27.12. Cathartic abuse. Loss of haustration to right half of colon and prolonged spasm in ascending colon (*arrow*).The patient had become dependant on using senna. Small arrows mark the caecal pole

observed (URSO et al. 1975). Polyps may form and in some cases differentiation from burnt out ulcerative colitis can be difficult, with the only pointer being the relative sparing of the rectosigmoid as compared to more proximal colon (URSO et al. 1975).

27.3
The Rectum

27.3.1
Mucosal and Submucosal Lesions

Haemorrhoids are dilatations of one or more of the three anal vascular cushions and are a common finding at barium enema. They may display a range of appearances (Fig. 27.13) but the one with the highest endoscopic correlation (77%) is that resembling a small cluster of submucosal nodules, like grapes. Other findings include lobulated mucosal folds extending up to 3 cm from the anorectal margin, which is a less sensitive marker (50%) but consistent with benign disease. However, extension beyond 3 cm with thickened folds should raise suspicion of more serious pathology including proctitis and adenocarcinoma (LEVINE et al. 1990). Further recognised findings include a polypoid mass arising from the anorectal margin or a varicoid mass in the distal

rectum (THOENI and VENBRUX 1982). Clearly these appearances may simulate malignant disease and require direct visualisation to clarify the diagnosis.

Hypertrophied anal papilla, colitis cystica profunda, solitary rectal ulcer syndrome and cloacogenic polyp are all believed to be related to chronic mucosal intussusception of the distal rectal mucosa when straining at defecation. This leads to prolapse of mucosa that is damaged as it enters the anal canal and it is because of this that these conditions are sometimes found to coexist.

Hypertrophied anal papillae are lobulated masses arising from the anal verge. They arise from the base of the columns of Morgagni and only occasionally grow large enough to prolapse into the distal rectum. They can be single or multiple and may measure over 2 cm in size (HEIKEN et al. 1984). Characteristic endoscopic appearances confirm this benign condition, but distinction from a rectal polyp is not possible by radiological findings alone (Fig. 27.14). A history of chronic anal irritation or infection may suggest the diagnosis.

Colitis cystica profunda is an uncommon condition caused by submucosal mucus cysts that result from implantation of mucosal cells in the healing phase of ulcerating colonic conditions. As it is often associated with solitary rectal ulcer syndrome it usually affects the rectum but other parts of the colon may be involved (BARNER 1967). The radiological appearances are of multiple intramural filling defects or

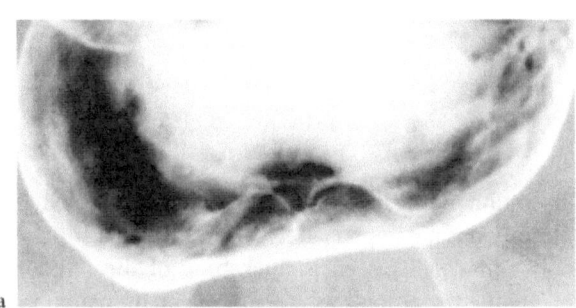

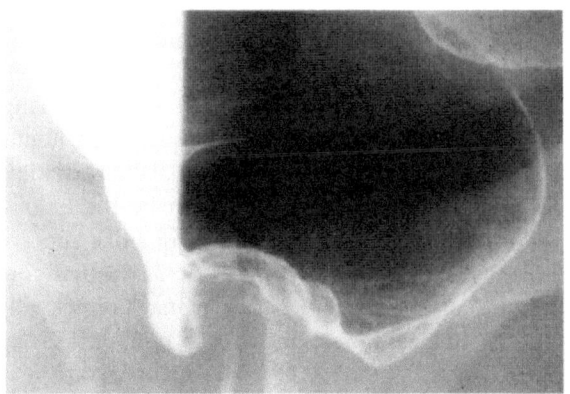

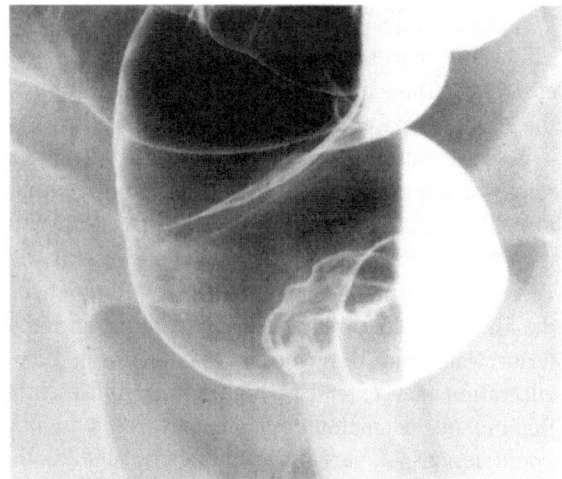

Fig. 27.13a–c. Haemorrhoids. **a** Typical appearance with prominence of the three anal vascular cushions. **b** Enlarged internal haemorrhoid. **c** Polypoid nodular mass arising from the anal margin simulating carcinoma

Fig. 27.14a–d. a Hypertrophied anal papilla prolapsing into the rectum and resembling a rectal polyp. b Nodularity of distal rectal mucosa and nodularity and thickening of middle rectal valve. Colitis cystica profunda and solitary rectal ulcer syndrome. c Pronounced thickening of rectal valve. Superficial ulceration was evident at endoscopy. Solitary rectal ulcer syndrome. d Rectal stricture in a patient with a long history of solitary rectal ulcer syndrome

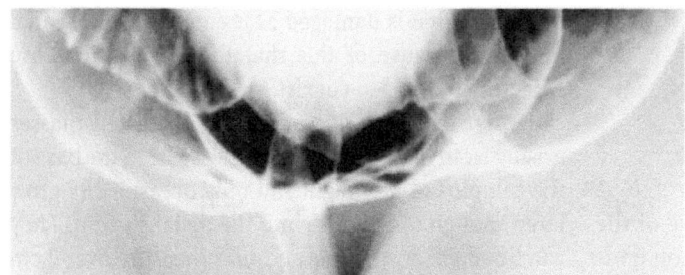
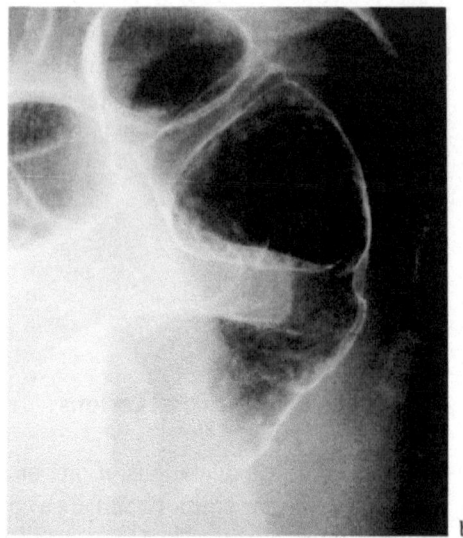

a   b

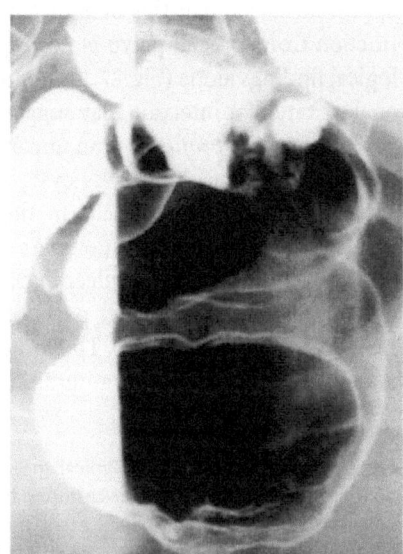
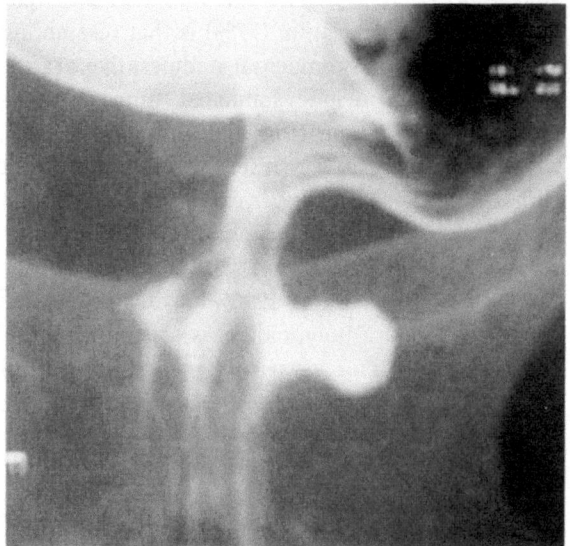

c   d

nodular polypoid masses extending into the rectum (MARSHACK et al. 1980; GRANT and ROLLER 1967; WALKER et al. 1986). Occasionally the only finding is of a thickened mucosal fold pattern (Fig. 27.14) (WALKER et al. 1986). There may also be associated thickening of the presacral space (LEDESMA-MEDINA et al. 1978).

Solitary rectal ulcer syndrome (SRUS) displays a range of appearances on barium enema examination. These have been classified by correlation with the endoscopic appearances (MILLWARD et al. 1985). Ulceration is usually superficial and typically effects the anterior rectal wall, although the lateral and posterior walls may be involved (FECZKO et al. 1980). Ulceration may extend as high as the mid-rectum. Redundant oedematous mucosa may result in polypoid lesions of varying size, often related to the inferior rectal valve (FECZKO et al. 1980). Superficial

ulceration may result in mucosal granularity but often ulceration is not appreciated at barium enema and the only abnormality seen is thickening of the inferior or middle rectal folds as a result of inflammation or involvement by colitis cystica profunda (Fig. 27.14).

Cloacogenic carcinoma is a rare malignancy arising from transitional cells at the anorectal junction. The typical finding is of a plaque-like mass extending along one wall into the distal rectum with or without accompanying superficial ulceration. Differentiation from rectal carcinoma is suggested by the lesions smaller size, distal position and plaque-like appearance (KYAW et al. 1972). However, occasionally atypical cases of cloacogenic carcinoma may present with a polypoid mass mimicking a rectal tumour (GLICKMAN and MARGULIS 1969). The main feature that distinguishes cloacogenic carcinoma from an anal squamous cell tumour is visualisation of the lower border of the mass, although adequate radiographic technique is essential to demonstrate this.

Rectal varices are a rare sequelae of portal hypertension effecting around 3.6% of cases (McCORMACK et al. 1984) at the site of shunting from the superior to inferior and middle hemorrhoidal veins. Typical appearances are of a polypoid mass arising from the lower rectum (LEE 1994), but varices may mimic haemorrhoids or tumour if there is circumferential luminal narrowing (FLEMING and SEAMAN 1968). A history of portal hypertension should suggest the diagnosis and endoscopic ultrasound can offer confirmation and avoid potentially fatal haemorrhage that can follow endoscopic biopsy (LEE 1994).

27.3.2
Strictures

Chronic ulcerative colitis, adenocarcinoma and Crohn's disease (Fig. 27.15) are all causes of rectal stricture. Barium enemas can often be performed in such cases but to minimise trauma and patient discomfort it is necessary to use a soft catheter (such as a 24-F Foley) to introduce the barium.

Solitary rectal ulcer syndrome may produce strictures in the distal and mid rectum, often in association with the other findings related to the condition (Fig. 27.14d). They can be smooth and tapered or shouldered and indistinguishable from carcinoma (MILLWARD et al. 1985; FECZKO et al. 1980). Strictures are caused by progressive fibrosis from chronic inflammation and represent the end stage of the condition.

Lymphogranuloma venereum is a sexually transmitted disease affecting the rectum through direct inoculation with *Chlamydia trachomatis*. The disease process results in mucosal ulceration and inflammation. When chronic this inflammatory process leads to granuloma production, fistula formation to skin or adjacent organs and stricturing which can progress confluently from the anus proximally and may even involve the whole of the sigmoid colon (SIDER et al. 1982; MARSHAK et al. 1980; SIMPKINS 1988). In the context of fistula formation alternative diagnoses such as Crohn's disease and Actinomycosis should be considered.

Gonococcal proctitis often displays no abnormality on barium enema examination. However, the most common abnormalities demonstrated are mucosal oedema with a granular appearance and superficial ulceration, limited to the rectum. Some cases display rectal spasm, or stricture formation with associated widening of the presacral space (SIMPKINS 1988;

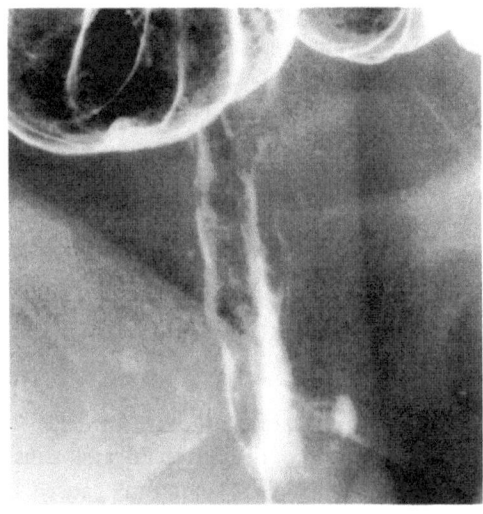

Fig. 27.15. Crohn's disease usually spares the rectum but in this case is causing rectal stricturing, ulceration and a small left-sided ischiorectal abscess

SIDER et al. 1982). However, there are no distinctive radiographic features that reliably distinguish this from other forms of proctitis.

Intracavity and external beam radiotherapy used in the treatment of pelvic malignancies cause, in the early period following treatment, cell death and damage which may manifest as mucosal granularity or thumb printing. An endarteritis may subsequently develop after a latent period of at least a year and produce more chronic changes. In mild cases there is a generalised rectal volume loss, shortening of the rectum and widening of the presacral space (Fig. 27.16). More severe cases can develop spasm, severe mucosal oedema

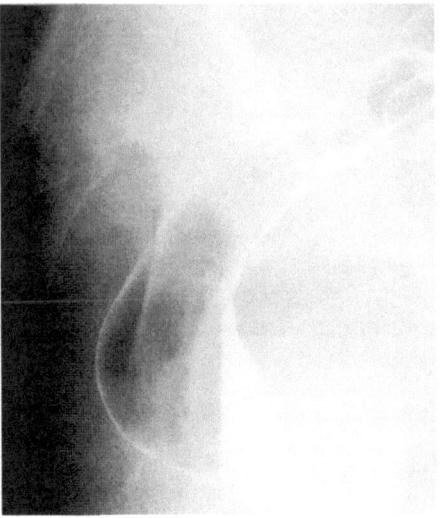

Fig. 27.16. Chronic colitis with narrowing of the radiation rectum, loss of rectal valves and a widened presacral space

and superficial or deep ulceration with associated fistula formation, particularly to bladder and vagina (Fig. 27.17) (MEYER 1981). This may be difficult to differentiate from recurrent disease. Smooth strictures sometimes develop (SIMPKINS 1988), particularly at a level adjacent to the site of intracavity treatment. The sigmoid colon may be affected similarly by virtue of its proximity to the radiation field.

27.3.3
The Stretched Rectum

Pelvic lipomatosis is a rare condition characterised by fibrofatty infiltration of the perirectal fat. It sometimes produces urinary tract symptoms caused by compression of the neck of the bladder or ureteric obstruction but is often asymptomatic (MOSS et al. 1972; FOGG and SMYTH 1968). On plain film there is an increased lucency to the pelvis from the increased fat that is present. Barium enema examination reveals a smooth, symmetrically narrowed rectum with intact mucosa. There is widening of the presacral space from fat deposition and the rectum is elongated, with the sigmoid colon displaced out of the pelvis (Fig. 27.18) (FOGG and SMYTH 1968; MORRETIN and WILSON 1971). Differentiation from other causes

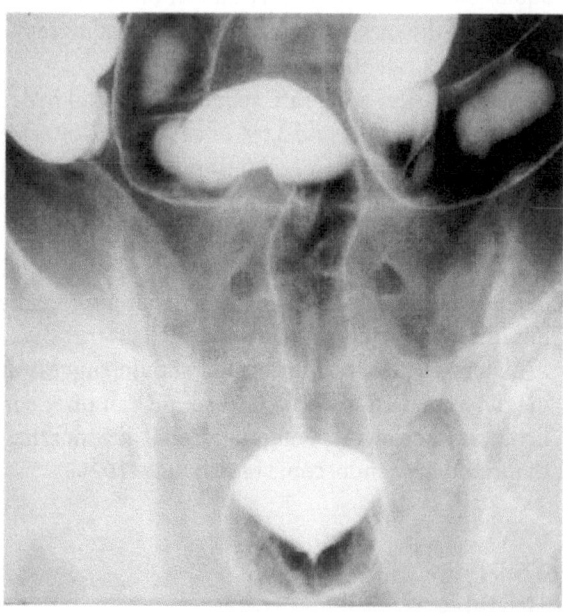

Fig. 27.18. Pelvic lipomatosis. Stretched upper rectum and distal sigmoid

of rectal distortion such as abscess, malignancy or hematoma can be made as the rectum maintains a midline position, the mucosa remains intact and there is concentric luminal narrowing (MORRETIN and WILSON 1971). An accurate radiological diagnosis should preclude further invasive investigations, and CT scanning is most helpful in this regard.

Enlarged internal iliac lymph nodes from lymphoma or metastatic disease spread from within the pelvis can lead to discrete extrinsic rectal indentations and thickening of the presacral space (Fig. 27.19) (SIMPKINS 1988).

Inferior vena cava or deep pelvic vein thrombosis results in collateralisation of pelvic vein tributaries, which can result in widening of the presacral space.

27.3.4
Anterior Indentation

A distended bladder on barium examination should be considered when there is a homogeneous soft tissue density in the pelvis. A lateral rectal film shows a biconcave, tapering compression of the upper rectum and distal sigmoid where the colon is compressed against the sacral promontory (Fig. 27.20). However, frontal views may demonstrate narrowing and an irregular outline to the recto-sigmoid from poor distension and this can simulate colorectal carcinoma (Fig. 27.20) (KLEINHAUS and KAFTORI 1979).

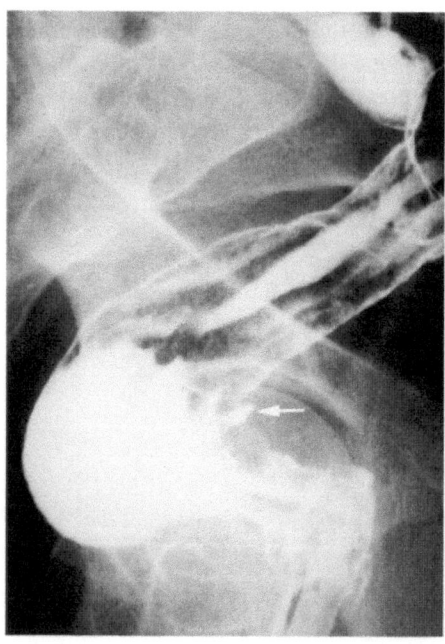

Fig. 27.17. Radiotherapy affecting rectum 9 months after treatment for carcinoma of the cervix. Mucosal oedema producing longitudinal folds in the rectum. Note the deep anterior wall ulcer (*arrow*). The patient subsequently developed a rectovaginal fistula

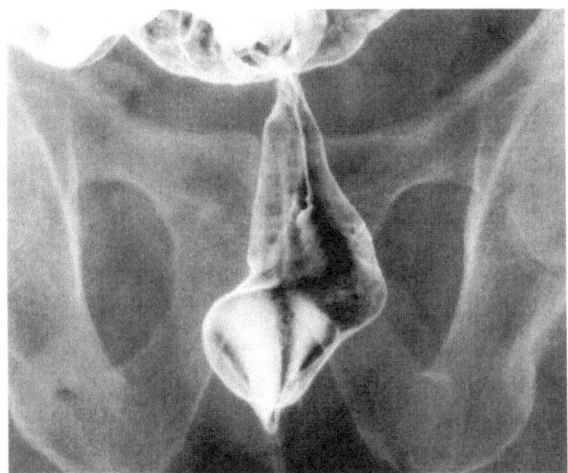

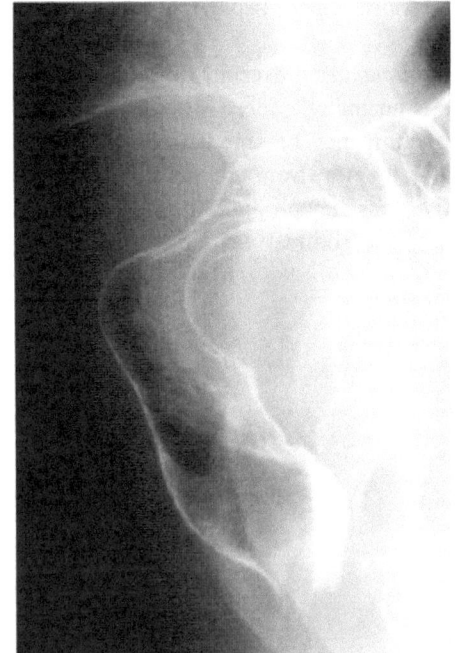

Fig. 27.19a,b. Carcinoma of prostate with pelvic lymphadenopathy. **a** AP view. Extrinsic indentation on rectum and distal sigmoid from enlarged pelvic lymph nodes. **b** Widened presacral space

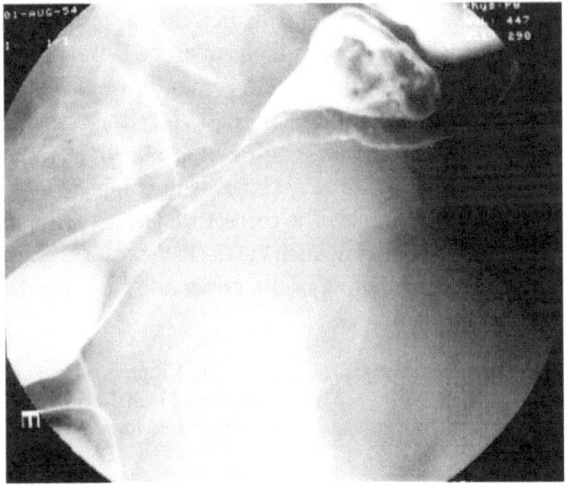

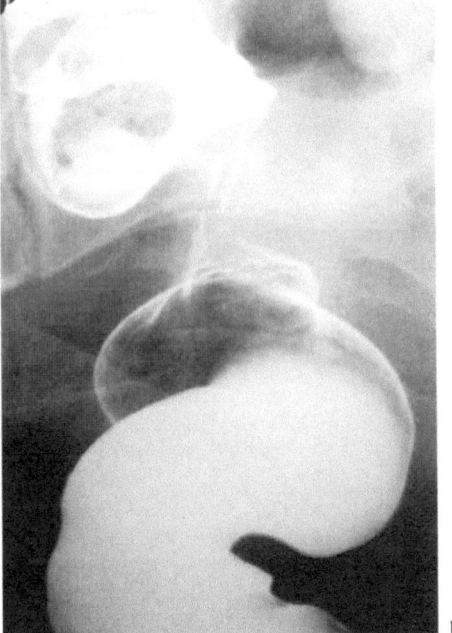

Fig. 27.20a,b. Enlarged bladder. **a** The upper rectum and distal sigmoid are compressed against the sacral promontory. **b** Another case in which chronic bladder enlargement is obstructing the distal sigmoid. Compression of the sigmoid against the sacral promontory is simulating a carcinoma

In a female patient an enlarged *fibroid uterus* can also compress the upper rectum and distal sigmoid (BRYK 1967). With large fundal fibroids, the uterus often indents the inferior surface of the distal sigmoid but again the mucosa remains intact.

Benign prostatic hypertrophy in men can produce a smooth tapering anterior rectal indentation without mucosal changes (GENGLER et al. 1975).

Peritoneal metastases from ovarian, pancreatic, gastric and other cancers may produce masses arising in the pouch of Douglas, which in the early stages may merely indent rather than invade the rectosigmoid. As the disease progresses a desmoplastic reaction ensues resulting in tethering of the bowel, a fixed transverse fold pattern and occasionally mucosal infiltration with nodularity and ulceration

(MARSHAK et al. 1980). *Direct neoplastic infiltration* and endometriosis may display similar features (Fig. 27.21).

Pelvic hematoma usually results from major pelvic trauma and is normally associated with pelvic fractures. The rectum may be smoothly indented and displaced laterally, away from the site of injury.

Perirectal abscess may produce any of a number of features on double contrast examination. Generally there is a soft tissue mass visible next to the rectum which may contain gas or an air fluid level and displace the bowel lumen (Fig. 27.22). There is compression or circumferential narrowing with a variety of mucosal patterns displayed including a crenulated appearance, irregular crumpling of folds or diffusely nodular mucosa. Rarely there may be evidence of intramural gas or direct filling of the abscess cavity via a fistulous track (CHENNELS and SIMPKINS 1981).

27.3.5
Extrinsic Infiltration

Prostatic carcinoma may involve the distal, anterior rectum (Fig. 27.23). However, if the disease extends to the seminal vesicles (RUBESIN et al. 1989) then the upper rectum may initially be involved. This may progress to circumferential involvement of the rectosigmoid junction, in preference to the mid rectum, along with associated thickening of the presacral space (Fig. 27.24). At this stage there is often submucosal involvement with tethering and spiculation of the mucosa. The bowel mucosa may display prominent longitudinal folds or a nodular pattern (RUBESIN et al. 1989). Disease progression results in frank ulceration and an intraluminal mass indistinguishable from rectal carcinoma (GENGLER et al. 1975; FRY et al. 1979). Some cases may progress to complete large bowel obstruction and a correct diagnosis prior to surgery is essential in such cases (FRY et al. 1979). In this instance widening of the presacral space may be

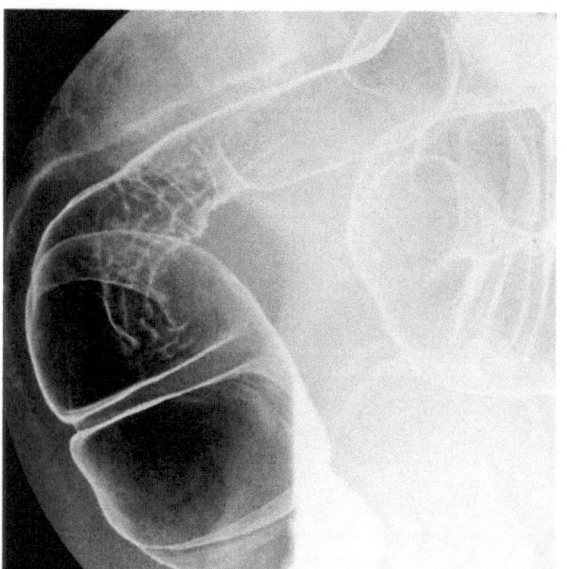

Fig. 27.21. Endometriosis of rectovaginal pouch involving upper rectum. A similar appearance may be produced by peritoneal metastases

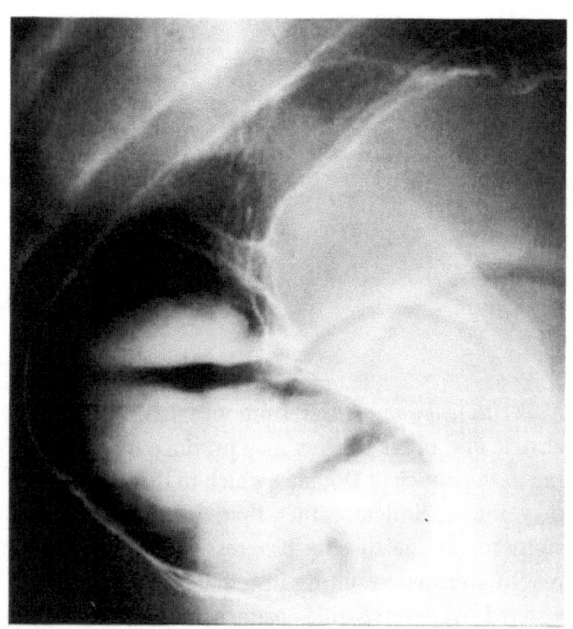

a

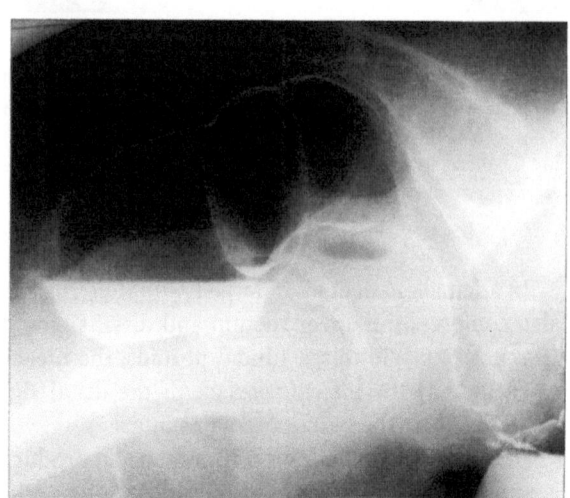

Fig. 27.22a,b. Perirectal abscess. **a** Extrinsic impression extending down to middle rectal valve denotes a mass in the rectovaginal pouch. **b** Decubitus film shows an air-fluid level

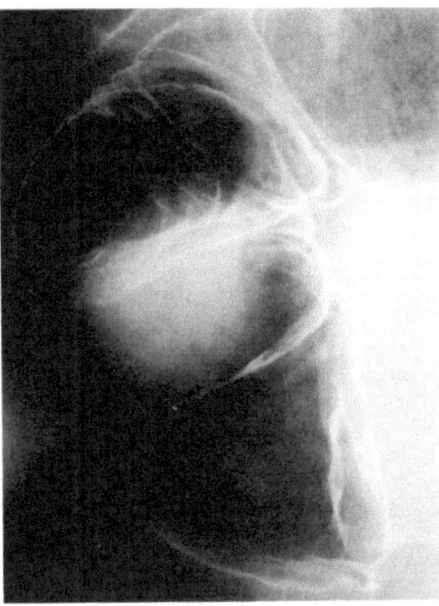

Fig. 27.23. Anterior indentation on distal rectum produced by an enlarged prostate (prostatitis)

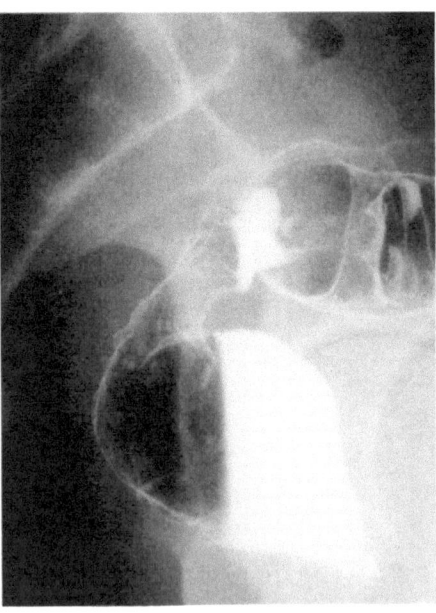

Fig. 27.24. Prostatic carcinoma stricturing upper rectum and distal sigmoid. The presacral space is widened

helpful in differentiating prostatic from rectal primary disease, where widening is seldom present (GENGLER et al. 1975). In a few cases the radiological evidence of disease may be anterior indentation at the rectosigmoid junction by metastatic peritoneal deposits in the pouch of Douglas.

Cervical carcinoma displays a similar range of appearances, from a smooth long stricture of the upper rectum and distal sigmoid with intact mucosa, to widening of the presacral space, to infiltration and ulceration of the bowel mucosa (MARSHAK 1947; MEYER 1981). These changes can be particularly difficult to differentiate from benign disease in the context of radiotherapy (MEYER 1981).

27.4
The Colon

27.4.1
Mucosal and Submucosal Nodularity

Pneumatosis coli manifests as cystic subserosal collections of air predominantly along the mesenteric border of the colon (Fig. 27.25) (KEYTING et al. 1961). The changes are usually centred on the left colon with sparing of the rectum and produce a scalloped appearance with intact overlying mucosa (MARSHAK et al. 1980). Cysts may vary in size from a few millime-

tres to several centimetres and can on rare occasions obstruct the colon (Fig. 27.25b).

Neurofibromatosis produces two main patterns of abnormality on double contrast examination. Large single intramural lesions may be present or there may be more diffuse involvement of the large bowel with multiple submucosal and intramural filling defects in which case the appearance may mimic familial adenomatous polyposis coli, although individual lesions tend to be greater in size (MARSHAK et al. 1980).

27.4.2
Pseudodiverticula (Pseudosacculations)

Pseudodiverticula are formed in both Crohn's disease and ischemic colitis by mucosal projection through weak post inflammatory fibrous tissue or contraction and ulceration of one side of the bowel causing the opposite side to form a redundant sac. The pseudodiverticula may either have a wide or narrow neck and can occur at the site of a previous ulcer (BRUNTON and GUYER 1979). Those related to Crohn's disease may affect any part of the colon (Fig. 27.26), whereas ischemic pseudodiverticula tend to centre on the splenic flexure (Fig. 27.27). When one wall of the colon is involved by the desmoplastic reaction associated with extrinsic neoplastic invasion, the wall shortens and so may also cause redundancy of the mucosa of the opposite wall and the formation of pseudodiverticula.

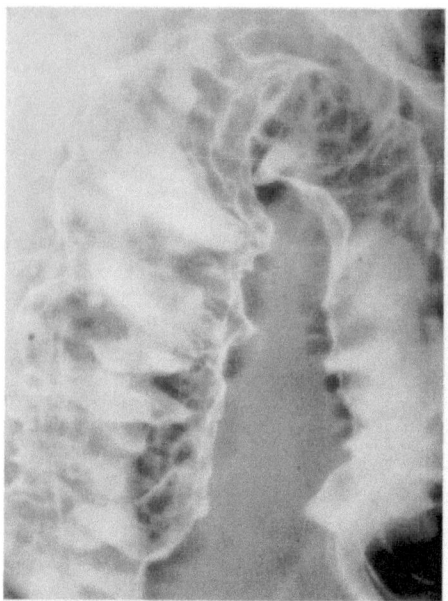
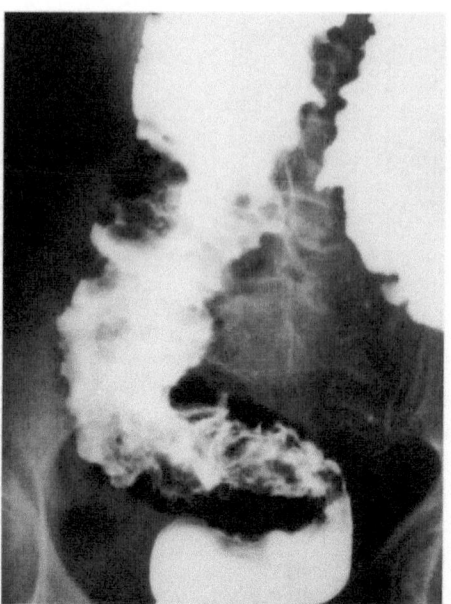

Fig. 27.25a,b. Pneumatosis coli. **a** Mucosal scalloping from submucosal blebs of air. **b** Pronounced pneumatosis causing obstruction to the rectosigmoid junction

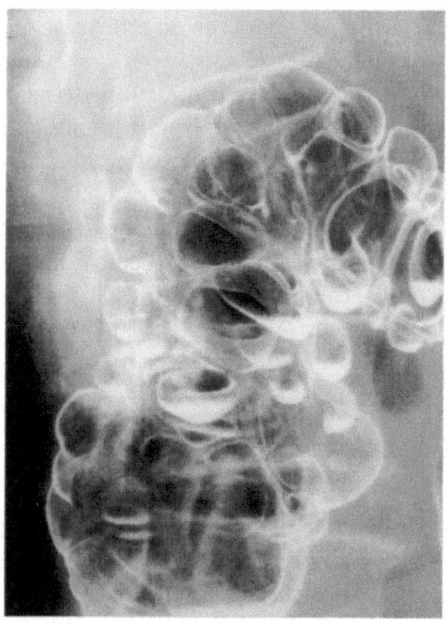

Fig. 27.26. Pseudodiverticula produced by scarring following healing in Crohn's disease

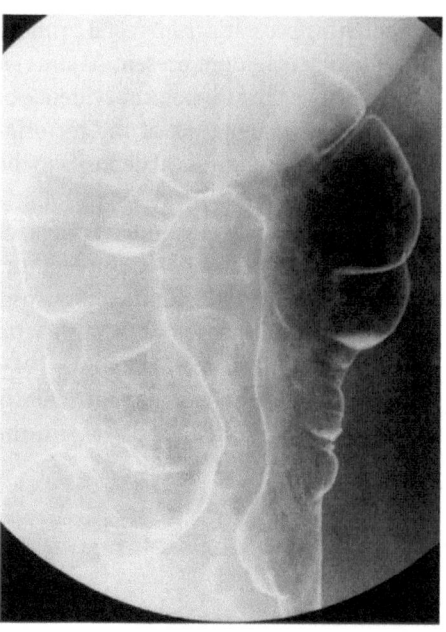

Fig. 27.27. Ischaemic colitis which has healed to produce a stricture with pseudodiverticula

Scleroderma affects the bowel in 50% of patients and in the colon vasculitis damages and weakens the muscularis propria leading to the formation of large wide mouthed pseudodiverticula (KEMP HARPER and JACKSON 1965). There is accompanying loss of the normal haustral pattern, but without the shortening seen in inactive chronic ulcerative colitis (MARTEL et al. 1976).

27.4.3
Extrinsic Infiltration

There are three patterns of spread of disease to involve the bowel. Direct spread may occur from contiguous tumours or from non-contiguous primary tumours when spread takes place along mesenteric reflections. Tumour may also reach the colon by peritoneal seeding or by embolic spread (Fig. 27.28) (MEYERS 1981). Apart from the stomach and pancreas, the ovary, prostate, uterus and kidney are other primary sites of disease that may directly invade the colon.

Renal cell carcinoma typically invades the left colon, causing extrinsic compression of the distal transverse, descending or proximal sigmoid colon. A broad based lobulated mass develops that projects into the lumen from the posterior wall (KHILNANI and WOLF 1960; MEYERS 1981). The tumour may represent extension of the primary disease, or recurrence at the site of a previous nephrectomy.

Ovarian and uterine carcinomas both cause displacement of sigmoid loops out of the pelvis by mass effect and stimulate an intense desmoplastic response, leading to tethering of the adjacent colon and a spiculated appearance to the mucosa (Fig. 27.29) (MEYERS 1981; WIGH and TAPLEY 1958; MARSHAK et al. 1980). Eventually the segment may become circumferentially involved in tumour, producing an annular malignant stricture (MEYERS 1981).

Mesenteric spread along peritoneal reflections produces characteristic patterns of involvement of the colon (Fig. 27.28). The superior border of the transverse colon is invaded when gastric carcinoma spreads along the gastrocolic ligament. This causes an intense inflammatory response, leading to tethering of the superior part of the transverse colon and redundancy of the inferior border, with a pseudodiverticula appearance. The mucosa may take on a cobblestone appearance,

with severe distortion of mucosal folds similar to that seen in Crohn's colitis, and this is the main differential diagnosis. There is abrupt termination of infiltration at the splenic flexure where the gastrocolic ligament ceases but disease may spread proximally to involve the ascending colon (MEYERS 1981).

Pancreatic carcinoma may spread along the transverse mesocolon, to affect the postero-inferior border of the transverse colon. A similar appearance to that seen in gastric cancer results, but with sparing of the superior aspect of the colon, and this again may lead to the formation of pseudodiverticula (MEYERS 1981).

Ovarian tumours may spread up the greater omentum to affect the inferior border of the transverse colon (Fig. 27.29) (RUBESIN and LEVINE 1985).

Metastatic disease may spread intraperitoneally to involve the colon and primary tumours responsible for this include the colon, ovary, stomach and pancreas. Four sites are recognised as common places for deposits to develop, influenced by the flow of peritoneal fluid (MEYERS 1973). The pouch of Douglas is the most frequently involved site in the peritoneal cavity, followed by the distal small bowel mesentery and the adjacent inferio-medial border of the caecum, then the sigmoid colon along its superior aspect and finally the colon along the right paracolic gutter. In each case the desmoplastic reaction produces mucosal tethering and spiculation (MEYERS 1981).

Peritoneal implants of endometriosis that invade through to the submucosa produce an identical radiological appearance to malignant disease (Fig. 27.30) (GORDON et al. 1982). Further recognised patterns

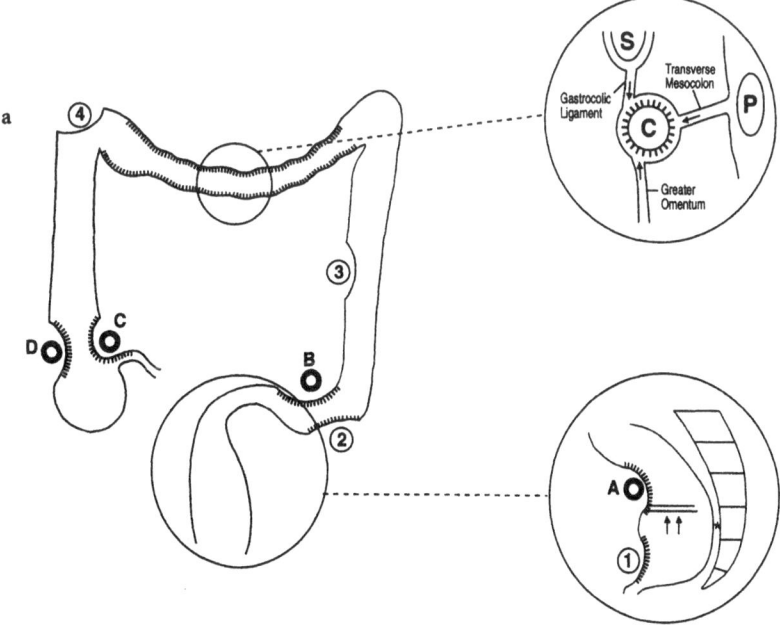
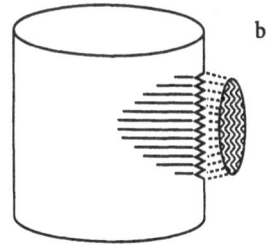

Fig. 27.28a,b. a Line drawing illustrating the common sites of extrinsic neoplastic invasion. Direct invasion: *1*, cervix and prostate; *2*, ovary; *3*, left kidney; *4*, gall bladder. Peritoneal metastases: *A*, pouch of Douglas; *B*, sigmoid mesocolon; *C*, ileocolic junction; *D*, right paracolic gutter; *S*, stomach; *C*, colon; *P*, pancreas **b** Desmoplastic reaction from extrinsic neoplastic invasion tethers wall to form multiple parallel folds which in profile produce a crenulated margin

Fig. 27.29a–c. Ovarian carcinoma. **a** Direct involvement of the inferior border of the sigmoid colon. The desmoplastic reaction has produced a crenulated margin (*arrows*) and multiple parallel lines when viewed en face (*small arrows*) **b** A similar appearance (c) with omental involvement (omental cake) extending to affect the transverse colon

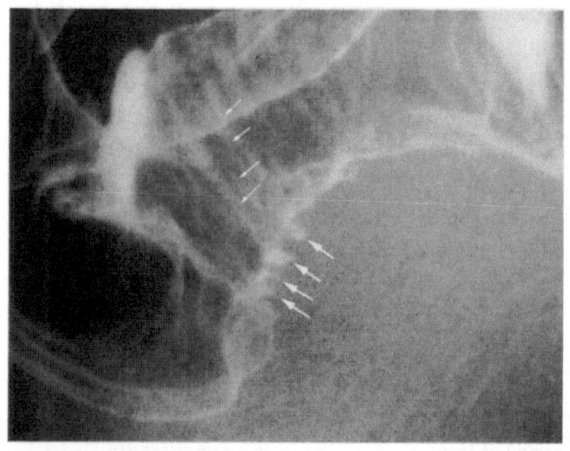

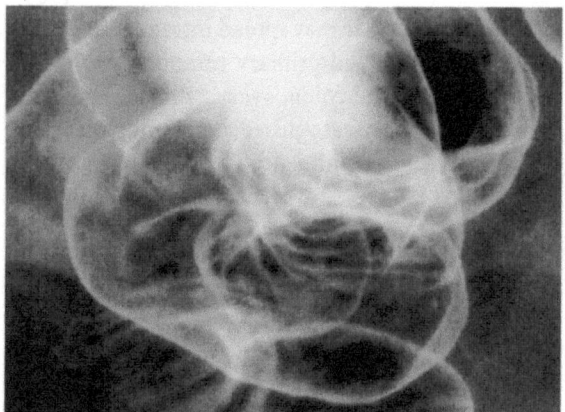

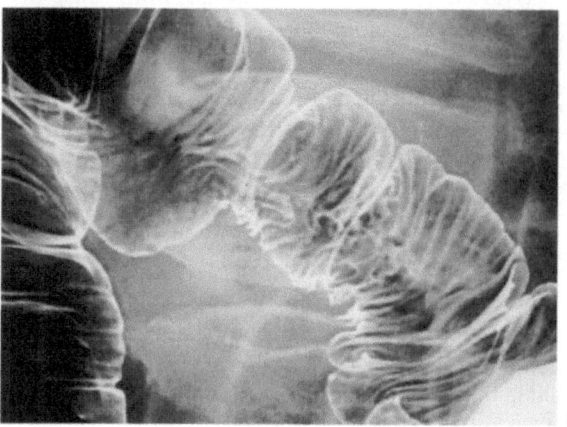

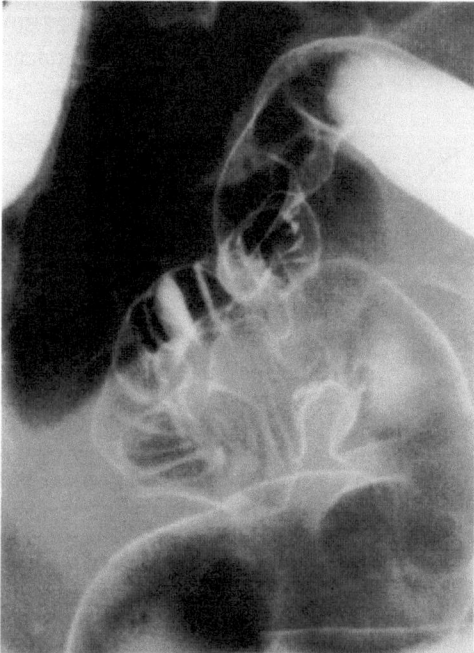

Fig. 27.30. Endometriosis involving the anti-mesenteric border of the sigmoid colon

of disease include polypoid intraluminal masses, short annular strictures, longer tapered strictures (SIEVERT et al. 1989) and intramural lesions.

27.4.4
Hematogenous Disease Spread

Carcinoma of the breast and lung along with melanoma are the commonest tumours to spread to the colon from the blood stream. *Melanoma* classically forms *bulls eye lesions*, which are submucosal masses that develop central ulceration that is large compared to the size of the mass (MEYERS and MCSWEENEY 1972). A *spoke wheel* appearance may be produced by small linear mucosal defects radiating from the ulcer crater (MEYERS and MCSWEENEY 1972). These submucosal deposits may be numerous and normally affect the antimesenteric border of the colon (MEYERS and MCSWEENEY 1972) and may progress to become large polypoid intraluminal masses. *Breast carcinoma* may involve the whole colon or target the right side or rectum. It causes *submucosal infiltration* appearing as nodular mucosa and discrete submucosal masses that may progress to strictures (MEYERS 1981). The mucosa itself is often intact. Barium enema appearances mimic inflammatory bowel disease and differentiation can be difficult without histology. *Lung tumours* produce submucosal deposits that may be small and ulcerating or progress to infiltrate and distort the bowel lumen and mucosal pattern (MEYERS 1981).

Schistosomiasis invades the colonic wall producing mucosal thickening and irregular submucosal nodularity (Fig. 27.31). The disease process may

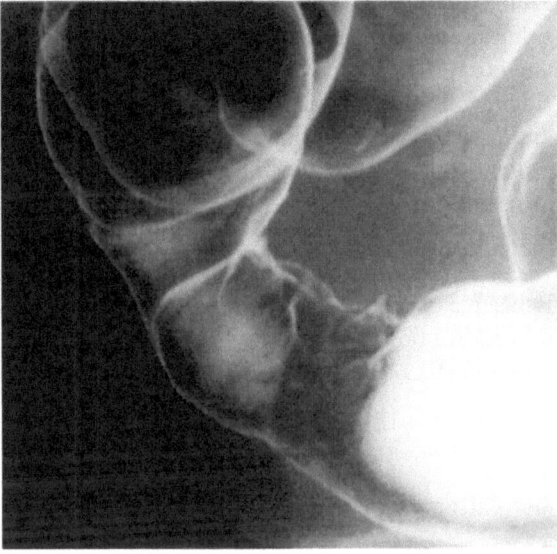

Fig. 27.31. Schistosomiasis producing a plaque of nodular mucosa in the sigmoid colon. (Courtesy of Dr. T. Blakeborough)

progress with time to produce strictures and polyp formation (MEDINA et al. 1965). Laminar colonic wall calcification, similar to that observed in the bladder wall, is not commonly seen (LEHMAN et al. 1971) but if seen differentiate the radiographic appearances from inflammatory bowel disease and malignancy.

27.4.5
Mucosal Oedema

Urticaria of the colon describes a flat mosaic mucosal pattern of polygonal and oval shapes. Initially this was thought to be the manifestation of an allergic response in the large bowel (BERK and MILLMAN 1971). However, this has, been disputed and it is now thought that this appearance is due to the submucosal oedema seen in many conditions including ischaemia, obstruction and ileus (Fig. 27.32) (SEAMAN and CLEMENTS 1982).

Herpes zoster may involve a segment of the colon, not necessarily corresponding to the cutaneous dermatome affected. It produces small polygonal filling defects in the mucosa, with a similar appearance to urticaria (MENUCK et al. 1976). These then progress to produce fine mucosal ulcerations and focal colonic narrowing may ensue in the affected segment (MENUCK et al. 1976). The changes resolve fully after an interval of a few weeks, mirroring the cutaneous manifestations.

Pseudomembranous colitis classically demonstrates a pancolitis with multiple sub-centimetre

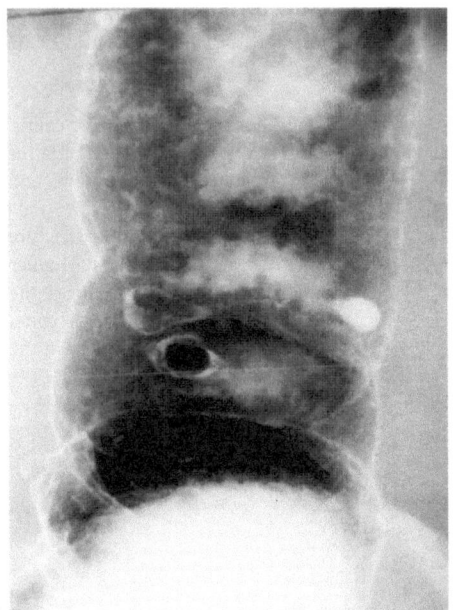

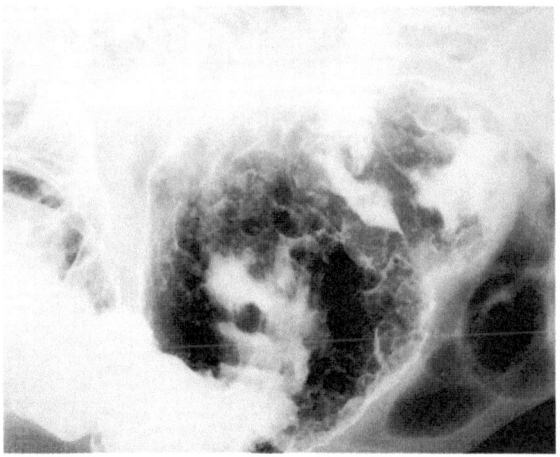

Fig. 27.32a,b. a Nodularity to the mucosa from oedema proximal to an obstructing sigmoid carcinoma. **b** Urticaria-like appearance as a result of ischaemia involving the caecum

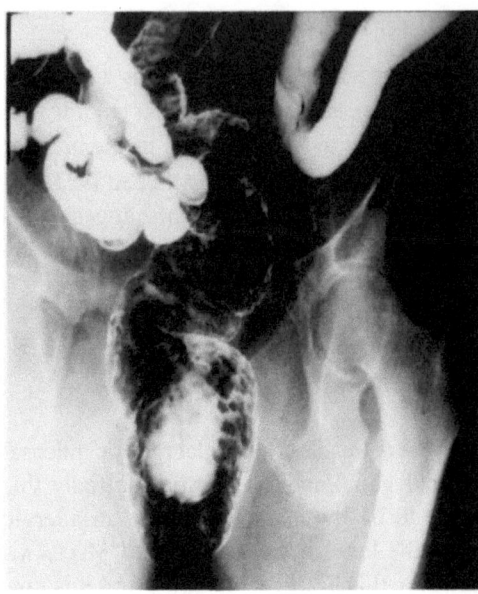

Fig. 27.33. Urticaria-like appearance to the rectum and sigmoid as a result of pseudomembranous colitis

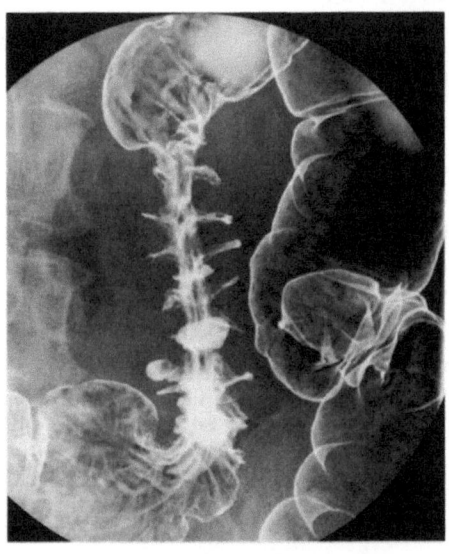

oval or rounded flat mucosal plaques (Fig. 27.33). Thumbprinting and toxic dilatation may be present in severe cases (GARDINER and STEVENSON 1982). Characteristic findings may not be present due to confluence of the pseudomembrane or mucus. The radiographic changes may be confused with pseudopolyp formation in ulcerative colitis, but flat plaques are more suggestive of pseudomembranous colitis.

Ischaemia shows a range of radiographic features according to the severity and time from the onset of symptoms. Thumb printing is characteristic of ischaemia and present in up to 75% of cases, but may be less obvious in double compared with single-contrast examinations (Fig. 27.34) (IIDA et al. 1986). Ulceration is linear and longitudinal, appearing in 60% of cases, and is a relatively acute finding along with transverse ridging of mucosal folds (IIDA et al. 1986). Strictures and pseudodiverticula may form several weeks after presentation (Fig. 27.27) and the association of mucosal ischaemia secondary to obstructing colonic neoplasms makes vigilance for other lesions in the colon essential. A barium enema is not attempted if severe ischaemia is suspected but plain films may show progressive bowel dilatation and loss of haustration (GORE et al. 1979) which may progress to perforation.

27.4.6
Fistulation

Any colonic disease process that involves deep ulceration or the formation of an abscess may fistulate to the skin or an adjacent viscus. In the pelvis fistulation is most often to the bladder or vagina (Fig. 27.35).

Fistulation may be to the colon when there is adjacent sepsis such as an empyema of the gall bladder or

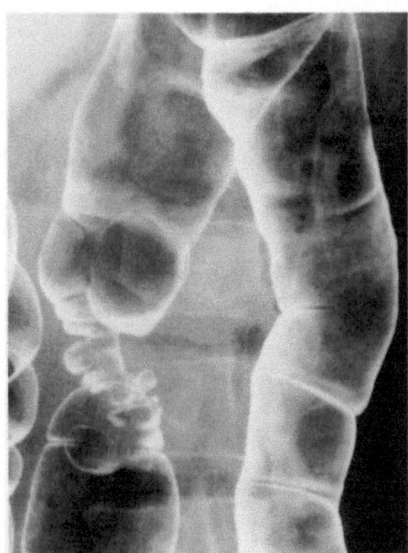

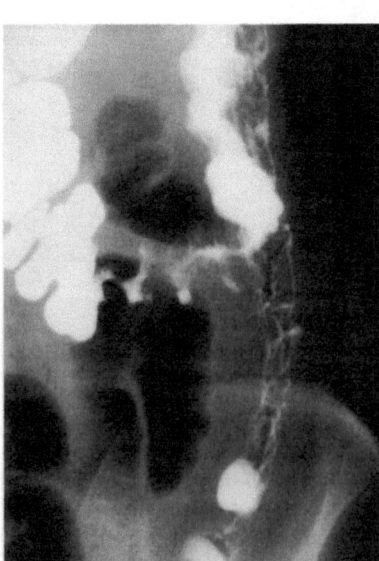

Fig. 27.34a–c. Ischaemic colitis. **a** Thumb printing left side of transverse colon from oedema and haemorrhage into the bowel wall. **b** Healed to leave a short stricture with pseudodiverticula. **c** Another patient with thumb printing of the left side of the transverse colon and longitudinal ulceration in the descending colon

a pyonephrosis. Iatrogenic gastrocolic fistula result from the ingestion of nonsteroidal anti-inflammatory drugs (NSAIDs) or steroids and gastric carcinomas may fistulate to the colon. When the fistulation is from small bowel Crohn's disease involvement of the colon is localised and surgery to the colon can be limited to the site of fistulation (Fig. 27.36).

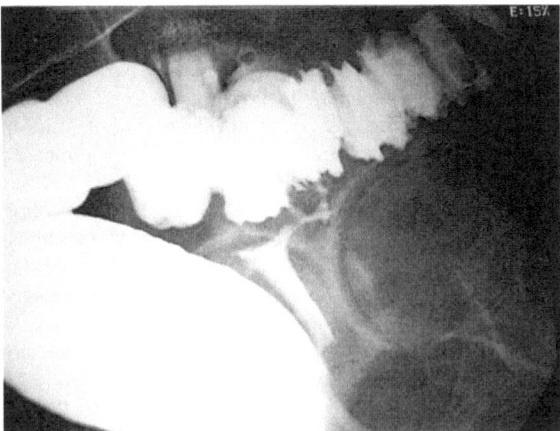

Fig. 27.35. Diverticulitis with fistulation between two diverticula and the vault of the vagina

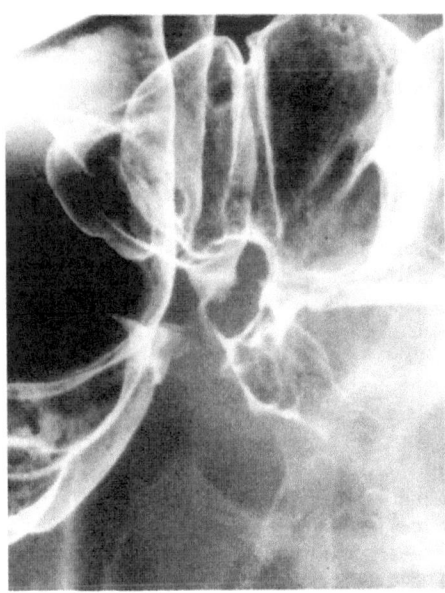

Fig. 27.36. Fistulation to the transverse colon from an adjacent loop of distal ileum (not shown) involved by Crohn's disease. The colonic involvement is localised to the site of fistulation

27.4.7
Diaphragm

Iatrogenic colonic diaphragms consist of submucosal fibrous tissue and are associated with the use of NSAIDs. They are usually asymptomatic and an incidental finding but may cause obstructive symptoms (Fig. 27.37). They appear as short smooth strictures in the colon with intact mucosa (FELLOWS et al. 1992; NICHOLSON and BENNETT 1995). There may be associated diaphragms in the proximal small bowel (FELLOWS et al. 1992).

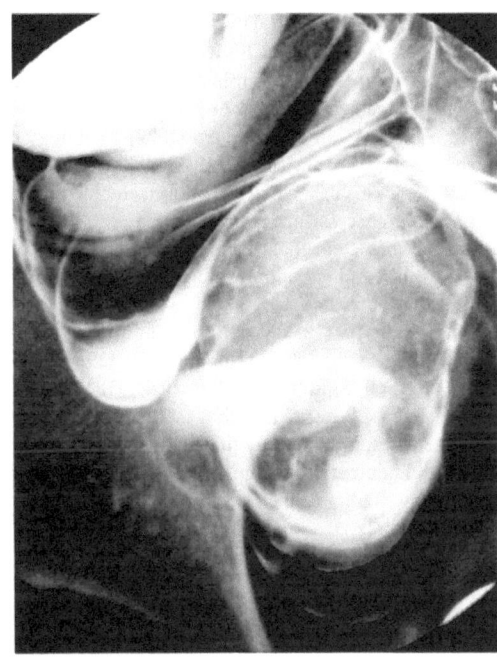

Fig. 27.37. Caecal diaphragm with a caecal faecalith. A fibrotic diaphragm was present, caused by excessive intake of the nonsteroidal anti-inflammatory drug ibuprofen

To be differentiated from a diaphragm is a congenital pericolic peritoneal band of fibrous tissue that is usually an incidental surgical finding but can rarely lead to colonic obstruction (MARSHAK et al. 1980).

References

Abramson SJ, Berdon WE, Baker DH (1983) Childhood typhlitis: its increasing association with Acute Myelogenous Leukemia. Radiology 146:61-64

Balikian JP, Uthman SM, Khouri NF (1974) Intestinal amebiasis: a roentgen analysis of 19 cases including 2 case reports. AJR 122:245-256

Balthazar EJ, Megibow AJ, Opulencia JF et al (1985) Cytomegalovirus colitis in AIDS: radiographic findings in 11 patients. Radiology 155:585-589

Barner JL (1967) Colitis Cystica Profunda. Radiology 89:435-437

Berk RN, Millman SJ (1971) Urticaria of the colon. Radiology 99:539-540

Berk RN, Davis GB, Cholhassey EB (1973) Lipomatosis of the ileocaecal valve. AJR 119:323-328

Brodley PA, Hill RP, Barron S (1977) Benign ulceration of the cecum. Radiology 122:323-327

Brunton FJ, Guyer PB (1979) Diverticulum formation in Crohn's disease of the colon. Clin Radiol 20:39-44

Bryk D (1967) Barium enema examination in the evaluation of large pelvic masses. AJR 101:970-977

Cardoso JM, Kimura K, Stoopen M et al (1977) Radiology of invasive amoebiasis of the colon. AJR 128:935-941

Chennels PM, Simpkins KC (1981) The barium enema diagnosis of paracolic abcess. Clin Radiol 32:73-84

Dackman AH, Lichtenstein JE, Friedman AC (1985) Mucocele of the appendix and pseudomyxoma peritonei. AJR 144:923-929

Del Fava RL, Cronin TG (1977) Typhlitis complicating leukemia in an adult: barium enema findings. AJR 129:347-348

El-Amin LC, Levine MS, Rubensin SE et al (2003) Ileocaecal valve: spectrum of normal findings at double-contrast barium enema examination. Radiology 227:52-58

Fagan CJ (1974) Endometriosis: clinical and roentgenographic manifestations. Radiol Clin North Am 12:109-125

Feczko PJ, O'Connell DJ, Riddell RH et al (1980) Solitary rectal ulcer syndrome: radiologic manifestations. AJR 135:499-506

Feldman M, Scarschmidt BF, Sleisenger MH (eds) (1998) Sleisenger and Fordtran's gastrointestinal and liver disease, pathology/diagnosis/management, 6th edn. Saunders, Philadelphia

Fellows IW, Clarke JMF, Roberts PF (1992) Non-steroidal anti-inflammatory drug-induced jejunal and colonic diaphragm disease: a report of two cases. Gut 33:1424-1426

Fleming RJ, Seaman WB (1968) Roentgenographic demonstration of unusual extra-oesophageal varices. AJR 103:281-290

Fogg LB, Smyth WJ (1968) Pelvic lipomatosis: a condition simulating pelvic neoplasm. Radiology 90:558-564

Fowler RC, Simpkins KC (1983) Abdominal actinomycosis: a report of three cases. Clin Radiol 34:301-307

Freedman E, Radwin MH, Linsman JF (1956) Roentgen simulation of polypoid neoplasms by invaginated appendiceal stumps. AJR 75:380-385

Fry DE, Amin M, Harbrecht PJ (1979) Rectal obstruction secondary to carcinoma of the prostate. Ann Surg 189:488-492

Gardiner GA, Bird CR (1980) Nonspecific ulcers of the colon resembling annular carcinoma. Radiology 137:331-334

Gardiner R, Stevenson GW (1982) The colitides. Radiol Clin North Am 20:797-817

Gengler L, Baer J, Finby N (1975) Rectal and Sigmoid involvement secondary to carcinoma of the prostate. Radiology 125:911-917

Glickman MG, Margulis AJR (1969) Cloacogenic carcinoma. AJR 107:175-180

Gordon RL, Evers K, Kressel HY et al (1982) Double-contrast enema in pelvic endometriosis. AJR 138:549-552

Gore RM, Calenoff L, Rogers LF (1979) Roentgenographic manifestations of ischemic colitis. JAMA 241:1171-1173

Grant KB, Roller GJ (1967) Colitis cystica profunda. Radiology 89:110-111

Heiken JP, Zuckerman GR, Balfe DM (1984) The hypertrophied anal papilla: recognition on air-contrast barium enema examinations. Radiology 151:315-318

Heilbrun N, Bernstein C (1955) Roentgen abnormalities of the large and small intestine associated with prolonged cathartic ingestion. Radiology 65:549-556

Iida M, Matsui T, Fuchigami T et al. (1986) Ischemic colitis: serial changes in double-contrast barium enema examination. Radiology 159:337-341

Kemp Harper RA, Jackson DC (1965) Progressive systemic sclerosis. Br J Radiol 38:825-834

Keyting WS, McCarver RR, Kovarik JL et al (1961) Pneumatosis intestinalis: a new concept. Radiology 76:733-741

Khilnani MT, Wolf BS (1960) Late involvement of the alimentary tract by carcinoma of the kidney. Am J Dig Dis 5:529-540

Kleinhaus U, Kaftori J (1979) Rectosigmoid pseudostenosis due to urinary retention. Radiology 127:645-647

Kolawole TM, Lewis EA (1974) Radiologic observations on intestinal amebiasis. AJR 122:257-265

Kolawole TM, Lewis EA (1975) A radiologic study of tuberculosis of the abdomen (gastrointestinal tract). AJR 123:348-358

Kyaw MM, Gallagher T, Haines JO (1972) Cloacogenic carcinoma of the anorectal junction. AJR 115:384-391

Ledesma-Medina J, Reid BS, Girdany BR (1978) Colitis cystica profunda. AJR 131:529-530

Lee SH (1994) Case report: transrectal ultrasound in the diagnosis of Ano-rectal varices. Clin Radiol 49:69-70

Lehman JS Jr, Farid Z, Bassily S et al (1971) Colonic calcification and polyposis in schistosomiasis. Report of a case. Radiology 98:379-380

Levine MS, Kam LW, Rubensin SE et al (1990) Internal haemorrhoids: diagnosis with double-contrast barium enema examinations. Radiology 177:141-144

Levitt RG, Koehler RE, Sagel SS et al (1982) Metastatic disease of the mesentery and omentum. Radiol Clin North Am 20:501-510

Madwed D, Mindelzun R, Jeffrey RB Jr (1992) Mucocele of the appendix: imaging findings. AJR 159:69-72

Marshak RH (1947) Extrinsic lesions affecting the rectosigmoid. AJR 58:439-450

Marshak RH, Lindner AE, Maklansky D (1980) Radiology of the colon. Saunders, Philadelphia

Martel W, Chang SF, Abell MR (1976) Loss of colonic haustration in progressive systemic sclerosis. AJR 126:704-713

McCormack TT, Bailey HR, Simms JM et al (1984) Rectal varices are not piles. Br J Surg 71:163

Medina JT, Seaman WB, Guzman-Acosta C (1965) The roentgen appearance of schistosomiasis Mansoni involving the colon. Diaz-Bonnet RB. Radiology 85:682-688

Menuck LS, Brahme F, Amberg J et al (1976) Colonic changes of herpes zoster. Am J Roentgenol 127:273-276

Meyer JE (1981) Radiography of the distal colon and rectum after irradiation of carcinoma of the cervix. AJR 136:691-699

Meyers MA (1973) Distribution of intra-abdominal malignant seeding: dependency on dynamics of flow of ascitic fluid. AJR 119:198-206

Meyers MA (1981) Intraperitoneal spread of malignancies and its effect on the bowel. Clin Radiol 32:129-146

Meyers MA, McSweeney J (1972) Secondary neoplasms of the bowel. Radiology 105:1-11

Millward SF, Bayjoo P, Dixon MF et al (1985) The barium enema appearances in solitary rectal ulcer syndrome. Clin Radiol 36:185-189

Morretin LB, Wilson M (1971) Pelvic lipomatosis. AJR 113: 181-184

Moss AA, Clark RE, Goldberg HI et al (1972) Pelvic lipomatosis: a roentgenographic diagnosis. AJR 115:411-419

Nicholson AA, Bennett JR (1995) Case report: radiological appearance of colonic stricture associated with the use of nonsteroidal ant-inflammatory drugs. Clin Radiol 50:268-269

Rubesin SE, Levine MS (1985) Omental cakes: colonic involvement by omental metastases. Radiology 154:593-596

Rubesin SE, Levine MS, Bezzi M et al (1989) Rectal involvement by prostatic carcinoma: Barium enema findings. AJR 152:53-57

Seaman WB, Clements JL (1982) Urticaria of the colon: a nonspecific pattern of mucosal oedema. AJR 138:545-547

Shallman RW, Kuehner M, Williams GH et al (1985) Benign caecal ulcers. Dis Colon Rectum 28:732-737

Sider L, Mintzer RA, Mendelson EB et al (1982) Radiographic findings of infectious proctitis in homosexual men. AJR 139:667-671

Sievert W, Sellin JH, Stringer AC (1989) Pelvic endometriosis simulating colonic malignant neoplasm. Arch Intern Med 149:935-938

Simpkins KC (1988) A textbook of radiological diagnosis: the alimentary tract, the hollow organs and salivary glands, 5th edn. Lewis, London

Teixidor HS, Honig CL, Norsdoph E et al (1987) Cytomegalovirus infection of the alimentary canal: radiologic findings with pathologic correlation. Radiology 163: 317-323

Thoeni RF, Venbrux AC (1982) Work in progress. The anal canal: distinction of internal haemorrhoids from small cancers by double-contrast barium enema examination. Radiology 145:17-19

Urso FP, Urso MJ, Lee CH (1975) The cathartic colon: pathological findings and radiological/pathological correlation. Radiology 118:557-559

Vaidya MG, Sodhi JS (1978) Gastrointestinal tract tuberculosis: a study of 102 cases including 55 hemicolectomies. Clin Radiol 29:189-195

Walker JP, Wiener I, Rowe EB (1986) Colitis cystica profunda. South Med J 79:1167-1170

Werdeloff L, Novis BH, Bank S et al (1973) The radiology of tuberculosis of the gastrointestinal tract. Br J Radiol 46: 329-336

Wigh R, Tapley N duV (1958) Metastatic lesions to the large intestine. Radiology 70:222-229

28 New Developments in Colonoscopy

Brian P. Saunders

CONTENTS

28.1   Introduction *301*
28.2   Historical Perspective *301*
28.3   Colonoscopy vs. Barium Enema/
        Virtual Colonoscopy *302*
28.4   New Technologies in Colonoscopy:
        Improving Insertion *302*
28.4.1 Magnetic Endoscope Imaging *302*
28.4.2 Variable-Stiffness Colonoscopes *306*
28.5   Improved Lesion Detection *307*
28.5.1 Video Systems *307*
28.5.2 Mucosal Dye *308*
28.5.3 In Vivo Diagnosis *309*
28.6   Future Possibilities *310*
28.7   Conclusions *312*
        References *312*

28.1
Introduction

Colonoscopy has revolutionised our understanding and management of colorectal disease by providing direct, in vivo, colour images of the mucosal surface. In expert hands the procedure can be performed with little or no sedation and can inspect the entire colorectal mucosa with up to 50 cm of the terminal ileum in 95%–99% of patients. Most importantly it also provides biopsy diagnosis and access for direct therapy, which often precludes the need for surgery. The all-round capability of the procedure makes it the optimal investigation for suspected colonic neoplasia, colonic bleeding, suspected inflammatory mucosal disease and for surveillance of those at increased risk for colorectal cancer. Radiologists should be aware that conventional colonoscopy is constantly developing as a technique. Recent developments have seen better instruments that are easier to pass to the caecum and better visualisation and identification of mucosal abnormalities thus increasing diagnostic accuracy. Colonoscopy provides internal access for therapy and is enabling a new form of minimally invasive surgery with endoscopic resection of very large polyps, early cancers, treatment of colonic stenoses with dilatation and stenting and mucosal ablation to treat bleeding lesions.

28.2
Historical Perspective

Total fibre-optic colonoscopy was first described in 1969 (Wolff and Shinya 1971). In the early 1970s instruments were short (90 cm in length), relatively inflexible with stiff shafts and had restricted bending sections. This resulted in only a limited application of the technique and not infrequent complications. By the mid 1970s diathermy polypectomy was developed expanding the indications for colonoscopy (Wolff and Shinya 1973). In the early days, colonoscopy was performed in the X-ray suite with the benefit of fluoroscopy to identify colonoscope looping and the anatomical position of the colonoscope tip. However by the 1980s endoscopists had moved away from the X-ray department to dedicated endoscopy suites. Instruments were now longer (160 cm) and had greater shaft flexibility. Insertion to the caecum or beyond could be achieved reliably in well over 90% of patients. Rapid expansion in colonoscopy services has occurred throughout the late 1980s and 1990s coinciding with the introduction of video colonoscopes in 1985. Colonoscopy workload has increased by nearly 100% in the UK in the last 6 years and looks set to increase further, particularly if colorectal cancer screening is introduced. The success of the procedure has brought problems in that there are insufficient numbers of "expert" colonoscopists. The British Society of Gastroenterology recently performed an extensive audit of colonoscopic practice and found completion rates across the board to be as low as 57%–77% (O. Epstein, personal communication). Procedural facilities and training in colonoscopy were also inadequate, highlighting the need for investment in these key areas.

B. P. Saunders, MD, FRCP
Senior Lecturer in Endoscopy, St. Mark's Hospital, Harrow, Middlesex, London, HA1 3UJ, UK

28.3
Colonoscopy vs. Barium Enema/Virtual Colonoscopy

Radiologists and endoscopists have long argued over the relative merits of barium enema and colonoscopy. Recently the debate has focused on the new technology of virtual colonoscopy. Any direct comparison of the techniques will greatly depend upon the experience and skill of the radiologist and endoscopist performing the procedures, but all things being equal a direct, real colour image with biopsy and therapeutic capability would seem intuitively to be diagnostically superior to any indirect imaging technique for mucosal disease (there speaks the endoscopist!). Several studies have confirmed the diagnostic superiority of colonoscopy to barium enema in polyp and cancer detection (SMITH and O'DWYER 2001; WINAWER et al. 2000; REX et al. 1997b; REX 2002), and early studies comparing virtual colonoscopy to colonoscopy have mainly shown virtual to be inferior to conventional colonoscopy for the detection of polyps <1 cm in size (LAGHI et al. 2002a,b; KAY et al. 2000; FENLON et al. 1999; REX et al. 1999). Virtual colonoscopy now appears to be as accurate as conventional colonoscopy in detecting large polyps and exophytic cancer, but, at this point in time, is probably less accurate in detecting flat lesions such as flat adenomas and early, flat cancers. However, colonoscopy, by definition, is more invasive, expensive and has a higher procedural complication rate. Therefore, there is a balance between diagnostic accuracy and cost/risk in deciding on which test to use. With improving virtual colonoscopy software and automation it seems likely that virtual colonoscopy will replace barium enema as a substitute when conventional colonoscopy has failed or is contraindicated or facilities for colonoscopy can not meet demand, but whether it will seriously rival conventional colonoscopy as the primary diagnostic investigation remains to be seen.

28.4
New Technologies in Colonoscopy: Improving Insertion

For the last 30 years the "holy grail" for the colonoscopist has been to consistently pass the instrument to the caecum without complication or undue discomfort. The last 5 years has seen the introduction of two complimentary technologies, magnetic imaging and

variable-stiffness colonoscopes, which have made this wish a near reality.

Magnetic imaging produces a real-time three-dimensional view of the entire colonoscope shaft during insertion allowing the endoscopist to appreciate looping and the correct manoeuvres to straighten the instrument whilst variable stiffness instruments, as the name suggests, allow the shaft rigidity to be altered according to the degree of fixation of the colon, to counter recurrent looping once the scope has been straightened.

28.4.1
Magnetic Endoscope Imaging

The clear advantage of being able to see what is happening and the inadequacies of fluoroscopy (cost, radiation exposure, two-dimensional view), has been the impetus for the development of a new, non-X-ray method of endoscope imaging, so-called magnetic endoscope imaging (MEI) (BLADEN et al. 1993a; WILLIAMS et al. 1993). MEI works by the generation of very low strength magnetic fields (1 millionth that of a magnetic resonance scanner) by a series of tiny wire coils positioned at regular intervals along the length of the colonoscope (Fig. 28.1) (BLADEN et al. 1993b). Originally, these coils were fitted in a plastic catheter which was introduced down the biopsy channel; however, dedicated imager colonoscopes are now available with the coils and electronics in-built, underneath the metal casing of the shaft. Each coil along the colonoscope shaft sequentially generates a magnetic field, which induces a current in larger receiver coils contained within a box, positioned alongside the patient (Fig. 28.2). By calculating the

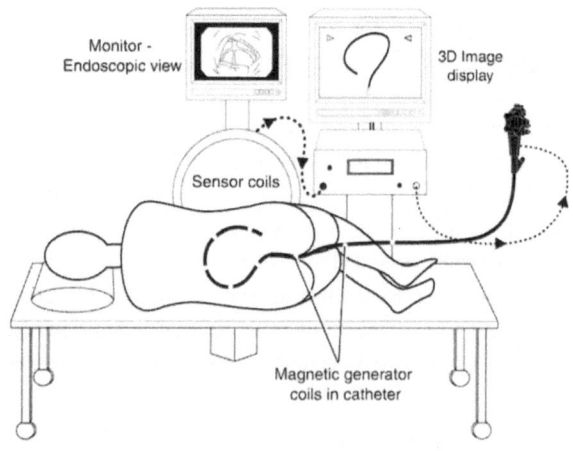

Fig. 28.1. Schematic representation of magnetic endoscope imaging

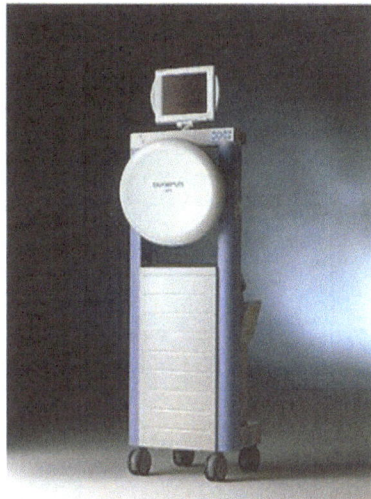

Fig. 28.2. "Scope-guide" stand-alone, magnetic imaging unit (Olympus optical company)

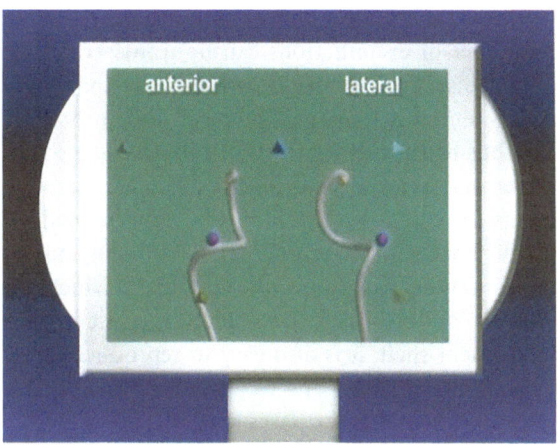

Fig. 28.3. Magnetic imager views showing simultaneous antero-posterior and lateral views. Note the purple sphere which correlates to the hand marker (see Fig. 28.5)

strength of the current in each sensor coil, the exact distance from sensor coils to generator coils can be determined. Hence the position in space is known of each generator coil within the colonoscope. The generator coils are positioned only 10 cm apart so that when a smooth line is drawn between each calculated point there is only one possible solution for the configuration of the colonoscope shaft. This is displayed on a separate computer monitor, or more conveniently can be placed adjacent to the endoscopic image on the video monitor using a video card and mixer. The on-screen view is updated five times a second so that the system is effectively real time. Polygon rendering gives a cylindrical, colonoscope-like image and differential shading (light grey, nearest the viewer; dark grey, furthest away) gives a three-dimensional effect. The system automatically produces an anteroposterior view of the scope within the abdomen but can also give a simultaneous lateral view (Fig. 28.3). Three marker coils, contained within a triangular plate and attached to the patient at the beginning of the procedure, provide anatomical reference points which correct the on-screen imager view if the patient changes position (Fig. 28.4). An additional sensor coil is contained within a plastic button and can be attached to the endoscopy assistant's hand when applying abdominal compression, so that the hand can be seen in relation to the scope (Fig. 28.5).

The data from each examination performed using the imager is stored and can be reviewed thereafter for purposes of review of technique and measurement of anatomic relationships or instrument movements,

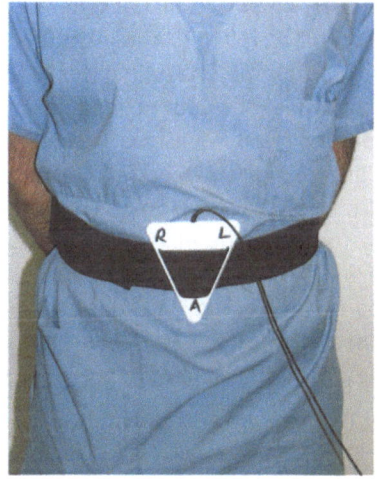

Fig. 28.4. Patient marker plate for MEI

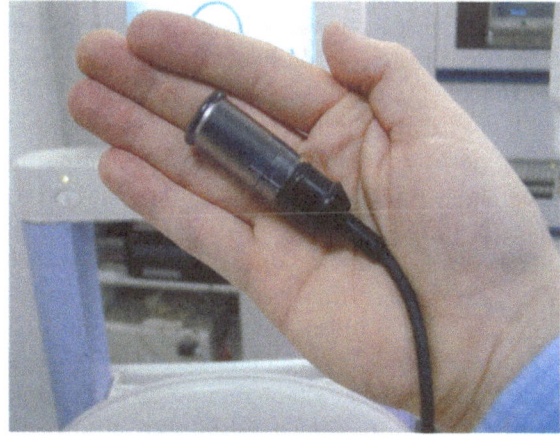

Fig. 28.5. Hand pressure marker used by the endoscopy assistant to identify correct application of abdominal hand pressure

which could lead to better academic understanding of flexible endoscopy. The complete data record of a number of examinations can be transferred onto floppy disc for analysis elsewhere. The loops and straightening manoeuvres involved in a procedure can thus be reviewed retrospectively on the monitor screen and from any view. Precise anatomic measurements (to within a few millimetres) can be made of the distance between any chosen sensor coil and any body marker, illustrating the degree to which the intestine and its attachments can be modified by the instrument shaft. It is also easy to reproduce three-dimensional graphics of selected endoscope configurations for teaching purposes (Fig. 28.6).

28.4.1.1
Impact on Colonoscopy Practice

The results of the first clinical trials of magnetic endoscope imaging were reported in 1993 (BLADEN et al. 1993a; WILLIAMS et al. 1993). In a small number of patients an early prototype imaging system was shown to accurately display the entire configuration of the colonoscope in three dimensions with close correlation with fluoroscopic images taken simultaneously. Since these early reports experience has been gained using the magnetic imaging system in over 3000 cases. This has provided a unique insight into the procedure of colonoscopy and has allowed comprehensive assessment of the likely benefits of magnetic imaging when it becomes more widely available.

28.4.1.2
Understanding Looping

In an audit of 100 consecutive colonoscopy cases performed by expert colonoscopists blinded to the magnetic imager view, the range of looping configurations that occur during routine practice were documented (SHAH et al. 2000b). Typical and atypical loops were encountered and have been described using new terminology to accurately indicate the looping state and likely straightening manoeuvres (Figs. 28.6, 28.7) (REX et al. 1999; BLADEN et al. 1993b). Despite application of the general principles of good insertion technique, loops occurred in most patients and in the sigmoid colon in 79%. The overall frequency of looping was similar in male and female patients although atypical loops were more common in women. Loops were incorrectly diagnosed in 69% of cases and unusual loops such as the anti-clockwise spiral loops (reverse splenic

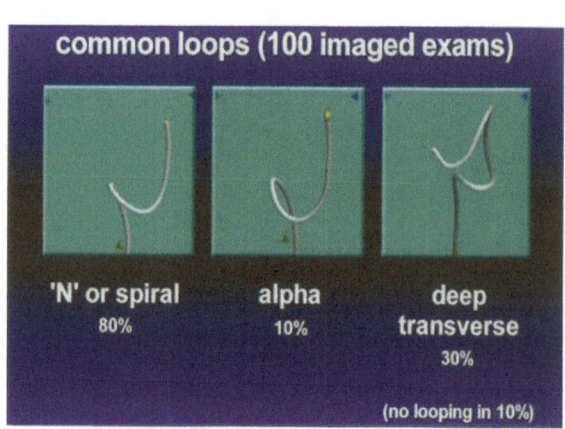

Fig. 28.6. MEI views showing common loops encountered during colonoscopy

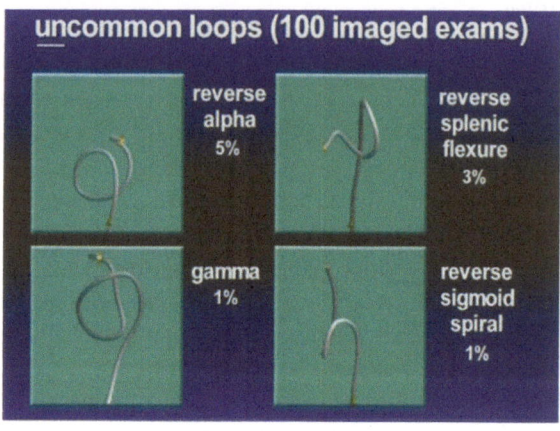

Fig. 28.7. MEI views showing atypical loops

flexure, reverse alpha loop) and transverse gamma loop were always incorrectly diagnosed. Complete colonoscopy was always achieved, but in 6% the full 160 cm of the colonoscope was inserted to push through an uncontrollable loop prior to endoscope straightening. In the majority of cases, however, with good technique and frequent loop straightening, less than 100 cm was inserted at any one time. Abdominal compression when applied was generally inaccurate due to either hand misplacement away from the apex of the loop or inaccessible looping deep within the abdomen. In a separate study pain episodes were documented to correspond directly with looping as seen utilising magnetic imaging (SHAH et al. 2002a). Looping in the sigmoid colon was most painful, particularly in female patients.

28.4.1.3
Accuracy of Tip Location

The imaging system accurately locates the colono-scope tip to aid in lesion recognition and caecal intubation. Comparison of contrast studies following imager-guided application of endoclips to predefined anatomical locations during insertion showed good correlation between the imager-defined and actual anatomical clip locations (SHAH et al. 2002b). Imager snap-shot views with corresponding endoscopic photos (with or without endoscopic tattooing with India ink) represents the best and most convenient method of documenting colonic pathology to guide future endoscopic examinations or surgical interven-tion (Fig. 28.8).

28.4.1.4
Colonoscopy Performance

A series of randomised studies have now been pub-lished assessing the impact of magnetic imaging on colonoscopy performance. An early study of 55 con-secutive patients undergoing colonoscopy by a single experienced endoscopist (1000 previous cases) with or without the imager view (early prototype), showed a reduction in the number of straightening attempts when the colonoscope shaft was looped, but without a corresponding decrease in the duration of loop for-mation or time taken to reach the caecal pole (SAUN-DERS et al. 1995). Abdominal hand compression was significantly improved when the endoscopist and endoscopy assistant were able to visualise the imager view, the lateral view giving increased information as to the depth of looping and correct site for application of assistant hand compression. In a more recent study the effect of magnetic imaging was assessed on the colonoscopy performance of both trainee (200 previ-ous cases) and expert endoscopists (>5000 previous cases) (SHAH et al. 2000a). Significant improvements in caecal completion rate, insertion time, duration of colonoscope looping, number of straightening attempts and accuracy of hand pressure were seen with the imaging system when used by the trainees. Similar though less marked benefits were recorded with the expert endoscopists who found the imag-ing system dramatically shortened insertion times in technically difficult cases. No differences were seen in patient pain scores or sedation requirements – a finding that is not surprising given the univer-sally low pain scores despite only low dose sedation given, usually as bolus medication at the start of the procedures.

28.4.1.5
Magnetic Imaging and Colonoscopy Training

Colonoscopy training has changed little in the last 30 years and still relies heavily on an apprenticeship scheme where an experienced colonoscopist hands down the "tricks of the trade" to the inexperienced trainee. Training is highly frustrating and unsatisfac-tory for all parties concerned. For the trainee it is difficult to appreciate why certain manoeuvres are apparently beneficial and for the trainer it is dif-ficult to assess why the trainee is stuck unless the scope is taken over by the trainer and manipulated appropriately, by which time the teaching oppor-tunity has often been lost. Magnetic imaging may address many of these frustrations by allowing a structured interaction between trainer and trainee, allowing the trainee to complete cases under supervi-sion where previously the trainer would have needed to take over, thus accelerating the trainee's learning

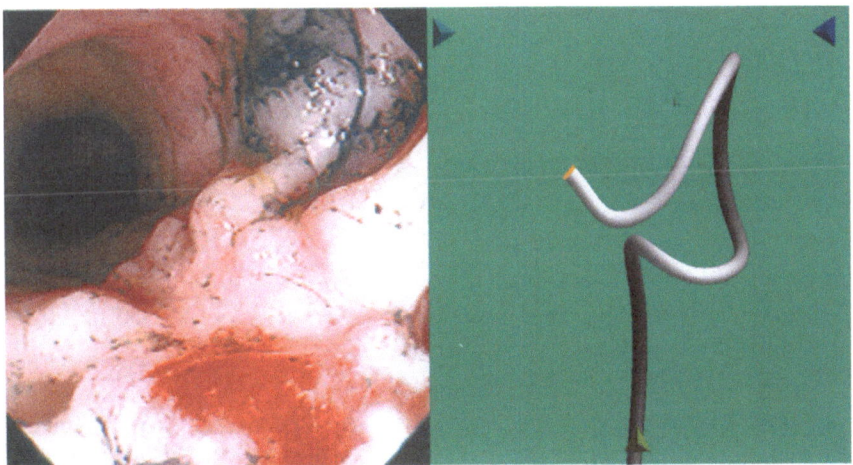

Fig. 28.8. Endoscopic view of small, early, flat cancer with India ink tattoo. MEI snapshot is recorded alongside endo-scopic view accurately placing the lesion in the proximal transverse colon

curve and acquisition of hand-skills. In an initial pilot study a single beginner colonoscopist (only 15 previous colonoscopies) performed procedures under supervision with examinations randomised to either with or without the imaging system (SHAH et al. 2002). Benefits in terms of loop management were seen with the imaging system in the initial stages of training with a plateau seen at approximately 50 cases, when a 90% completion rate to the caecum was seen. Thereafter no demonstrable difference was seen comparing cases with or without the imager suggesting that imaging is particularly valuable early during the learning curve. Further work is required to define the longer term impact on skill acquisition; however, it seems logical that future computer simulators teaching basic colonoscope hand-skills will incorporate simulated imager views which will lay the foundations for hands-on training with the imager in live cases. Performance assessment utilising a specific score from a combined video and magnetic imaging recorder may prove a robust tool for ensuring standards and charting trainee's progress (Fig. 28.9) (SHAH et al. 2002c).

28.4.2
Variable-Stiffness Colonoscopes

As mentioned above, variable-stiffness colonoscopes have recently been introduced which allow the endoscopist to change the shaft characteristics of the colonoscope at any time during insertion. Variable-stiffness scopes contain a graduated dial situated just below the head of the colonoscope (Fig. 28.10), which can be turned manually to vary shaft stiffness. Turning the dial straightens or relaxes an internal "stiffening" cable, which runs along the length of the colonoscope, stopping 20 cm short of the tip. Insertion through the sigmoid colon is generally conducted with the scope in the floppy paediatric mode with maximal stiffening applied to prevent recurrent looping once the tip has reached the descending colon and the scope has been straightened. In an early-randomised trial the variable-stiffness scope compared to a conventional instrument speeded insertion times and caused less discomfort (BROOKER et al. 2000). Subsequent studies have confirmed the benefit of the variable-stiffness instrument in reducing the perceived difficulty of the procedure and in reducing the need for ancillary manoeuvres such as change in patient position and application of abdominal hand pressure (REX 2001; ODORI et al. 2001).

Without shaft imaging, however, precise utilisation of the variable-stiffness function is difficult to ascertain during insertion and its use is often by best guess and trial and error. It is therefore logical to combine the variable-stiffness function with the magnetic imaging system and variable-stiffness/ imaging colonoscopes are now available. Two studies have assessed the impact of magnetic imaging on use of the variable-stiffness colonoscope (SHAH et al. 2002). In the first, MEI was used to evaluate the success of scope insertion during back-to-back proximal colon randomised insertions with and without the colonoscope maximally stiffened. Stiffening resulted in a more rapid proximal colon inser-

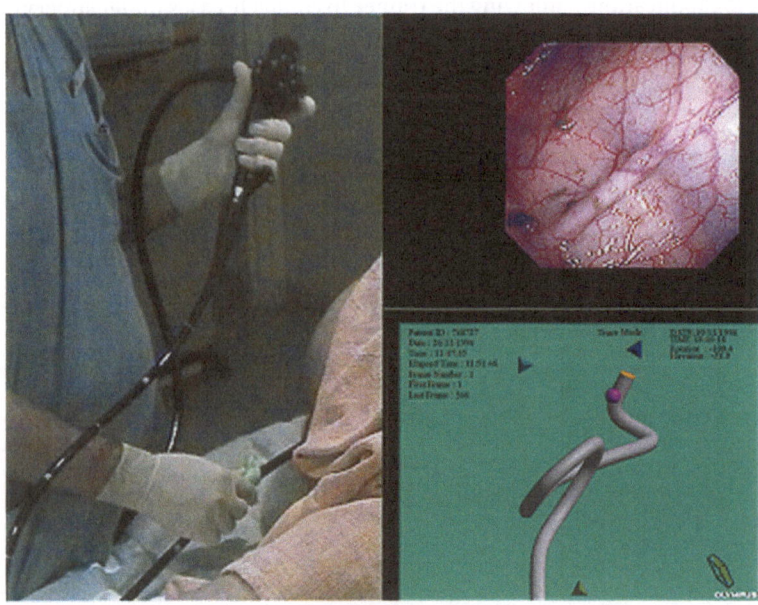

Fig. 28.9. Tri-split video recording of room, endoscope and imager views

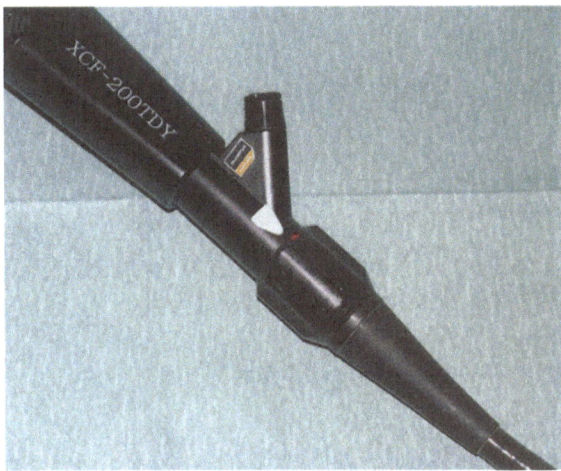

Fig. 28.10. Head of variable-stiffness colonoscope. Note the dial just below the head for increasing or decreasing shaft rigidity

tion, particularly around the splenic flexure and with less recourse to ancillary manoeuvres such as hand pressure or position change. In the second study an experienced endoscopist was randomised to perform consecutive examinations with a VS scope with or without the benefit of the imager view in addition. Not unsurprisingly successful use of the variable-stiffness function was significantly more likely when the imager could be seen. The new generation variable-stiffness/imager colonoscopes (CF-240DL, Olympus Optical Company) appear to have major advantages over conventional colonoscopes, the new modalities in combination amounting to a greater overall benefit than the sum of the halves.

28.5
Improved Lesion Detection

Rapid insertion to the caecum with a straight scope lays the foundation for the most crucial part of colonoscopy, the examination during withdrawal. Recently considerable attention has focused on the quality of the withdrawal examination. Adenoma detection rates, particularly for small polyps, vary considerably between different endoscopists, depending on a variety of "quality criteria" such as re-examination of the proximal sides of folds, time spent viewing and determination of the endoscopist to improve the view with adequate distension and suctioning and washing to remove retained stool (Postic et al. 2002; Rex et al. 1997a; Rex 2000). Provided position change, use of anti-spasmodics and anti-foaming

agents are used liberally and good examination technique is adhered to polypoid lesions are unlikely to be missed. However, there is an increasing awareness of the presence of flat adenomas and early, small flat cancers (Fig. 28.11). In colonoscopic series from Western countries flat adenomas have been reported to account for between 10%–36% of all adenomas, depending on the definitions of what constitutes a "flat" rather than a sessile lesion (Rembacken et al. 2000; Tsuda et al. 2002; Saitoh et al. 2001). Small flat cancers (<2 cm in size) have now been described in many Western populations and appear to constitute approximately 10% of all cancer detected at colonoscopy (Rembacken et al. 2000; Tsuda et al. 2002). It seems biologically likely that certain flat adenomas may go on to develop rapidly into flat cancers and therefore detection of these lesions is important. Flat adenomas that are flush with the mucosal surface (type 11b, Japanese classification) (Kudo et al. 2000) or depressed below the mucosal surface (type 11c) appear to be particularly prone to malignant transformation, whereas minimally elevated (type 11a) lesions may have no increased malignant potential compared to sessile and polypoid adenomas. It is important to appreciate that even in Japanese series type 11b and 11c flat adenomas are a relatively rare finding accounting for only approximately 2% of all adenomas. A major challenge for barium radiology and virtual colonoscopy is to be able to detect these lesions, which may even be missed during direct mucosal inspection at colonoscopy! With experience, good bowel preparation and careful examination at colonoscopy flat lesions can, in fact, be detected reliably. Visual clues of an abnormality include a break in the mucosal vessel pattern, a disruption of the haustral fold, or a colour change, usually an increase in vascularity. Understandably there has been considerable interest in methods that improve detection of subtle abnormalities at colonoscopy.

28.5.1
Video Systems

Video colonoscopes contain a charge coupled device (CCD) chip at their tip, behind the lens, which contains multiple, linear, photoelectric picture elements or pixels. These pixels produce a tiny electrical signal dependent on reflected light from the mucosal surface, which is interpreted by the video processor, and a composite image is built up and displayed on the monitor. With miniaturisation and improvements in electrical processing CCD chips with twice

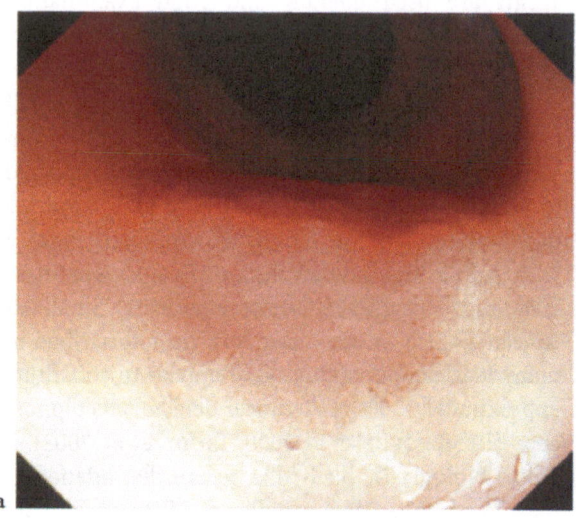
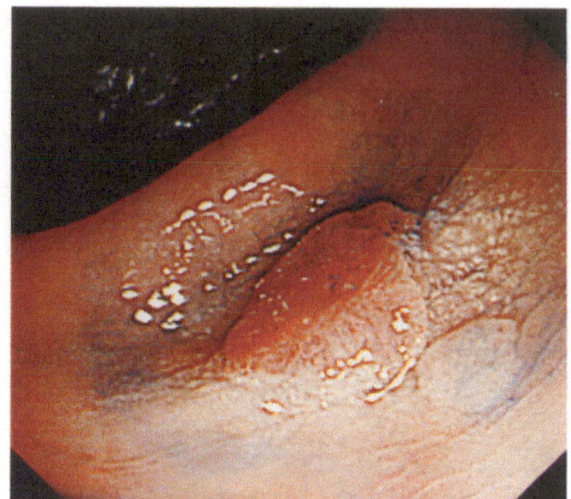

Fig. 28.11a,b. a Type 11b, flat adenoma. **b** Small flat cancer

or even three times the number of pixels (in excess of 400,000) are now standard, improving the degree of fine resolution of the final video image. Digital enhancement is also possible, which increases the definition between edges making subtle mucosal detail stand out (Fig. 28.12).

28.5.2
Mucosal Dye

Despite these advances in video technology the application of mucosal dye, particularly indigo carmine (0.1%–0.8%) greatly improves surface definition. The blue dye is not absorbed and sits on the mucosal surface defining the surface architecture, with pooling in depressions and the innominate grooves (Fig. 28.12). Most endoscopists use dye spray only when standard video assessment suggests a subtle abnormality. Dye can be pushed easily through the biopsy channel of the scope using a 30 ml syringe onto the mucosal surface. In certain conditions such as familial adenomatous polyposis dye spray can be used electively to demonstrate microadenomas. Pancolonic dye spray, utilising a dye spray catheter or dye capsule (100 mg indigo carmine) taken with the bowel preparation is certainly feasible and has been described for routine colonoscopy and resulted in an increased detection of small adenomas, particularly in the right colon (BROOKER et al. 2002). However,

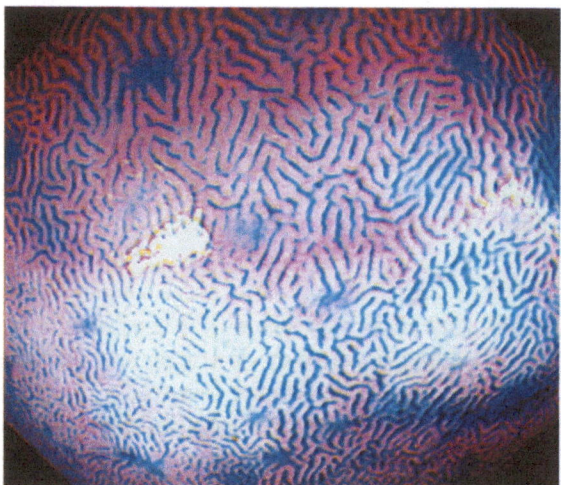
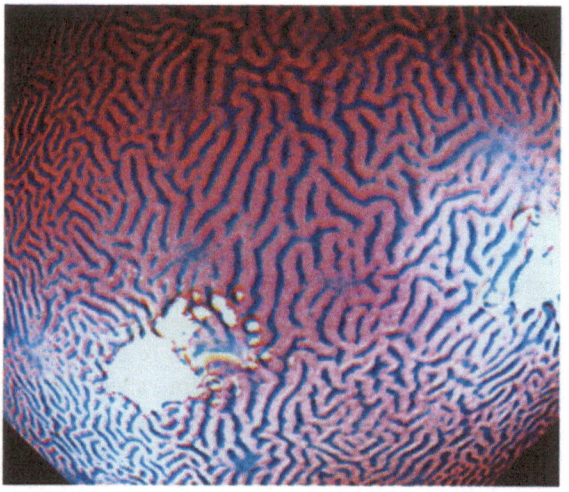

Fig. 28.12a,b High resolution chromoendoscopy (indigo carmine 0.2%) showing the normal mucosal surface (innominate grooves) with (**a**) normal view and (**b**) digital enhanced view

this approach is time-consuming and doubles withdrawal time. It may well have a role in assessment of known high-risk groups such as those with multiple sporadic adenomas, hereditary non-polyposis colorectal cancer syndromes and in those with long-standing extensive ulcerative colitis. Dye spraying appears to be without patient risk and a major advance in accuracy of colonoscopy.

28.5.3
In Vivo Diagnosis

The major advantage of colonoscopy and also the greatest potential for morbidity comes from therapeutic intervention. Having detected an abnormality at colonoscopy it is therefore vital that an appropriate assessment is made and choice of therapeutic intervention. Metaplastic polyps for instance, particularly small left-sided lesions may have no neoplastic potential and removal of these lesions puts the patient at risk of complications from polypectomy with no benefit in terms of cancer risk reduction. Endoscopists have long pondered on the ability to distinguish reliably neoplastic from non-neoplastic lesions at colonoscopy. Japanese authors have described five, basic mucosal pit patterns, as seen under the low power light microscope which correspond to different types of polyp (Fig. 28.13) (KUDO et al. 2001a). To some extent pit pattern can be seen with existing video technology, augmented by indigo carmine dye spray; however, prospective trials have only demonstrated sensitivity and specificity for differentiating adenomatous from non-adenomatous polyps of around 80% (EISEN et al. 2002).

28.5.3.1
Magnifying Colonoscopes

Sensitivity and specificity for determining neoplastic from non-neoplastic polyps can be improved by also using a specific magnifying instrument (TUNG et al. 2001; TAMURA et al. 2002). These colonoscopes contain a complex lens system at their tip, which provides up to 100 times magnification and gives views similar to those seen with a low power light microscope (Fig. 28.13b). However there are fundamental problems with the routine use of magnifying endoscopes. Although of standard length (160 cm) they tend to be stiffer and more difficult to pass than modern variable-stiffness colonoscopes and have a longer bending section, making steering around acute bends more difficult (Fig. 28.14). When high magnification is attempted any slight patient movement, such as aortic pulsation tends to blur the image making interpretation difficult. This can be countered to some extent by using a plastic cap to suck and hold the mucosa onto the colonoscope tip, at the cost of a slight reduction in the overall view. Therefore, many Western endoscopists who have tried using magnifying instruments have come to the conclusion that they are time-consuming to use with little realistic gain in terms of improved diagnosis. This view is further augmented by the growing literature that suggests that some metaplastic polyps, particularly large lesions in the right colon may have neoplastic potential (JASS et al. 2002). A primary goal of the colonoscopist is to remove all potentially cancerous lesions, therefore many have the pragmatic approach that all lesions above the recto-sigmoid should be

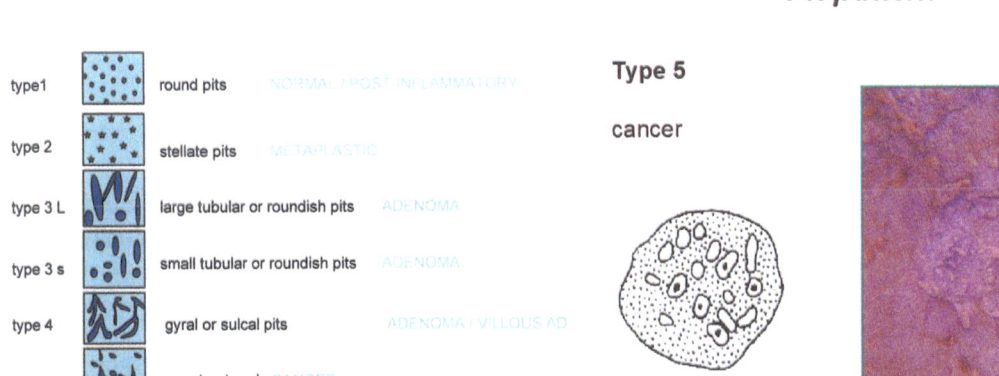

Pit pattern

type1	round pits	NORMAL / POST-INFLAMMATORY
type 2	stellate pits	METAPLASTIC
type 3 L	large tubular or roundish pits	ADENOMA
type 3 s	small tubular or roundish pits	ADENOMA
type 4	gyral or sulcal pits	ADENOMA / VILLOUS AD
type 5	non-structured	CANCER

Type 5

cancer

Fig. 28.13a,b. a Diagram of the five basic "pit patterns" seen with the magnifying colonoscope corresponding to neoplastic and non-neoplastic lesions. **b** Amorphous pit pattern typical of a cancer

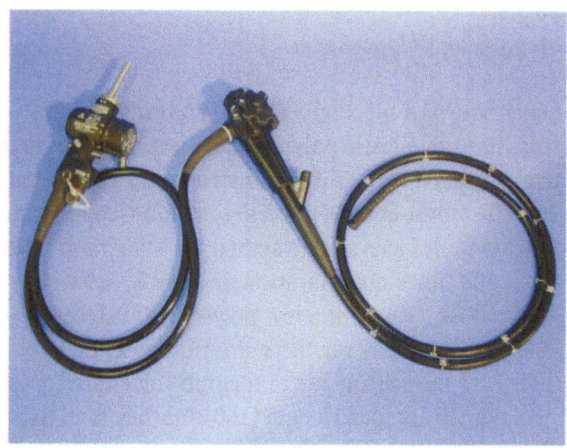
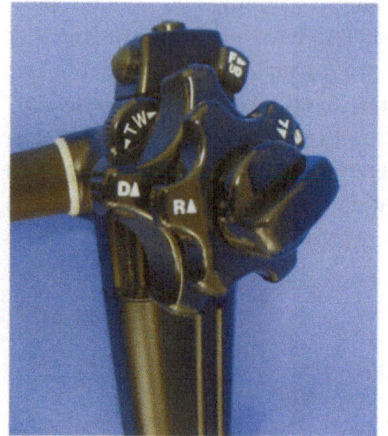

a   b

Fig. 28.14a,b. a Overview of the Olympus 200ZL magnifying colonoscope. **b** Close-up view of magnifying colonoscope showing "bridge-control" for magnifying onto lesions

removed anyway, and if multiple tiny metaplastic rectal polyps are seen (too numerous to practically remove), a representative sample should be cold biopsied (no risk) to confirm the diagnosis. One role of magnification, which may be beneficial, is in selecting which early flat cancers are amenable to endoscopic mucosal resection (EMR). Severe disruption to the pit pattern has been described as a poor prognostic factor and associated with an increased risk of lymph node metastases (MATSUMOTO et al. 2002).

28.5.3.2
Colonoscopic Ultrasound

Perhaps a more elegant approach to determine depth of invasion of early cancer is the use of endoscopic ultrasound. Dedicated, axial EUS scopes are available for colon cancer staging; however, most cancers at the time of diagnosis invade the muscularis propria, are not amenable to endoscopic therapy and will be treated surgically regardless. In this context EUS adds little to the management algorithm. Early cancers and sessile polyps pose a different problem as endoscopic therapy is the optimal choice of therapy for mucosal lesions or very early cancers that just invade into the first third of the submucosa (KUDO et al. 2000, 2001b). Mini-probes (12.5, 20, 30 Mhz) passed down the biopsy channel of conventional endoscopes offer a good alternative for immediate ultrasound assessment at the time of a conventional colonoscopic examination (Fig. 28.15). High definition of the submucosal layer (hyperechoic) can be achieved and disruption of this layer suggests invasion to at least the second third of the submucosa, a point at which the risk of lymph node metastases

and the need for a formal surgical resection becomes the optimal treatment. An intact submucosa would encourage the endoscopist to perform an endoscopic mucosal resection with the potential for cure without surgery (Fig. 28.15c). Studies suggest that high frequency EUS, in experienced hands can be fairly accurate (80%–90% sensitivity) in predicting local depth of invasion of early cancer (MATSUMOTO et al. 2002; AKAHOSHI et al. 2001; YOSHIDA et al. 1995). In reality few endoscopists have access to either magnification or EUS and will make an empirical decision on the endoscopic resectability of a lesion by its visual appearance, gentle palpation with the biopsy forceps and its lifting state; if a lesion lifts completely after submucosal saline injection it is unlikely to involve the submucosa and can therefore be removed endoscopically with an excellent prospect of cure (ISHIGURO et al. 1999). Partial lifting usually deters the endoscopist unless the patient is unlikely to be a surgical candidate.

28.6
Future Possibilities

It seems likely that magnetic imaging will become a standard for colonoscopy practice. Initially teaching units will incorporate the technology as training lists are immediately transformed and become enjoyable, interactive and more logical. Once the next generation of endoscopists become familiar with the imager it will be seen as essential technology to improve completion rates in difficult cases and help document total colonoscopy. In particular, imager

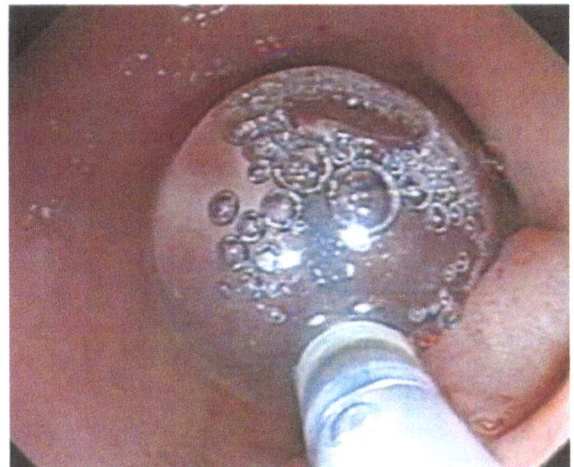

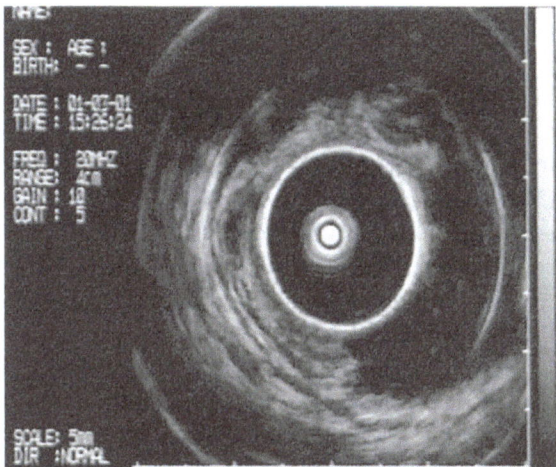

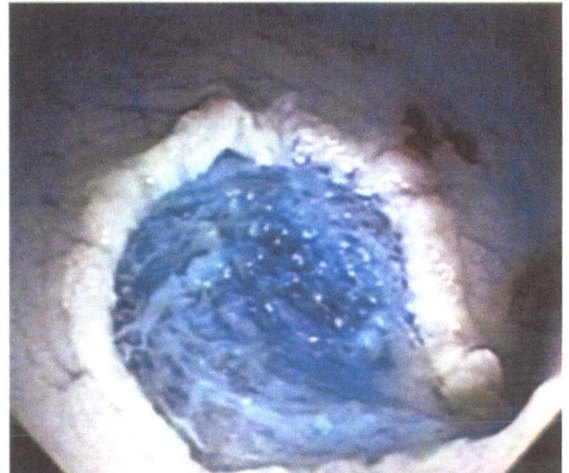

Fig. 28.15a–c. a Endoscopic view of 20-MHz EUS mini-probe. **b** A 20-MHz probe view of benign colonic polyp. **c** Endoscopic appearance of polyp base after endoscopic mucosal resection

records will help endoscopists to assess their own performance and maintain standards within each Endoscopy Unit. A simple and potentially important future improvement will be to increase the degree of stiffness that can be imparted to the shaft of the new generation of variable-stiffness imager scopes. The ability to see that the colonoscope shaft is straight will mean that the increased stiffening function can be applied entirely safely. Using data from the imager will help in future colonoscope design and it is not beyond comprehension to envisage a semi-automatic endoscope which adapts to the degree of looping or which suggests manoeuvres to help the endoscopist depending on shaft configuration.

Mucosal definition and endoscopic detection of neoplasia is likely to be improved considerably in the next 5–10 years, keeping colonoscopy "ahead of the game" compared to virtual colonoscopy. New technologies include advanced video manipulation to highlight vascular areas (flat adenomas, angiodyspla-sias) by so-called haemoglobin enhancement. Here the video processor preferentially responds to light of the same wavelength as haemoglobin enhancing any red structure within the field of view. Tissue autofluores-cence, the real-time interrogation of the mucosa with light of a known wavelength and subsequent capture of the reflected spectral pattern to characterise mucosal tissue types, is still in its infancy, but preliminary clinical trials are underway (WANG et al. 1999; MYCEK et al. 1998). Early prototypes have been based around fibre-optic scopes, a clear limiting factor; however, it can not be long before equipment manufacturers produce "conventional handling", video scopes with two video systems – standard white light video colonoscopy and a second video autofluorescence mode which allows switching from one to the other at the press of a button. Along similar lines "optical biopsy" is likely to become a standard procedure to augment conventional colonoscopy and reduce the demands on already over-stretched histopathology departments.

Prototype systems utilising optical biopsy forceps (conventional hot biopsy forceps with a central laser exciter and receiver fibre) are under evaluation and have the potential to allow, if necessary, hundreds of biopsies per examination. Recently there has been much interest in "capsule colonoscopy". This video pill (11 mm × 22 mm) relays images to a set of remote sensors on a jacket worn by the patient (Fig. 28.16). The entire patient record is downloaded to a purpose-built workstation for subsequent analysis (FRITSCHER-RAVENS and SWAIN 2002). The primary indication for a capsule examination is examination of the small bowel; however, it has been proposed as a non-invasive method for colonoscopy. Preliminary experience suggests that there are many problems with the capsule if used primarily for colonoscopy. Small bowel transit time varies considerably and battery time may not be sufficient to view the colon. The main problem however is that the colon is a large and capacious organ and only very limited, uncontrolled views are seen as the capsule is passed by peristalsis through the colon. If a method for steering the capsule becomes available then capsule colonoscopy may have a place where conventional colonoscopy has failed. However the lack of biopsy or therapeutic potential also make it unlikely to rival a conventional examination.

28.7
Conclusions

Magnetic endoscope imaging in conjunction with variable-stiffness instruments is making colonoscope insertion easier and probably safer and allowing more time for detailed mucosal analysis. Simple techniques such as selective use of indigo carmine dye-spray help to define subtle mucosal irregularities. Optimal assessment of early, flat cancers involves

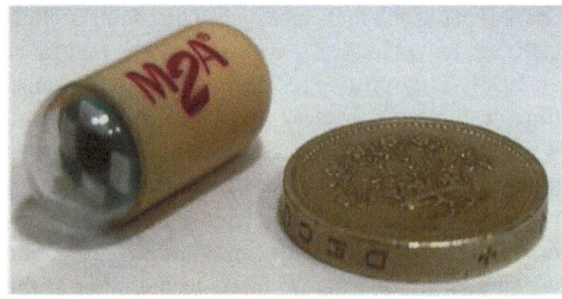

Fig. 28.16. The video pill, which relays images to a set of remote sensors on a jacket worn by the patient, is used primarily to examine the small bowel but it has been proposed as a non-invasive method of examining the colon

magnification to assess pit pattern and EUS, although the "lifting state" of the lesion on submucosal injection is equally important and requires no additional equipment or expertise. In the future new imaging modalities such as video autofluorescence are likely to keep conventional colonoscopy ahead of other imaging techniques as the most accurate modality in the colon.

References

Akahoshi K, Yoshinaga S, Soejima A, Nagaie T, Koyanagi N, Nakanishi K, Harada N, Nawata H (2001) Transit endoscopic ultrasound of colorectal cancer using a 12 MHz catheter probe. Br J Radiol 74:1017–1022

Bladen JS, Anderson AP, Bell GD, Heatley DJ (1993a) A non-radiological technique for the real time imaging of endoscopes in 3 dimensions. Conference record of the 1993 IEEE nuclear science symposium and medical imaging conference, 1891–1894

Bladen JS, Anderson AP, Bell GD, Heatley DJ (1993b) Non-radiological technique for three-dimensional imaging of endoscopes. Lancet 341:719

Brooker JC, Saunders BP, Shah SG, Williams CB (2000) A new variable stiffness colonoscope makes colonoscopy easier: a randomised controlled trial. Gut 46:801–805

Brooker JC, Saunders BP, Shah SG, Thapar CJ, Thomas HJ, Atkin WS, Cardwell CR, Williams CB (2002) Total colonic dye-spray increases the detection of diminutive adenomas during routine colonoscopy: a randomized controlled trial. Gastrointest Endosc 56:333–338

Eisen GM, Kim CY, Fleischer DE, Kozarek RA, Carr-Locke DL, Li TC, Gostout CJ, Heller SJ, Montgomery EA, Al-Kawas FH, Lewis JH, Benjamin SB (2002) High-resolution chromoendoscopy for classifying colonic polyps: a multicenter study. Gastrointest Endosc 55:687–694

Fenlon HM, Nunes DP, Schroy PC 3rd, Barish MA, Clarke PD, Ferrucci JT (1999) A comparison of virtual and conventional colonoscopy for the detection of colorectal polyps. N Engl J Med 341:1496–1503

Fritscher-Ravens A, Swain CP (2002) The wireless capsule: new light in the darkness. Dig Dis 20:127–133 (Gastroenterology 2001, 120:1657–1665)

Ishiguro A, Uno Y, Ishiguro Y, Munakata A, Morita T (1999) Correlation of lifting versus non-lifting and microscopic depth of invasion in early colorectal cancer. Gastrointest Endosc 50:329–333

Jass JR, Whitehall VL, Young J, Leggett BA (2002) Emerging concepts in colorectal neoplasia. Gastroenterology 123: 862–876

Kay CL, Kulling D, Hawes RH, Young JW, Cotton PB (2000) Virtual endoscopy-comparison with colonoscopy in the detection of space-occupying lesions of the colon. Endoscopy 32:226–232

Kudo S, Kashida H, Tamura T, Kogure E, Imai Y, Yamano H, Hart AR (2000) Colonoscopic diagnosis and management of nonpolypoid early colorectal cancer. World J Surg 24: 1081–1090

Kudo S, Rubio CA, Teixeira CR, Kashida H, Kogure E (2001a)

Pit pattern in colorectal neoplasia: endoscopic magnifying view. Endoscopy 33:367–373

Kudo S, Tamegai Y, Yamano H, Imai Y, Kogure E, Kashida H (2001b) Endoscopic mucosal resection of the colon: the Japanese technique. Gastrointest Endosc Clin North Am 11:519–535

Laghi A, Iannaccone R, Carbone I, Catalano C, Di Giulio E, Schillaci A, Passariello R (2002a) Detection of colorectal lesions with virtual computed tomographic colonography. Am J Surg 183:124–131

Laghi A, Iannaccone R, Carbone I, Catalano C, Panebianco V, Di Giulio E, Schillaci A, Passariello R (2002b) Computed tomographic colonography (virtual colonoscopy): blinded prospective comparison with conventional colonoscopy for the detection of colorectal neoplasia. Endoscopy 34:441–446

Matsumoto T, Hizawa K, Esaki M, Kurahara K, Mizuno M, Hirakawa K, Yao T, Iida M (2002) Comparison of EUS and magnifying colonoscopy for assessment of small colorectal cancers. Gastrointest Endosc 56:354–360

Mycek MA, Schomacker KT, Nishioka NS (1998) Colonic polyp differentiation using time-resolved autofluorescence spectroscopy. Gastrointest Endosc 48:390–394

Odori T, Goto H, Arisawa T, Niwa Y, Ohmiya N, Hayakawa T (2001) Clinical results and development of variable-stiffness video colonoscopes. Endoscopy 33:65–69

Postic G, Lewin D, Bickerstaff C, Wallace MB (2002) Colonoscopic miss rates determined by direct comparison of colonoscopy with colon resection specimens. Am J Gastroenterol 97:3182–3185

Rembacken BJ, Fujii T, Cairns A, Dixon MF, Yoshida S, Chalmers DM, Axon AT (2000) Flat and depressed colonic neoplasms: a prospective study of 1000 colonoscopies in the UK. Lancet 355:1211–1214

Rex DK (2000) Colonoscopic withdrawal technique is associated with adenoma miss rates. Gastrointest Endosc 51:33–36

Rex DK (2001) Effect of variable stiffness colonoscopes on cecal intubation times for routine colonoscopy by an experienced examiner in sedated patients. Endoscopy 33:60–64

Rex DK (2002) Rationale for colonoscopy screening and estimated effectiveness in clinical practice. Gastrointest Endosc Clin North Am 12:65–75

Rex DK, Cutler CS, Lemmel GT, Rahmani EY, Clark DW, Helper DJ, Lehman GA, Mark DG (1997a) Colonoscopic miss rates of adenomas determined by back-to-back colonoscopies. Gastroenterology 112:24–28

Rex DK, Rahmani EY, Haseman JH, Lemmel GT, Kaster S, Buckley JS (1997b) Relative sensitivity of colonoscopy and barium enema for detection of colorectal cancer in clinical practice. Gastroenterology 112:17–23

Rex DK, Vining D, Kopecky KK (1999) An initial experience with screening for colon polyps using spiral CT with and without CT colography (virtual colonoscopy). Gastrointest Endosc 50:309–313

Saitoh Y, Waxman I, West AB, Popnikolov NK, Gatalica Z, Watari J, Obara T, Kohgo Y, Pasricha PJ (2001) Prevalence and distinctive biologic features of flat colorectal adenomas in a North American population. Gastroenterology 120:1657–1665

Saunders BP, Bell GD, Williams CB, Bladen JS, Anderson AP (1995) First clinical results with a real time, electronic imager as an aid to colonoscopy. Gut 36:913–917

Shah SG, Brooker JC, Williams CB, Thapar C, Saunders BP (2000a) Effect of magnetic endoscope imaging on colonoscopy performance: a randomised controlled trial. Lancet 356:1718–1722

Shah SG, Saunders BP, Brooker JC, Williams CB (2000b) Magnetic imaging of colonoscopy: an audit of looping, accuracy and ancillary maneuvers. Gastrointest Endosc 52:1

Shah SG, Brooker JC, Thapar C, Williams CB, Saunders BP (2002a) Patient pain during colonoscopy – an analysis using real-time magnetic endoscope imaging. Endoscopy 34:435–440

Shah SG, Pearson HJ, Moss S, Kweka E, Jalal PK, Saunders BP (2002b) Magnetic endoscope imaging: a new technique for localizing colonic lesions. Endoscopy 34:900–904

Shah SG, Thomas-Gibson S, Brooker JC, Suzuki N, Williams CB, Thapar C, Saunders BP (2002c) Use of video and magnetic endoscope imaging for rating competence at colonoscopy: validation of a measurement tool. Gastrointest Endosc 56:568–573

Shah SG, Brooker JC, Williams CB, Thapar C, Suzuki N, Saunders BP (2002d) The variable stiffness colonoscope: assessment of efficacy by magnetic endoscope imaging. Gastrointest Endosc 56:195–201

Shah SG, Lockett M, Thomas-Gibson S, Brooker JC, Vance M, Thapar CJ, Saunders BP (2002e) Effect of magnetic endoscope imaging (MEI) on acquisition of colonoscopy skills. Gut 50 [Suppl 2]:A41

Smith GA, O'Dwyer PJ (2001) Sensitivity of double contrast barium enema and colonoscopy for the detection of colorectal neoplasms. Surg Endosc 15:649–652

Tamura S, Ookawauchi K, Onishi S, Yokoyama Y, Yamada T, Higashidani Y, Tadokoro T, Onishi S (2002) The usefulness of magnifying chromoendoscopy: pit pattern diagnosis can predict histopathological diagnosis precisely. Am J Gastroenterol 97:2934–2935

Tsuda S, Veress B, Toth E, Fork FT (2002) Flat and depressed colorectal tumours in a southern Swedish population: a prospective chromoendoscopic and histopathological study. Gut 51:550–555

Tung SY, Wu CS, Su MY (2001) Magnifying colonoscopy in differentiating neoplastic from nonneoplastic colorectal lesions. Am J Gastroenterol 96:2628–2632

Wang TD, Crawford JM, Feld MS, Wang Y, Itzkan I, van Dam J (1999) In vivo identification of colonic dysplasia using fluorescence endoscopic imaging. Gastrointest Endosc 49:447–455

Williams CB, Guy C, Gillies DF, Saunders B (1993) Electronic three-dimensional imaging of intestinal endoscopy. Lancet 341:724

Winawer SJ, Stewart ET, Zauber AG, Bond JH, Ansel H, Waye JD, Hall D, Hamlin JA, Schapiro M, O'Brien MJ, Sternberg SS, Gottlieb LS (2000) A comparison of colonoscopy and double-contrast barium enema for surveillance after polypectomy. National Polyp Study Work Group. N Engl J Med 342:1766–1772

Wolff WI, Shinya H (1971) Colonofiberoscopy. JAMA 217:1509–1512

Wolff WI, Shinya H (1973) Polypectomy via the fiberoptic colonoscope. Removal of neoplasms beyond reach of the sigmoidoscope. N Engl J Med 288:329–332

Yoshida M, Tsukamoto Y, Niwa Y, Goto H, Hase S, Hayakawa T, Okamura S (1995) Endoscopic assessment of invasion of colorectal tumors with a new high-frequency ultrasound probe. Gastrointest Endosc 41:587–592

Subject Index

A

Accordion sign   187, 194
Actinomycosis   284
Acute contrast enema   264–265
Adenoma
– classification   33
– colon (*see* colon-adenoma)
– duodenal   16
– dysplasia   33
– flat   (*see* flat adenoma)
– grading   33
– micro-adenoma   32
– pathology   32-36
– serrated   35
– tubular   33
– tubulovillous   33
– villous   33, 271
Adenoma-like DALM (ALD)   36
Adenomatous polyposis coli (*see* familial adenomatous
   polyposis)
Adhesions   207, 267
Amoebiasis   41, 178, 191, 281, 284
Amphetamine   193
Amsterdam criteria (*see* Hereditary Non-Polyposis Colorectal
   Cancer)
Angiodysplasia   235
Angiography
– colonic bleeding   235–240
– embolization   238–239
– provocative   237
– therapeutic   238–240
Appendicitis
– abscess   159, 279
– chronic   157
– classification   161
– clinical findings   147, 158
– computer tomography (CT)   157–162
– epidemiology   158
– phlegmon   159
– technique   148
– ultrasound   147–155
Appendix
– anatomy   157, 159
– duplication   157
– mucocoele   150, 279
– myxoglobulosis   279
Apthous ulcers   173, 178
Artery
– inferior mesenteric   230
– superior mesenteric   230
Aster-Collier staging   98

B

Backwash ileitis   186
Bannayan-Reilly-Ruvalcaba polyposis syndrome   37, 46
Barium enema (BE)
– acuracy   52
– Crohn's disease   172
– inflammatory bowel disease   171–175
– intussusception   271
– merits   51
– safety   53
– sensitivity   6, 19, 29
– single contrast (SCBE)   55, 56
Behçet's syndrome   188, 193
Benign lymphoid polyp   41
Benign lymphoid polyposis syndrome   44
Bernoulli equation   269
Bethesda criteria (*see* Hereditary Non-Polyposis Colorectal
   Cancer)
Bisacodyl   284
Bladder   288
Blastomycosis   196
Bleeding (intestinal)
– angiographic diagnosis   235–237
– embolization   238–239
– management   238–240
– provocative angiography   237
– scintigraphic diagnosis   216 218
– vasopressin   239–240
Breast carcinoma   45, 46, 293
Bulls eye lesions   294

C

Campylobacteriosis   150, 188
Candidiasis   191
Carcinoembryonic antigen (CEA)   142–143, 223
Carcinoid   38
Carcinoma (*see* under specific organ)
Carthartic abuse   284
Cascara   284
Caustic colitis   195
Cervical carcinoma   291
Cholelithiasis   207
Cholangiocarcinoma   207
Chordoma   102
Churg-Strauss syndrome   193
Cloacogenic
– carcinoma   286
– polyp   42, 285
Cobblestone ulceration   173
Cocaine   193

Colitis (*see* Crohn's disease, Ulcerative Colitis)
- accordion sign   187, 194
- amoebic   41, 178, 191, 281, 284
- backwash ileitis   186
- bacterial colitis   188–190
- Behçet's colitis   188, 193
- blastomycosis   196
- campylobacteriosis   150, 188
- candidiasis   191
- caustic colitis   195
- computer tomography (CT)   185–197
- cryptosporidiosis   190
- cystica profunda   102, 285
- cytomegalovirus (CMV) colitis   190, 284
- eosinophilic colitis   192
- escherichia coli coitis   188
- fungal colitis   190
- graft-versus-host disease   192
- herpes zoster   295
- histioplasmosis colitis   191
- indeterminate colitis   202
- inflammatory polyps   41
- ischaemic   179, 182, 192, 238, 296
- magnetic resonance imaging (MRI)   201–212
- mucormycosis   191
- neutropenic (typhlitis)   182
- risk of neoplasia   19
- parasitic colitis   190
- pseudomembranous   179, 182, 194, 249, 295
- radiation   111, 196, 287
- salmonellosis   150, 178, 189
- schistosomiasis   41, 249, 295
- shigellosis   178, 189
- strongyloidiasis   196
- toxic magacolon   186, 249
- tuberculous colitis   189, 196, 280, 283
- typhlitis   182, 192, 284
- ultrasound   171–183
- viral colitis   190
- yersinia colitis   150, 189, 280
Colon
- adenoma
- - classification   25, 307
- - flat (*see* flat adenoma)
- - right sided   6, 9
- - risk of neoplasia   3
- - surveillance   19
- adhesions   276
- anatomy   177
- benign ulcer   280
- bull's eye lesions   294
- capsule colonoscopy   312
- carcinoma
- - adenoma-carcinoma sequence   2, 18, 35, 47
- - risk factors   2, 5, 13
- - immuno-scintigraphy   222–224
- - incidence   1
- - polypoid   38
- - right sided   6, 9
- - staging   126–127
- - surveillance   3, 19, 28, 127–132
- - survival rates   2, 127–129
- computer tomographic angiography (CTA)   227–232

- diaphragm   297
- infiltration (extrinsic)   293
- intussusception   270
- obstruction   263–267
- perforation   251–256
- pneumatosis   43, 249, 291
- polyp
- - risk of neoplasia   2, 51
- - small   51
- pseudo-obstruction   267–270
- scintigraphy   215–225
- surgery   267
- transit studies   220–222
- trauma   252–260
- - blunt   257
- - foreign body   256
- - penetrating   259
- - perforation   251–256
- ultrasound   177
- urticaria   295
- volvulus   273
Colonoscopy
- capsule   312
- cost   8
- developments   301
- endoscopic mucosal resection (EMR)   310
- endoscopic ultrasound   310
- haemaglobin engancement   311
- incomplete   57
- looping   304
- magnetic endoscope imaging (MAI)   302
- magnifying   309
- merits   51, 302
- mucosal dye spray   308
- optical biopsy forceps   312
- safety   53
- screening   6
- sensitivity   6
- tissue autofluorescence   311
- training   305
- variable stiffness colonoscopes   306
- video systems   307
Congenital hypertrophy of retinal pigment epithelium
   (CHRPE)   16
Contraceptives (oral)   193
Cowden syndrome   13, 17, 37
Comb sign   188
Computed Tomography (CT)
- angiography   227–232
- appendicitis   157–162
- colitis   189–197
- intussusception   272
- obstruction   266
Computed Tomography Colonography (CTC)   61–69
- automatic segmentation   64
- bowel preparation   61
- cancer staging   54, 63
- completeness   54
- computer aided detection (CAD)   64
- 2D axial imaging   63
- 3D endoluminal imaging   64
- faecal tagging   56, 62, 71–79
- normal findings   64–66

– radiation dose   54, 63
– safety   54
– screening   6, 68
– sensitivity   19, 29, 53, 64, 67
– specificity   67
– technique   61–64
– reading   63
Crohn's disease   13, 171, 280
– activity   209
– apthous ulcers   173, 178
– barium enema   172, 283
– cobblestone ulceration   173
– comb sign   188
– complications   204–207
– computer tomography (CT)   187
– differential diagnosis   210–212
– magnetic resonance imaging (MRI)   204–209
– rose-thorn ulcers   173
Cronkite-Canada syndrome   46
Cryptosporidiosis   190
Cystic fibrosis   157, 249
Cytomegalovirus (CMV) colitis   190, 284

D
Dermoid   102
Desmoid tumours   16, 44
Devon polyposis syndrome   46
Diaphragm   297
Diverticultits
– aetiology   165
– bleeding   235
– clinical findings   166
– computer tomography (CT)   165–170
– differential diagnosis   169
– epidemiology   165
– pathology   165
– staging   169
– ultrasound   152
Dukes staging system   97, 126
DNA based stool tests   7
Duodenum
– adenoma   16, 44
– carcinoma   17
Dysplasia   28, 32
Dysplasia associated lesion or mass (DALM)   36

E
Embolization   238–239
Endoscopic mucosal resection (EMR)   310
Endometrial carcinoma   14, 47
Endometriosis   43, 102, 271, 282, 293
Endorectal Ultrasound (ERUS)
– anatomy of rectum   99
– biopsy   106
– equipment   97–98
– follow-up   105
– rectal carcinoma   100–105
– recurrent rectal carcinoma   105
– staging   103, 113
– surveillance   131
– technique   98–99
Endoscopic polypectomy   3

– complications   8
Endoscopic ultrasound   310
Eosinophilic colitis   192
Epiploic appendagitis   152, 195
Escherichia coli coitis   188
Extrinsic infiltration   293

F
Faecal occult blood test (FOBT)   3, 19
– compliance   7
– complications   8
– cost-effectiveness   9
– Haemoccult   3
– screening trials   5
Faecal tagging   56, 62, 71–79
Familial adenomatous polyposis (FAP)   13, 16, 249
– genetics   16, 4
– screening   16
– pathology   44
Familial polyposis coli (see familial adenomatous polyposis)
Fistulae   173, 297
Flat adenoma
– classification   25, 307
– diagnosis   28
– pathology   34
– pit pattrn   309
– relevance   27
– risk of neoplasia   28, 51
Flexible sigmoidoscopy (FS)   5
– complications   8
– cost   8
– cost-effectiveness   9
– screening   5

G
Gallstone ileus   276
Gall bladder empyema   296
Ganglioneuroma   36, 46
Gardner syndrome   13, 17, 44
Gastric cancer   45, 47, 293
Gastrointestinal stromal tumours (GIST)   36, 39
Giant hyperplastic polyposis syndrome   45
Glutaraldehyde   195
Gonoccocal proctitis   287
Gorlin syndrome   13, 17
Graft-versus-host disease   192
Granular cell tumours   36

H
Haemangioma   36, 37
Haemorrhage (see bleeding)
Haemorrhoids   285
Hamartomas   39, 40
Hartmann procedure   267
Hepatobiliary carcinoma   14
Hepatoblastoma   16, 44
Hereditary Non-Polyposis Colorectal Cancer (HNPCC)
   2, 13, 309
– Amsterdam criteria   14
– Bethesda criteria   14
– Genetics   15, 46
– Pathology   46
– Screening   16

Hernias 276
Herpes zoster 295
Heterotopic gastric mucosa 43
Histioplasmosis colitis 191
Hyperplastic polyp (*see* metaplastic)
Hyperplastic polyposis syndrome 41
Hypersensitivity reaction 195
Hypertrophied anal papilla 285

I
Ileitis
– backwash 186
Ileocaecal valve 280
Immunochemical tests (*see* DNA based stool tests)
Indeterminate colitis 202
Inflammatory bowel disease (*see* Colitis) 171–175, 185–197
Inflammatory fibroid polyp 43
Infliximab (anti-TNF- alpha) 209
Intra-abdominal fibromatosis (*see* desmoid tumours)
Intussusception 270–273
– rectal mucosa 285
Inverted diverticula 63
Ischaemic colitis 179, 182, 192, 238, 296

J
Juvenile polyposis syndrome 13, 17, 40, 44
Juvenile polyp 40

L
Laplace's law 263–264
Leiomyoma 36, 102, 271
Leiomyosarcoma 39
Lipohyperplasia of ileocaecal valve 36
Lipoma 36, 63
Lipomatosis (pelvic) 277, 288
Lipomatous ileocaecal valve 280
Lipomatous polyposis 36, 46
Lung carcinoma 294
Lymphocytic phlebitis 193
Lymphogranuloma venereum 287
Lymphoid hyperplasia 249
Lymphoid polyp (*see* benign lymphoid polyp)
Lymphoma 39, 102, 187, 243–249, 288
– B cell non-Hodgkin's 244, 249
– Burkitt's 244
– Hodgkin's 244
– large B cell 244
– mantle cell 244, 248
– T cell 244
Lymphomatous polyposis 46
Lynch syndrome (*see* Hereditary Non-Polyposis Colorectal Cancer)

M
Magnetic endoscope imaging (MAI) 302
Magnetic Resonance Colonography (MRC) 81–88
– bowel preparation 82, 86
– cancer staging 84
– colonic distension 82
– compared to CT 85
– data acquisition 83

– faecal tagging 55, 86
– safety 85
– screening 57
– sensitivity 55, 85
– technique 81
Magnetic Resonance Imaging (MRI)
– colitis 201–212
– contrast agents 203
– rectum 111–123
– rectal tumour extent 116
– staging 113–117
– technique 202–204
Medulloblastoma 16
Megacolon
– toxic 186
Melanoma 39
Mesenchymal tumours 36, 39
Mesenteric panniculitis 277
Mesorectal fascia 111
Metaplastic polyp 40
Metaplastic polyposis syndrome 44
Metastasis 39, 102
– chemotherapy 129
– dissemination 125
– liver resection 127
– peritoneal 283, 289
– survival 127
– thermal ablation 127
– thoroscopic surgery 128
Micro-adenoma 32, 44
Mucocoele of appendix 150, 279
Mucormycosis 191
Multiple endocrine neoplasia syndrome 37
Myxoglobulosis of appendix 279

N
Nasal decongestants 193
National polyp study 28, 29
Neuroendocrine carcinomas 38
Neurofibromas 36
Neurofibromatosis 36, 291
Neutropenic typhlitis 150, 182
Non steroidal anti-inflammatory drugs (NSAIDS) 297
Non-syndromic familial colorectal cancer 8
Non-polypoid adenoma (*see* flat adenoma)

O
Obstipation 276
Obstruction
– acute contrast enema 264
– complications 267
– computed tomography (CT) 266
– emergency surgery 89
– gallstone ileus 276
– stenting 89–96, 267
– surgery 267
– ultrasound 266
Oesophageal carcinoma 45
Ogilvie's syndrome 269
Osteoma 16, 44
Ovarian carcinoma 14, 45, 47, 293

P

Pancreatic carcinoma 45, 293
Pancreatitis 207
Pelvic
– haematoma 290
– lipomatosis 277, 288
– vein thrombosis 288
Perforation
– barium enema 253–256
– endoscopic 251–253
– intraperitoneal 253
– retroperitoneal 253
Peri-ampullary carcinoma 44
PET scanning (*see* Positron Emission Tomography)
Peutz-Jegher syndrome (PJS) 13, 18, 45
– surveillance 18
Phenobarbital 193
Phenolphthalein 284
Pneumatosis coli 43, 249, 291
Polyp
– benign lymphoid 41
– cap 42
– classification 31
– cloacogenic 42, 285
– endometriosis 43
– hamartomatous 17, 39
– heterotopic gastric mucosa 43
– hyperplastic (*see* metaplastic)
– inflammatory 41, 172
– inflammatory fibroid 42
– juvenile 17, 39, 40
– lymphoid (*see* benign lymphoid)
– metaplastic 40
– myoglandular 42
– Peutz-Jeghers 39
– post inflammatory 41, 172, 249
– prolapsing 42
– pseudopolyps 41, 172
– risk of neoplasia 2, 68, 172
Polypectomy (*see* endoscopic polypectomy)
Polyposis syndromes
– Bannayan-Reilly-Ruvelcaba 46
– benign lymphoid 44
– Cowden syndrome 13, 17, 37, 46
– Cronkite-Canada syndrome 46
– Devon polyposis syndrome 46
– familial adenomatous polyposis (FAP) 13, 16, 44
– Gardner syndrome 13, 17, 44
– giant hyperplastic 45
– Gorlin syndrome 13, 17
– hereditary non-polyposis colorectal cancer syndrome 2, 13–16, 46, 309
– hyperplastic polyposis 41
– juvenile polyposis syndrome 13, 17, 40, 44
– lipomatous polyposis 36, 46
– Lynch syndrome (*see* Hereditary Non-Polyposis Colorectal Cancer Syndrome)
– non-syndromic familial colorectal cancer 8
– lymphomatous 46
– metaplastic 44
– Peutz-Jegher syndrome (PJS) 13, 18, 45
– Ruvalcaba-Myhre-Smith syndrome 13, 17
– Turcot's syndrome 44

Polyethylene Glycol (PEG) 203
Positron Emission Tomography (PET) 137–146
– CEA levels 142–143
– FDG 137
– follow-up 144
– pelvic recurrence 141
– primary disease 143
– screening 143
– staging 127, 138
– technique 138
Pouchitis 209
Proctitis
– gonoccocal 287
– lymphogranuloma venereum 287
Prostate
– benign hypertrophy 289
– cancer 102, 290
Pseudodiverticula 291
Pseudomembranous colitis 179, 182, 194, 249, 295
Pseudomyxoma peritonei 150
Pseudo-obstruction 267–270
– differential diagnosis 264

R

Radiotherapy 111, 196, 287
Radionuclide imaging (*see* scintigraphy)
Rectum
– carcinoma
– – biopsy 106
– – MRI 111–123
– – staging with EUS 100–105
– – staging with MRI 113–116
– – recurrence 105
– – resection margin 118–119
– – treatment 111
– – ultrasound (*see* endorectal ultrasound, EUS) 97–109
Renal
– adenocarcinoma 293
– hydronephrosis 207
– pyonephrosis 297
– transitional cell carcinoma 14, 16, 47
Rose-thorn ulceration 172
Ruvalcaba-Myhre-Smith syndrome 13, 17

S

Salmonelliasis 150, 178, 189
Schistosomiasis 41, 249, 295
Schwannoma 36
Scintigraphy 215–225
– carcinoma 222–224
– colitis 218–220
– immuno-scintigraphy 222–224
– – guided surgery 224
– intestinal bleeding 216–218
– – labelled red blood cells 216, 236
– – labelled colloid 217–218
– colonic transit 220–222
Scleroderma 292
Sclerosing cholangitis 207
Senna 284
Serrated polyp (*see* hyperpalstic polyp)

Shigellosis 178, 189
Sinuses 173
Strongyloidiasis 196
Surgery
– abdominoperineal excision 97
– low anterior excision 97
– transanal excision (TAE) 97
Small bowel
– carcinoma 14, 45, 47
Solitary rectal ulcer syndrome (SRUS) 42, 102, 285
Sonography (see ultrasound)
Staging 125–135
– Aster-Collier 98
– Dukes 97
– rectal carcinoma 100–105
– TNM 97, 98
Stents 89–96, 267
– aftercare 94
– complications 94
– indications 90
– results 94–95
– technique 91–94
– types 93
Stool subtraction 75
Strictures 173, 287–288
Strongyloidiasis 196
Superparamagnetic contrast agents 203
Systemic lupus erythematosis 193

T
Tail gut cysts 102
Teratoma 102
Testicular carcinoma 45
Thyroid carcinoma 44, 46
TNM staging system 97, 126
Total mesorectal excision 111
– Dutch trial 112
Toxic Megacolon 186, 249
Transit studies 220–222
Trauma 251–260
– blunt 257
– foreign body 256
– penetrating 259
– perforation 251–256
Tuberculosis 189, 196, 280, 283
Tuberous sclerosis 40
Turcot's syndrome 44
Typhlitis 150, 182, 284

U
Ulceration
– apthous ulcers 173, 178

– cobblestone ulceration 173
– rose-thorn ulcers 173
Ulcerative colitis 171
– adenoma-like DALM (ALD) 36
– computer tomography (CT) 185
– differential diagnosis 210–212
– dysplasia associated lesion or mass (DALM) 36
– magnetic resonance imaging (MRI) 209
– risk of neoplasia 13, 35
– ultrasound 180
Ultrasound
– colitis 171–183
– – activity 181
– – sensitivity 181
– – specificity 181
– endorectal 97–109, 183
– hydrocolonic 182
– intussusception 271
– obstruction 266
– transabdominal
– – anatomy 148
– – appendicitis 147–155
– – indications 152
– – technique 148
Ureter
– transitional cell carcinoma 14, 16
Uterine carcinoma 293
Ureterosigmoidostomy 41
Urticaria 295

V
Varices (rectal) 287
Vasopressin 239–240
Veins
– inferior mesenteric 231
– portal 231
– splenic 231
– superior mesenteric 231
Veterans Affairs Study 28
Video pill 312
Villous tumours
– staging with EUS 104
Virtual colonoscopy (see CT colonography)
Volvulus 273
– caecal 275
– compound 275
– double 275
– ileo-sigmoid knot 275
– sigmoid 273–274
Von Recklinghausen's disease 36

Y
Yersinia enterocolitica 150, 189, 280

List of Contributors

WENDY ATKIN, MD
Deputy Director, Colorectal Cancer Unit
Cancer Research UK
Honorary Reader in Epidemiology
Imperial College of Science,
Technology and Medicine, London
St Mark's Hospital
Northwick Park, Watford Road
Harrow, Middlesex HA1 3UJ
UK

ISABELLA BAELI, MD
Department of Radiology
University of Rome "La Sapienza"
Policlinicio Umberto I
Viale Regina Elena 324
00161 Rome
Italy

GEERARD L. BEETS, MD, PhD
Department of Surgery
University Hospital Maastricht
P Debyelaan 25
PO Box 5800
6202 AZ Maastricht
The Netherlands

REGINA G. H. BEETS-TAN, MD, PhD
Department of Radiology
University Hospital Maastricht
P Debyelaan 25
PO Box 5800
6202 AZ Maastricht
The Netherlands

JOHN BRUZZI, FFRRCSI, FRCR
Department of Radiology
Mater Misericordiae Hospital
Eccles Street
Dublin 7
Ireland

DINA F. CAROLINE, MD
Department of Diagnostic Imaging
Temple University Hospital
3401 Broad and Ontario Streets
Philadelphia, PA 19140-5189
USA

ANTHONY H. CHAPMAN, MD, FRCP, FRCR
Clinical Director of Radiology
Department of Clinical Radiology
Leeds Teaching Hospitals Trust
St. James's University Hospital
Beckett Street
Leeds, West Yorkshire LS9 7TF
UK

ETIENNE M. DANSE, MD
Department of Medical Imaging
Saint-Luc University Hospital
Université Catholique de Louvain
Avenue Hippocrate 10
1200 Brussels
Belgium

GEORGIA P. ECONOMOU, MD
Iaso Hospital
Voutsina 1A
Ekali
Athens 145–78
Greece

RICHARD EDWARDS, MD
Consultant Interventional Radiologist
Gartnavel General Hospital
North Glasgow University Hospitals Trust
1053 Great Western Road
Glasgow G12 0YN
UK

HELEN FENLON, FFRRCSI, FRCR
Department of Radiology
Mater Misericordiae Hospital
Eccles Street
Dublin 7
Ireland

RICARDO FERRARI, MD
Department of Radiology
University of Rome "La Sapienza"
Policlinicio Umberto I
Viale Regina Elena 324
00161 Rome
Italy

ABRAHAM A. GHIATAS, MD
Director of Medical Imaging
Iaso Hospital
Voutsina 1A
Ekali
Athens 145–78
Greece

ALISON GILLAMS, MD
Department of Medical Imaging
The Middlesex Hospital
Mortimer Street
London, W1T 3AA
UK

STEFAN GRYSPEERDT, MD
Stedelijk Ziekenhuis
Bruggesteenweg 90
8800 Roeselare
Belgium

J. ASHLEY GUTHRIE, MRCP, FRCR
Consultant Radiologist
Department of Clinical Radiology
St James's University Hospital
Lincoln Wing
Beckett Street
Leeds LS9 7TF
UK

STEPHEN HALLIGAN, MD, MRCP, FRCR
Intestinal Imaging Centre, Level 4V
St Mark's Hospital
Northwick Park
Watford Road
Harrow, Middlesex HA1 3UJ
UK

NIKLAS HENNESSY, MRCP, FRCR
Specialist Registrar in Radiology
Southampton University Hospital
Tremona Road
Southampton S016 6YD
UK

MICHAEL C. HILL, MB
Department of Radiology
The George Washington University Hospital
Medical Center
900 23rd Street, NW
1st Floor Suite Room 11104
Washington, DC 20037
USA

SHIRLEY HODGSON, MD
Professor of Cancer Genetics
Division of Medical and Molecular Genetics
St. George's Hospital
Tooting
London SW17 ORE
UK

FRANCO IAFRATE, MD
Department of Radiology
University of Rome "La Sapienza"
Policlinicio Umberto I
Viale Regina Elena 324
00161 Rome
Italy

NICK KRITIKOS, MD
Iaso Hospital
Voutsina 1A, Ekali
Athens 145–78
Greece

ANDREA LAGHI, MD
Department of Radiology
University of Rome "La Sapienza"
Policlinicio Umberto I
Viale Regina Elena 324
00161 Rome
Italy

PHILIPPE LEFERE, MD
Stedelijk Ziekenhuis
Bruggesteenweg 90
8800 Roeselare
Belgium

ANDREW LOWE, BSc, MB ChB (Hons), MRCP, FRCR
St. James's University Hospital
Beckett Street
Leeds, West Yorkshire LS9 7TF
UK

FRANCESCA MACCIONI, MD
Istituto di Radiologia
III piano, Policlinico Umberto I
University "La Sapienza"
Viale Regina Elena 324
161 Rome
Italy

JENNY MACPHERSON, MRCP, FRCR
Fellow in Abdominal Radiology
Vancouver Hospital and Health Sciences Centre
855 West 12th Avenue
Vancouver, British Columbia V5Z 1M9
Canada

FILIPPO MANGIAPANE, MD
Department of Radiology
University of Rome "La Sapienza"
Policlinicio Umberto I
Viale Regina Elena 324
00161 Rome
Italy

DANIELE MARIN, MD
Department of Radiology
University of Rome "La Sapienza"
Policlinicio Umberto I
Viale Regina Elena 324
00161 Rome
Italy

CARLO MIGLIO, MD
Department of Radiology
University of Rome "La Sapienza"
Policlinicio Umberto I
Viale Regina Elena 324
00161 Rome
Italy

JOHN NORTHOVER, MD
Professor of Intestinal Surgery
Imperial College of Science,
Technology and Medicine, London
Director, Colorectal Cancer Unit
Cancer Research UK
Chair, Department of Surgey
St Mark's Hospital
Northwick Park, Watford Road
Harrow, Middlesex HA1 3UJ
UK

PASQUALE PAOLANTONIO, MD
Department of Radiology
University of Rome "La Sapienza"
Policlinicio Umberto I
Viale Regina Elena 324
00161 Rome
Italy

ROBERTO PASSARIELLO, MD
Professor and Director of Department of Radiology
University of Rome "La Sapienza"
Policlinicio Umberto I
Viale Regina Elena 324
00161 Rome
Italy

ROBERT JAMES PECK, MD
Consultant Radiologist
Department of Clinical Radiology
Royal Hallamshire Hospital
Glossop Road
Sheffield, South Yorkshire S10 2JF
UK

BJORN REMBACKEN, MD
Consultant Gastroenterologist
The General Infirmary at Leeds
Great George Street
15 Wayland Close, Adel
Leeds LS1 3EX
UK

IAIN ROBERTSON, MD
Consultant Interventional Radiologist
Gartnavel General Hospital
North Glasgow University Hospitals Trust
1053 Great Western Road
Glasgow G12 0YN
UK

PHILIP J. A. ROBINSON, MD
Professor of Radiology
Department of Clinical Radiology
St James's University Hospital
Lincoln Wing, Beckett Street
Leeds LS9 7TF
UK

BRIAN P. SAUNDERS, MD, FRCP
Senior Lecturer in Endoscopy
St. Mark's Hospital
Northwick Park, Watford Road
Harrow, Middlesex HA1 3UJ
UK

NIGEL SCOTT, MD, MRC Path
Consultant Pathologist
St James's University Hospital
Beckett Street
Leeds, West Yorkshire LS9 7TF
UK

MARIA SHERIDAN, MRCP, FRCR
Consultant Radiologist
Department of Clinical Radiology
St. James's University Hospital
Lincoln Wing, Beckett Street
Leeds LS9 7TF
UK

STEPHEN J. SKEHAN, MD
Consultant Radiologist
St. Vincent's University Hospital
Elm Park
Dublin 4
Ireland

PATRICE TAOUREL, MD
Service de Radiologie
Hôpital la Peyronie
CHU de Montpellier
2 Avenue Berlin Sans
34295 Montpellier Cedex 5
France

RUEDI F. THOENI, MD
Professor of Radiology
University of California, San Francisco
PO Box 0628
San Francisco, CA 94143
USA

MARC TISCHKOWITZ, MD
Clinical Research Fellow
Division of Medical and Molecular Genetics
Guy's Hospital
St. Thomas Street
London, SE1 9RT
UK

DAMIAN TOLAN, MB, MRCP
St. James's University Hospital
Beckett Street
Leeds, West Yorkshire LS9 7TF
UK

SIMONE TRENNA, MD
Department of Radiology
University of Rome "La Sapienza"
Policlinicio Umberto I
Viale Regina Elena 324
00161 Rome
Italy

KEN TUNG, FRCP, FRCR
Consultant Radiologist
Southampton University Hospital
Tremona Road
Southampton S016 6YD
UK

BERNHARD E. VAN BEERS, MD, PhD
Department of Medical Imaging
Saint-Luc University Hospital
Université Catholique de Louvain
Avenue Hippocrate 10
1200 Brussels
Belgium

MEDICAL RADIOLOGY Diagnostic Imaging and Radiation Oncology

Titles in the series already published

DIAGNOSTIC IMAGING

Innovations in Diagnostic Imaging
Edited by J. H. Anderson

Radiology of the Upper Urinary Tract
Edited by E. K. Lang

The Thymus - Diagnostic Imaging, Functions, and Pathologic Anatomy
Edited by E. Walter, E. Willich, and W. R. Webb

Interventional Neuroradiology
Edited by A. Valavanis

Radiology of the Pancreas
Edited by A. L. Baert, co-edited by G. Delorme

Radiology of the Lower Urinary Tract
Edited by E. K. Lang

Magnetic Resonance Angiography
Edited by I. P. Arlart, G. M. Bongartz, and G. Marchal

Contrast-Enhanced MRI of the Breast
S. Heywang-Köbrunner and R. Beck

Spiral CT of the Chest
Edited by M. Rémy-Jardin and J. Rémy

Radiological Diagnosis of Breast Diseases
Edited by M. Friedrich and E.A. Sickles

Radiology of the Trauma
Edited by M. Heller and A. Fink

Biliary Tract Radiology
Edited by P. Rossi

Radiological Imaging of Sports Injuries
Edited by C. Masciocchi

Modern Imaging of the Alimentary Tube
Edited by A. R. Margulis

Diagnosis and Therapy of Spinal Tumors
Edited by P. R. Algra, J. Valk, and J. J. Heimans

Interventional Magnetic Resonance Imaging
Edited by J.F. Debatin and G. Adam

Abdominal and Pelvic MRI
Edited by A. Heuck and M. Reiser

Orthopedic Imaging
Techniques and Applications
Edited by A. M. Davies and H. Pettersson

Radiology of the Female Pelvic Organs
Edited by E. K.Lang

Magnetic Resonance of the Heart and Great Vessels
Clinical Applications
Edited by J. Bogaert, A.J. Duerinckx, and F. E. Rademakers

Modern Head and Neck Imaging
Edited by S. K. Mukherji and J. A. Castelijns

Radiological Imaging of Endocrine Diseases
Edited by J. N. Bruneton
in collaboration with B. Padovani and M.-Y. Mourou

Trends in Contrast Media
Edited by H. S. Thomsen, R. N. Muller, and R. F. Mattrey

Functional MRI
Edited by C. T. W. Moonen and P. A. Bandettini

Radiology of the Pancreas
2nd Revised Edition
Edited by A. L. Baert
Co-edited by G. Delorme and L. Van Hoe

Emergency Pediatric Radiology
Edited by H. Carty

Spiral CT of the Abdomen
Edited by F. Terrier, M. Grossholz, and C. D. Becker

Liver Malignancies
Diagnostic and Interventional Radiology
Edited by C. Bartolozzi and R. Lencioni

Medical Imaging of the Spleen
Edited by A. M. De Schepper and F. Vanhoenacker

Radiology of Peripheral Vascular Diseases
Edited by E. Zeitler

Diagnostic Nuclear Medicine
Edited by C. Schiepers

Radiology of Blunt Trauma of the Chest
P. Schnyder and M. Wintermark

Portal Hypertension
Diagnostic Imaging-Guided Therapy
Edited by P. Rossi
Co-edited by P. Ricci and L. Broglia

Recent Advances in Diagnostic Neuroradiology
Edited by Ph. Demaerel

Virtual Endoscopy and Related 3D Techniques
Edited by P. Rogalla, J. Terwissscha Van Scheltinga, and B. Hamm

Multislice CT
Edited by M. F. Reiser, M. Takahashi, M. Modic, and R. Bruening

Pediatric Uroradiology
Edited by R. Fotter

Transfontanellar Doppler Imaging in Neonates
A. Couture and C. Veyrac

Radiology of AIDS
A Practical Approach
Edited by J.W.A.J. Reeders and P.C. Goodman

CT of the Peritoneum
Armando Rossi and Giorgio Rossi

Magnetic Resonance Angiography
2nd Revised Edition
Edited by I. P. Arlart, G. M. Bongratz, and G. Marchal

Pediatric Chest Imaging
Edited by Javier Lucaya and Janet L. Strife

Applications of Sonography in Head and Neck Pathology
Edited by J. N. Bruneton
in collaboration with C. Raffaelli and O. Dassonville

Imaging of the Larynx
Edited by R. Hermans

3D Image Processing
Techniques and Clinical Applications
Edited by D. Caramella and C. Bartolozzi

Imaging of Orbital and Visual Pathway Pathology
Edited by W. S. Müller-Forell

Pediatric ENT Radiology
Edited by S. J. King and A. E. Boothroyd

Radiological Imaging of the Small Intestine
Edited by N. C. Gourtsoyiannis

Imaging of the Knee
Techniques and Applications
Edited by A. M. Davies and V. N. Cassar-Pullicino

Perinatal Imaging
From Ultrasound to MR Imaging
Edited by Fred E. Avni

Radiological Imaging of the Neonatal Chest
Edited by V. Donoghue

Diagnostic and Interventional Radiology in Liver Transplantation
Edited by E. Bücheler, V. Nicolas, C. E. Broelsch, X. Rogiers, and G. Krupski

Radiology of Osteoporosis
Edited by S. Grampp

Imaging Pelvic Floor Disorders
Edited by C. I. Bartram and J. O. L. DeLancey
Associate Editors: S. Halligan, F. M. Kelvin, and J. Stoker

Imaging of the Pancreas
Cystic and Rare Tumors
Edited by C. Procassi and A. J. Megibow

High Resolution Sonography of the Peripheral Nervous System
Edited by S. Peer and G. Bodner

Imaging of the Foot and Ankle
Techniques and Applications
Edited by A. M. Davies, R. W. Whitehouse, and J. P. R. Jenkins

Radiology Imaging of the Ureter
Edited by F. Joffre, Ph. Otal, and M. Soulie

Imaging of the Shoulder
Techniques and Applications
Edited by A. M. Davies and J. Hodler

Radiology of the Petrous Bone
Edited by M. Lemmerling and S. S. Kollias

Interventional Radiology in Cancer
Edited by A. Adam, R. F. Dondelinger, and P. R. Mueller

Duplex and Color Doppler Imaging of the Venous System
Edited by G. H. Mostbeck

Multidetector-Row CT of the Thorax
Edited by U. J. Schoepf

Functional Imaging of the Chest
Edited by H.-U. Kauczor

Radiology of the Pharynx and the Esophagus
Edited by O. Ekberg

Radiological Imaging in Hematological Malignancies
Edited by A. Guermazi

Imaging and Intervention in Abdominal Trauma
Edited by R. F. Dondelinger

Multislice CT
2nd Revised Edition
Edited by M. F. Reiser, M. Takahashi, M. Modic, and C. R. Becker

Intracranial Vascular Malformations and Aneurysms
From Diagnostic Work-Up to Endovascular Therapy
Edited by M. Forsting

Radiology and Imaging of the Colon
Edited by A. H. Chapman

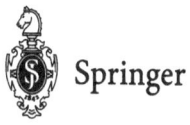 Springer

RADIATION ONCOLOGY

Lung Cancer
Edited by C.W. Scarantino

**Innovations in
Radiation Oncology**
Edited by H. R. Withers
and L. J. Peters

**Radiation Therapy
of Head and Neck Cancer**
Edited by G. E. Laramore

**Gastrointestinal Cancer –
Radiation Therapy**
Edited by R.R. Dobelbower, Jr.

**Radiation Exposure
and Occupational Risks**
Edited by E. Scherer, C. Streffer,
and K.-R. Trott

**Radiation Therapy
of Benign Diseases**
A Clinical Guide
S. E. Order and S. S. Donaldson

**Interventional Radiation Therapy
Techniques – Brachytherapy**
Edited by R. Sauer

**Radiopathology
of Organs and Tissues**
Edited by E. Scherer, C. Streffer,
and K.-R. Trott

**Concomitant Continuous Infusion
Chemotherapy and Radiation**
Edited by M. Rotman
and C. J. Rosenthal

**Intraoperative Radiotherapy –
Clinical Experiences and Results**
Edited by F. A. Calvo, M. Santos,
and L.W. Brady

**Radiotherapy of Intraocular
and Orbital Tumors**
Edited by W. E. Alberti and
R. H. Sagerman

**Interstitial and Intracavitary
Thermoradiotherapy**
Edited by M. H. Seegenschmiedt
and R. Sauer

Non-Disseminated Breast Cancer
Controversial Issues
in Management
Edited by G. H. Fletcher and
S.H. Levitt

**Current Topics in
Clinical Radiobiology of Tumors**
Edited by H.-P. Beck-Bornholdt

**Practical Approaches to Cancer
Invasion and Metastases**
A Compendium of Radiation
Oncologists' Responses
to 40 Histories
Edited by A. R. Kagan with the
Assistance of R. J. Steckel

**Radiation Therapy
in Pediatric Oncology**
Edited by J. R. Cassady

Radiation Therapy Physics
Edited by A. R. Smith

Late Sequelae in Oncology
Edited by J. Dunst and R. Sauer

Mediastinal Tumors. Update 1995
Edited by D. E. Wood
and C. R. Thomas, Jr.

**Thermoradiotherapy
and Thermochemotherapy**
Volume 1:
Biology, Physiology, and Physics
Volume 2:
Clinical Applications
Edited by M.H. Seegenschmiedt,
P. Fessenden, and C.C. Vernon

Carcinoma of the Prostate
Innovations in Management
Edited by Z. Petrovich, L. Baert,
and L.W. Brady

**Radiation Oncology
of Gynecological Cancers**
Edited by H.W. Vahrson

Carcinoma of the Bladder
Innovations in Management
Edited by Z. Petrovich, L. Baert,
and L.W. Brady

**Blood Perfusion and Micro-
environment of Human Tumors**
Implications for
Clinical Radiooncology
Edited by M. Molls and P. Vaupel

**Radiation Therapy
of Benign Diseases**
A Clinical Guide
2nd Revised Edition
S. E. Order and S. S. Donaldson

**Carcinoma of the Kidney and Testis,
and Rare Urologic Malignancies**
Innovations in Management
Edited by Z. Petrovich, L. Baert,
and L.W. Brady

**Progress and Perspectives in the
Treatment of Lung Cancer**
Edited by P. Van Houtte,
J. Klastersky, and P. Rocmans

**Combined Modality Therapy of
Central Nervous System Tumors**
Edited by Z. Petrovich, L. W. Brady,
M. L. Apuzzo, and M. Bamberg

Age-Related Macular Degeneration
Current Treatment Concepts
Edited by W. A. Alberti, G. Richard,
and R. H. Sagerman

**Radiotherapy of Intraocular
and Orbital Tumors**
2nd Revised Edition
Edited by R. H. Sagerman,
and W. E. Alberti

**Biological Modification
of Radiation Response**
Edited by C. Nieder, L. Milas,
and K. K. Ang

Palliative Radiation Oncology
R. G. Parker. N. A. Janjan,
and M. T. Selch

**Clinical Target Volumes in
Conformal and Intensity Modulated
Radiation Therapy**
A Clinical Guide to Cancer
Treatment
Edited by V. Grégoire, P. Scalliet,
and K. K. Ang

Springer

Printing and Binding: Stürtz AG, Würzburg